Prostaglandins:
Physiological, Pharmacological and Pathological Aspects

Advances in Prostaglandin Research

Prostaglandins: Physiological, Pharmacological and Pathological Aspects

Edited by
S. M. M. Karim

MTP

Published by

MTP Press Ltd
St Leonard's House
St Leonardgate
Lancaster
England

Copyright © 1976 MTP Press Ltd

ISBN 0 85200143 6

First Published 1976

Printed in Great Britain by
R & R Clark Ltd,
Newhaven Road, Edinburgh

Contents

1 Prostaglandins and the central nervous system   1
  Flavio Coceani and Cecil R. Pace-Asciak

2 Effects of prostaglandins on autonomic neurotransmission   37
  Per Hedqvist

3 Prostaglandins and the eye   63
  Kenneth E. Eakins

4 Prostaglandins and the respiratory system   83
  Alexander P. Smith

5 Cardiovascular actions of prostaglandins   103
  Kafait U. Malik and John C. McGiff

6 Renal prostaglandins   201
  John C. McGiff and Kafait U. Malik

7 Prostaglandins and the alimentary tract   247
  Alan Bennett

8 Prostaglandins and blood coagulation   277
  Peter W. Howie

9 Prostaglandins and inflammation   293
  M. W. Greaves

10 Prostaglandins and tumours   303
  Sultan M. M. Karim and Bhashini Rao

11 Pharmacology of some prostaglandins analogues   327
  Sultan M. M. Karim and P. Ganesan Adaikan

Index   361

Advances in Prostaglandin Research

This book is one of three books on the Prostaglandins edited by Professor Karim which together are designed to represent a comprehensive, critical and entirely up-to-date review of prostaglandin research. The contents of the other two books in the series are shown below:

Prostaglandins and Reproduction
Edited by S. M. M. Karim

GENERAL INTRODUCTION AND COMMENTS
S. M. M. Karim and B. Rao

PHYSIOLOGICAL ROLES AND PHARMACOLOGICAL ACTIONS OF PROSTAGLANDINS IN RELATION TO HUMAN REPRODUCTION
S. M. M. Karim and K. Hillier

INTERRUPTION OF PREGNANCY WITH PROSTAGLANDINS
S. M. M. Karim and J.-J. Amy

INDUCTION OF LABOUR WITH PROSTAGLANDINS
M. Thiery and J.-J. Amy

PROSTAGLANDINS AND REPRODUCTION IN SUB-HUMAN PRIMATES
K. T. Kirton

PROSTAGLANDINS AND STUDIES RELATED TO REPRODUCTION IN LABORATORY ANIMALS
A. P. Labhsetwar

PROSTAGLANDINS AND REPRODUCTIVE PROCESSES IN FEMALE SHEEP AND GOAT
A. P. Flint and K. Hillier

PRACTICAL APPLICATION OF PROSTAGLANDINS IN ANIMAL HUSBANDRY
M. J. Cooper and A. L. Walpole

Prostaglandins: Chemical and Biochemical Aspects
Edited by S. M. M. Karim

THE CHEMISTRY OF THE PROSTAGLANDINS
W. P. Schneider

METHODS FOR ANALYSIS OF PROSTAGLANDINS
J. A. Salmon and S. M. M. Karim

INHIBITION OF PROSTAGLANDIN BIOSYNTHESIS
W. E. M. Lands and L. H. Rome

PROSTAGLANDIN ANTAGONISTS
J. H. Sanner and K. E. Eakins

PROSTAGLANDIN–CYCLE NUCLEOTIDE INTERACTIONS IN MAMMALIAN TISSUES
F. A. Kuehl, V. J. Cirillo and H. G. Olen

List of Contributors

P. Ganesan Adaikan, L.I.Biol.
Research Assistant,
Department of Obstetrics and Gynaecology,
University of Singapore,
Kandang Kerbau Hospital, Hampshire Road,
Singapore 8, Republic of Singapore.

Alan Bennett, Ph.D.
Reader in Pharmacology,
Department of Surgery,
King's College Hospital Medical School,
Denmark Hill, London SE5 8RX,
England.

Flavio Coceani, M.D.
Associate Professor,
Department of Physiology,
University of Toronto, Canada.

K. E. Eakins, Ph.D.
Associate Professor of Pharmacology,
Ophthalmology Research,
College of Physicians and Surgeons,
Columbia University,
New York, N.Y. 10032, U.S.A.

M. W. Greaves, M.D., Ph.D., F.R.C.P.
Professor of Dermatology,
The Institute of Dermatology,
St. John's Hospital for Diseases of the Skin,
Lisle Street, Leicester Square,
London WC2H 7BJ, England.

P. Hedqvist, M.D.
Department of Physiology,
Karolinska Institutet,
104 01 Stockholm 60,
Sweden.

P. W. Howie, M.D., M.R.C.O.G.
Senior Lecturer,
University Department of Obstetrics and Gynaecology,
Royal Maternity Hospital,
Rottenrow, Glasgow G4 0NA,
Scotland.

S. M. M. Karim, Ph.D., D.Sc.
Research Professor of Obstetrics and Gynaecology,
Department of Obstetrics and Gynaecology, University of Singapore,
Kandang Kerbau Hospital, Hampshire Road,
Singapore 8, Republic of Singapore.

K. U. Malik, D.Sc., Ph.D.
Associate Professor of Pharmacology,
Department of Pharmacology,
The University of Tennessee Center for the Health Sciences,
College of Basic Medical Sciences,
800 Madison Avenue, P.O. Box CR 301,
Memphis, Tennessee 38163, U.S.A.

J. C. McGiff, M.D.
Professor and Chairman,
Department of Pharmacology,
School of Medicine, University of Tennessee,
800 Madison Avenue, P.O. Box CR 301,
Memphis, Tennessee 38163, U.S.A.

Cecil R. Pace-Asciak, Ph.D.
Assistant Professor,
Department of Pharmacology,
University of Toronto,
Canada.

Bhashini Rao, Ph.D.
Research Fellow,
Department of Obstetrics and Gynaecology,
University of Singapore, Kandang Kerbau Hospital,
Hampshire Road, Singapore 8, Republic of Singapore.

Alexander P. Smith, M.R.C.P.
Lecturer in Medicine,
King's College Hospital Medical School,
Denmark Hill, London SE5 9RS,
England.

Preface

This is the third in a series of three books on advances in prostaglandin research. In recent years there has been unparalleled interest in these compounds and as a result a vast amount of research data has accumulated since the publication of my earlier book in 1972. At that time it was possible to present a fairly comprehensive review of the various aspects of prostaglandin research in one volume. This is no longer possible and the contents are now divided into three volumes; the first one dealing with prostaglandins and reproduction was published in October 1975; the second volume dealing with chemical and biochemical aspects of prostaglandin research was published in March 1976 and the present one dealing with physiological, pharmacological and pathological aspects is to be published in April 1976.

The authorship of the volume represents international scientists consisting of physiologists, pharmacologists, biochemists and medical specialists in various disciplines actively engaged in prostaglandin research. An attempt has been made to provide a total coverage of advances relating to prostaglandins. For the sake of completeness and continuity, material covered in the 1972 book is either briefly summarised or reference made to that edition.

In recent years there have been notable advances in the physiological, pharmacological and pathological aspects of prostaglandin research and these are discussed by various authorities in the chapters that follow.

The need for rapid publication in a fast expanding field is obvious. Attempts have been made to cover work published until the middle of 1975 (and in some areas until the end of 1975, although some omissions are inevitable) and publication date set for April 1976. This has only been possible as a result of co-operation of the contributors in submitting their manuscripts on time and the efforts of the publishers in bringing out the book within a few months of receiving the manuscript.

Tables and figures previously published are in general acknowledged by a reference in the legends and I am grateful to the respective authors, editors and publishers for their permission.

My thanks are due to my various colleagues, particularly Dr Bhashini Rao, Mr P. G. Adaikan, Miss Lo Pia Yong, Miss Tai Mei Yoon for proof reading and cross-checking journal references. Miss Lily Koh has provided excellent secretarial assistance. I am grateful to Professor S. S. Ratnam, Head of Department of Obstetrics and Gynaecology, University of Singapore for his support and encouragement.

Singapore, January 1976   Sultan M. M. Karim

1

Prostaglandins and the
Central Nervous System

FLAVIO COCEANI and CECIL R. PACE-ASCIAK

1.1	INTRODUCTION	2
1.2	BIOSYNTHESIS	2
	1.2.1 *Inhibition of prostaglandin biosynthesis*	6
1.3	METABOLISM	6
1.4	RELEASE	9
	1.4.1 *Prostaglandins in cerebrospinal fluid*	10
1.5	ACTION OF PROSTAGLANDINS	11
	1.5.1 *Behaviour*	11
	1.5.2 *Hypothalamus*	12
	1.5.2.1 Regulation of body temperature	12
	1.5.2.2 Regulation of food intake	17
	1.5.3 *Brain stem*	17
	1.5.4 *Spinal cord and motor pathways*	18
	1.5.5 *Effects on single neurons*	19
1.6	PROSTAGLANDINS, CYCLIC NUCLEOTIDES AND NEUROTRANSMITTERS	20
1.7	CEREBRAL CIRCULATION	24
1.8	CONCLUSION	25
	ACKNOWLEDGEMENTS	26
	REFERENCES	26

1.1 INTRODUCTION

About 10 years have elapsed since Samuelsson's original discovery of a prostaglandin in ox brain. Subsequently, a wealth of data have accrued on the occurrence, release and action of different types of prostaglandins in the central nervous system of many species. From these studies it has become apparent that prostaglandins are implicated in neural function, and particularly in the mediation or modulation of humoral and other stimuli to neurons.

1.2 BIOSYNTHESIS

It is well established that prostaglandins are formed from certain C-20 unsaturated fatty acids (Bergström *et al.*, 1964a, b; Hamberg and Samuelsson, 1966, 1967; Nugteren *et al.*, 1966; Struijk *et al.*, 1966; Beerthuis *et al.*, 1968, 1971). In mammals, arachidonic acid is the most common precursor. The biosynthetic sequence (Figure 1.1) is initiated by the cleavage of the appropriate fatty acid from a membrane lipid. This step is rate-limiting because fatty acids esterified to lipids cannot act as a substrate (Lands and Samuelsson, 1968; Vonkeman and Van Dorp, 1968). Although phospholipids (and a phospholipase A) have been commonly implicated in prostaglandin

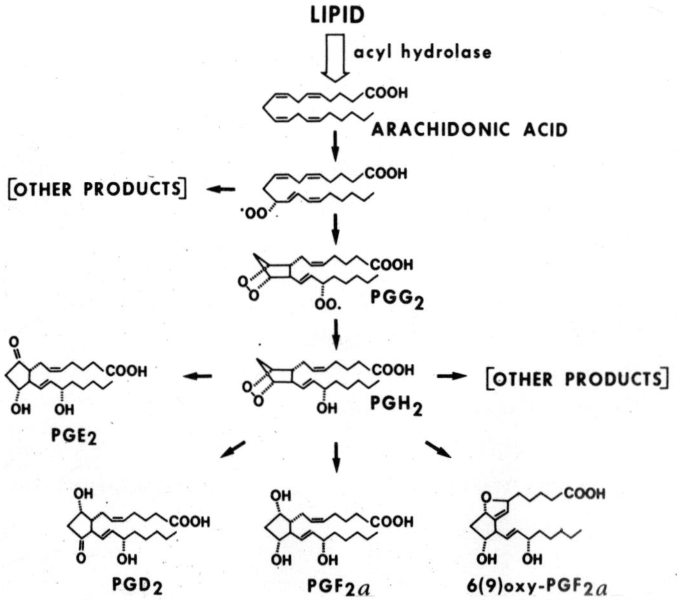

Figure 1.1 The pathway for prostaglandin biosynthesis from arachidonic acid. The initial step in the sequence (open arrow) is rate-limiting. The biological activity of the endoperoxide intermediates and the prostaglandin end-products varies with the test system, whereas non-prostanoate derivatives are inactive

biosynthesis (Kunze and Vogt, 1971), theoretically other lipids can be the source of the precursor acid. Conversion of the fatty acid to prostaglandins is effected by a membrane-bound (plasma membrane and/or endoplasmic reticulum) multienzyme complex conveniently termed prostaglandin synthetase. The nature of the enzymes forming this complex can best be defined through the description of the reaction sequence. Briefly, biosynthesis is initiated by a stereo-selective elimination of the 13-L hydrogen atom from the precursor fatty acid, followed by isomerization of the Δ^{11} double bond into the Δ^{12} position and stereospecific hydroperoxidation at the 11α position (Hamberg and Samuelsson, 1967). The 11α-hydroperoxide can then attack the 9α position of the Δ^8 double bond with concomitant conrotatory cyclization between C-8 and C-12, isomerization of the Δ^{12} double bond into the Δ^{13} position and another stereospecific hydroperoxidation at the 15(S) position. This process requires molecular oxygen (Samuelsson, 1965; Klenberg and Samuelsson, 1965; Nugteren and Van Dorp, 1965) and is catalyzed by a mono-oxygenase and a dioxygenase (cyclo-oxygenase, Hamberg et al., 1974b). The resulting compound, 15(S)-hydroperoxy-9, 11α-cyclic prostaglandin endoperoxide, is reduced enzymatically to 15(S)-hydroxy-9, 11α-cyclic prostaglandin endoperoxide. Both endoperoxides have been recently isolated (Nugteren and Hazelhof, 1973; Hamberg and Samuelsson, 1973; Hamberg et al., 1974a; Willis et al., 1974; Pace-Asciak and Nashat, 1975a) and named respectively PGG and PGH (Nelson, 1974). The PGH endoperoxide acts as the substrate for several reactions that are both enzymatic and non-enzymatic. The end-products are listed below (see also Figure 1.1).

  (i) PGE, formed by an endoperoxide isomerase (Nugteren and Hazelhof, 1973; Hamberg and Samuelsson, 1973)

 (ii) PGF_α formed by an endoperoxide reductase (Nugteren and Hazelhof 1973; Hamberg and Samuelsson, 1973)

(iii) PGD, formed by a PGH–PGD isomerase (Nugteren and Hazelhof, 1973)

(iv) 6(9)oxy-$PGF_{2\alpha}$, formed by a specific cyclase (Pace-Asciak and Wolfe, 1971; Pace-Asciak and Nashat, 1975b)

 (v) malonaldehyde, 12-hydroxyheptadecatrienoic and 12-hydroxyheptadecadienoic acids (Niehaus and Samuelsson, 1968; Nugteren and Hazelhof, 1973; Hamberg and Samuelsson, 1974a, b; Hamberg et al., 1974b)

(vi) 12-hydroxyeicosatetraenoic acid (Hamberg and Samuelsson, 1974a, b; Hamberg et al., 1974b)

(vii) PHD, a hemiacetal derivative of 8-(1-hydroxy-3-oxopropyl)-9,12-dihydroxy-5, 10-heptadecadienoic acid (Hamberg and Samuelsson, 1974a, b; Hamberg et al., 1974b)

Several other prostaglandin-like products (cyclic ethers) have been isolated (Pace-Asciak, 1971), but it is not yet known whether they are formed enzymatically via the endoperoxide(s) or via an entirely separate pathway.

  A central feature of this process is that prostaglandins are not accumulated in stores, but are formed continuously as required by the functional state of the tissue. Also, the direction of prostaglandin biosynthesis can be modified by a number of factors. In the tissue homogenate, PGE biosynthesis is stimulated by reduced glutathione (Nugteren *et al.*, 1966). Conversely, PGFs are formed preferentially in the presence of tetrahydrofolate (Hamberg and Samuelsson, 1967), copper-dithiol mixtures (Lands *et al.*, 1971; Maddox, 1973) and catecholamines (Sih *et al.*, 1970); although an increase in both PGE_2 and $6(9)oxy-PGF_{2\alpha}$ rather than $PGF_{2\alpha}$ is reported by Pace-Asciak (1972) in the rat stomach. The relative amounts of PGEs and PGFs formed may also change in the intact tissue (*in vitro* and *in vivo*), particularly with brain (see Section 1.4).

The biosynthetic sequence, as outlined here, has been verified with seminal vesicles and some other tissues but information is lacking about the sequence in the central nervous system. Prostaglandins of E- and F-type have been isolated from brain of several species (for a summary, see Coceani, 1974). PGE_2 and $PGF_{2\alpha}$ are found more commonly in mammals, and in some cases they have been unequivocally identified (Samuelsson, 1964; Pappius *et al.*, 1974; Pace-Asciak, 1975b). Reported values of prostaglandin content are inconsistent (0.01 to 0.3 $\mu g/g$ tissue for $PGF_{2\alpha}$), which is not surprising because biosynthesis is stimulated by a variety of physiological and unphysiological factors (for a summary, see Piper and Vane, 1971), including dissection of specimens (Wolfe, 1975) and tissue homogenization at low temperature (Pace-Asciak *et al.*, 1968). Thus, these values reflect the biosynthetic capacity of the tissue rather than the actual endogenous level of the compounds. This is a well-recognized phenomenon, and explains why the early line of research which aimed at determining prostaglandin content of tissues has been abandoned in favour of the more meaningful measurement of prostaglandin biosynthesis. One method commonly employed in the measurement of the biosynthetic activity of tissues (whole homogenate or microsomal fraction) involves the conversion of a labelled precursor fatty acid into prostaglandin. While this method works well with some tissues (e.g. seminal vesicles, renal papilla and stomach fundus), it cannot be used with most tissues, and particularly with brain. In brain, only 1–2% of the exogenous labelled substrate is converted to the prostaglandins; yet, significant amounts of prostaglandins are formed from the endogenous substrate. The dilution of the added precursor by the endogenous fatty acid pool probably explains this apparent anomaly (Pace-Asciak *et al.*, 1968). Relevant to this point is the demonstration in brain of both calcium-sensitive and calcium-insensitive phospholipases that can be activated by many conditions (Gatt, 1968; Webster and Cooper, 1968; Bazan, 1970; Price and Rowe, 1972; Woelk and Porcellati, 1973). Alternatively, the exogenous fatty acid normally used in trace quantities in the incubation system may bind non-specifically to proteins, thus remaining inaccessible to the synthetic enzymes. Both difficulties are overcome by measuring biosynthesis from the endogenous substrate in the presence or the absence of relatively large amounts of exogenous unlabelled precursor. This approach has been used with several organs, including brain, and the results are summarized in Table 1.1. The values for biosynthetic activity of brain are similar to those of most organs and show no obvious variation with the maturity of the tissue. The data presented in Table 1.1 require a comment with regard to the time-course of the biosynthetic reaction in the intact tissue (slice) versus

Table 1.1 Biosynthesis of PGE₂ and PGF₂ₓ by several organs

Organ	Species	Age	Amount of exogenous arachidonic acid added ($\mu g/g$ tissue)	Incubation time (min)	*Prostaglandin formed ($\mu g/g$ tissue) E_2	$F_{2\alpha}$	Reference
KIDNEY							
Medulla	Rabbit	Adult	1000	60	20–24	8–14	Crowshaw (1971)
Medulla	Rabbit	Adult	0	60	10–14	5–7	Crowshaw (1971)
†‡Medulla	Rabbit	Adult	10	30	12–16	—	Larsson and Änggård (1973)
Medulla	Rabbit	Adult	98	30	22	7	Hamberg (1969)
†‡Papilla	Rabbit	Adult	10	30	16–28	—	Larsson and Änggård (1973)
Papilla (slice)	Rat	Adult	0	30	10	—	Danon and Chang (1973)
Papilla	Rat	Adult	100	10	9	23	Pace-Asciak (1975b)
Papilla	Rat	20 days	100	10	5	18	Pace-Asciak (1975b)
LUNG	Guinea pig	Adult	40	30	0.4–2.0	0.8–2.0	Vane (1971)
†‡SPLEEN	Dog	Adult	20	20	1.7–3.0	—	Flower et al. (1972)
BRAIN							
†‡Whole brain	Rabbit	Adult	60	20	1.36	—	Flower and Vane (1972)
Whole brain	Rat	Adult	100	10	1.6–1.9	0.40–0.44	Pace-Asciak (unpublished)
Whole brain	Rat	1 day	100	10	1.90	0.23	Pace-Asciak (unpublished)
Whole brain	Lamb	Fetus at term	100	10	0.50	0.10	Pace-Asciak (1975b)
Whole brain	Lamb	2 days	100	10	0.53	0.13	Pace-Asciak (1975b)
§Cerebral cortex (slice)	Rat	Adult	0	60	0.26	0.71	Wolfe (1975)
§Cerebral cortex (slice)	Rat	Adult	0	60	0.12	0.56	Wolfe (1975)
§Cerebral cortex (slice)	Cat	Adult	0	60	0.53	1.52	Wolfe (1975)

* Incubation of the whole homogenate or a tissue slice at 37 °C. Phosphate buffer used unless indicated otherwise
† Incubation of the microsomal fraction at 37 °C
‡ Reduced glutathione and hydroquinone added
§ Incubation in Ringer–bicarbonate–glucose medium

tissue fractions (whole homogenate or microsomal fraction). Biosynthetic enzymes remain active for a long period (up to 2 h at 37 °C) in the intact tissue (Tan and Privett, 1973; Wolfe, 1975), whereas their activity is terminated within a 10-min period (37 °C) in the homogenate (Struijk et al., 1966). Thus, the two sets of values are not strictly comparable.

A novel method for measuring the capacity of part of the biosynthetic pathway is afforded by the recent isolation of the endoperoxide intermediates (Nugteren and Hazelhof, 1973; Hamberg and Samuelsson, 1973; Hamberg et al., 1974a; Willis et al., 1974). PGG_2 and PGH_2 endoperoxides are converted in good yield (50–70%) to PGE_2 and $PGF_{2\alpha}$ in the total homogenate of rat brain (Pace-Asciak and Nashat, 1975c), thus indicating a high activity of the endoperoxide reductase and isomerase. This finding supports the view expressed earlier that low conversion of labelled arachidonic acid to prostaglandins in nervous tissue is due largely, if not exclusively, to dilution by the endogenous substrate.

1.2.1 Inhibition of prostaglandin biosynthesis

Several compounds of diverse chemical structure are known to inhibit prostaglandin biosynthesis (for a review, see Flower, 1974). Among these, aspirin and related drugs are particularly important and have been used extensively in brain (see Section 1.5) and elsewhere, to investigate the functional role of the prostaglandins. These compounds have unequal potency on the prostaglandin synthetase from various sources (see Flower, 1974). For example, paracetamol (4-acetamidophenol), an antipyretic drug devoid of anti-inflammatory activity, is about 10 times more active on the brain than on the spleen synthetase (Flower and Vane, 1972; Willis et al., 1972). While this finding may have important implications therapeutically (see Section 1.5.2.1), it also raises some intriguing questions about the molecular form and the cellular localization of the prostaglandin synthetase. Flower and Vane (1974) have proposed that the synthetase may exist in multiple molecular forms. Alternatively, the same synthetase may be located in different regions of the plasma membrane (or the endoplasmic reticulum) and may then be unevenly accessible to the inhibitor. Consistent with the latter concept is the finding (Raz et al., 1973) that indomethacin effectively blocks prostaglandin synthesis in homogenates but not in slices of seminal vesicles. More work is needed to settle this point.

1.3 METABOLISM

Prostaglandins are metabolized by tissues to a variety of products. The sequence of reactions that take place in vitro and in vivo is mainly known through the elegant and extensive studies of the investigators at the Karolinska Institutet (Änggård and Samuelsson, 1964; Änggård et al., 1965, 1971; Änggård and Larsson, 1971; Granström et al., 1965; Granström and Samuelsson, 1969a, b; 1971; Granström, 1972; Gréen, 1969, 1971; Gréen and Samuelsson, 1971; Hamberg, 1968, 1973, 1974; Hamberg and

Israelsson, 1970; Hamberg and Samuelsson, 1969a, b). Their work complemented with that of other groups has led to the definition of several enzymatic reactions. These are shown in Figure 1.2. Among the various enzymes, the 15-hydroxy dehydrogenase (15-PGDH) is most important because of its wide occurrence and its rate-limiting function in the main metabolic pathway.

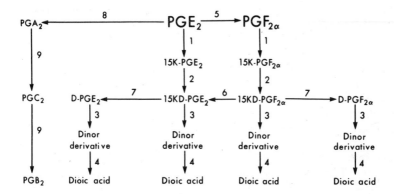

1. 15-hydroxy dehydrogenase (Anggard et al., 1971)

2. Δ^{13}-reductase (Anggard et al., 1971)

3. β-oxidation (Hamberg, 1968; Hamberg and Samuelsson, 1969; Granstrom and Samuelsson, 1971)

4. ω-oxidation (Hamberg, 1968; Hamberg and Samuelsson, 1969; Granstrom and Samuelsson, 1971)

5. *PGE 9-keto(α)-reductase (Hensby, 1974; Lee and Levine, 1974)

6. 15-keto-13,14-dihydro PGF$_\alpha$ 9α-hydroxy dehydrogenase (Pace-Asciak, 1975)

7. 15-keto-13,14-dihydro PG 15-keto reductase (Anggard and Samuelsson, 1964)

8. Dehydratase (Kantor et al., 1974; Polet and Levine, 1975)

9. Isomerase (Jones et al., 1972)

Figure 1.2 Steps in the metabolism of E-type and F-type prostaglandins. This is a comprehensive scheme, and some of the references pertaining to the identification, distribution and subcellular localization of individual enzymes are given in parentheses. 15K-PG, 15-keto prostaglandin; 15KD-PG, 15-keto-13,14-dihydro prostaglandin; D-PG, 13-14-dihydro prostaglandin.
*PGE 9-keto(β)-reductase has also been reported (Hamberg, 1968; Hamberg and Israelsson, 1970)

The activity and distribution of metabolic enzymes in the central nervous system are peculiar. Although Änggård et al. (1971) reported originally that porcine brain contains some 15-PGDH and high levels of 13-PGR (Δ^{13}-reductase), subsequent studies in several mammalian species (rat, guinea pig, lamb, rabbit, dog, cat) have been essentially negative (Nakano et al., 1972; Pappius et al., 1974; Pace-Asciak, 1975b and unpublished). In all such studies, the conversion of labelled prostaglandins to less polar (15K or 15KD) products, whether in the intact tissue or in tissue homogenates, is at the most around 4%. Interestingly, the brain of two of four species examined (lamb and rabbit, but not rat and guinea pig) shows significant 15-PGDH and 13-PGR activities during the fetal period (Pace-Asciak et al., 1974; Pace-Asciak, unpublished). In this respect, results with the lamb (Pace-Asciak *et al.*, 1974) are particularly striking and demonstrate an inverse relation between metabolic activity and brain maturity. The activity of the 15-PGDH and 13-PGR is seemingly related not only to ontogenesis but also to the phylogenetic condition of the animal. Support for this concept comes from work of Bishai and Coceani (1975), who found significant activities of both enzymes in the spinal cord of mature frogs.

A third enzyme, PGE 9-keto(α)-reductase (9K-PGR), has recently been described in the brain of various mammals (Leslie and Levine, 1973; Lee and Levine, 1974) and has been unequivocally identified in the frog spinal cord (Bishai and Coceani, 1975). This enzyme is responsible for the direct conversion of E to F prostaglandins (Figure 1.2). Interestingly, the capacity of the enzyme of the frog spinal cord, whether in the intact tissue or tissue fractions, is conspicuously higher (100 times in the tissue homogenate) than that of the 15-PGDH or the 13-PGR (Bishai and Coceani, 1975). However, the time-course of the reaction, at least with tissue homogenates, is slower (Bishai and Coceani, 1975; see also Lee and Levine, 1974).

Species and age differences in the activity of these enzymes are not easily explained. High activity of the 15-PGDH and 13-PGR at an early stage of development could be important to the postulated role (see Section 1.6) of prostaglandins in neuronal growth and differentiation (protection against the premature induction of cell differentiation?), but this concept is not easily reconciled with the observed species differences. The significance of these findings is further complicated by the more general question of the mechanism of prostaglandin inactivation in the central nervous system. Although it has been suggested (Wolfe, 1975) that, in the absence of catabolizing enzymes, the action of prostaglandins may be terminated through their removal by the circulation and/or the cerebrospinal fluid (Holmes and Horton, 1968b; Bito and Davson, 1974), the efficiency of such mechanism(s) is somewhat questionable especially in those instances where prostaglandins are implicated in synaptic processes (see Section 1.6). Alternative ways for rapid prostaglandin inactivation are then required, and clues as to their identity are afforded by studies in the central nervous system and elsewhere. High turnover of prostaglandins may be confined to certain types of cells. The metabolic enzymes of such cells escape detection when large sections of the brain (or the whole brain) are analysed. Consistent with this view is the finding of Siggins *et al.* (1971b) that Purkinje cells are unique among other neuronal types, within and without the cerebellum, for their high 15-PGDH activity. Alternatively, inactivation could be attained through a shift of the direction of prostaglandin biosynthesis towards inactive compounds (see Section 1.2) and/or through the direct interconversion of the prostaglandins. The conversion of PGEs to PGFs may well be an inactivation step, because, of the different sensitivity of the adenylate cyclase system, a major target for prostaglandin action, to the two classes of compounds (see Section 1.6). Interestingly, PGFs rather than PGEs are formed in the stimulated, intact tissue (see Section 1.4). Finally, recent work proving the high biological activity of the labile endoperoxide intermediates in some tissues (Hamberg *et al.*, 1974b; Willis *et al.*, 1974; Hamberg *et al.*, 1975) raises the possibility that such intermediates, and not the classical prostaglandins, are the active species of the prostaglandin system. Transformation of the endoperoxide intermediates to the prostaglandins would represent a de-activation. All of the mechanisms considered here are not mutually exclusive. In fact, they may well function together and provide a flexible and efficient means of prostaglandin inactivation in the central nervous system.

1.4 RELEASE

There are a number of studies showing that PGEs and PGFs (or, in most cases, PGE- and PGF-like compounds) are released from various regions of the central nervous system both *in vivo* and *in vitro*. (Coceani and Wolfe, 1965; Ramwell and Shaw, 1966; Ramwell *et al.*, 1966; Bradley *et al.*, 1969; Matsuura *et al.*, 1969; Holmes, 1970; Beleslin and Myers, 1971; Beleslin *et al.*, 1971; Coceani *et al.*, 1971; Samuels, 1972; Feldberg and Gupta, 1973; Feldberg *et al.*, 1973; Dey *et al.*, 1974a, b; Wolfe and Mamer, 1975) as well as from cultured neuroblastoma and glial cells (Hamprecht *et al.*, 1973). In general, the rate of release correlates with the level of neuronal activity. Several stimuli (Table 1.2), that may or may not be physiological, can accelerate such release and their action is likely exerted on the rate-limiting step in the biosynthetic pathway (see Figure 1.1). Consistent with this view is the finding (Price and Rowe, 1972) that some neurohormones (e.g. 5-hydroxytryptamine) increase the concentration of unesterified fatty acids, including arachidonic acid, in brain synaptosomes.

The site of prostaglandin release cannot be defined under the conditions of the experiments, and it may well vary with the kind of stimulus applied. While stimulation of neural pathways conceivably affects only neurons, neurohormones may act on both neurons and glia. Pyrogens may elicit prostaglandin release from neurons and leucocytes, whereas multiple loci—neurons, vessels, platelets—probably contribute to the prostaglandin release under ischaemic conditions.

Table 1.2   Stimuli for prostaglandin release in the central nervous system

Stimulus	Species	Reference
Neural	Cat	Ramwell and Shaw (1966); Bradley *et al.* (1969)
	Frog	Ramwell *et al.* (1966); Coceani *et al.* (1971)
Neurohormones	Dog	Holmes (1970)
	Frog	Ramwell *et al.* (1966)
Analeptics	Cat	Ramwell and Shaw (1966); Samuels (1972)
Pyrogens	Cat	Feldberg and Gupta (1973); Feldberg *et al.* (1973); Dey *et al.* (1974a)
Trauma	Man	Wolfe and Mamer (1975)
	Cat	Dey *et al.* (1974b)
Ischaemia	Man	La Torre *et al.* (1974); Wolfe and Mamer (1975)

An interesting feature of prostaglandin release in the central nervous system is that F compounds are formed preferentially, if not exclusively, upon stimulation (Ramwell *et al.*, 1966; Bradley *et al.*, 1969; Coceani *et al.*, 1971). This event may reflect a change in the direction of prostaglandin biosynthesis at the endoperoxide step and/or the direct conversion of E to F prostaglandins, and it may be important to the termination of prostaglandin effects (see Section 1.3).

1.4.1 Prostaglandins in cerebrospinal fluid

It has been known for some time that prostaglandin-like material is normally present in the cerebrospinal fluid (c.s.f.) of humans and various experimental animals (Holmes, 1970; see also Ramwell, 1964; Buckell, 1964; Wilkins *et al.*,

Table 1.3   PGF$_{2\alpha}$ in human cerebrospinal fluid

Condition	Mean concentration (pg/ml)	No. of samples
*Normal	72 (range: 30–139)	16
Epilepsy before surgery	559 (range: 124–1230)	11
Epilepsy after surgery	1197 (range: 118–2500)	13
Meningitis–encephalitis	954 (range: 252–2196)	5

Modified after Wolfe and Mamer (1975). PGF$_{2\alpha}$ measured by the gas chromatographic–mass spectrometric technique
* Patients with no evidence of organic disease. Normal c.s.f. and pneumogram

1967). Only recently, however, one prostaglandin component of the c.s.f. (PGF$_{2\alpha}$) has been unequivocally identified (Wolfe and Mamer, 1975) and its levels have been measured in normal human subjects and in patients suffering from a variety of pathological conditions (La Torre *et al.*, 1974; Wolfe and Mamer, 1975). Table 1.3 provides a partial summary of the findings of Wolfe and Mamer (1975). PGF$_{2\alpha}$ levels, which are normally below 100 pg/ml, are elevated when neuronal activity is pathologically enhanced, and as a result of inflammatory states and brain damage. All these conditions are known to stimulate prostaglandin synthesis (for a review, see Piper and Vane, 1971). Values in the control group are in good agreement with those obtained by radioimmunoassay (La Torre *et al.*, 1974). La Torre *et al.* (1974) have analysed in detail the PGF$_{2\alpha}$ content of c.s.f. in patients with ruptured aneurysms on the assumption that the prostaglandin is responsible for the arterial vasospasm commonly associated with this condition (see Section 1.7). Indeed, most of these patients showed a severalfold elevation of PGF$_{2\alpha}$ levels, but the prostaglandin activity did not correlate with the presence or severity of the vasospasm. Comparable results are found in the report of Wolfe and Mamer (1975).

Prostaglandin activity of the c.s.f. has been also studied in pyrogen fever. As mentioned elsewhere (Section 1.5.2.1), c.s.f. collected during febrile episodes contains high amounts of a prostaglandin with the properties of PGE_2 (Feldberg et al., 1973). This prostaglandin is thought to be an essential link in the action of pyrogens on neurons, but its identity needs to be confirmed by chemical means.

Another aspect of prostaglandin research of relevance here concerns migraine. Some years ago, Barrie and Jowett (1967) reported that c.s.f. of migranous patients contains at times an active material which may be identified with the prostaglandins. This has not been confirmed (Sandler, 1972). Still, the idea that prostaglandins might be implicated in the pathogenesis of migraine remains particularly appealing because of the vasoactive properties of these compounds (see Section 1.7) and their ability to induce a migraine-like attack (Bergström et al., 1965; Carlson et al., 1968). A systematic study of c.s.f. from migranous patients employing chemical or immunologic assay techniques is required to settle this point.

1.5 ACTION OF PROSTAGLANDINS

1.5.1 Behaviour

Prostaglandins have a depressant action on behaviour, which varies in intensity from mild sedation to catatonia depending on the route of administration and the compound used. PGEs are most active (Horton, 1964; Horton and Main, 1965; Holmes and Horton, 1968a, b; Asakawa and Yoshida, 1971; Potts and East, 1971a; Gilmore and Shaikh, 1972; Desiraju, 1973; Haubrich et al., 1973; Nisticó and Marley, 1973; Potts et al., 1973, Wellmann and Schwabe, 1973), but little or no effect is seen with $PGF_{2\alpha}$ (Horton and Main, 1965; Gilmore and Shaikh, 1972; Desiraju, 1973; Wellmann and Schwabe, 1973). Results with PGA_2 are inconsistent (Potts and East, 1971b; Gilmore and Shaikh, 1972; Dobrin et al., 1973). Behavioural changes are particularly striking after intraventricular injection of PGE_1 or PGE_2 (7–20 µg/kg in the cat; 25–50 µg/kg in the monkey) and consist of a reduction in spontaneous locomotion and of unresponsiveness to stimuli, followed by stupor and eventually catatonia. Symptoms are persistent, and a varying degree of sedation may still be detected in animals 48 h after the injection. By contrast, a short-lived sedation (30–60 min) follows administration of PGEs by the parenteral route, even at higher doses (0.5 mg/kg or more). The substantial degradation of circulating prostaglandins in lungs and other organs explains the different intensity of responses.

The depressant effect of prostaglandins is also manifested by their interaction with other drugs. In particular, they enhance the action of barbiturates (Holmes and Horton, 1968a; Gilmore and Shaikh, 1972) and oppose the convulsive effects of pentylenetetrazol and strychnine (Holmes and Horton, 1968a; Duru and Türker, 1969).

Electrocorticographic activity changes inconsistently during prostaglandin-induced sedation. A slow-wave pattern prevails in some cases (Desiraju,

1973; Nisticó and Marley, 1973), while in others the electroencephalogram is reminiscent of that recorded during activated sleep (Haubrich et al., 1973). The two patterns may also occur in different phases of the same sedation period (Desiraju, 1973). Lyneham et al. (1973) have reported electro-encephalographic abnormalities of epileptic type in some patients treated with $PGF_{2\alpha}$ for termination of pregnancy, but the finding has not been confirmed (Fraser and Gray, 1974a, b; Van der Plaetsen et al., 1974).

The mechanism for the sedative action remains uncertain. Experiments with labelled PGE_1 (Holmes and Horton, 1968b) indicate that only minute amounts of compound are taken up by nervous tissue, even after intra-ventricular injection. In some way, however, this little prostaglandin causes a long-lasting change of neuronal function. According to Haubrich et al. (1973), prostaglandin effects are exerted through an increase of the turnover of 5-hydroxytryptamine. Cholinergic (Haubrich et al., 1973) and nor-adrenergic (Bergström et al., 1973) mechanisms may also be modified by the compounds. Some evidence links the sedative action to the stimulation of adenylate cyclase (Wellmann and Schwabe, 1973). Conceivably, several factors, including possibly an alteration in the cerebral circulation (see Section 1.7), contribute to the behavioural change. The low or absent 15-PGDH and 13-PGR activities (see Section 1.3) may account for the persistence of effects.

1.5.2 Hypothalamus

1.5.2.1 Regulation of body temperature

For some time, it was thought that the constancy of body temperature depends solely on the interplay between monoamines (5-hydroxytryptamine and norepinephrine) and acetylcholine at hypothalamic sites (Feldberg and Myers, 1964; Lomax, 1970; Myers, 1971; Bligh et al., 1971). Two recent findings—the demonstration that prostaglandins are potent pyretic agents (Milton and Wendlandt, 1970) and that antipyretics block prostaglandin synthesis in tissues (Vane, 1971)—have brought the prostaglandins into the field of thermoregulation and have stimulated a great deal of research on these compounds. To date, the concept that prostaglandins are implicated in temperature responses is well-established, and questions pertinent to their function can be formulated as follows:

    (a) Are prostaglandins involved in the pathogenesis of pyrogen fever?
    (b) If so, are they also involved in other forms of fever?
    (c) Do prostaglandins play a role in normal thermoregulation?
    (d) Are the prostaglandins functionally related to the monoaminergic, cholinergic and adenylate cyclase systems?

It is somewhat paradoxical that this review should dwell first upon the pathology rather than the physiology of thermoregulation. However, impressive advances in fever research justify this curious 'cart-before-the-horse' approach. Supporting evidence for a role of prostaglandins in pyrogen fever is summarized below.

(i) E and F prostaglandins are normal constituents of hypothalamic tissue (Holmes and Horton, 1968a, c), and their identity has been unequivocally determined by mass spectrometric analysis (Pappius et al., 1974; Wolfe, 1975)

(ii) Administration of prostaglandins by the ventricular route or by local injection into the hypothalamus produces a prompt elevation of body temperature (Milton and Wendlandt, 1971b; Feldberg and Saxena, 1971a; Potts and East, 1972; Hales et al., 1973; Nisticó and Marley, 1973; Lipton and Fossler, 1974; Pittman et al., 1975). PGE_1 and PGE_2 are generally most effective (threshold: 100pg; see Veale and Cooper, 1974), although species differences in the relative activity of E versus F prostaglandins have been reported. For example, it has been shown that $PGF_{2\alpha}$ is almost as active as PGE_2 in the sheep (Hales et al., 1973). The same may apply to humans, judging from the frequent occurrence of pyrexia during the clinical use of $PGF_{2\alpha}$ (Hendricks et al., 1971; Gillett et al., 1972). Unlike the monoamines (Veale and Cooper 1973), prostaglandins are hyperthermic agents in all but one (Baird et al., 1974) of the several species examined. In this respect, prostaglandins mimic the pyrogens. Yet, an important difference between prostaglandin and pyrogen fever is that only the latter is susceptible to antipyretic treatment (Milton and Wendlandt, 1970; Milton and Wendlandt, 1971a; Milton, 1973)

(iii) Arachidonic acid, the precursor to PGE_2 and $PGF_{2\alpha}$, causes a rise in body temperature when injected into the cerebral ventricles (Girault et al., 1973; Splawinski et al., 1974). Unlike the prostaglandin fever, the arachidonic acid fever shows delayed onset and slow time-course, and also it is abolished by antipyretics. These findings not only confirm the presence of prostaglandin synthetase in hypothalamic tissue but also suggest that the fatty acid acquires pyretic activity upon conversion to a prostaglandin

(iv) Microinjection (Feldberg and Saxena, 1971b; Stitt, 1973; Veale and Cooper, 1975) and ablation (Veale and Cooper, 1975) experiments have proved that the anterior hypothalamic preoptic area is the target of PGE action. Pyrogens act most intensely at the same site (Cooper et al., 1967; Veale and Cooper, 1975; Myers et al., 1974). Probably, the same region is involved with the antipyretic effect of drugs (Cranston and Rawlins, 1972; Avery and Penn, 1974)

(v) The magnitude and time-course of PGE fever are identical at low and high ambient temperatures (Stitt, 1973; Bligh and Milton, 1973; Hales et al., 1973; Hori and Harada, 1974; Veale and Cooper, 1975). However, the mechanism whereby the febrile response is brought about differs in the two conditions. Thus, heat production is maximal in the cold and reduction of heat loss predominates during heat exposure. Findings are similar with the pyrogens (Palmes and Park, 1965)

(vi) Although the site and mode of action are seemingly the same for PGEs and pyrogens, PGE fever has a quicker onset (Stitt, 1973; Lipton and Fossler, 1974; Schoener and Wang, 1974; Veale and

Cooper, 1975; Pittman *et al.*, 1975). This may mean that prostaglandin has a more direct action on the thermogenic mechanism

(vii) Pyrogen fever is associated with the appearance of, or increase in, prostaglandin activity in the c.s.f. (Feldberg and Gupta, 1973; Feldberg *et al.*, 1973; Dey *et al.*, 1974a). The prostaglandin has the chromatographic, immunologic and biological properties of PGE_2 (Feldberg *et al.*, 1973). Prostaglandin levels parallel the course of the febrile episode, and antipyretic treatment is effective in reducing both fever and prostaglandin synthesis (Feldberg and Gupta, 1973; Feldberg *et al.*, 1973; Dey *et al.*, 1974a). The action of pyrogens (as PG-releasing agents) is not confined to the hypothalamus but extends to the whole brain (Feldberg *et al.*, 1973)

(viii) Microiontophoretic studies with PGEs (PGE_1 and PGE_2) have demonstrated a greater incidence of responses among thermosensitive versus non-thermosensitive cells of the hypothalamus (Ford, 1974; Jell, 1975; see also Section 1.5.5). Both excitation and inhibition have been described, but according to Ford (1974) cold-sensitive cells respond exclusively with excitation. The latter result is reminiscent of findings with pyrogens (Cabanac *et al.*, 1968; Eisenman, 1969).

All these findings are consistent with the idea that prostaglandins endogenous to the anterior hypothalamus mediate the fever response to pyrogens. According to a current model, pyrogens act at some step in the prostaglandin biosynthetic process to accelerate or trigger the *ex novo* formation of an E-type compound, which, in turn, produces fever by resetting the 'hypothalamic thermostat' at higher body temperatures. Whether the action of PGEs is direct or mediated, at least in part, by the monoaminergic, cholinergic or adenylate cyclase systems (see below) is an open question. Also, it is not known whether the site of pyrogen-induced PGE synthesis is neuronal, as generally implied, or extra-neuronal (leucocytes?). A final question concerns the significance of pyrogen action outside the hypothalamus. According to Feldberg *et al.* (1973), some of the symptoms occurring with high fever (e.g. malaise) could result from the exaggerated formation of PGEs through brain.

Prostaglandins might also be involved in the pathogenesis of non-infective fever (question b above). This possibility has been recently examined with some forms of experimental fever (Dey *et al.*, 1974b) and with a variety of clinical conditions (Hanson *et al.*, 1975). Two criteria have been used, at least in the experimental situation, to identify a prostaglandin fever, namely occurrence of high prostaglandin activity in the c.s.f. and sensitivity to antipyretic treatment (Dey *et al.*, 1974b). According to Dey *et al.* (1974b) the fever which follows injection of artificial c.s.f. into the cerebral ventricles satisfies both criteria. In contrast, acute pyrexia occurring during perfusion of the cerebral ventricles with calcium-free artificial c.s.f. appears not to be mediated by the prostaglandins. A single criterion (e.g. effectiveness of antipyretics) can be applied to the clinical situation. Despite the limitation, findings suggest that prostaglandins may indeed be implicated in the fever associated with neoplastic disorders and with acute myocardial infarction

(Hanson *et al.*, 1975). Conceivably, prostaglandins have no role in febrile states where central thermoregulation is not impaired (e.g. thyrotoxicosis).

The question of whether prostaglandins are concerned with normal thermoregulation (question c above) is intimately connected to that of the relation of the prostaglandins to other neurohumoral agents (question d), and the two problems are best examined together. The literature on the subject is not easily appraised, because of the many inconsistencies and the species differences in the (postulated) humoral control of body temperature (for a review, see Veale and Cooper, 1973). Therefore, it is convenient to define the conditions for a prostaglandin role in thermoregulation, and then examine whether the experimental data agree with the theoretical postulate. Since the participation of the monoamines in thermoregulatory processes is well established (Feldberg and Myers, 1964; Lomax, 1970; Myers, 1971; Bligh *et al.*, 1971), the first condition is that prostaglandins either mediate the action of monoamines (or rather the monoamine that happens to be thermogenic depending on the species) on thermosensitive cells or act through the monoaminergic pathways to produce appropriate temperature adjustments. Secondly, prostaglandins need to be synthesized continuously in the hypothalamic control centres to maintain body temperature within the physiological range. As a corollary it has to be postulated that fever and normal thermoregulation are different states of activity of the same process, which involves the prostaglandins and the monoamines. The experimental evidence is negative or inconclusive on either point.

Some years ago, Holmes (1970) found that infusion of 5-hydroxytryptamine into the cerebral ventricles of the dog stimulated the release of PGE compounds. In contrast, catecholamines had no effect. Since 5-hydroxytryptamine and catecholamines are respectively thermogenic and thermolytic in this species (see Veale and Cooper, 1973), these findings might suggest that prostaglandins are mediators of monoamine action. The work of Milton and Wendlandt (1968, 1971a) showing inhibition of the late phase of 5-hydroxytryptamine (cat) and epinephrine (rat) hyperthermia by paracetamol is consistent with this idea. However, the recent demonstration (Dey *et al.*, 1974b) that perfusion of the cerebral ventricles with artificial c.s.f. leads *per se* (injury?) to a gradual rise in PGE synthesis and fever casts serious doubts on the validity of the above results (see also Milton and Harvey, 1975). This proposal is further weakened by the report (Kandasamy *et al.*, 1975) that antipyretics have inconsistent effects on monoamine fever in the rabbit.

The alternative proposal of a mediation of prostaglandin effects by monoamines is equally controversial. Several years ago, it was shown (Cooper *et al.*, 1967) that depletion of brain monoamines with reserpine, while severely impairing the thermoregulatory mechanisms, is without effect on the fever induced by pyrogens. A recent extension of that work (Cooper and Veale, 1974; see also Cooper *et al.*, 1975) differs somewhat in the conclusions for it proves that fever responses to both pyrogens and PGE_1 are delayed in onset and development in the reserpinized animal. The problem of monoamine function in PGE_1 fever has been also approached though the use of specific inhibitors of noradrenergic or serotoninergic pathways, and again results have been inconsistent. Thus, Harvey and Milton (1974; see also Milton and Harvey, 1975, and Laburn *et al.*, 1974) have found that febrile responses to PGE_1 are substantially reduced following depletion of 5-hydroxytryptamine (cat) or norepinephrine (rabbit) stores in brain. Accordingly, phenoxybenzamine (an α-adrenergic blocking agent) attenuated PGE_1 fever in the rabbit (Laburn et al., 1974) and methysergide (a 5-hydroxytryptamine blocker) lowered normal body temperature in the cat (Milton and Harvey, 1975). However, other investigators have reported negative (Sinclair and Chaplin, 1974; Veale and Cooper, 1975) or inconclusive (Kandasamy et al., 1975) results under similar experimental conditions. An additional point against this proposal is that PGE_1 hyperthermia (Stitt, 1973; Bligh and Milton, 1973; Hales et al., 1973; Hori and Harada, 1974; Veale and Cooper, 1975), unlike monoamine hyperthermia (Bligh et al., 1971), is independent of ambient temperature. Finally, it must be pointed out that the concept of monoamines being 'messengers' of prostaglandin action on hypothalamic cells runs counter to an accepted model of norepinephrine (and 5-hydroxytryptamine?)–prostaglandin relationship elsewhere (Hedqvist, 1973; see also Bergström et al., 1973; and Section 1.6).

The second condition for a prostaglandin role in normal thermoregulation, i.e., continuous prostaglandin synthesis in the afebrile state, has not been verified experimentally. Antipyretics, whether administered systemically (Milton, 1973; Pittman et al., 1974b; Kandasamy et al., 1975) or applied topically to the anterior hypothalamus (Cranston and Rawlins, 1972; Avery and Penn, 1974), have no effect on normal body temperature, and the few exceptions (Satinoff, 1972; Milton, 1973) can be explained without implicating the prostaglandin system (Milton, 1973).

In conclusion, it seems that prostaglandins are involved marginally or not at all with normal thermoregulation. No conclusion can be made on the role of monoamines in prostaglandin action and the pathogenesis of pyrogen fever. The available data strongly suggest that fever and normal thermoregulation are separate states, involving different neurohumoral mechanisms. Recent work of Cooper, Veale and associates (Pittman et al., 1974a; Cooper et al., 1975) is relevant to the last point. In brief, these authors have demonstrated that the newborn lamb does not develop fever when challenged first with pyrogens. The absence of pyrogen action contrasts sharply with the quasi-complete maturation of central thermoregulatory mechanisms, thus re-affirming the fundamental difference between physiological and pathological temperature responses.

A final comment concerns the significance of the cholinergic and adenylate cyclase systems to the hyperthermic action of prostaglandins. Cooper and Veale (1974; see also Veale and Cooper, 1975) have reported that fever responses to either pyrogen or PGE_1 are blocked by atropine, and their data suggest that the cholinergic link is located outside the anterior hypothalamic preoptic area. This finding has not been confirmed (Sinclair and Chaplin, 1974; Vishwanathan and Rudy, 1974). Stronger evidence implicates adenosine 3',5'-cyclic monophosphate (cyclic AMP) in PGE_1 fever (see also Section 1.6). First, it has been shown that cyclic AMP (or the dibutyryl derivative) causes hyperthermia when injected into the anterior hypothalamus (Breckenridge and Lisk, 1969; Laburn et al., 1974). The response is dose-dependent, and has been obtained with two of the three species examined (no response in the monkey; see Lipton and Fossler, 1974).

Secondly, pharmacologic manipulation of the adenylate cyclase modifies the magnitude of pyrogen and PGE_1 fever (Dascombe and Milton, 1972; Laburn et al., 1974). The two findings suggest (Laburn et al., 1974) that cyclic AMP is an essential intermediate in PGE (and pyrogen) action on hypothalamic neurons. Potentially relevant to this hypothesis is the finding that morphine, a hypothermic agent in low doses, antagonizes PGE stimulation of brain adenylate cyclase (Collier and Roy, 1974a, b).

1.5.2.2 Regulation of food intake

Scaramuzzi et al. (1971) were the first to report that prostaglandins given subcutaneously inhibit food intake in the rat. Among the prostaglandins tested, PGE_1 and PGE_2 were most active (effective dose 0.1 mg/kg,) followed by PGA_1, $PGF_{1\alpha}$ and $PGF_{2\alpha}$ (effective dose 1 mg/kg). PGB_1 has a small and delayed effect. Subsequent studies (Baile et al., 1973, 1974) proved that prostaglandins may also modify feeding behaviour when injected directly into the hypothalamus, but the interpretation of the results is made difficult by species differences in the location of the responsive sites, the dual action of prostaglandins in the same species and the possible interference of injected prostaglandins with thermoregulatory mechanisms. PGE_1 (2 μg), but not PGB_1, decreases food intake in the rat when injected into the lateral hypothalamus and the anterior commissure region (Baile et al., 1974). Opposite results were obtained in the ewe where microinjection of PGE_1, 5 or 10 μg, may either suppress (anterior and medial hypothalamus) or enhance (lateral hypothalamus) feeding (Baile et al., 1974). Surprisingly, PGE_2 is without effect (Baile et al., 1974). Additional findings in the ewe are that PGE_1 inhibits the norepinephrine-induced feeding (Baile, 1974) and that polyphloretin phosphate, a prostaglandin antagonist in some tissues, elicits eating when applied to sites where PGE_1 has suppressive action (Baile et al., 1974). These results have led Baile and associates (Baile et al., 1973, 1974) to propose that prostaglandins play a role in the hypothalamic control of food intake, and consequently in the maintenance of energy balance. In their view, prostaglandin action is exerted through the modulation of a noradrenergic mechanism. These findings and their interpretation have been challenged by Whishaw and Veale (1974).

1.5.3 Brain stem

Although changes of respiratory and cardiac function of possible central origin have been often described as a side-effect of the intravascular (Carlson and Orö, 1966; Carlson et al., 1969; White et al., 1971; Steiner et al., 1972) and intraventricular (or intracisternal) (Pennink et al., 1972; Emerson et al., 1974) administration of prostaglandins, few studies have dealt specifically with this topic. Kaplan et al. (1969) were the first to provide direct evidence of a centrally-mediated cardiovascular response to a prostaglandin. Using a cross-circulation procedure, they found that PGE_1 (5 or 10 μg/kg, by the intracarotid route) has a hypertensive effect in the dog.

Under normal conditions, such an effect would be masked by the hypotension resulting from stimulation of carotid sinus receptors and peripheral vasodilatation. A pressor response is also observed in the intact animal during infusion of prostaglandins into the vertebral artery (Lavery *et al.*, 1970; Sweet *et al.*, 1971; Gyang *et al.*, 1973). Results differ somewhat with the species and the experimental conditions. $PGF_{2\alpha}$ is the most potent prostaglandin in the dog and produces a dose-dependent rise of systemic arterial blood pressure in the range of 4 to 64 ng/kg per min (Lavery *et al.*, 1970). Hypertension is associated with tachycardia in the anaesthetized animal (Lavery *et al.*, 1970, 1971), but not in the unanaesthetized animal (Sweet *et al.*, 1971). PGE_1 causes only tachycardia in the anaesthetized dog (4–360 ng/kg per min) (Lavery *et al.*, 1970) and hypertension with tachycardia in the anaesthetized cat (1–20 ng/kg per min) (Gyang *et al.*, 1973). While the possibility cannot be ruled out that the prostaglandin effects may be due, at least partly, to vascular changes in the autonomic centres (see Section 1.7), the experimental evidence favours a neuronal site of action (Lavery *et al.*, 1970). Still, there is no agreement on the mechanism of such an action, and both depression of the parasympathetic tone (Lavery *et al.*, 1970) and stimulation of the sympathetic tone (Kaplan *et al.*, 1969; Sweet *et al.*, 1971) have been implicated in these responses.

Experiments with dogs suffering from sinus arrhythmia provide another example of prostaglandin action on brain stem mechanisms. In brief, McQueen and Ungar (1969) have found that PGE_1 injected rapidly into the common carotid artery (1.5–10 μg/kg) causes a substantial reduction or suppression of the arrhythmia. The effect may last up to 20 min, and is attributed to the release from a tonic control of the respiratory on the cardioinhibitory centres. PGE_1 also shortens the expiration time and this results in a marked increase (up to 100%) in pulmonary ventilation.

Synaptic transmission through the cuneate nucleus is depressed by $PGF_{2\alpha}$ applied topically (10 μg/ml) to the surface of the medulla oblongata (Coceani *et al.*, 1969). A post-synaptic site is the likely target of $PGF_{2\alpha}$ action. In contrast, PGE_1 is without effect (Coceani *et al.*, 1971), whether tested by local superfusion of the medulla or by microiontophoresis (see also Section 1.5.5).

1.5.4 Spinal cord and motor pathways

In a series of investigations, Horton and associates (for a review, see Horton, 1972) have proved that spinal reflexes and postural mechanisms are profoundly affected by the prostaglandins. Their findings, however, vary with the species, the preparation and the prostaglandin, and consequently they are not easily integrated into a consistent framework.

$PGF_{2\alpha}$ given intravenously (25–450 μg/kg) enhances extensor muscle tone and the crossed extensor reflex in the intact and spinal chick (Horton and Main, 1965). The same prostaglandin is without effect in the intact cat (Horton and Main, 1965), but it enhances the rigidity of the decerebrate animal (Horton and Main, 1967). Results with PGE_1 (1–32 μg/kg, intravenously or intra-arterially) are more complex (Horton and Main, 1967;

Duda *et al.*, 1968; Horton and Main, 1969). The crossed extensor reflex is facilitated, depressed or undergoes a biphasic change (facilitation to depression) depending on the preparation. Facilitation and depression occur respectively in the spinal and intact animal, whereas the decerebrate animal may respond in either way. In this respect, cat and chick behave similarly. An increase of the extensor tone is associated with facilitation of the crossed extensor reflex. With either prostaglandin, changes of monosynaptic reflexes are inconsistent (Horton and Main, 1967; Duda *et al.*, 1968; Horton and Main, 1969). Prostaglandin action may last up to several hours and is prone to tachyphylaxis.

According to Horton and associates, prostaglandin excitation is exerted on spinal neurons. Experiments with topically (Phillis and Tebēcis, 1968; Coceani *et al.*, 1971) and iontophoretically (Coceani and Viti, 1973, 1975; see Section 1.5.5.) applied PGE_1 in the frog spinal cord provide support for this view. Conversely, prostaglandin inhibition is attributed to the activation of pathways from supraspinal centres. It is an open question whether local circulatory changes (see Section 1.7) contribute to the responses.

1.5.5 Effects on single neurons

The microiontophoretic technique of applying drugs has been used extensively to determine effects of PGEs and PGFs on single neurons. PGE_1 has been tested more often. The action of prostaglandins, as reported originally by Avanzino *et al.* (1966) and subsequently confirmed by other investigators (Siggins *et al.*, 1971b; Coceani and Viti, 1973, 1975; Poulain and Carette, 1974), is mainly excitatory, regardless of the prostaglandin type, the animal species and the brain region examined (cerebral cortex, hypothalamus, brain stem, cerebellar cortex and spinal cord). According to Ford (1974), the pattern of responses of hypothalamic thermosensitive cells to PGE_1 accords with the postulated role of the compound in fever-producing mechanisms (see Section 1.5.2.1). Mixed responses to PGE_1, with a predominance of inhibition, have been reported with unidentified hippocampal neurons (Siggins *et al.*, 1971b). Cuneate neurons (in the cat) stand out for their unresponsiveness to PGE_1 (Coceani *et al.*, 1971; see Section 1.5.3).

Prostaglandin effects have a rapid time-course, and occasionally they outlast the application by more than 1 min (Poulain and Carette, 1974). Tachyphylaxis is a common feature of these responses and, characteristically, it is specific for the prostaglandin tested and it is not associated with changes in the reactivity of neurons to synaptic or chemical (glutamate) stimuli. Interestingly, quiescent cells can be provoked into activity by iontophoretic applications of prostaglandins (Coceani and Viti, 1973; 1975; Poulain and Carette, 1974), which is reminiscent of findings with putative neurotransmitters.

An inhibitory effect of $PGF_{2\alpha}$ on cerebrocortical neurons has been demonstrated by intracellular recording (Marazzi and Huang, 1975). $PGF_{2\alpha}$ was given by the intra-carotid route and, even though vascular effects were ruled out, the precise site of action of the compound remains to be defined.

According to some authors, direct effects of the prostaglandins do not reflect the prime (and physiological) action of the compounds. Prostaglandins are envisaged rather as modulators of transmitter action, and a pertinent model of transmitter–prostaglandin relationship is presented in Section 1.6.

1.6 PROSTAGLANDINS, CYCLIC NUCLEOTIDES AND NEUROTRANSMITTERS

There is now considerable evidence that the prostaglandin and the adenylate cyclase systems are linked together in the control of cell function (for recent reviews, see Hittelman and Butcher, 1973; Kuehl, 1974). According to an accepted scheme, cyclic AMP formed within the plasma membrane serves as the 'messenger' of external stimuli (e.g. hormonal stimuli) to intracellular effector sites, whereas the prostaglandins (PGEs in particular) modulate cell responses primarily through their action on the adenylate cyclase. An alternative proposal suggests PGEs, like cyclic AMP, function as inter-mediates in the cellular activation sequence (Kuehl, 1974). These models of PGE–cyclic AMP relationship are based on work with non-neural tissues, but they probably apply to the central nervous system as well.

Several investigators have demonstrated that prostaglandins are capable of raising cyclic AMP levels in different preparations of nervous tissue *in vitro* (Table 1.4). The effect is seen with PGEs (PGE_1 and PGE_2), but not with

Table 1.4   Effect of E-type prostaglandins on cyclic AMP concentrations of neural tissue *in vitro*

Tissue preparation	Species	Effect		Reference
		Increase	No change	
Cerebral cortex slice	Rat	+		Berti *et al.* (1973)
Whole brain homogenate	Rat	+		Collier and Roy (1974a)
Cultured fetal brain	Rat	+		Gilman and Schrier (1972)
Cerebral cortex slice	Guinea pig		+	Shimizu *et al.* (1970)
Cerebral cortex slice	Rabbit		+	Berti *et al.* (1973)
Cerebral cortex slice	Pig		+	Sato *et al.* (1974)
Medial hypothalamus slice	Pig		+	Sato *et al.* (1974)
Cerebral cortex slice	Man		+	Berti *et al.* (1973)
*Cultured neuroblastoma (C-1300)	Mouse	+		Gilman and Nirenberg (1971a); Hamprecht and Schultz (1973); Schultz and Hamprecht (1973); Sheppard and Prasad (1973)
Cultured glioma (C-6; C-2_1)	Rat	†(+)	+	Gilman and Nirenberg (1971b)
Cultured glioma (lines CHB, 118132 and 1181N1)	Man	+		Gilman and Nirenberg (1971b); Perkins (1973)

* Neuroblastoma cells have the morphological and functional properties of a differentiated neuron (Gilman 1972)
† Marginal increase with the clonal line C-6

PGFs ($PGF_{1\alpha}$ and $PGF_{2\alpha}$), and is attributed to the activation of the adenylate cyclase. Surprisingly, the response of mature nervous tissue is species-related. As shown in Table 1.4, PGEs are inactive in all of the animals examined but the rat. With the rat, stimulation occurs both *in vitro* and *in vivo* (Wellman and Schwabe, 1973). This finding suggests that the PGE-sensitive adenylate cyclase is unevenly distributed between species. Alternatively, the apparent lack of PGE effects could be explained, at least in some instances, by a rapid breakdown of the newly formed cyclic AMP. In fact, there is evidence of phosphodiesterase activation (in addition to the known activation of the adenylate cyclase) in neuroblastoma cells treated with PGE_1 (Prasad and Kumar, 1973). Furthermore, work with certain lines of neuroblastoma (Hamprecht and Schultz, 1973; Schultz and Hamprecht, 1973) has proved that PGE_1 may be inactive by itself, but it markedly increases cyclic AMP levels if tested with a phosphodiesterase inhibitor.

PGE action, whether *in vitro* or *in vivo*, has a rapid time-course (Gilman and Nirenberg, 1971a; Hamprecht and Schultz, 1973; Wellmann and Schwabe, 1973). In this respect, the response of neuroblastoma cells is particularly striking because it occurs within 1 s of the application (Gilman and Nirenberg, 1971a). Also, changes of cyclic AMP concentration can be detected after application of as little as 1 ng/ml of PGE_1 (Gilman and Nirenberg, 1971a). These two findings are consistent with the concept that the PGE–cyclic AMP complex plays a key role in neural function. Evidence of such a role is found in two processes, neuronal growth and synaptic transmission.

1 Neuronal growth and differentiation

Work with different lines of cultured cells has shown that endogenous levels of cyclic AMP are inversely related to the growth rate and that the growth rate can be stimulated or depressed by pharmacologic manipulation of the adenylate cyclase system (Burger *et al.*, 1972; Sheppard, 1972). These findings indicate that cyclic AMP might be concerned with cell differentiation. Evidence supporting this concept has been also obtained in neural tissue.

Prasad and Hsie (1971) and Furmanski *et al.* (1971) first reported that cyclic AMP (or the dibutyryl derivative) stimulates nuclear (and overall cellular) growth and neurite formation in cultured neuroblastoma cells. These morphologic changes are considered an expression of maturation and differentiation, and are associated with an increase of acetylcholinesterase activity (Furmanski *et al.*, 1971). Identical responses are obtained with inhibitors of the phosphodiesterase (Furmanski *et al.*, 1971; Prasad and Sheppard, 1972; Sheppard and Prasad, 1973) and with E-type prostaglandins (Prasad, 1972). By contrast, $PGF_{2\alpha}$ is without effect (Prasad, 1972). Since PGEs stimulate adenylate cyclase in the same test system (see Table 1.4), it is thought that PGEs act via cyclic AMP to induce neuronal differentiation. This would be an instance of a 'messenger' role of the prostaglandins to the adenylate cyclase system. Maturation of tumour glial cells (human line, see Table 1.4) might be controlled by the same mechanism (Edström *et al.*, 1974). It remains an open question whether normal cells behave as the tumour cells in their response to the two agents. Experiments with cultured brain cells (Shapiro, 1973; see also Werner *et al.*, 1971) suggest that this is indeed the case. Both prostaglandins (see Section 1.2) and cyclic AMP (Schmidt *et al.*, 1970; Perkins, 1973) are present in the immature brain.

2 Synaptic transmission

Work from several laboratories has proved that many chemical agents, including neurotransmitters, produce a substantial elevation of cyclic AMP levels in isolated brain slice preparations (for a summary, see Daly, 1975). Effects of different neurotransmitters or those of neurotransmitters and PGEs are additive or more than additive depending on the tissue (Daly, 1975; see also Berti *et al.*, 1973). Although these results are indicative of a link between cyclic AMP and synaptic processes, their interpretation is a hard task because of the heterogeneity of the test system and the multiple sites of action of the compounds. Some of these difficulties are overcome by using microiontophoresis to apply substances to single neurons. This technique (supplemented with cytochemical and pharmacological techniques) has been instrumental in establishing a model of neurotransmitter–cyclic AMP–prostaglandin interaction (Siggins *et al.*, 1971a, b; Siggins *et al.*, 1973; Hoffer *et al.*, 1973). The model has been developed with cerebellar Purkinje cells but, according to the proponents, it also applies to other cell types in brain. As shown in Figure 1.3(A), the model states that activation of a noradrenergic pathway to Purkinje (and other) neurons elicits the post-synaptic formation of cyclic AMP. The nucleotide is ultimately responsible for the appropriate response of the cell (in this case, depression). As a corollary, it is postulated that E-type prostaglandins formed within the

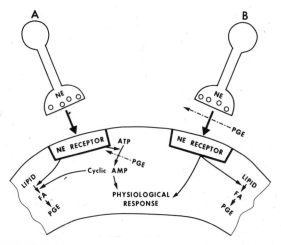

Figure 1.3 Possible mechanisms of prostaglandin action in noradrenergic synapses. A. Model proposed by Bloom and associates. B. Model proposed by Hedqvist. NE, norepinephrine; FA, fatty acid

Purkinje cell in response to norepinephrine, cyclic AMP, or both, exert a modulatory control on the synaptic process through a negative feedback action on the adenylate cyclase. A recent extension of this work (Stone et al., 1975) suggests that the intracellular action of cyclic AMP is normally opposed by cyclic GMP. While cyclic AMP is under adrenergic control, cyclic GMP is under cholinergic control. The scheme is supported by data obtained in a peripheral synapse (McAfee and Greengard, 1972), and is also consistent with findings in non-neural tissues (Kuehl, 1974). Interestingly, the idea of an opposing action of the two cyclic nucleotides could be extended to the prostaglandins because there is evidence linking F-type prostaglandins to cyclic GMP (Kuehl, 1974). Although in many ways attractive, this proposal is presently subject to vigorous controversy. Different investigators (Godfraind and Pumain, 1971; Jordan et al., 1972; Lake et al., 1972; Lake et al., 1973; Lake and Jordan, 1974) have been unable to confirm, in the cerebellum or elsewhere, a consistent correlation between effects of exogenous cyclic AMP (or the dibutyryl derivative) and norepinephrine. Furthermore, findings with phosphodiesterase inhibitors and prostaglandins have been questioned (Lake et al., 1972; Lake et al., 1973). According to Bloom and associates, the action of exogenous (and endogenous) norepinephrine is antagonized by concurrently applied E-type prostaglandins. Results of others in the cerebral cortex (Lake et al., 1972; Lake et al., 1973), brain stem (Anderson et al., 1973; see also Avanzino et al., 1966) and spinal cord (Caulford and Coceani, unpublished) under comparable experimental conditions have been negative or inconclusive. In this context, it should be emphasized that the model proposed by Bloom and associates (Siggins et al., 1971a, b; Siggins et al., 1973; Hoffer et al., 1973) implies that PGEs have an inhibitory rather than an excitatory action on cyclic AMP-generating mechanism(s). This concept is at variance with experimental data (see Table 1.4) and while this does not necessarily contradict their postulate, it certainly argues against its general applicability. Unfortunately, Bloom and associates did not test PGEs in experiments where the cyclic AMP content of Purkinje cells at rest or under noradrenergic stimulation was directly monitored by a cytochemical procedure (Siggins et al., 1973). Technical factors may explain the inconsistencies (Bloom et al., 1974) and more information on the subject is certainly forthcoming.

An alternative model of neurotransmitter–prostaglandin relationship originates from work with peripheral noradrenergic synapses (Hedqvist, 1973). As shown in Figure 1.3(B), the site of prostaglandin formation and the type of prostaglandin formed are the same as in the former proposal. Unlike the former proposal, however, prostaglandin action is thought to be presynaptic. According to Hedqvist (1973), PGEs inhibit the release of the transmitter possibly by interfering with the Ca^{2+} uptake mechanism. Evidence of a similar mechanism in brain has been presented (Bergström et al., 1973).

With either model, prostaglandins are envisaged in the role of modulators of noradrenergic transmission. It is an open question whether prostaglandins play a similar role in other synapses.

1.7 CEREBRAL CIRCULATION

A number of reports have appeared in the recent literature concerning the action of prostaglandins on the cerebral circulation. $PGF_{2\alpha}$ and PGE_1 have been examined more often, and findings are summarized in Table 1.5.

Table 1.5   The response of cerebral vessels to $PGF_{2\alpha}$ and PGE_1

Prostaglandin	Species	Route	Response	Reference
IN VIVO $F_{2\alpha}$	Dog	Intracarotid	Constriction	Denton et al. (1972); Yamamoto et al. (1972); Emerson et al. (1974)
	*Monkey	Intracarotid	Constriction	White et al. (1971); Denton et al. (1972); Pickard (1973); Welch et al. (1974)
	Dog	Subarachnoid	Constriction	Pennink et al. (1972)
	Dog	Ventricular	Constriction	Emerson et al. (1974)
	Cat	†Topical	Constriction	Handa et al. (1974)
E_1	Dog	Intracarotid	Dilation	Denton et al. (1972); Nakano et al. (1973)
			Constriction	Yamamoto et al. (1972)
	Monkey	Intracarotid	Dilation	Pelofsky et al. (1972)
	Dog	Subarachnoid	No response	Pennink et al. (1972)
	Cat	†Topical	Constriction	Handa et al. (1974)

Prostaglandin	Species	Artery	Response	Reference
IN VITRO $F_{2\alpha}$	Dog	Middle cerebral, basilar	Constriction	Allen et al. (1974a)
E_1	Dog	Middle cerebral, basilar	Biphasic, constriction to dilatation	Allen et al. (1974a)

* *Macaca mulatta, Macaca nemestrina, Papio cynocephalus* or *Papio anubis*
† Basilar artery
In any experiment, effects of PGE_2, PGA_1 and PGA_2 mimic those of PGE_1 (Nakano et al., 1973; Handa et al., 1974)

All studies, whether performed *in vivo* or *in vitro*, are consistent in showing that $PGF_{2\alpha}$ is a constrictor agent. Effective doses *in vivo* differ with the route of administration and the recording procedure; however, in the same experimental set-up, responses are more intense when the compound is given by the carotid route than by the ventricular route (Emerson et al., 1974). The active removal of prostaglandins from the c.s.f. (Holmes and Horton, 1968; Bito and Davson, 1974) may explain this observation. According to Yamamoto et al. (1972), $PGF_{2\alpha}$ action is exerted only on the arterial side of the circulation and particularly on the small ($< 200\mu$) vessels (see also Emerson et al., 1974).

Results with PGE_1 are contradictory, even in comparable experimental conditions. For example, constrictor (Yamamoto *et al.*, 1972) and dilator (Denton *et al.*, 1972; Nakano *et al.*, 1973) responses have been obtained in the dog following intra-carotid administration of the compound. In the same species, PGE_1 is without effect when given by the subarachnoid route (Pennink *et al.*, 1972). Technical differences in recording intracerebral vascular changes may explain the inconsistencies. Relevant to this point is the recent demonstration in the monkey (not included in Table 1.5) that PGE_1, although not active by itself on the internal carotid vessels, reduces cerebral blood flow through its vasodilator action on the external carotid bed (Welch *et al.*, 1974). Furthermore, findings *in vitro* (Allen *et al.*, 1974a) prove that PGE_1 action is biphasic, and consequently the varying response *in vivo* may well result from a different concentration of the compound at the target site(s). It must also be stressed that cerebral blood flow is reduced by indomethacin (Pickard and Mackenzie, 1973), and this implies a vasodilator action for the endogenous prostaglandin(s).

Prostaglandin action is not mediated by norepinephrine or 5-hydroxy-tryptamine receptor sites (White *et al.*, 1971; Allen *et al.*, 1974b), and probably the effect is exerted directly on the vascular smooth muscle. Experiments with exogenous prostaglandin suggest that a change of cerebral oxygen consumption may precede (and determine) the vascular change (Pickard, 1973), but results with indomethacin do not support this idea (Pickard and Mackenzie, 1973).

In spite of the uncertainties on the site and mode of action of prostaglandins, it has been speculated that endogenous prostaglandins in the vascular smooth muscle and/or the nervous tissue play a role in the control of cerebral haemodynamics under normal and pathological conditions (for a review, see Wolfe, 1975). Of special interest is the possibility that a constrictor prostaglandin may contribute to the arterial spasm often associated with a bleeding aneurysm. Such prostaglandin would originate from the ischaemic brain tissue, and also possibly from platelets. Consistent with this hypothesis is the finding of high levels of $PGF_{2\alpha}$ in c.s.f. of such patients (La Torre *et al.*, 1974; see also Wolfe and Mamer, 1975). Conceivably, $PGF_{2\alpha}$ may also be responsible for the brain ischaemia associated with head injury, for the vascular changes occurring around areas of cerebral infarction and for certain forms of migraine, e.g., hemiplegic migraine (for a model of PGE action, see Welch *et al.*, 1974).

1.8 CONCLUSION

Prostaglandins are normally present in the central nervous tissue and exert potent and varied actions on diverse neuronal types. Their mechanism of action is not fully understood, but several lines of evidence link prostaglandins with cyclic nucleotides and neurotransmitters. Prostaglandins may also act directly on neurons, possibly through a change in the cell membrane permeability to ions. A number of processes, whether physiological or pathological, are likely to be mediated or influenced by the prostaglandins. Fever affords the best-documented example of one of their functions. Two concepts emerge from this review. First, prostaglandins are formed at multiple sites, both neuronal and extraneuronal, and they may interact in a varied manner to control neuronal function. Second, the prostaglandin system is complex, and it generates several products of varying biological activity that may or may not retain the original prostanoate structure. Thus, the system is potentially very flexible and lends itself admirably to the control of the ever-changing neuron.

Acknowledgements

Experimental work of the authors reported in this article was supported by the Medical Research Council of Canada and the Ontario Heart Foundation.

Since the completion of this chapter, a novel pathway of arachidonic acid metabolism has been identified in platelets, which involves the enzymatic conversion of the endoperoxide intermediates to an active non-prostaglandin product named thromboxane A_2 (Hamberg, M., Svensson, J., and Samuelsson, B. (1975). Thromboxanes: a new group of biologically active compounds derived from prostaglandin endoperoxides. *Proc. Nat. Acad. Sci. (USA)*, **72**, 2994). Thromboxane A_2 is exceedingly labile in aqueous medium (half-life at 37 °C is about 30 s) and yields an inactive derivative, thromboxane B_2 or PHD (see Section 1.2). This pathway may well occur in the central nervous system, and data on this subject will undoubtedly be forthcoming.

References

Allen, G. S., Henderson, L. M., Chou, S. N. and French, L. A. (1974a). Cerebral arterial spasm. Part 1: *In vitro* contractile activity of vasoactive agents on canine basilar and middle cerebral arteries. *J. Neurosurg.*, **40**, 433

Allen, G. S., Henderson, L. M., Chou, S. N. and French, L. A. (1974b). Cerebral arterial spasm. Part 2: *In vitro* contractile activity of serotonin in human serum and CSF on the canine basilar artery, and its blockage by methyl-sergide and phenoxybenzamine. *J. Neurosurg.*, **40**, 422

Anderson, E. G., Haas, H. L. and Hösli, L. (1973). Comparison of effects of noradrenaline and histamine with cyclic AMP on brain stem neurones. *Brain Res.*, **49**, 471

Änggård, E. and Samuelsson, B. (1964). Metabolism of prostaglandin E_1 in guinea-pig lung: the structure of two metabolites. *J. Biol. Chem.*, **239**, 4097

Änggård, E., Gréen, K. and Samuelsson, B. (1965). Synthesis of tritium-labelled prostaglandin E_2 and studies on its metabolism in guinea-pig lung. *J. Biol. Chem.*, **240**, 1932

Änggård, E. and Larsson, C. (1971). The sequence of the early steps in the metabolism of prostaglandin E_1. *Eur. J. Pharmacol.*, **14**, 66

Änggård, E., Larsson, C. and Samuelsson, B. (1971). The distribution of 15-hydroxy prostaglandin dehydrogenase and prostaglandin-Δ^{13}-reductase in tissues of the swine. *Acta Physiol. Scand.*, **81**, 396

Asakawa, T. and Yoshida, H. (1971). Studies on the functional role of adenosine 3′,5′-monophosphate, histamine and prostaglandin E_1 in the central nervous system. *Jap. J. Pharmacol.*, **21**, 569

Avanzino, G. L., Bradley, P. B. and Wolstencroft, J. H. (1966). Actions of prostaglandins E_1, E_2 and $F_{2\alpha}$ on brain stem neurones. *Br. J. Pharmac.*, **27**, 157

Avery, D. D. and Penn, P. E. (1974). Blockage of pyrogen induced fever by intrahypothalamic injections of salicylate in the rat. *Neuropharmacology*, **13**, 1179

Balie, C. A. (1974). Putative neurotransmitters in the hypothalamus and feeding. *Fed. Proc.*, **33**, 1166

Balie, C. A., Simpson, C. W., Bean, S. M., McLaughlin, C. L. and Jacobs, H. L. (1973).

Prostaglandins and food intake of rats: a component of energy balance regulation? *Physiol. Behav.*, **10**, 1077

Baile, C. A., Martin, F. H., Forbes, J. M., Webb, R. L. and Kingsbury, W. (1974). Intra-hypothalamic injections of prostaglandins and prostaglandin antagonists and feeding in sheep. *J. Dairy Sci.*, **57**, 81

Baird, J. A., Hales, J. R. S. and Lang, W. J. (1974). Thermoregulatory responses to the injection of monoamines, acetylcholine and prostaglandins into a lateral ventricle of the echidna. *J. Physiol. (Lond.)*, **236**, 539

Barrie, M. and Jowett, A. (1967). A pharmacological investigation of cerebro-spinal fluid from patients with migraine. *Brain*, **90**, 785

Bazan, J. G., Jr. (1970). Effects of ischemia and electroconvulsive shock on free fatty acid pool in the brain. *Biochim. Biophys. Acta*, **218**, 1

Beerthuis, R. K., Nugteren, D. H., Pabon, H. J. J. and Van Dorp, D. A. (1968). Biologically active prostaglandins from some new odd-numbered essential fatty acids. *Recl. Trav. Chim. Pays-Bas Belg.*, **87**, 461

Beerthuis, R. K., Nugteren, D. H., Pabon, H. J. J., Steenhoek, A. and Van Dorp, D. A. (1971). Synthesis of a series of polyunsaturated fatty acids. Their potencies as essential fatty acids and as precursors of prostaglandins. *Recl. Trav. Chim. Pays-Bas Belg.*, **90**, 943

Beleslin, D. B. and Myers, R. D. (1971). Release of an unknown substance from brain structures of unanaesthetized monkeys and cats. *Neuropharmacology*, **10**, 121

Beleslin, D. B., Radmanović, B. Z. and Rakić, M. M. (1971). Release during convulsions of an unknown substance into the cerebral ventricles of the cat's brain. *Brain Res.*, **35**, 625

Bergström, S., Carlson, L. A., Ekelund, L.-G. and Orö, L. (1965). Cardiovascular and metabolic response to infusions of prostaglandin E_1 and to simultaneous infusions of noradrenaline and prostaglandin E_1 in man. *Acta Physiol. Scand.*, **64**, 332

Bergström, S., Danielsson, H., Klenberg, D. and Samuelsson, B. (1964a). The enzymatic conversion of essential fatty acids into prostaglandins. *J. Biol. Chem.*, **239**, 4006

Bergström, S., Danielsson, H. and Samuelsson, B. (1964b). The enzymatic formation of prostaglandin E_2 from arachidonic acid. *Biochim. Biophys. Acta*, **90**, 207

Bergström, S., Farnebo, L. O. and Fuxe, K. (1973). Effect of prostaglandin E_2 on central and peripheral catecholamine neurons. *Eur. J. Pharmacol.*, **21**, 362

Berti, F., Trabucchi, M., Bernareggi, V. and Fumagalli, R. (1973). Prostaglandins on cyclic AMP formation in cerebral cortex of different mammalian species. *Adv. Biosci.*, **9**, 475

Bishai, I. and Coceani, F. (1975). Demonstration of two pathways for prostaglandin (PG) metabolism in the frog spinal cord. *Proc. Can. Fed. Biol. Soc.*, **18**, 67

Bito, L. Z. and Davson, H. (1974). Carrier-mediated removal of prostaglandins from cerebrospinal fluid. *J. Physiol. (Lond.)*, **234**, 39P

Bligh, J., Cottle, W. H. and Maskrey, M. (1971). Influence of ambient temperature on the thermoregulatory responses to 5-hydroxytryptamine, noradrenaline and acetylcholine injected into the lateral cerebral ventricles of sheep, goats and rabbits. *J. Physiol. (Lond.)*, **212**, 377

Bligh, J. and Milton, A. S. (1973). The thermoregulatory effects of prostaglandin E_1 when infused into a lateral cerebral ventricle of the Welsh mountain sheep at different ambient temperatures. *J. Physiol. (Lond.)*, **229**, 30P

Bloom, F. E., Siggins, G. R. and Hoffer, B. J. (1974). Interpreting the failures to confirm the depression of cerebellar Purkinje cells by cyclic AMP. *Science*, **185**, 627

Bradley, P. B., Samuels, G. M. R. and Shaw, J. E. (1969). Correlation of prostaglandin release from the cerebral cortex of cats with electrocorticogram, following stimulation of the reticular formation. *Br. J. Pharmac.*, **37**, 151

Breckenridge, B. McL. and Lisk, R. D. (1969). Cyclic adenylate and hypothalamic regulatory functions. *Proc. Soc. Exp. Biol. Med.*, **131**, 934

Buckell, M. (1964). Demonstration of substances capable of contracting smooth muscle in the haematoma fluid from certain cases of ruptured cerebral aneurysm. *J. Neurol. Neurosurg. Psychiat.*, **27**, 198

Burger, M. M., Bombik, B. M. Breckenridge, B. McL. and Sheppard, J. R. (1972). Growth control and cyclic alterations of cyclic AMP in the cell cycle. *Nature (Lond.)*, **239**, 161

Cabanac, M., Stolwijk, J. A. J. and Hardy, J. D. (1968). Effect of temperature and pyrogens on single unit activity in the rabbit's brain stem. *J. Appl. Physiol.*, **24**, 645

Carlson, L. A., Ekelund, L.-G. and Orö, L., (1968). Clinical and metabolic effects of different doses of prostaglandin E_1 in man. *Acta Med. Scand.*, **183**, 423

Carlson, L. A., Ekelund, L.-G. and Orö, L. (1969). Circulatory and respiratory effects of different doses of prostaglandin E_1 in man. *Acta Physiol. Scand.*, **75**, 161

Carlson, L. A. and Orö, L. (1966). Effect of prostaglandin E_1 on blood pressure and heart rate in the dog. *Acta Physiol. Scand.*, **67**, 89

Coceani, F. (1974). Prostaglandins and the central nervous system. *Arch. Intern. Med.*, **133**, 119

Coceani, F., Dreifuss, J. J., Puglisi, L. and Wolfe, L. S. (1969). Prostaglandins and membrane function. In *Prostaglandins, Peptides and Amines*, Mantegazza, P., and Horton, E. W. (eds.), pp. 73–84 (London: Academic Press)

Coceani, F., Puglisi, L. and Lavers, B. (1971). Prostaglandins and neuronal activity in spinal cord and cuneate nucleus. *Ann. N.Y. Acad. Sci.*, **180**, 289

Coceani, F. and Viti, A. (1973). Actions of prostaglandin E_1 on spinal neurons in the frog. *Adv. Biosci.*, **9**, 481

Coceani, F. and Viti, A. (1975). Responses of spinal neurons to iontophoretically applied prostaglandin E_1 in the frog. *Can. J. Physiol. Pharmacol.*, **53**, 273

Coceani, F. and Wolfe, L. S. (1965). Prostaglandins in brain and the release of prostaglandin-like compounds from the cat cerebellar cortex. *Can. J. Physiol. Pharmacol.*, **43**, 445

Collier, H. O. J. and Roy, A. C. (1974a). Morphine-like drugs inhibit the stimulation by E prostaglandin of cyclic AMP formation by rat brain homogenate. *Nature (Lond.)*, **248**, 24

Collier, H. O. J. and Roy, A. C. (1974b). Inhibition of E prostaglandin-sensitive adenylcyclase as the mechanism of morphine analgesia. *Prostaglandins*, **7**, 361

Cooper, K. E., Cranston, W. I. and Honour, A. J. (1967). Observations on the site and mode of action of pyrogens in the rabbit brain. *J. Physiol. (Lond.)*, **191**, 325

Cooper, K. E., Pittman, Q. J. and Veale, W. L. (1975). Observations on the development of the 'fever' mechanism in the fetus and newborn. In *Temperature Regulation and Drug Action*, Lomax, P., Schönbaum, E., and Jacob, J. (eds.), pp. 43–50 (Basel: Karger)

Cooper, K. E. and Veale, W. L. (1974). The effects of reserpine and atropine, injected into the lateral cerebral ventricle, on fever due to intravenous leucocyte pyrogen and hypothalamic injection of prostaglandin E_1 in the unanaesthetized rabbit. *J. Physiol. (Lond.)*, **241**, 25P

Cranston, W. I. and Rawlins, M. D. (1972). Effects of intracerebral micro-injection of sodium salicylate on temperature regulation in the rabbit. *J. Physiol. (Lond.)*, **222**, 257

Crowshaw, K. (1971). Prostaglandin biosynthesis from endogenous precursors in rabbit kidney. *Nature (New Biology)*, **231**, 240

Daly, J. W. (1975). Cyclic adenosine $3',5'$-monophosphate role in the physiology and pharmacology of the central nervous system. *Biochem. Pharmacol.*, **24**, 159

Danon, A. and Chang, L. C. T. (1973). Release of prostaglandins from the rat renal papilla *in vitro*: effects of arachidonic acid and angiotensin II. *Fed. Proc.*, **32**, 788

Dascombe, M. J. and Milton, A. S. (1972). The effect of caffeine on the antipyretic action of aspirin administered during endotoxin induced fever. *Br. J. Pharmac.*, **46**, 548P

Denton, I. C. Jr., White, R. P. and Robertson, J. T. (1972). The effects of prostaglandins E_1, A_1 and $F_{2\alpha}$ on the cerebral circulation of dogs and monkeys. *J. Neurosurg.*, **36**, 34

Desiraju, T. (1973). Effect of intraventricularly administered prostaglandin E_1 on the electrical activity of cerebral cortex and behaviour in the unanaesthetized monkey. *Prostaglandins*, **3**, 859

Dey, P. K., Feldberg, W. and Wendlandt, S. (1974a). Lipid A and prostaglandin. *J. Physiol. (Lond.)*, **239**, 102P

Dey, P. K., Feldberg, W., Gupta, K. P., Milton, A. S. and Wendlandt, S. (1974b). Further studies on the role of prostaglandins in fever. *J. Physiol. (Lond.)*, **241**, 629

Dobrin, E. I., Bloss, J. L. and Potts, W. J. (1973). Neuropharmacological and behavioural toxicity studies with prostaglandin A_2. *Toxicol. Appl. Pharmacol.*, **25**, 460

Duda, P., Horton, E. W. and McPherson, A. (1968). The effects of prostaglandins E_1, $F_{1\alpha}$ and $F_{2\alpha}$ on monosynaptic reflexes. *J. Physiol. (Lond.)*, **196**, 151

Duru, S. and Türker, R. K. (1969). Effect of prostaglandin E_1 on the strychnine-induced convulsion in the mouse. *Experientia*, **25**, 275

Edström, A., Kanje, M. and Walum, E. (1974). Effects of dibutyryl cyclic AMP and prostaglandin E_1 on cultured human glioma cells. *Exptl. Cell Res.*, **85**, 217

Eisenman, J. S. (1969). Pyrogen-induced changes in the thermosensitivity of septal and preoptic neurons. *Am. J. Physiol.*, **216**, 330

Emerson, T. E. Jr., Radawski, D., Veenendaal, M. and Daugherty, R. M. Jr. (1974). Effects of cerebral ventricular, systemic, and local administration of prostaglandin $F_{2\alpha}$ on canine cerebral hemodynamics. *Prostaglandins*, **8**, 521

Feldberg, W. and Gupta, K. P. (1973). Pyrogen fever and prostaglandin-like activity in cerebrospinal fluid, *J. Physiol. (Lond.)*, **228**, 41

Feldberg, W., Gupta, K. P., Milton, A. S. and Wendlandt, S. (1973). Effect of pyrogen and antipyretics on prostaglandin activity in cisternal c.s.f. of unanaesthetized cats. *J. Physiol. (Lond.)*, **234**, 279

Feldberg, W. and Myers, R. D. (1964). Effects on temperature of amines injected into the cerebral ventricles: a new concept of temperature regulation. *J. Physiol. (Lond.)*, **173**, 226

Feldberg, W. and Saxena, P. N. (1971a). Fever produced by prostaglandin E_1. *J. Physiol. (Lond.)*, **217**, 547

Feldberg, W. and Saxena, P. N. (1971b). Further studies on prostaglandin E_1 fever in cats. *J. Physiol. (Lond.)*, **219**, 739

Flower, R. J. (1974). Drugs which inhibit prostaglandin biosynthesis, *Pharmac. Rev.*, **26**, 33

Flower, R., Gryglewski, R., Herbaczynska-Cedro, K. and Vane, J. R. (1972). Effects of anti-inflammatory drugs on prostaglandin biosynthesis. *Nature (New Biology)*, **238**, 104

Flower, R. J. and Vane, J. R. (1972). Inhibition of prostaglandin synthetase in brain explains the antipyretic activity of paracetamol (4-acetamidophenol). *Nature (Lond.)*, **240**, 410

Flower, R. J. and Vane, J. R. (1974). Some pharmacologic and biochemical aspects of prostaglandin biosynthesis and its inhibition. In *Prostaglandin synthetase inhibitors— their effects on physiological functions and pathological states*, Robinson, H. J. and Vane, J. R. (eds.), pp. 9–18 (New York: Raven Press)

Ford, D. M. (1974). A selective action of prostaglandin E_1 on hypothalamic neurones in the cat which respond to brain cooling. *J. Physiol. (Lond.)*, **242**, 142P

Fraser, I. S. and Gray, C. (1974a). Electroencephalogram changes after prostaglandin. *Lancet*, **i**, 360

Fraser, I. S. and Gray, C. (1974b). Prostaglandin $F_{2\alpha}$ and electroencephalogram changes. *Lancet*, **ii**, 49

Furmanski, P., Silverman, D. J. and Lubin, M. (1971). Expression of differentiated functions in mouse neuroblastoma mediated by dibutyryl-cyclic adenosine monophosphate. *Nature (Lond.)*, **233**, 413

Gatt, S. (1968). Purification and properties of phospholipase A_1 from rat and calf brain. *Biochim. Biophys. Acta*, **159**, 304

Gillett, P. G., Kinch, R. A. H., Wolfe, L. S. and Pace-Asciak, C. R. (1972). Therapeutic abortion with the use of prostaglandin $F_{2\alpha}$. A study of efficacy, tolerance and plasma levels with intravenous administration. *Am. J. Obstet. Gynecol.*, **112**, 330

Gilman, A. G. (1972). Regulation of cyclic AMP metabolism in cultured cells of the nervous system. In *Advances in Cyclic Nucleotide Research, Vol. 1*, Greengard, P., Paoletti, P. and Robison, G. A. (eds.), pp. 389–410 (New York: Raven Press)

Gilman, A. G. and Nirenberg, M. (1971a). Regulation of adenosine 3′,5′-cyclic monophosphate metabolism in cultured neuroblastoma cells. *Nature (Lond.)*, **234**, 356

Gilman, A. G. and Nirenberg, M. (1971b). Effect of catecholamines on the adenosine 3′,5′-cyclic monophosphate concentrations of clonal satellite cells of neurons. *Proc. Nat. Acad. Sci. (USA)*, **68**, 2165

Gilman, A. G., and Schrier, B. K. (1972). Adenosine cyclic 3′,5′-monophosphate in fetal rat brain cell cultures: I. Effect of catecholamines. *Molec. Pharmacol.*, **8**, 410

Gilmore, D. P. and Shaikh. A. A. (1972). The effect of prostaglandin E_2 in inducing sedation in the rat. *Prostaglandins*, **2**, 143

Girault, J-M., Kandasamy, B. et Jacob, J. (1973). Actions de l'indomètacine et de la phénoxybenzamine sur les hyperthermies produites par un pyrogène bactérieu purifié, l'acide arachidonique et la prostaglandin E_1 administrés par voie intracérèbroventriculaire au lapin éveillé. *J. Pharmacol. (Paris)*, **4**, 423

Godfraind, J. M. and Pumain, R. (1971). Cyclic adenosine monosphosphate and norepinephrine: effect on Purkinje cells in rat cerebellar cortex. *Science*, **174**, 1257

Granström, E. (1972). On the metabolism of prostaglandin $F_{2\alpha}$ in female subjects. Structure of two C-14 metabolites. *Eur. J. Biochem.*, **25**, 581

Granström, E., Inger, U. and Samuelsson, B. (1965). The structure of a urinary metabolite of prostaglandin $F_{1\alpha}$ in the rat. *J. Biol. Chem.*, **240**, 457

Granström, E. and Samuelsson, B. (1969a). The structure of a urinary metabolite of prostaglandin $F_{2\alpha}$ in man. *J. Am. Chem. Soc.*, **91**, 3398

Granström, E. and Samuelsson, B. (1969b). The structure of the main urinary metabolite of prostaglandin $F_{2\alpha}$ in the guinea-pig. *Eur. J. Biochem.*, **10**, 411

Granström, E. and Samuelsson, B. (1971). On the metabolism of prostaglandin $F_{2\alpha}$ in female subjects. *J. Biol. Chem.*, **246**, 5254

Gréen, K. (1969). Structure of urinary metabolites of prostaglandin $F_{2\alpha}$ in the rat. *Acta Chem. Scand.*, **23**, 1453

Gréen, K. (1971). Metabolism of prostaglandin E_2 in the rat. *Biochemistry*, **10**, 1072

Gréen, K. and Samuelsson, B. (1971). Quantitative studies on the synthesis *in vivo* of prostaglandins in the rat—cold stress induced stimulation of synthesis. *Eur. J. Biochem.*, **22**, 391

Gyang, E. A., Deuben, R. R. and Buckley, J. P. (1973). Interaction of prostaglandin E_1 and angiotensin II on centrally mediated pressor activities in the cat. *Proc. Soc. Exp. Biol. Med.*, **142**, 532

Hales, J. R. S., Bennett, J. W., Baird, J. A. and Fawcett, A. A. (1973). Thermoregulatory effects of prostaglandins E_1, E_2, $F_{1\alpha}$ and $F_{2\alpha}$ in the sheep. *Pflügers Arch.*, **339**, 125

Hamberg, M. (1968). Metabolism of prostaglandins in rat liver mitochondria. *Eur. J. Biochem.*, **6**, 135

Hamberg, M. (1969). Biosynthesis of prostaglandins in the renal medulla of the rabbit. *FEBS Lett.*, **5**, 127

Hamberg, M. (1973). Quantitative studies on prostaglandin synthesis in man. II. Determination of the major urinary metabolite of prostaglandins $F_{1\alpha}$ and $F_{2\alpha}$. *Anal. Biochem.*, **55**, 368

Hamberg, M. (1974). Quantitative studies on prostaglandin synthesis in man. III. Excretion of the major urinary metabolite of prostaglandins $F_{1\alpha}$ and $F_{2\alpha}$ during pregnancy. *Life Sci.*, **14**, 247

Hamberg, M., Hedqvist, P., Strandberg, K., Svensson, J. and Samuelsson, B. (1975). Prostaglandin endoperoxides IV. Effects on smooth muscle. *Life Sci.*, **16**, 451

Hamberg, M. and Israelsson, U. (1970). Metabolism of prostaglandin E_2 in guinea-pig liver. I. Identification of seven metabolites. *J. Biol. Chem.*, **245**, 5107

Hamberg, M. and Samuelsson, B. (1966). Novel biological transformations of 8,11,14-eicosatrienoic acid. *J. Am. Chem. Soc.*, **88**, 2349

Hamberg, M. and Samuelsson, B. (1967). On the mechanism of the biosynthesis of prostaglandins E_1 and $F_{1\alpha}$. *J. Biol. Chem.*, **242**, 5336

Hamberg, M. and Samuelsson, B. (1969a). The structure of a urinary metabolite of prostaglandin E_2 in the guinea-pig. *Biochem. Biophys. Res. Comm.*, **34**, 22

Hamberg, M. and Samuelsson, B. (1969b). The structure of the major urinary metabolite of prostaglandin E_2 in man. *J. Am. Chem. Soc.*, **91**, 2177

Hamberg, M. and Samuelsson, B. (1973). Detection and isolation of an endoperoxide intermediate in prostaglandin biosynthesis. *Proc. Nat. Acad. Sci. (USA)*, **70**, 889

Hamberg, M. and Samuelsson, B. (1974a). Prostaglandin endoperoxides. Novel transformations of arachidonic acid in human platelets. *Proc. Nat. Acad. Sci. (USA)*, **71**, 3400

Hamberg, M. and Samuelsson, B. (1974b). Prostaglandin endoperoxides VII. Novel transformation of arachidonic acid in guinea pig lung. *Biochem. Biophys. Res. Comm.*, **61**, 942

Hamberg, M., Svensson, J. and Samuelsson, B. (1974a). Prostaglandin endoperoxides. A new concept concerning the mode of action and release of prostaglandins. *Proc. Nat. Acad. Sci. (USA)*, **71**, 3824

Hamberg, M., Svensson, J., Wakabayashi, T. and Samuelsson, B. (1974b). Isolation and structure of two prostaglandin endoperoxides that cause platelet aggregation. *Proc. Nat. Acad. Sci. (USA)*, **71**, 345

Hamprecht, B., Jaffe, B. M. and Philpott, G. W. (1973). Prostaglandin production by neuroblastoma, glioma and fibroblast cell lines; stimulation by N^6,O^2-dibutyryl adenosine 3′,5′-cyclic monophosphate. *FEBS Lett.*, **36**, 193

Hamprecht, B. and Schultz, J. (1973). Stimulation by prostaglandin E_1 of adenosine 3′,5′-cyclic monophosphate formation in neuroblastoma cells in the presence of phosphodiesterase inhibitors. *FEBS Lett.* **34**, 85

Handa, J., Yoneda, S., Matsuda, M. and Handa, H. (1974). Effects of prostaglandins A_1, E_1, E_2 and $F_{2\alpha}$ on the basilar artery of cats. *Surg. Neurol.*, **2**, 251

Hanson, A., Johansson, B., Malmquist, J. and Tönesson, M. (1975). The effect of paracetamol on fever in various non-infectious diseases. In *Temperature Regulation and Drug Action*, Lomax, P., Schönbaum, E. and Jacob, J. (eds.), pp. 227–232 (Basel: Karger)

Harvey, C. A. and Milton, A. S. (1974). The effect of parachlorophenylalanine on the response of the conscious cat to intravenous and intraventricular bacterial pyrogen and to intraventricular prostaglandin E_1. *J. Physiol. (Lond.)*, **236**, 14P

Haubrich, D. R., Perez-Cruet, J. and Reid, W. D. (1973). Prostaglandin E_1 causes sedation and increases 5-hydroxytryptamine turnover in rat brain. *Br. J. Pharmac.*, **48**, 80

Hedqvist, P. (1973). Autonomic neurotransmission. In *The Prostaglandins, Vol. 1*, Ramwell, P. W. (ed.), pp. 101–131 (New York: Plenum Press)

Hendricks, C. H., Brenner, W. E., Ekbladh, L., Brotanek, V. and Fishburne, J. I. Jr. (1971). Efficacy and tolerance of intravenous prostaglandin $F_{2\alpha}$ and E_2. *Am. J. Obstet. Gynecol.*, **111**, 564

Hensby, C. N. (1974). Reduction of prostaglandin E_2 to prostaglandin $F_{2\alpha}$ by an enzyme in sheep blood. *Biochim. Biophys. Acta*, **348**, 145

Hittelman, K. J. and Butcher, R. W. (1973). Cyclic AMP and the mechanism of action of the prostaglandins. In *The Prostaglandins, Pharmacological and Therapeutic Advances*, Cuthbert, M. F. (ed.), pp. 151–165 (London: William Heinemann Medical Books)

Hoffer, B. J., Siggins, G. R., Oliver, A. P. and Bloom, F. E. (1973). Activation of the pathway from locus coeruleus to rat cerebellar Purkinje neurons: pharmacological evidence of noradrenergic central inhibition. *J. Pharmac. exp. Ther.*, **184**, 553

Holmes, S. W. (1970). The spontaneous release of prostaglandins into the cerebral ventricles of the dog and the effect of external factors on this release. *Br. J. Pharmac.*, **38**, 653

Holmes, S. W. and Horton, E. W. (1968a). Prostaglandins and the central nervous system. In *Prostaglandin Symposium of the Worcester Foundation for Experimental Biology*, Ramwell, P. W. and Shaw, J. E. (eds.), pp. 21–38 (New York: John Wiley and Sons Ltd.)

Holmes, S. W. and Horton, E. W. (1968b). The distribution of tritium-labelled prostaglandin E_1 injected in amounts sufficient to produce central nervous effects in cats and chicks. *Br. J. Pharmac.*, **34**, 32

Holmes, S. W. and Horton, E. W. (1968c). The identification of four prostaglandins in dog brain and their regional distribution in the central nervous system. *J. Physiol. (Lond.)*, **195**, 731

Hori, T. and Harada, Y. (1974). The effects of ambient and hypothalamic temperatures on the hyperthermic responses to prostaglandins E_1 and E_2. *Pflügers Arch.*, **350**, 123

Horton, E. W. (1964). Actions of prostaglandins E_1, E_2 and E_3 on the central nervous system. *Br. J. Pharmac.*, **22**, 189

Horton, E. W. (1972). Prostaglandins. *Monographs on Endocrinology*, **7**, (New York: Springer-Verlag)

Horton, E. W. and Main, I. H. M. (1965). Differences in the effects of prostaglandin $F_{2\alpha}$, a constituent of cerebral tissue, and prostaglandin E_1 on conscious cats and chicks. *Int. J. Neuropharmac.*, **4**, 65

Horton, E. W. and Main, I. H. M. (1967). Further observations on the central nervous action of prostaglandins $F_{2\alpha}$ and E_1. *Br. J. Pharmac.*, **30**, 568

Horton, E. W. and Main, I. H. M. (1969). Actions of prostaglandin E_1 on spinal reflexes in the cat. In *Prostaglandins, Peptides and Amines*, Mantegazza, P. and Horton, E. W. (eds.), pp. 121–122 (London: Academic Press)

Jell, R. M. (1975). Amine–prostaglandin modulation of activity of thermoregulatory neurones. In *Temperature Regulation and Drug Action*, Lomax, P., Schönbaum, E. and Jacob, J. (eds.), pp. 119–123 (Basel: Karger)

Jones, R. L., Cammock, S. and Horton, E. W. (1972). Partial purification and properties of cat plasma prostaglandin A isomerase. *Biochim. Biophys. Acta*, **280**, 588

Jordan, L. M., Lake, N. and Phillis, J. W. (1972). Mechanisms of noradrenaline depression of cortical neurones: a species comparison. *Eur. J. Pharmacol.*, **20**, 381

Kandasamy, B., Girault, J.-M. and Jacob, J. (1975). Central effects of a purified bacterial pyrogen, prostaglandin E_1 and biogenic amines on the temperature in the awake rabbit. In *Temperature Regulation and Drug Action*, Lomax, P., Schönbaum, E. and Jacob, J. (eds.), pp. 124–132 (Basel: Karger)

Kantor, H. S., Johnson, C. R. and Kiefer, H. C. (1974). Cyclic AMP dependent conversion of prostaglandin E_1 to prostaglandin A_1 in intestinal epithelial cells. *Clin. Res.*, **22**, 604A

Kaplan, H. R., Grega, G. J., Sherman, G. P. and Buckley, J. P. (1969). Central and reflexogenic cardiovascular actions of prostaglandin E_1. *Int. J. Neuropharmac.*, **8**, 15

Klenberg, D. and Samuelsson, B. (1965). The biosynthesis of prostaglandin E_1 studied with specifically ^{3}H-labelled 8,11,14-eicosatrienoic acids. *Acta Chem. Scand.*, **19**, 534

Kuehl, F. A., Jr. (1974). Prostaglandins, cyclic nucleotides and cell function. *Prostaglandins*, **5**, 325

Kunze, H. and Vogt, W. (1971). Significance of phospholipase A for prostaglandin formation. *Ann. N.Y. Acad. Sci.*, **180**, 123

Laburn, H. P., Rosendorff, C., Willies, G. and Woolf, C. (1974). A role for noradrenaline and cyclic AMP in prostaglandin E_1 fever. *J. Physiol. (Lond.)*, **240**, 49P

Lake, N., Jordan, L. M. and Phillis, J. W. (1972). Mechanism of noradrenaline action in cat cerebral cortex. *Nature (Lond.)*, **240**, 249

Lake, N., Jordan, L. M. and Phillis, J. W. (1973). Evidence against cyclic adenosine 3′,5′ monophosphate (AMP) mediation of noradrenaline depression of cerebral corticaneurones. *Brain Res.*, **60**, 411

Lake, N. and Jordan, L. M. (1974). Failure to confirm cyclic AMP as second messenger for norepinephrine in rat cerebellum. *Science*, **183**, 663

Lands, W., Lee, R. and Smith, W. (1971). Factors regulating the biosynthesis of various prostaglandins. *Ann. N.Y. Acad. Sci.*, **180**, 107

Lands, W. E. M. and Samuelsson, B. (1968). Phospholipid precursor of prostaglandins. *Biochim. Biophys. Acta*, **164**, 426

Larsson, C. and Änggård, E. (1973). Regional differences in the formation and metabolism of prostaglandins in the rabbit kidney. *Eur. J. Pharmacol.*, **21**, 30

La Torre, E., Patrono, C., Fortuna, A. and Grossi-Belloni, D. (1974). Role of prostaglandin $F_{2\alpha}$ in human cerebral vasospasm. *J. Neurosurg.*, **41**, 293

Lavery, H. A., Lowe, R. D. and Scroop, G. C. (1970). Cardiovascular effects of prostaglandins mediated by the central nervous system of the dog. *Br. J. Pharmac.*, **39**, 511

Lavery, H. A., Lowe, R. D. and Scroop, G. C. (1971). Central autonomic effects of prostaglandin $F_{2\alpha}$ on the cardiovascular system of the dog. *Br. J. Pharmac.*, **41**, 454

Lee, S-C. and Levine, L. (1974). Prostaglandin metabolism. I. Cytoplasmic reduced nicotinamide adenine dinucleotide phosphate-dependent and microsomal reduced nicotinamide adenine dinucleotide-dependent prostaglandin E 9-ketoreductase activities in monkey and pigeon tissues. *J. Biol. Chem.*, **249**, 1369

Leslie, C. A. and Levine, L. (1973). Evidence for the presence of a prostaglandin E_2-9-keto reductase in rat organs. *Biochem. Biophys. Res. Comm.*, **52**, 717

Lipton, J. M. and Fossler, D. E. (1974). Fever produced in the squirrel monkey by intravenous and intracerebral endotoxin. *Am. J. Physiol.*, **226**, 1022

Lomax, P. (1970). Drugs and body temperature. *Int. Rev. Neurobiol.*, **12**, 1

Lyneham, R. C., McLeod, J. G., Smith, I. D., Low, P. A., Shearman, R. P. and Korda, A. R. (1973). Convulsions and electroencephalogram abnormalities after intra-amniotic prostaglandin $F_{2\alpha}$. *Lancet*, **ii**, 1003

Maddox, I. S. (1973). The role of copper in prostaglandin synthesis. *Biochim. Biophys. Acta*, **306**, 74

Marrazzi, M. A. and Huang, C. C. (1975). Prostaglandin cerebral inhibition, membrane potentials. *Fed. Proc.*, **34**, 764

Matsuura, S., Kawaguchi, S., Ichiki, M., Sorimachi, M., Kataoka, K. and Inouye, A. (1969). Perfusion of frog's spinal cord as a convenient method for neuropharmacological studies. *Eur. J. Pharmacol.*, **6**, 13

McAfee, D. A. and Greengard, P. (1972). Adenosine 3′,5′-monophosphate: electrophysiological evidence for a role in synaptic transmission. *Science*, **178**, 310

McQueen, D. S. and Ungar, A. (1969). The modification by prostaglandin E_1 of central nervous interaction between respiratory and cardio-inhibitor pathways. In *Prostaglandins, Peptides and Amines*, Mantegazza, P. and Horton E. W. (eds.), pp. 123–124 (London: Academic Press)

Milton, A. S. (1973). Prostaglandin E_1 and endotoxin fever, and the effects of aspirin, indomethacin, and 4-acetamidophenol. *Adv. Biosci.*, **9**, 495

Milton, A. S. and Harvey, C. A. (1975). Prostaglandins and monoamines in fever. In *Temperature Regulation and Drug Action*, Lomax, P., Schönbaum, E. and Jacob, J. (eds.), pp. 133–142 (Basel: Karger)

Milton, A. S. and Wendlandt, S. (1968). The effect of 4-acetamidophenol in reducing fever produced by the intracerebral injection of 5-hydroxytryptamine and pyrogen in the conscious cat. *Br. J. Pharmac.*, **34**, 215P

Milton, A. S. and Wendlandt, S. (1970). A possible role for prostaglandin E_1 as a modulator for temperature regulation in the central nervous system of the cat. *J. Physiol. (Lond.)*, **207**, 76P

Milton, A. S. and Wendlandt, S. (1971a). The effects of 4-acetamidophenol (paracetamol) on the temperature response of the conscious rat to the intracerebral injection of prostaglandin E_1, adrenaline and pyrogen. *J. Physiol. (Lond.)*, **217**, 33P

Milton, A. S. and Wendlandt, S. (1971b). Effects on body temperature of prostaglandin of the A, E and F series on injection into the third ventricle of unanaesthetized cats and rabbits. *J. Physiol. (Lond.)*, **218**, 325

Myers, R. D. (1971). Hypothalamic mechanisms of pyrogen action in the cat and monkey. In *Ciba Foundation Symposium on Pyrogens and Fever*, Wolstenholme, G. E. W. and Birch, J. (eds.), pp. 131–153 (Edinburgh: Churchill Livingstone)

Myers, R. D., Rudy, T. A. and Yaksh, T. L. (1974). Fever produced by endotoxin injected into the hypothalamus of the monkey and its antagonism by salicylate. *J. Physiol. (Lond.)*, **243**, 167

Nakano, J., Chang, A. C. K. and Fisher, R. G. (1973). Effects of prostaglandins E_1, E_2, A_1, A_2 and $F_{2\alpha}$ on canine carotid arterial blood flow, cerebrospinal fluid pressure, and intraocular pressure. *J. Neurosurg.*, **38**, 32

Nakano, J., Prancan, A. V. and Moore, S. E. (1972). Metabolism of prostaglandin E_1 in the cerebral cortex and cerebellum of the dog and rat. *Brain Res.*, **39**, 545

Nelson, N. A. (1974). Prostaglandin nomenclature. *J. Med. Chem.*, **17**, 911

Niehaus, W. G., Jr. and Samuelsson, B. (1968). Formation of malonaldehyde from phospholipid arachidonate during microsomal lipid peroxidation. *Eur. J. Biochem.*, **6**, 126

Nisticó, G. and Marley, E. (1973). Central effects of prostaglandin E_1 in adult fowls. *Neuropharmacology*, **12**, 1009

Nugteren, D. H., Beerthuis, R. K. and Van Dorp, D. A. (1966). The enzymic conversion of all-cis 8,11,14-eicosatrienoic acid into prostaglandin E_1. *Recl. Trav. Chim. Pays-Bas Belg.*, **85**, 405

Nugteren, D. H. and Hazelhof, E. (1973). Isolation and properties of intermediates in prostaglandin biosynthesis. *Biochim. Biophys. Acta*, **326**, 448

Nugteren, D. H. and Van Dorp, D. A. (1965). The participation of molecular oxygen in the biosynthesis of prostaglandins. *Biochim. Biophys. Acta*, **98**, 654

Pace-Asciak, C. (1971). Polyhydroxy cyclic ethers formed from tritiated arachidonic acid by acetone powders of sheep seminal vesicles. *Biochemistry*, **10**, 3664

Pace-Asciak, C. (1972). Prostaglandin synthetase activity in the rat stomach fundus. Activation by L-norepinephrine and related compounds. *Biochim. Biophys. Acta*, **280**, 161

Pace-Asciak, C. R. (1975a). Prostaglandin 9-hydroxy dehydrogenase activity in the adult rat kidney. Identification, pathway and some enzyme properties. *J. Biol. Chem.*, **250**, 2789

Pace-Asciak, C. R. (1975b). Biosynthesis and catabolism of prostaglandins during animal development. In *Advances in Prostaglandin and Thromboxane Research, Vol. 1*, Samuelsson, B. and Paoletti, R. (eds.), (New York: Raven Press). In press.

Pace-Asciak, C. R., Coceani, F. and Olley, P. M. (1974). Age-dependent decrease in the *in vitro* inactivation of prostaglandin $F_{2\alpha}$ by foetal lamb brain. *Trans. Am. Soc. Neurochem.*, **5**, 120

Pace-Asciak, C. R., Morawska, K., Coceani, F. and Wolfe, L. S. (1968). The biosynthesis of prostaglandins E_2 and $F_{2\alpha}$ in homogenates of the rat stomach. In *Prostaglandin Symposium of the Worcester Foundation for Experimental Biology*, Ramwell, P. W., and Shaw J. E. (eds.), pp. 371–378 (New York: Interscience Publishers)

Pace-Asciak, C. R. and Nashat, M. (1975a). Catabolism of an isolated, purified intermediate of prostaglandin biosynthesis by regions of the adult rat kidney. *Biochim. Biophys. Acta.*, **388**, 243

Pace-Asciak, C. R. and Nashat, M. (1975b). Mechanism of formation of 6(9)oxy-$PGF_{2\alpha}$. Deuterium-labelled arachidonic acid and endoperoxide studies. In *Advances in Prostaglandin and Thromboxane Research, Vol. 1*, Samuelsson, B. and Paoletti, R. (eds.), (New York: Raven Press). In press.

Pace-Asciak, C. R. and Nashat, M. (1975c). Catabolism of 15-hydroxy-9,11-cyclic prostadienoate endoperoxide by homogenates of rat kidney, brain and stomach. In *Advances in Prostaglandin and Thromboxane Research, Vol. 1*, Samuelsson, B. and Paoletti, R. (eds.), (New York: Raven Press). In press.

Pace-Asciale, C. R. and Wolfe, L. S. (1971). A novel prostaglandin derivative formed from arachidonic acid by rat stomach homogenates. *Biochemistry*, **10**, 3657

Palmes, E. D. and Park, C. R. (1965). The regulation of body temperature during fever. *Arch. Env. Hlth.*, **11**, 749

Pappius, H. M., Rostworowski, K. and Wolfe, L. S. (1974). Biosynthesis of prostaglandin $F_{2\alpha}$ and E_2 by brain tissue *in vitro*. *Trans. Am. Soc. Neurochem.*, **5**, 119

Pelofsky, S., Jacobson, E. D. and Fisher, R. G. (1972). Effects of prostaglandin E_1 on experimental cerebral vasospasm. *J. Neurosurg.*, **36**, 634

Pennink, M., White, R. P., Crockarell, J. R. and Robertson, J. T. (1972). Role of prostaglandin $F_{2\alpha}$ in the genesis of experimental cerebral vasospasm: angiographic study in dogs. *J. Neurosurg.*, **37**, 398

Perkins, J. P. (1973). Adenyl cyclase. In *Advances in Cyclic Nucleotide Research, Vol. 3*, Greengard, P. and Robison, G. A. (eds.), pp. 1–64 (New York: Raven Press)

Phillis, J. W. and Tebēcis, A. K. (1968). Prostaglandins and toad spinal cord responses. *Nature (Lond.)*, **217**, 1076

Pickard, J. D. (1973). The mechanism of action of prostaglandin $F_{2\alpha}$ on cerebral flow in the baboon. *J. Physiol. (Lond.)*, **234**, 46P

Pickard, J. D. and Mackenzie, E. T. (1973). Inhibition of prostaglandin synthesis and the response of baboon cerebral circulation to carbon dioxide. *Nature (New Biology)*, **245**, 187

Piper, P. and Vane, J. (1971). The release of prostaglandins from lung and other tissues. *Ann. N.Y. Acad. Sci.*, **180**, 363

Pittman, Q. J., Cooper, K. E., Veale, W. L. and Van Petten, G. R. (1974a). Observations on the development of the febrile response to pyrogens in sheep. *Clin. Sci. Mol. Med.*, **46**, 591

Pittman, Q. J., Veale, W. L. and Cooper, K. E. (1974b). Prostaglandin in normal thermoregulation. *Proc. 4th Meeting Soc. Neurosciences (USA)*, 375

Pittman, Q. J., Veale, W. L. and Cooper, K. E. (1975). Effect of prostaglandin E_1 and bacterial pyrogen on body temperature in the chicken. *Canada Physiology*, **6**, 45

Polet, H. and Levine, L. (1975). Metabolism of prostaglandin E, A, and C in serum. *J. Biol. Chem.*, **250**, 351

Potts, W. J. and East, P. F. (1971a). The effects of prostaglandin E_2 on conditioned avoidance response performance in rats. *Archs. int. Pharmacodyn. Ther.*, **191**, 74

Potts, W. J. and East, P. F. (1971b). Effects of prostaglandins and prostaglandin precursors on the conditioned avoidance response (CAR) in rats. *Pharmacologist*, **13**, 292

Potts, W. J. and East, P. F. (1972). Effects of prostaglandin E_2 on the body temperature of conscious rats and cats. *Archs. int. Pharmacodyn. Ther.*, **197**, 31

Potts, W. J., East, P. F., Landry, D. and Dixon, J. P. (1973). The effects of prostaglandin E_2 on conditioned avoidance behaviour and the electroencephalogram. *Adv. Biosci.*, **9**, 489

Poulain, P. and Carette, B. (1974). Iontophoresis of prostaglandins on hypothalamic neurons. *Brain Res.*, **79**, 311

Prasad, K. N. (1972). Morphological differentiation induced by prostaglandin in mouse neuroblastoma cells in culture. *Nature (Lond.)*, **236**, 49

Prasad, K. N. and Hsie, A. W. (1971). Morphologic differentiation of mouse neuroblastoma cells induced *in vitro* by dibutyryl adenosine $3',5'$-cyclic monophosphate. *Nature (Lond.)*, **233**, 141

Prasad, K. N. and Kumar, S. (1973). Cyclic $3',5'$-AMP phosphodiesterase activity during cyclic AMP-induced differentiation of neuroblastoma cells in culture. *Proc. Soc. Exp. Biol. Med.*, **142**, 406

Prasad, K. N. and Sheppard, J. R. (1972). Inhibitors of cyclic nucleotide-phosphodiesterase induce morphological differentiation of mouse neuroblastoma cell culture. *Exptl. Cell Res.*, **73**, 436

Price, C. J. and Rowe, C. E. (1972). Stimulation of the production of unesterified fatty acids in nerve endings of guinea-pig brain *in vitro* by noradrenaline and 5-hydroxytryptamine. *Biochem. J.*, **126**, 575

Ramwell, P. W. (1964). The action of cerebrospinal fluid on the frog rectus abdominis muscle and other isolated tissue preparations. *J. Physiol. (Lond.)*, **170**, 21

Ramwell, P. W. and Shaw, J. E. (1966). Spontaneous and evoked release of prostaglandins from cerebral cortex of anaesthetized cats. *Am. J. Physiol.*, **211**, 125

Ramwell, P. W., Shaw, J. E. and Jessup, R. (1966). Spontaneous and evoked release of prostaglandins from frog spinal cord. *Am. J. Physiol.*, **211**, 998

Raz, A., Stern, H. and Kenig-Wakshal, R. (1973). Indomethacin and aspirin inhibition of prostaglandin E_2 synthesis by sheep seminal vesicles microsome powder and seminal vesicles slices. *Prostaglandins*, **3**, 337

Samuels, G. M. R. (1972). Factors influencing the release of prostaglandins from the cerebral cortex. *Progr. Brain Res.*, **36**, 167

Samuelsson, B. (1964). Identification of a smooth muscle-stimulating factor in bovine brain. *Biochim. Biophys. Acta*, **84**, 218

Samuelsson, B. (1965). On the incorporation of oxygen in the conversion of 8,11,14-eicosatrienoic acid to prostaglandin E_1. *J. Am. Chem. Soc.*, **87**, 3011

Sandler, M. (1972). Migraine: a pulmonary disease? *Lancet*, **i**, 618

Satinoff, E. (1972). Salicylate: action on normal body temperature in rats. *Science*, **176**, 532

Sato, A., Onaya, T., Kotani, M., Harada, A. and Yamada, T. (1974). Effects of biogenic amines on the formation of adenosine 3′,5′-monophosphate in porcine cerebral cortex, hypothalamus and anterior pituitary slices. *Endocrinology*, **94**, 1311

Scaramuzzi, O. E., Baile, C. A. and Mayer, J. (1971). Prostaglandins and food intake of rats. *Experientia*, **27**, 256

Schmidt, M. J., Palmer, E. C., Dettbarn, W.-D. and Robison, G. A. (1970). Cyclic AMP and adenyl cyclase in the developing rat brain. *Developmental Psychobiology*, **3**, 53

Schoener, E. P. and Wang, S. C. (1974). Sodium acetylsalicylate effectiveness against fever induced by leukocytic pyrogen and prostaglandin E_1 in the cat. *Experientia*, **30**, 383

Schultz, J. and Hamprecht, B. (1973). Adenosine 3′,5′-monophosphate in cultured neuroblastoma cells: effect of adenosine, phosphodiesterase inhibitors and benzazepines. *Naunyn-Schmiedeberg's Arch. Pharmacol.*, **278**, 215

Shapiro, D. L. (1973). Morphological and biochemical alterations in fetal rat brain cells cultured in the presence of monobutyryl cyclic AMP. *Nature (Lond.)*, **241**, 203

Sheppard, J. R. (1972). Difference in the cyclic adenosine 3′,5′-monophosphate levels in normal and transformed cells. *Nature (New Biology)*, **236**, 14

Sheppard, J. R. and Prasad, K. N. (1973). Cyclic AMP levels and the morphological differentiation of mouse neuroblastoma cells. *Life Sci.*, **12**, 431

Shimizu, H., Creveling, C. R. and Daly, J. W. (1970). Effect of membrane depolarization and biogenic amines on the formation of cyclic AMP in incubated brain slices. In *Advances in Biochemical Pharmacology, Vol. 3*, Greengard, P. and Costa, E. (eds.), pp. 135–154 (New York: Raven Press)

Siggins, G. R., Hoffer, B. J. and Bloom, F. E. (1971a). Studies of norepinephrine-containing afferents to Purkinje cells of rat cerebellum: III. Evidence for mediation of norepinephrine effects by cyclic 3′,5′-adenosine monophosphate. *Brain Res.*, **25**, 535

Siggins, G., Hoffer, B. and Bloom, F. (1971b). Prostaglandin–norepinephrine interactions in brain: microelectrophoretic and histochemical correlates. *Ann. N.Y. Acad. Sci.*, **180**, 302

Siggins, G. R., Battenberg, E. F., Hoffer, B. J., Bloom, F. E. and Steiner, A. L. (1973). Noradrenergic stimulation of cyclic adenosine monophosphate in rat Purkinje neurons: an immunocytochemical study. *Science*, **179**, 585

Sih, C. J., Takeguchi, C. and Foss, P. (1970). Mechanism of prostaglandin biosynthesis. III. Catecholamines and serotonin as coenzymes. *J. Am. Chem. Soc.*, **92**, 6670

Sinclair, J. G. and Chaplin, M. F. (1974). Effects of *p*-chlorophenylalanine, α-methyl-*p*-tyrosine, morphine and chlorpromazine on prostaglandin E_1 hyperthermia in the rabbit. *Prostaglandins*, **8**, 117

Splawinski, J. A., Reichenberg, K., Vetulani, J., Marchaj, J. and Kaluza, J. (1974). Hyperthermic effect of intraventricular injections of arachidonic acid and prostaglandin E_2 in the rat. *Pol. J. Pharmacol. Pharm.*, **26**, 101

Steiner, L., Forster, D. M. C., Bergvall, U. and Carlson, L. A. (1972). Effect of prostaglandin E_1 on cerebral circulatory disturbances following subarachnoid haemorrhage in man. *Neuroradiology*, **4**, 20

Stitt, J. T. (1973). Prostaglandin E_1 fever induced in rabbits. *J. Physiol. (Lond.)*, **232**, 163

Stone, T. W., Taylor, D. A. and Bloom, F. E. (1975). Cyclic AMP and cyclic GMP may mediate opposite neuronal responses in the rat cerebral cortex. *Science*, **187**, 845

Struijk, C. B., Beerthuis, R. K., Pabon, H. J. J. and Van Dorp, D. A. (1966). Specificity in the enzymic conversion of polyunsaturated fatty acids into prostaglandins. *Recl. Trav. Chim. Pays-Bas Belg.*, **85**, 1233

Sweet, C. S., Kadowitz, P. J. and Brody, M. J. (1971). A hypertensive response to infusion of prostaglandin $F_{2\alpha}$ into the vertebral artery of the conscious dog. *Eur. J. Pharmacol.*, **16,** 229

Tan, W. C. and Privett, O. S. (1973). Studies on detection and synthesis of prostaglandins in tail skin of the rat. *Lipids*, **8,** 166

Van Der Plaetsen, L., Thiery, M., Amy, J. J. and De Hemptinne, D. (1974). Effect of prostaglandin E_2 therapy on the cerebral cortex. *Lancet*, **i,** 1226

Vane, J. R. (1971). Inhibition of prostaglandin synthesis as a mechanism of action for aspirin-like drugs. *Nature (New Biology)*, **231,** 232

Veale, W. L. and Cooper, K. E. (1973). Species differences in the pharmacology of temperature regulation. In *The Pharmacology of Thermoregulation*, Schönbaum, E. and Lomax, P. (eds.), pp. 289–301 (Basel: Karger)

Veale, W. L. and Cooper, K. E. (1974). Evidence for the involvement of prostaglandins in fever. In *Recent Studies of Hypothalamic Function*, Lederis, K. and Cooper, K. E. (eds.), pp. 359–370 (Basel: Karger)

Veale, W. L. and Cooper, K. E. (1975). Comparison of sites of action of prostaglandin E and leucocyte pyrogen in brain. In *Temperature Regulation and Drug Action*, Lomax, P., Schönbaum, E. and Jacob, J. (eds.), pp. 218–226 (Basel: Karger)

Vishwanathan, C. T. and Rudy, T. A. (1974). Modulation of central cholinergic function as a possible basis for prostaglandin-evoked hyperthermia in the rat. *Fed. Proc.*, **33,** 286

Vonkeman, H. and Van Dorp, D. A. (1968). The action of prostaglandin synthetase on 2-arachidonyl-lecithin. *Biochim. Biophys. Acta*, **164,** 430

Webster, G. R. and Cooper, M. (1968). On the site of action of phosphatide acyl-hydrolase activity of rat brain homogenates on lecithin. *J. Neurochem.*, **15,** 795

Welch, K. M. A., Spira, P. J. Knowles, L. and Lance, J. W. (1974). Effects of prostaglandins on the internal and external carotid blood flow in the monkey. *Neurology*, **24,** 711

Wellman, W. and Schwabe, U. (1973). Effects of prostaglandins E_1, E_2 and $F_{2\alpha}$ on cyclic AMP levels in brain *in vivo*. *Brain Res.*, **59,** 371

Werner, I., Peterson, G. R. and Shuster, L. (1971). Choline acetyltransferase and choline acetylcholinesterase in cultured brain cells from chick embryo. *J. Neurochem.*, **18,** 141

Whishaw, I. Q. and Veale, W. L. (1974). Comparison of the effect of prostaglandin E_1 and norepinephrine injected into the brain on ingestive behaviour in the rat. *Pharmac. Biochem. Behav.*, **2,** 421

White, R. P., Heaton, J. A. and Denton, I. C. (1971). Pharmacological comparison of prostaglandin $F_{2\alpha}$, serotonin and norepinephrine on cerebrovascular tone of monkey. *Eur. J. Pharmacol.*, **15,** 300

Wilkins, R. H., Wilkins, G. K., Gunnells, J. C. and Odom, G. (1967). Experimental studies of intracranial arterial spasm using aortic strip assays. *J. Neurosurg.*, **27,** 490

Willis, A. L., Davison, P., Ramwell, P. W., Brockelhurst, W. E. and Smith, B. (1972). Release and actions of prostaglandins in inflammation and fever: inhibition by anti-inflammatory and antipyretic drugs. In *Prostaglandins in Cellular Biology*, Ramwell, P. W. and Pharriss, B. B. (eds.), pp. 227–268 (New York: Plenum Press)

Willis, A. L., Vane, F. M., Kuhn, D. C., Scott, C. G. and Petrin, M. (1974). An endoperoxide aggregator (LASS), formed in platelets in response to thrombotic stimuli-purification, identification and unique biological significance. *Prostaglandins*, **8,** 453

Woelk, H. and Porcellati, G. (1973). Subcellular distribution and kinetic properties of rat brain phospholipase A_1 and A_2. *Hoppe-Seyler's Z. Physiol. Chem.*, **354,** 90

Wolfe, L. S. (1975). Possible roles of prostaglandins in the nervous system. In *Advances in Neurochemistry*, *Vol. 1*, Aprison, M. and Agranoff, B. W. (eds.), pp. 1–49 (New York: Plenum Press)

Wolfe, L. S. and Mamer, O. A. (1975). Measurement of prostaglandin $F_{2\alpha}$ levels in human cerebrospinal fluid in normal and pathological conditions. *Prostaglandins*, **9,** 183

Yamamoto, Y. L., Feindel, W., Wolfe, L. S., Katoh, H. and Hodge, C. P. (1972). Experimental vasoconstriction of cerebral arteries by prostaglandins. *J. Neurosurg.*, **37,** 385

2
Effects of Prostaglandins on Autonomic Neurotransmission

PER HEDQVIST

2.1 INTRODUCTION   37

2.2 ADRENERGIC NEUROEFFECTOR JUNCTIONS   38
    2.2.1 *Spleen*   38
    2.2.2 *Heart*   39
    2.2.3 *Kidney*   41
    2.2.4 *Vascular tissue*   42
    2.2.5 *Vas deferens*   45
    2.2.6 *Other tissues*   46
    2.2.7 *Total catecholamine production and NA turnover*   47
    2.2.8 *Possible mechanisms of prostaglandin-induced*
         prejunctional inhibition   48

2.3 GANGLIONIC TRANSMISSION   50

2.4 CHOLINERGIC NEUROEFFECTOR JUNCTIONS   51
    2.4.1 *Heart*   51
    2.4.2 *Gastrointestinal tract*   52
    2.4.3 *Other tissues*   53

2.5 CONCLUSION   53
    REFERENCES   54

2.1 INTRODUCTION

The autonomic nervous system is an essential regulator of the physiological functions of a large number of organs and organ systems, and disturbances in the autonomic nervous system have been attributed a pivotal role in different pathological conditions. The discovery by Euler (1934, 1935, 1936, and 1939) that prostaglandins affect smooth muscle function in many organs evidently initiated an important research field. Especially during the last decade, after the elucidation of the prostaglandin structures (Bergström and Sjövall, 1960a, b; Bergström et al. 1963), total chemical synthesis (Corey, 1969), and the introduction of prostaglandin synthesis inhibitors (Downing et al., 1970; Vane, 1971), prostaglandins have been shown to possess distinct actions on a large number of biological systems. Physiological or pathophysiological functions have often been attributed to them. Although there is an impressive range of prostaglandin activities, few effects seem to be of such widespread significance as those on autonomic neuroeffector junctions. The purpose of this chapter is to review the large body of evidence indicating (1) that prostaglandins are probably released in the vicinity of autonomic neuroeffector junctions both spontaneously and in response to electrical, mechanical and chemical stimulations; (2) that released prostaglandins presumably influence both transmitter release from the nerve terminals and the response of the effector organ to the secreted transmitter; (3) that the overall effect of a given prostaglandin varies with the dose, organ and animal species chosen, and that the effect of different prostaglandins differs not only quantitatively but qualitatively as well; (4) that there seem to exist distinct differences between prostaglandin actions at adrenergic and cholinergic neuroeffector junctions.

2.2 ADRENERGIC NEUROEFFECTOR JUNCTIONS

2.2.1 Spleen

At an early stage of the prostaglandin era it was observed that the spleen was a rich source of prostaglandins inasmuch as large amounts (mostly PGE_2 and to a lesser extent $PGF_{2\alpha}$) were released in response to sympathetic nerve stimulation or catecholamine administration (Davies et al., 1967, 1968; Ferreira and Vane, 1967; Gilmore et al., 1968). It was therefore somewhat unexpected when Davies and Withrington (1968, 1969, 1971) found no effect of PGE_1, PGE_2 and PGA_2 on canine splenic responses to nerve stimulation and norepinephrine (NA), and but a weak potentiation with $PGF_{2\alpha}$ and PGA_1. On the other hand attempts with the cat spleen were more encouraging. It was found that PGE_1 and PGE_2 inhibited vascular and capsular responses as well as the NA overflow response to sympathetic nerve stimulation (Hedqvist, 1968, 1970a; Hedqvist and Brundin, 1969). With increasing doses of PGE_2, the outflow of NA progressively decreased and paralleled the inhibition of the effector responses, with regard to onset, intensity and recovery (Figure 2.1). The mechanical responses to NA were substantially inhibited by PGE_1, while PGE_2 only weakly inhibited the capsular response to NA and affected the vascular response to NA in a biphasic manner, causing inhibition at low doses and potentiation with high doses. From these observations it was concluded that PGE_2 inhibited the sympathetic neuromuscular transmission mainly as a consequence of a pre-

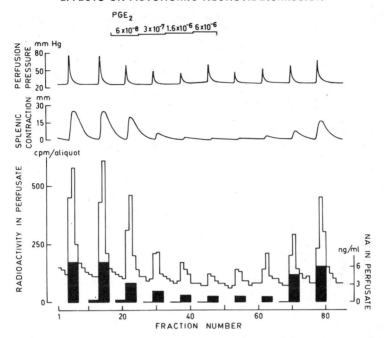

Figure 2.1 Isolated, perfused cat spleen loaded with ³H-NA. Lower panel: Outflow of radioactivity and fluorimetrically determined NA from the spleen, resting and in response to nerve stimulation (NS), 200 pulses, 10 Hz. Upper panels: Perfusion pressure and splenic contraction responses to NS. Effect of increasing doses of PGE_2 (molar conc.). (From Hedqvist, 1970a)

junctional action resulting in decreased transmitter release from the nerve terminals, whereas PGE_1 acted at both prejunctional and post-junctional levels. Furthermore, since the prostaglandin doses needed to substantially inhibit splenic neurotransmission were comparable to those known to be released from the organ, it was proposed that locally formed PGE might serve the function of controlling transmitter release from sympathetic nerve terminals (Hedqvist, 1970b). This hypothesis has gained considerably in weight by observations that prostaglandin synthesis inhibitors, such as eicosatetraynoic acid and indomethacin, increase transmitter release and effector responses to nerve stimulation, as well as responses to injected catecholamines (Hedqvist et al., 1971; Ferreira and Moncada, 1971; Ferreira et al., 1971, 1973). However, meclofenamic acid (also a PG synthesis inhibitor) has been reported not to enhance adrenergic responses in the cat spleen (Hoszowska and Panczenko, 1974).

2.2.2 Heart

PGEs have been shown to increase the rate of contraction of isolated guinea pig heart and atria (Berti et al., 1965; Bhagat et al., 1972). The isolated heart of most other laboratory animals appears to be insensitive, and the chronotropic effect often observed on intravenous injection of PGE_1 seems to be mediated through reflex sympathetic stimulation as a consequence of de-creased arterial blood pressure. The inotropic response is species-dependent since PGE increases the amplitude of contraction in the rat, frog, guinea pig and chicken heart (Berti *et al.*, 1965; Vergroeson *et al.*, 1967; Horton and Main, 1967) whilst it is ineffective in the rabbit and cat heart (Berti *et al.*, 1965).

In the perfused rabbit heart, PGE_1 and PGE_2 reversibly inhibit the chronotropic and inotropic responses to sympathetic nerve stimulation in a dose-dependent manner, but have no effect on responses to added NA (Hedqvist and Wennmalm, 1971; Wennmalm, 1971). Since the two com-pounds were found to inhibit NA overflow in response to nerve stimulation (at least to the same extent as they depressed the effector responses) the inhibition was concluded to be mainly prejunctional, consisting of reduction of the amount of transmitter released from the nerve terminals. Prostaglandin $F_{2\alpha}$ administered in the same concentrations as PGE_1 and PGE_2 did not affect the overflow of NA in response to nerve stimulation, nor did it alter the mechanical responses induced by nerve stimulation or by exogenous NA (Figure 2.2).

There appears to be a continuous low release of prostaglandin (probably mostly PGE_2) from the isolated perfused rabbit heart (Wennmalm, 1971; Block *et al.*, 1974). Increased prostaglandin release occurs as a result of sympathetic nerve stimulation (Wennmalm, 1971), NA (Junstad and Wennmalm, 1973) and hypoxia or arterial emboli (Minkes *et al.*, 1973; Wennmalm *et al.*, 1974; Block *et al.*, 1974). It is therefore of interest that

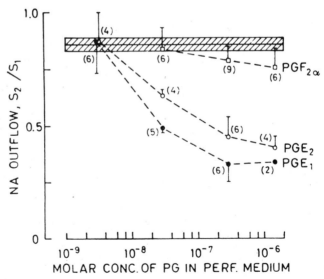

Figure 2.2 Perfused rabbit heart. Effect of PGE_1, PGE_2, and $PGF_{2\alpha}$ on outflow of NA in response to sympathetic nerve stimulation (10 Hz, 30 s). Values are presented as the ratio between a second stimulation with PGs present and a preceding control stimulation (S_2/S_1). Hatched area: Control experiment in which PGs were omitted. Vertical bars: Means $\pm$ SEM. Figures in parentheses: Number of experiments. From Hedqvist and Wennmalm, 1971)

inhibition of prostaglandin formation in the rabbit heart by means of eicosatetraynoic acid or indomethacin is associated with an increased overflow of NA in response to nerve stimulation (Wennmalm, 1971; Chanh *et al.*, 1972). These observations have led to the assumption that local prostaglandin formation serves the function of controlling the release of transmitter from adrenergic nerves in the heart.

2.2.3 Kidney

The rabbit kidney has a high capacity for both synthesis (predominantly in the medulla) and degradation (in the renal cortex) of prostaglandins (Hamberg, 1969; Crowshaw, 1971; Larsson and Änggård, 1973a). Prostaglandin E_2 is the most abundant renal prostaglandin and is a potent vasodilator (Lee *et al.*, 1967; Daniels *et al.*, 1967). Consequently, it has been postulated that PGE_2 has a physiological role in the blood flow regulation in the kidney (McGiff *et al.*, 1970; Lonigro *et al.*, 1973; McGiff and Itskowitz, 1973; Herbaczynska-Cedro and Vane, 1973, 1974; Larsson and Änggård, 1974; Needleman *et al.*, 1974). It has also been shown that both renal nerve stimulation and catecholamine administration increase the output of prostaglandins in the renal venous effluent of dogs and rabbits (Dunham and Zimmerman, 1970; Davis and Horton, 1972; Needleman *et al.*, 1974). It is therefore of considerable interest that, in the dog, PGE_2

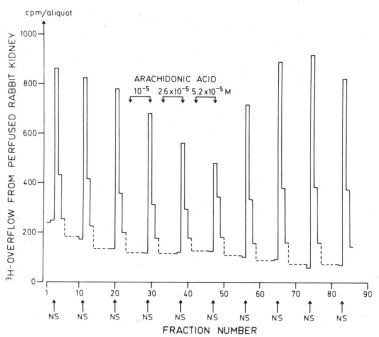

Figure 2.3 Isolated, perfused rabbit kidney, preloaded with ^{3}H-NA. Effect of cumulative doses of arachidonic acid on transmitter overflow resulting from renal nerve stimulation (NS), 150 pulses at 5 Hz. (From Frame and Hedqvist, 1975).

and PGA_2 reverse the actions of nerve stimulation on the kidney. The response of the kidney to administered NA is minimally affected (Lonigro et al., 1973). Prostaglandin E_1 has also been reported to inhibit vascular responses to NA in the dog kidney (Kadowitz et al., 1971a). In the rabbit kidney in vivo and in vitro PGE_2 inhibits vascular responses to nerve stimulation with very little effect on the responses to NA administrations (Frame et al., 1974). Furthermore, PGE_2 and arachidonic acid inhibit NA release resulting from nerve stimulation in a dose-dependent manner (Figure 2.3). Indomethacin and meclofenamic acid, which by themselves increase NA release induced by nerve stimulation, abolish the inhibitory effect of arachidonic acid, without reducing that of PGE_2 (Frame and Hedqvist, 1974, 1975). These observations indicate that exogenous as well as endogenously formed prostaglandin has the capacity to modulate transmitter release and ensuing vascular responses in the rabbit kidney. Further studies on actions of the different renal prostaglandins are of great interest, assuming that renal haemodynamics presumably have a key function in the development of hypertension.

2.2.4 Vascular tissue

Prostaglandins of the E series decrease blood pressure, and with a few exceptions relax vascular beds. Likewise, the PGAs relax vascular tissue, although they are less potent than the PGEs. The PGFs are depressor in cat and rabbit, whilst in dog, monkey and man they increase blood pressure, presumably because of increased cardiac output resulting from venoconstriction and an augmented venous return to the heart (for references see Karim and Somers, 1972; Nakano, 1973).

Following intravenous injection or continuous infusion of PGE_1 into the rat, cat and dog, the pressor responses to NA are diminished in a dose-dependent manner. Similarly, when the blood pressure is raised by NA infusion, administration of PGE_1, PGE_2 or PGE_3 produces a fall in blood pressure in the dog, rabbit, cat and rat (Steinberg et al., 1963; Holmes et al., 1963; Bergström, 1964). Furthermore, catecholamines, vasopressin and angiotensin are still pressor in dogs receiving PGE infusions, and ganglionic stimulation (chemically or electrically) causes increased pressure even in the presence of PGE infusion (Holmes et al., 1963; Nakano and McCurdy, 1967; Carlson and Orö, 1966). Observations such as these have led to the assumption that the antagonism between PGEs and catecholamines on the vascular tree represents the summation of opposite effects (vasodilatation–vasoconstriction) rather than adrenergic inhibition by PGEs.

This view, however, is an over-simplification and other mechanisms have to be considered as well. Thus, topical application of PGE_1 to mesenteric and cremasteric vessels in the rat results in a reduced responsiveness to NA which persists long after the disappearance of the direct vasodilator effect of PGE_1 (Weiner and Kaley, 1969; Messina et al., 1974). In the hindleg of the cat, PGEs inhibit vascular effects of sympathetic nerve stimulation without significantly affecting those due to administered NA (Hedqvist, 1970d, 1972a). In the canine gracilis muscle and paw, PGE_1 inhibits vascular responses to both nerve stimulation and NA (Hedwall *et al.*, 1971; Kadowitz *et al.*, 1971a). Greenberg (1974) found that PGE_2 inhibited the contractile responses to electrical stimulation in the rabbit portal vein without altering the responses to NA. Indomethacin and eicosatetraynoic acid enhanced the responses to low frequency stimulation, an effect which was attenuated by pretreatment of the preparation with α-methyl-*p*-tyrosine. It was therefore concluded that the two compounds increased the release of NA from the sympathetic nerve terminals as a consequence of inhibition of prostaglandin synthesis. Likewise, attenuation of pressor responses to NA in the perfused rabbit ear (which is assumed to be due to prostaglandin synthesis) is considerably reduced by indomethacin treatment (Gryglewski and Korbut, 1973). Simpson (1974) found spontaneous hypertensive rats to be more sensitive than normotensive rats to the blood pressure-reducing effect of PGE_2. On the other hand, after acute or chronic sympathectomy, the spontaneous hypertensive rats were less sensitive than normotensive rats to intravenous injection of PGE_2. This implies that at least part of the blood pressure-lowering effect of PGE_2 in spontaneous hypertensive rats could be due to an inhibitory action on NA release from the adrenergic nerve terminals.

Direct evidence for a prejunctional effect of PGEs on adrenergic neuro-effector transmission has recently been obtained in experiments with isolated vascular tissue. Thus, in mesenteric artery strips from cat and man, PGE_1 and PGE_2 inhibit NA release resulting from postganglionic nerve (transmural) stimulation in a dose-dependent manner (Stjärne and Gripe, 1973; Hedqvist, 1974c). On the other hand, administration of prostaglandin synthesis inhibitors substantially increase stimulated transmitter release, suggesting that locally formed prostaglandin might be of significance in the control of transmitter release by nerve action potentials (Figure 2.4).

Consequently, at least three mechanisms whereby PGEs may affect local blood flow and pressure must be considered:

(1) direct vasodilatation
(2) decreased responsiveness to circulating catecholamines and to locally released NA
(3) inhibition of NA release from sympathetic nerve terminals. However, as will be considered in more detail below, PGE compounds do not inhibit responses to sympathetic nerve stimulation in all vascular beds or even in the same vascular bed from different animal species. Rather, facilitation of adrenergic transmission can sometimes be demonstrated with PGEs, as well as with members of the PGF and PGB series.

Prostaglandin E_1 potentiates responses to NA in the rabbit aorta and mesenteric artery *in vitro* (Strong and Chandler, 1972; Tobian and Viets, 1970), and vasoconstrictor responses to NA in the canine uterus *in situ* (Clark *et al.*, 1973). In the latter tissue, pressor responses to nerve stimulation are either reduced or enhanced by PGE_1. On the other hand, PGE_1 has been reported to enhance the vasoconstrictor response to nerve stimulation and to reduce that due to NA (Mayer *et al.*, 1970). Prostaglandin E_2 facilitates vasoconstriction induced by nerve stimulation without affecting the response to NA (Kadowitz *et al.*, 1971b). Very high doses of PGE_1 have been

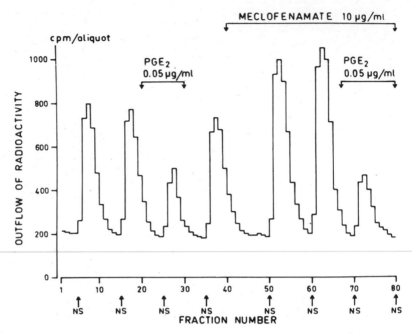

Figure 2.4 Isolated, superfused cat mesenteric artery preincubated with ³H-NA. Effect of PGE₂ and sodium meclofenamate on the outflow of tracer in response to transmural stimulation (NS), 5 Hz, 1 ms, 450 pulses. Fraction number is the time in minutes. (From Hedqvist, 1974c)

reported to increase the NA overflow response to nerve stimulation in the blood-perfused cat spleen, although in this case the effect of PGE_1 was probably due to inhibition of platelet thrombus formation which otherwise often terminated the experiment (Blakeley *et al.*, 1968).

A more consistent, mainly stimulant effect on neurotransmission in vascular tissue seems to occur with prostaglandins of the F-series. In the hindlimb of the dog, $PGF_{2\alpha}$ causes venoconstriction, and this effect is abolished after denervation (DuCharme *et al.*, 1968). Similarly, $PGF_{2\alpha}$ enhances reflex vasoconstriction in the dog paw and gracilis muscle (Brody and Kadowitz, 1974). $PGF_{2\alpha}$ also facilitates the vascular response to nerve stimulation but not to NA in the paw. In the gracilis muscle the response to nerve stimulation is unchanged, and that to NA is actually depressed by $PGF_{2\alpha}$ In the canine tibial artery, $PGF_{2\alpha}$ enhances the response to nerve stimulation without affecting that to NA. While all these observations strongly suggest that $PGF_{2\alpha}$ facilitates NA release in vascular tissue, a postjunctional stimulant action can also be demonstrated in some vascular beds. Thus, $PGF_{2\alpha}$ enhances vasoconstrictor responses to NA in the pulmonary lobar artery and vein, and to both nerve stimulation and NA in hindlimb superficial veins in the dog (Kadowitz *et al.*, 1973; Kadowitz *et al.*, 1971c).

PGA_1 and PGA_2 inhibit pressor responses to nerve stimulation and NA in the canine hindpaw (Kadowitz, Sweet and Brody, 1972). Both compounds inhibit NA release in response to nerve stimulation in the guinea pig vas deferens but they are considerably less effective than the corresponding PGEs (Hedqvist, unpublished). It is, however, of interest that PGA_2 might be converted to PGC_2 and subsequently to PGB_2 (Jones, 1972). Prostaglandin B_2 is a potent vasoconstrictor in superficial and pulmonary vasculature (Greenberg, Engelbrecht and Wilson, 1974;) Greenberg, Howard and Wilson, 1974; Robinson *et al.*, 1973). It enhances pressor responses to nerve stimulation but not to NA in the canine hind paw. Moreover, it produces an intense vasoconstriction which is blocked by reserpine pre-treatment or by decentralization. These observations therefore suggest a presynaptic stimulant effect on NA release from the nerve terminals.

It is evident from what has been discussed in this section that different prostaglandins do not unitarily influence neuroeffector transmission in vascular tissue. Not even within one particular prostaglandin group is the effect obvious and predictable. Rather, the effect of a given prostaglandin seems subject to a confusing variation depending on the dose used, and on selected stimulation parameters, organ and animal species. Further characterization of the vascular effects of different prostaglandins, with special regard to predominant pre- or post-junctional action is required before their possible implication in normal and disordered vascular function can be established.

2.2.5 Vas deferens

This male accessory genital tissue illustrates the complexity of prostaglandin action on autonomic neuroeffector junctions. Prostaglandins E_1, E_2 and A_1 have been shown to enhance contractile responses to nerve stimulation and catecholamines in the guinea pig vas deferens while having no effect on responses in the cat and rat, and actually depressing responses to both nerve stimulation and catecholamines in the rabbit (Holmes *et al.*, 1963; Mantegazza and Naimzada, 1965; Graham and Al Katib, 1967; Naimzada 1969a). In the guinea pig, Sjöstrand and Swedin (1968) found PGE_1 caused minor changes in the response to nerve stimulation, varying from slight inhibition to moderate potentiation. Several authors (Euler and Hedqvist, 1969; Ambache and Zar, 1970; Baum and Shropshire, 1971) have found that PGE_1 and PGE_2 inhibited nerve stimulation induced contractions and enhanced those to NA in the guinea pig vas deferens, while Bhagat *et al.* (1972) reported enhancement of nerve stimulation and inhibition of NA responses with PGE_2.

While these data may seem rather confusing, further studies have clearly shown that PGEs exert a prejunctional inhibitory and a postjunctional stimulatory action in the guinea pig vas deferens. Hedqvist and Euler (1972a) found that low doses of PGE_1 and PGE_2 reduce, and high doses enhance twitch contractions induced by nerve stimulation. Inhibition with high doses of PGEs was also seen after treatment of the vas deferens with the prostaglandin receptor blocker SC-19220. On the other hand, low as well as high doses of PGE invariably enhanced contractile responses to NA. Another characteristic of the inhibitory prejunctional effect was that it varied inversely with stimulation frequency, pulse duration and the number of pulses delivered. Furthermore, the PGEs also increased the latency of contraction (Stjärne, 1973c; Illes, Vizi and Knoll, 1974). Further support for a dual action on neuroeffector transmission are observations that PGE_2 inhibits the stimulated release of dopamine-β-hydroxylase (Johnson *et al.*, 1971), and that low doses of PGE_1 enhance the contractile response to direct electrical stimulation in the chronically denervated vas deferens (Sjöstrand and Swedin, 1974). Direct proof for a prejunctional inhibitory action has, however, also been obtained. Thus, PGE_1 and PGE_2 produce a dose-dependent, inverse frequency-dependent, and reversible inhibition of NA release induced by nerve stimulation in the guinea pig vas deferens (Hedqvist, 1973a, 1974a; Stjärne, 1973a, b). On the other hand, different and chemically unrelated inhibitors of prostaglandin synthesis (eicosatetraynoic acid, indomethacin, meclofenamic acid) all increase nerve stimulation induced NA release (Hedqvist, 1973b, 1974d; Fredholm and Hedqvist, 1973a; Stjärne, 1973a).

Since nerve stimulation presumably releases E prostaglandins from the guinea pig vas deferens (Hedqvist and Euler, 1972b; Swedin, 1971a), this implies that the prostaglandin synthesis inhibitors increase transmitter release by removing a control mechanism operating through local prostaglandin formation. It is questionable, however, if this mechanism is generally present in other animal species, since at least the rat and cat vasa deferentia seem to be rather insensitive to prostaglandin influence.

2.2.6 Other tissues

In the rabbit, intravenous injection of PGE_1 counteracts the rise in luminal pressure in the oviduct induced by nerve stimulation or NA (Brundin, 1968). An inhibitory effect on the adrenergic neuroeffector transmission is therefore suggested in this organ, although the level of action cannot be presently defined.

Guinea pig and rat seminal vesicles respond with contraction to catecholamines and to hypogastric nerve stimulation (Eliasson and Risley, 1966, 1967; Naimzada, 1969a, b; Sjöstrand and Swedin, 1970; Hedqvist, 1972b). However, with low doses of PGEs an inhibition of nerve-induced contractions is unmasked, while enhancement of responses to NA is still present (Hedqvist, 1972b). These observations, which closely resemble those seen in the guinea pig vas deferens, are consistent with a dual, prejunctional inhibitory and postjunctional stimulant action.

In the cat nictitating membrane, PGE_1 markedly reduces the duration of contractions induced by nerve stimulation (Holmes *et al.*, 1963). However, PGE_1 and $PGF_{2\alpha}$, have also been reported not to affect contractions of the cat nictitating membrane induced by transmural or postganglionic nerve stimulation (Illes *et al.*, 1974; Brody and Kadowitz, 1974).

In the epididymal fat pad of the rat and canine subcutaneous adipose tissue, lipolysis induced by sympathetic nerve stimulation is markedly depressed by low doses of PGE_1 and PGE_2 (Berti and Usardi, 1964; Fredholm and Rosell, 1970; Fredholm and Hedqvist, 1973b). In blood-perfused canine subcutaneous adipose tissue, NA release and vascular responses to nerve stimulation are, however, not normally influenced by PGE_2, although inhibition of NA release can be demonstrated after prior treatment with the α-receptor blocker phenoxybenzamine (Fredholm and Hedqvist, 1973b). Moreover, indomethacin and meclofenamic acid do not enhance basal or induce lipolysis in rat adipose tissue and isolated fat cells or in blood-perfused canine adipose tissue (Fain *et al.*, 1973; Fredholm and Hedqvist, 1975a). These observations seem to lend little support to the view that PGEs inhibit lipolysis by a prejunctional action on sympathetic neurotransmission in adipose tissue, or that endogenous prostaglandins are of consequence as modulators of lipolysis.

2.2.7 Total catecholamine production and NA turnover

Intravenous infusion of the prostaglandin precursor, arachidonic acid, lowers arterial blood pressure in the rabbit and spontaneously hypertensive rats (Ichikawa and Yamada, 1962; Larsson and Änggård, 1973b; Änggård and Larsson, 1974; Cohen *et al.*, 1973), an effect which is reduced or abolished by pretreatment of the animal with eicosatetraynoic acid or indomethacin. Furthermore, in the rabbit, prostaglandin synthesis inhibitors substantially increase arterial blood pressure (Davis and Horton, 1972; Änggård and Larsson, 1974).

Indomethacin has been reported to increase urinary excretion of NA in rats, the animals being either cold-stressed or kept at room temperature (Stjärne, 1972a; Junstad and Wennmalm, 1972). There is good reason to believe that this hyperexcretion of NA at least initially was due to increased release from the sympathetic nerves (Euler, 1956; Leduc, 1961), and was subsequently augmented by increased adrenomedullary secretory activity, as reflected by an increase in urinary epinephrine and a fall in NA content of the adrenal medulla.

More recently, Fredholm and Hedqvist (1975b) found that oral administration of indomethacin increased NA turnover rate in a number of different tissues in the rat. Since indomethacin did not affect monoamine oxidase (MAO) and catechole-O-methyltransferase (COMT) activities, or NA uptake in the different tissues the results are consistent with the hypothesis that indomethacin increased NA turnover in the rat by blockade of a locally operating feedback inhibition of transmitter release mediated by prostaglandins. However, the experiments do not exclude the possibility that indomethacin increased the impulse traffic in the adrenergic nerves.

2.2.8 Possible mechanisms of prostaglandin-induced prejunctional inhibition

The demonstration of a prejunctional inhibitory action of PGE_1 in several sympathetically innervated tissues has led to attempts at specifying the target for this effect. Admittedly, clarifying mechanisms underlying a presumed stimulant action should be indicated as well. However, presently no data seem to be available, and, although convincing indirect evidence is accumulating, a direct demonstration of facilitation of transmitter release is not forthcoming.

Theoretically, prostaglandins might reduce the effective outflow of NA from stimulated tissues by promoting its metabolic degradation or uptake. After labelling of the NA stores with tritiated NA in order to monitor the outflow of NA from the spleen, PGE_1 and PGE_2 treatment causes a simultaneous, closely parallel, and reversible reduction of the efflux of total radioactive material and of fluorimetrically determined NA in response to nerve stimulation (Hedqvist and Brundin, 1969; Hedqvist 1970a). Moreover, PGE_2 does not alter MAO and COMT activities in the guinea pig heart (Bhagat et al., 1972). The possibility that PGE depresses NA outflow on nerve stimulation by means of facilitated reuptake has been studied in the cat spleen (Hedqvist, 1970a). It was found that PGE_2 did not alter removal of tritium-labelled NA infused into the organ. It seems unlikely, therefore, that altered disposition of NA released from the nerve terminals could explain the inhibitory effect of the PGEs.

Available evidence seems to be against the view that prostaglandins reduce NA release by means of inhibition of NA synthesis. Nerve stimulation is believed to cause preferential release of newly formed NA (Kopin et al., 1968; Stjärne and Wennmalm, 1971). If prostaglandins inhibit NA synthesis, then stimulation of the spleen (after labelling of the stores with ^{3}H-NA) would be expected to result in a relative rise of the specific activity of NA in the effluent, and not a closely parallel reduction of the outflow of radioactive material and fluorimetrically determined NA, and as a consequence an unchanged specific activity. Moreover, PGEs do not seem to inhibit NA biosynthesis from tyrosine in bovine splenic nerves (Hedqvist and Stjärne, unpublished).

There is overwhelming evidence to suggest that the release of NA from sympathetic nerve terminals is critically Ca^{++}-dependent. It is believed that upon arrival of a nerve action potential, depolarization causes an inward movement of membrane Ca^{++}, which in turn promotes release of NA into the junctional cleft (cf. Simpson, 1968; Hubbard, 1970). Apparently, Ca^{++} interacts with the inhibitory effect of PGEs on transmitter release from adrenergic nerves. Thus, increasing the Ca^{++} concentration in the perfusion medium to the cat spleen counteracts the inhibitory action of PGE_2 on NA release and restores normal output (Hedqvist, 1970c). The same interaction between PGEs and Ca is seen in the guinea pig vas deferens, and in fact the inhibitory effect of PGE on NA release is markedly increased when environmental Ca^{++} concentration is reduced (Hedqvist, 1973b, 1974b; Stjärne, 1973c, d). (Figure 2.5). It is also worth noting that in the cat spleen NA release by tyramine (which is a calcium independent process) is not affected by PGE_2 (Hedqvist, 1970c). Influx of Ca^{++} and subsequent transmitter release probably depends not only on the depolarization of the axonal membrane but also on the pulse duration and pulse frequency. It is therefore interesting that PGE_1 and PGE_2 are more prone to inhibit NA release and adrenergic effector responses when the stimulation frequency is low and the pulse duration is kept short than at a high stimulation frequency or a long pulse duration (Hedqvist and Euler, 1972a; Hedqvist, 1973a; Stjärne, 1973b). Evidently, all these observations are consistent with PGEs inhibiting NA release by interfering with the accessibility to Ca^{++} of the axonal structures where it promotes NA secretion. Such an action can

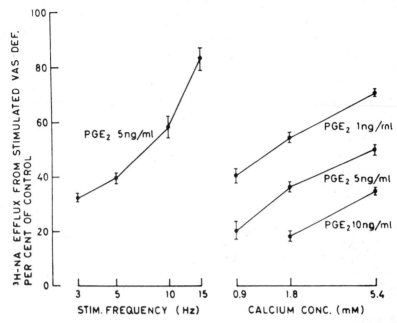

Figure 2.5 Inhibitory effect of PGE₂ on ³H-NA efflux from superfused guinea pig vas deferens, transmurally stimulated (450 pulses, 1 ms pulse duration, supramaximal voltage). To the left: Calcium in superfusion medium concentration 1.8 mM, stimulation frequency 3–15 Hz. To the right: Calcium concentration in superfusion medium 0.9–5.4 mM, stimulation frequency 5 Hz. Values presented in per cent of corresponding control stimulation without PGE₂ and given as means ± SEM, n=4–6. (From Hedqvist, 1973a)

be achieved by blockade of Ca^{++} transport in the axonal membrane.

It has been known for some time that in motor nerve junctions and synapses, transmitter release induced by nerve action potentials varies inversely with the polarization of the axonal membrane (Hubbard and Willis, 1962a, b; Miledi and Slater 1966). Since the change in nerve action potential amplitude has a shorter time constant than that in the junctional or synaptic potential, variations of membrane potential have been concluded to affect transmitter release by an action on membrane Ca^{++} (Hubbard and Schmidt, 1963; Miledi and Slater, 1966; Hubbard, 1970). Assuming that the same principle is operative in sympathetic nerve terminals, PGEs could, as an alternative, indirectly reduce the influx of Ca^{++} by bringing about a depolarization of the axonal membrane. At present it is not known whether PGEs exert such an action on adrenergic terminal C-fibres but it is well recognized that they depolarize smooth muscle cells in various species (Clegg *et al.*, 1966; Sjöstrand, 1972; Taylor and Einhorn, 1972). In the guinea pig, rat, rabbit and cat heart PGEs (20 ng/ml) have been reported to reduce resting potential and action potential overshoot, while lower doses (5 ng/ml) sometimes produce the reverse effect (Kecskemeti *et al.*, 1973, 1974). Independently of whether PGEs block Ca^{++} channels in the axonal membrane or alter the resting membrane potential, the result will be reduction of

Ca^{++} influx necessary for the ultimate release of transmitter into the junctional cleft.

In autonomically innervated tissues, prostaglandin release seems to be closely related to the function of the effector cell. Thus, nerve stimulation and injection of epinephrine cause contraction of the spleen and release of prostaglandin. Alpha adrenergic receptor blockade abolishes both types of response to adrenaline, while chronic denervation does not (Davies et al., 1967; Gilmore et al., 1968). Similarly phenoxybenzamine blocks the pressor response and release of prostaglandin induced by NA infusion in the perfused rabbit ear (Gryglewski and Korbut, 1973). In the rat stomach, vagal stimulation induces prostaglandin release, which is abolished by blockade of the motor response (Coceani et al., 1967; Bennett et al., 1967).

The possibility that nerve terminals represent a significant source of prostaglandin formation and release should, however, not be overlooked. Thus, prostaglandin formation has been noted in pure nerve tissue, such as vagus nerve (Karim et al., 1968) and splenic nerves (Hedqvist, unpublished). Furthermore, indomethacin increases the release of NA from the transmurally stimulated guinea pig vas deferens, even in the absence of contraction of the effector organ (Stjärne, 1972b). Similarly, propranolol (in a dose sufficient to block mechanical responses to NA) or phenoxybenzamine do not inhibit NA induced release of prostaglandins in the rabbit heart (Junstad and Wennmalm, 1973), although the authors did not assume the released prostaglandin to be neural in origin.

Independently of whether prostaglandins released from autonomically innervated tissues are derived from the nerves or from the effector cells, or from both, they should at least have the same chance to affect transmitter release as exogenously administered prostaglandins.

2.3 GANGLIONIC TRANSMISSION

The information about prostaglandin action on ganglionic transmission is sparse and even controversial. Kayaalp and McIsaac (1968) found no effect of PGE_1 or PGE_2 on postganglionic action potentials elicited by preganglionic stimulation of the cervical sympathetic chain in the cat. On the other hand, Swedin (1971b) reported that, in the guinea pig vas deferens, a given dose of PGE_1 was more apt to inhibit the contractile response to pre- than to postganglionic nerve stimulation, an observation which may be consistent with PGE_1 interfering with ganglionic transmission.

Cardiovascular effects elicited by intra-carotid infusion of PGE_1 in intact dogs or in cross-circulation experiments are abolished by ganglion blocking drugs (Carlson and Orö, 1966; Kaplan et al., 1969). At least part of these effects are presumably mediated by the central nervous system, where prostaglandins are capable of either stimulating or inhibiting ganglionic transmission (Duda et al., 1968; Coceani et al., 1969; Coceani and Viti, 1973). Whether or not PGE_1 may have also influenced transmission in peripheral ganglia is not known.

The adrenal medullary secretory cells are homologues to postganglionic nerve fibres, and the nerve–effector cell junction can therefore be regarded as a specialized type of ganglionic transmission. Miele (1969) found that PGE_1 and $PGF_{1\alpha}$ did not modify resting outflow or increased secretion of catecholamines induced by acetylcholine, potassium or splanchnic nerve stimulation. On the other hand, Brody and Kadowitz (1974) using vaso-constrictor responses in the canine paw as an indicator of catecholamine secretion from the animal's adrenal medulla, found that intravenous injection of small amounts of $PGF_{2\alpha}$ increased vasoconstrictor responses to splanchnic nerve stimulation. They concluded that $PGF_{2\alpha}$ had actually facilitated catecholamine secretion from the adrenal medulla. Further studies, including direct analysis of catecholamine secretion from the adrenal medulla, are needed to confirm this interesting observation.

2.4 CHOLINERGIC NEUROEFFECTOR JUNCTIONS

2.4.1 Heart

Wennmalm and Hedqvist (1971) found that PGE_1 blocked the effect of vagal nerve stimulation in the rabbit heart. Since the effect of acetylcholine was unaffected by PGE_1 they concluded that PGE_1 exerted its effect mainly prejunctionally, i.e. on acetylcholine release from nerve terminals (Figure 2.6). Since prostaglandin release from the rabbit heart can be brought about

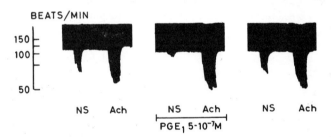

Figure 2.6 Perfused rabbit heart. Chronotropic responses to three consecutive periods of vagal nerve stimulation (10 pulses, 1 Hz) and infusion of acetylcholine (0.7 μg). Effect of PGE_1. (From Wennmalm and Hedqvist, 1971)

by means of vagal nerve stimulation and acetylcholine administration (the effect of the latter being blocked by atropine) prostaglandin could be sus-pected to control cholinergic neuroeffector transmission in the heart in a way similar to that proposed for the adrenergic system (Wennmalm, 1971; Junstad and Wennmalm, 1974). The prejunctional target for such a mech-anism has, however, been questioned by some authors. PGE_2 has been tested for effects on the chronotropic responses induced by electrical stimula-tion of autonomic nerves in the isolated rabbit sino-atrial node. PGE_2 did not affect negative chronotropic responses (in the presence of propranolol), while it heavily depressed positive chronotropic responses (in the presence of atropine) (Park *et al.*, 1973). In spontaneously beating guinea pig atria, PGE_1 was found to block negative chronotropic responses to both vagal nerve stimulation and to acetycholine (Hadhazy *et al.*, 1973).

Although a prostaglandin system might serve the function of controlling cholinergic neuroeffector transmission in the heart it does not seem to be a prerequisite for the muscarinic inhibition of NA release (Fuder and Muscholl, 1974).

2.4.2 Gastrointestinal tract

Prostaglandin formation and release (mainly PGE_1) occurs in the stomach both spontaneously and in response to nerve stimulation (Bennett et al., 1967; Coceani et al., 1967). PGE_1 inhibits gastric secretion in response to vagal nerve stimulation and various secretagogues in the rat (Shaw and Ramwell, 1968; Robert, 1968). The mechanism by which PGE_1 exerts its anti-secretory effect is largely unknown. At least part of it should be considered to be due to a postjunctional action, or an effect directly on the secretory cells.

In contrast to the antisecretory property, prostaglandins generally stimulate gastrointestinal smooth muscle, although a few exceptions have been noted (cf. Bennett, 1972). Moreover, prostaglandins in subspasmogenic doses potentiate contractions elicited by other stimulants and by stimulation of intestinal parasympathetic nerves (Clegg, 1966; Bennett et al., 1968; Baum and Shropshire, 1971; Eckenfels and Vane, 1972; Illes et al., 1974; Kadlec et al., 1974). Prostaglandin release from the intestine (both spontaneous, and nerve stimulation induced) has been reported (Radmanovic, 1968; Botting and Salzmann, 1974). Inhibition of prostaglandin formation is associated with a decrease in tone and contractions induced by nerve stimulation, and these effects can be reversed by the addition of small amounts of PGE (Ferreira et al., 1972; Davison et al., 1972; Botting and Salzmann, 1974; Kadlec et al., 1974). Apart from directly affecting intestinal smooth muscle, prosta-glandins have been suggested to stimulate cholinergic nerve fibres (Horton, 1965; Bennett et al., 1968; Sanner, 1971). Direct measurement of acetyl-choline release from intestinal preparations has, however, failed to disclose facilitation by PGE_2 or inhibition by indomethacin (Hadhazy et al., 1973; Illes et al., 1974; Botting and Salzmann, 1974). In this context it should be noted that PGE_1 and PGE_2 counteract the inhibition of gut motility resulting from electrical stimulation of the periarterial sympathetic nerves, without affecting inhibitory responses to NA (Persson and Hedqvist, 1973; Hedqvist, 1974d; Illes et al., 1974). These observations are consistent with a presynaptic inhibitory action on intestinal adrenergic neurotransmission, similar to that reported in several other sympathetically innervated tissues. Kadlec et al. (1974) found that pretreatment with guanethidine or α-methyl-p-tyrosine (in order to block adrenergic transmission) prevented the inhibitory effect of indomethacin on excitatory responses in the guinea pig ileum. These authors concluded that prostaglandins enhance gut motility by inhibiting the release of NA from sympathetic nerve endings. On the other hand, indomethacin has been reported to selectively inhibit contractions of the guinea pig ileum elicited by angiotensin, the effect of which is at least partly mediated by activation of cholinergic nerves (Chong and Downing, 1973). Ehrenpreis et al. (1973) have also concluded that prostaglandins may influence acetyl-choline release from cholinergic nerve terminals in the gut. The experimental basis for this assumption is that morphine- and indomethacin-induced failure of cholinergic transmission in the guinea pig ileum was restored by low doses of PGE_2 but not by exogenous acetylcholine.

There is thus considerable evidence to suggest that E-prostaglandins, apart from directly affecting the smooth muscle cells, may influence gut motility by means of effects on both cholinergic and adrenergic neurotransmission. Further studies on actions of the prostaglandins on these systems, as well as on other putative transmitters, are needed, however, before their significance in intestinal function can be established.

2.4.3 Other tissues

PGEs seem to inhibit adrenergic neurotransmission in the dilator muscle of the iris (Bergström et al., 1973). On the other hand, there is reason to believe that E prostaglandins have the opposite effect on cholinergic transmission in the sphincter muscle in this organ (Gustafsson et al., 1973, 1975; Gustafsson and Hedqvist, 1975). PGE_1, PGE_2 and the prostaglandin precursor, arachidonic acid, enhance contractions induced by cholinergic nerve stimulation, and the PGEs enhance contractions induced by acetylcholine as well (Figure 2.7). The effect of arachidonic acid is abolished by prostaglandin synthetase inhibitors, which in addition relax the muscle. Prostaglandin release, both spontaneous and in response to nerve stimulation has been noted (Posner, 1973). It is conceivable, therefore, that prostaglandins have the function of controlling tone and motor transmission (probably mostly postjunctionally) in the muscle.

A mediator role has also been attributed to prostaglandin in the cholinergic transmission of salivary glands (Hahn and Patil, 1972, 1974; Taira and Satoh, 1973). $PGF_{2\alpha}$, acetylcholine and stimulation of the corda tympani all induce salivation and increased blood flow in the canine submandibular gland. Tetrodotoxin abolishes the responses to $PGF_{2\alpha}$ and corda tympani stimulation while those to acetylcholine remain unaltered. These observations are compatible with the suggestion that $PGF_{2\alpha}$ facilitates acetylcholine release from the nerve terminals.

2.5 CONCLUSION

Prostaglandins of the E series have been found to inhibit NA release and ensuing effector responses resulting from adrenergic nerve stimulation in a

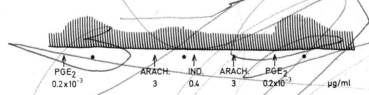

$$
\begin{array}{ccccc}
\text{PGE}_2 & \text{ARACH.} & \text{IND.} & \text{ARACH.} & \text{PGE}_2 \\
0.2 \times 10^{-3} & 3 & 0.4 & 3 & 0.2 \times 10^{-3} \quad \mu g/ml
\end{array}
$$

Figure 2.7 Isolated sphincter muscle from the bovine iris. Contraction responses to transmural stimulation (3 Hz, 1 ms, 15 pulses) at 1 min intervals. Effects of PGE_2, arachidonic acid (arach.) and indomethacin (ind.). Wash at dots. (From Gustafsson and Hedqvist, 1975)

great number of tissues. The prostaglandin doses needed to produce distinct effects are often comparable to those known to overflow from stimulated tissues. Furthermore, inhibition of prostaglandin synthesis is normally associated with increased transmitter release and effector responses to nerve activity. There is therefore considerable evidence to suggest that locally formed PGEs may serve the function of controlling NA release in sympathetically innervated tissues. Exceptions have, however, been noted, and with other prostaglandin series (PGF, PGB) facilitation is often seen. It is conceivable, therefore, that the spectrum of available prostaglandins influences adrenergic neuroeffector transmission in such a way that, depending on the specialized function of the effector organ and the prostaglandin predominantly synthesized, and the level of its synthesis, the effect will be either inhibitory or stimulant.

Numerous investigations have dealt also with prostaglandin action on cholinergic neuroeffector junctions. In contrast to the common observation in adrenergically innervated tissues, the effect is mainly stimulant. The heart and the secretion from the gastric mucosa seem, however, to constitute important exceptions. The level of action may be pre- or postjunctional although most investigations suggest that the latter is primarily affected. Release of substantial amounts of prostaglandins occurs from stimulated tissues, and prostaglandin synthesis inhibitors and prostaglandins seem to produce opposite effects on cholinergic neuroeffector junctions. Observations such as these merit the assumption that this system is also subject to control by locally formed prostaglandins.

References

Ambache, N. and Zar, M. A. (1970). An inhibitory effect of prostaglandin E_2 on neuromuscular transmission in the guinea-pig vas deferens. *J. Physiol. (Lond.)*, **208**, 30P

Änggård, E. and Larsson, C. (1974). Stimulation and inhibition of prostaglandin biosynthesis: opposite effects on blood pressure and intrarenal blood flow distribution. In *Prostaglandin Synthetase Inhibitors*, Robinson, H. J. and Vane, J. R. (eds.), pp. 311–316 (New York: Raven Press)

Baum, T. and Shropshire, A. T. (1971). Influence of prostaglandins on autonomic responses. *Am. J. Physiol.*, **221**, 1470

Bennett, A. (1972). Effects of prostaglandins on the gastrointestinal tract. In *The Prostaglandins, Progress in Research*, Karim, S. M. M. (ed.), pp. 205–221 (Oxford: MTP)

Bennett, A., Eley, K. G. and Scholes, G. B. (1968). Effects of prostaglandins E_1 and E_2 on human, guinea-pig and rat isolated small intestine. *Br. J. Pharmac.*, **34**, 630

Bennett, A., Friedmann, C. A. and Vane, J. R. (1967). Release of prostaglandin E_1 from the rat stomach. *Nature (Lond.)*, **216**, 873

Bergström, S. (1964). The prostaglandins and their role in lipid metabolism. *Abstracts 6th Int. Congr. Biochem. (New York)*, **7**, 559

Bergström, S., Farnebo, L. O. and Fuxe, K. (1973). Effect of prostaglandin E_2 on central and peripheral catecholamine neurons. *Eur. J. Pharmac.*, **21**, 362

Bergström, S., Ryhage, R., Samuelsson, B. and Sjövall, J. (1963). The structures of prostaglandin E_1, $F_{1\alpha}$ and $F_{1\beta}$. *J. Biol. Chem.*, **238**, 3555

Bergström, S. and Sjövall, J. (1960a). The isolation of prostaglandin F from sheep prostate glands. *Acta Chem. Scand.*, **14**, 1693

Bergström, S. and Sjövall, J. (1960b). The isolation of prostaglandin E from sheep prostate glands. *Acta Chem. Scand.*, **14**, 1701

Berti, F., Lentati, R. and Usardi, M. M. (1965). The species specificity of prostaglandin E_1 effects on isolated heart. *Med. Pharmac. Exp.*, **13**, 233

Berti, F. and Usardi, M. M. (1964). Investigations on a new inhibitor of free fatty acid mobilization. *G. Arterioscl.*, **2**, 261

Bhagat, B., Dhalla, N. S., Ginn, D., La Montagne, A. E. and Montier, A. D. (1972). Modification by prostaglandin $E_2(PGE_2)$ of the response of guinea-pig isolated vasa deferentia and atria to adrenergic stimuli. *Br. J. Pharmac.*, **44**, 689

Blakeley, A. G. H., Brown, G. L., Dearnaley, D. P. and Woods, R. I. (1968). The use of prostaglandin E_1 in perfusion of the spleen with blood. *J. Physiol. (Lond.)*, **198**, 31P

Block, A. J., Poole, S. and Vane, J. R. (1974). Modification of basal release of prostaglandins from rabbit isolated hearts. *Prostaglandins*, **7**, 473

Botting, J. H. and Salzmann, R. (1974). The effect of indomethacin on the release of prostaglandin E_2 and acetylcholine from guinea-pig isolated ileum at rest and during field stimulation. *Br. J. Pharmac.*, **50**, 119

Brody, M. J. and Kadowitz, P. J. (1974). Prostaglandins as modulators of the autonomic nervous system. *Fed. Proc.*, **33**, 48

Brundin, J. (1968). The effect of prostaglandin E_1 on the response of the rabbit oviduct to hypogastric nerve stimulation. *Acta Physiol. Scand.*, **73**, 54

Carlson, L. A. and Orö, L. (1966). Effect of prostaglandin E_1 on blood pressure and heart rate in the dog. *Acta Physiol. Scand.*, **67**, 89

Chanh, P. H., Junstad, M. and Wennmalm, Å. (1972). Augmented noradrenaline release following nerve stimulation after inhibition of prostaglandin synthesis with indomethacin. *Acta Physiol. Scand.*, **86**, 563

Chong, E. K. S. and Downing, O. A. (1973). Selective inhibition of angiotensin-induced contractions of smooth muscle by indomethacin. *J. Pharm. Pharmac.*, **25**, 170

Clark, K. E., Ryan, M. J. and Brody, M. J. (1973). Effects of prostaglandins E_1 and $F_{2\alpha}$ on uterine hemodynamics and motility. *Adv. Biosci.*, **9**, 779

Clegg, P. C. (1966). Antagonism by prostaglandins of the responses of various smooth muscle preparations to sympathomimetics *Nature (Lond.)*, **209**, 1137

Clegg, P. C., Hall, W. J. and Pickles, V. R. (1966). The action of ketonic prostaglandins on the guinea-pig myometrium. *J. Physiol. (Lond.)*, **183**, 123

Coceani, F., Dreifuss, J. J., Puglisi, L. and Wolfe, L. S. (1969). Prostaglandins and membrane function. In *Prostaglandins, Peptides and Amines*, Mantegazza, P. and Horton, E. W. (eds.), pp. 73–84 (London and New York: Academic Press).

Coceani, F., Pace-Asciak, C., Volta, F. and Wolfe, L. S. (1967). Effect of nerve stimulation on prostaglandin formation and release from the rat stomach. *Am. J. Physiol.*, **213**, 1056

Coceani, F. and Viti, A. (1973). Actions of prostaglandin E_1 on spinal neurons in the frog. *Adv. Biosci.*, **9**, 481

Cohen, M., Sztokalo, J. and Hinsch, E. (1973). The antihypertensive action of arachidonic acid in the spontaneous hypertensive rat and its antagonism by anti-inflammatory agents. *Life Sci.*, **13**, 317

Corey, E. J. (1969). Total syntheses of prostaglandins. In *Proc. of the Robert A. Welch Found. Conf. on Chem. Res. XII. Organic Synthesis*, Milligan, W. O. (ed.), pp. 51–79 (Houston)

Crowshaw, K. (1971). Prostaglandin biosynthesis from endogenous precursors in rabbit kidney. *Nature (New Biology)*, **231**, 240

Daniels, E. G., Hinman, J. W., Leach, B. E. and Muirhead, E. E. (1967). Identification of prostaglandin E_2 as the principal vasodepressor lipid of rabbit renal medulla. *Nature (Lond.)*, **215**, 1298

Davies, B. N., Horton, E. W. and Withrington, P. G. (1967). The occurrence of prostaglandin E_2 in splenic venous blood of the dog following splenic nerve stimulation. *J. Physiol. (Lond.)*, **188**, 38P

Davies, B. N., Horton, E. W. and Withrington, P. G. (1968). The occurrence of prostaglandin E_2 in splenic venous blood of the dog following splenic nerve stimulation. *Br. J. Pharmac.*, **32**, 127

Davies, B. N. and Withrington, P. G. (1968). The effects of prostaglandin E_1 and E_2 on the smooth muscle of the dog spleen and on its responses to catecholamines, angiotensin and nerve stimulation. *Br. J. Pharmac.*, **32**, 136

Davies, B. N. and Withrington, P. G. (1969). Actions of prostaglandins A_1, A_2, E_1, E_2, $F_{1\alpha}$, $F_{2\alpha}$ on splenic vascular and capsular smooth muscle and their interactions with sympathetic nerve stimulation, catecholamines and angiotensin. In *Prostaglandins, Peptides and Amines*, Mantegazza, P. and Horton, E. W. (eds.), pp. 53–56 (London and New York: Academic Press)

Davies, B. N. and Withrington, P. G. (1971). Actions of prostaglandin $F_{2\alpha}$ on the splenic vascular and capsular smooth muscle in the dog. *Br. J. Pharmac.*, **41**, 1

Davis, H. A. and Horton, E. W. (1972). Output of prostaglandins from the rabbit kidney, its increase on renal nerve stimulation and its inhibition by indomethacin. *Br. J. Pharmac.*, **46**, 658

Davison, P., Ramwell, P. W. and Willis, A. L. (1972). Inhibition of intestinal tone and prostaglandin synthesis by 5,8,11,14-tetraynoic acid. *Br. J. Pharmac.*, **46**, 547P

Downing, D. T., Ahern, D. G. and Bachta, M. (1970). Enzyme inhibition by acetylenic compounds. *Biochem. Biophys. Res. Comm.* **40**, 218

DuCharme, D. W., Weeks, J. R. and Montgomery, R. G. (1968). Studies on the mechanism of the hypertensive effect of prostaglandin $F_{2\alpha}$. *J. Pharmac. Exp. Ther.*, **160**, 1

Duda, P., Horton, E. W. and McPherson, A. (1968). The effects of prostaglandins E_1, $F_{1\alpha}$ and $F_{2\alpha}$ on monosynaptic reflexes. *J. Physiol. (Lond.)*, **196**, 151

Dunham, E. W. and Zimmerman, B. G. (1970). Release of prostaglandin-like material from dog kidney during renal nerve stimulation. *Am. J. Physiol.*, **219**, 1279

Eckenfels, A. and Vane, J. R. (1972). Prostaglandins, oxygen tension and smooth muscle tone. *Br. J. Pharmac.*, **45**, 451

Ehrenpreis, S., Greenberg, J. and Belman, S. (1973). Prostaglandins reverse inhibition of electrically-induced contractions of guinea-pig ileum by morphine, indomethacin and acetylsalicylic acid. *Nature (New Biology)*, **245**, 280

Eliasson, R. and Risley, P. L. (1966). Potentiated response of isolated seminal vesicles to catecholamines and acetylcholine in the presence of PGE_1. *Acta Physiol. Scand.*, **67**, 253

Eliasson, R. and Risley, P. L. (1967). Potentiated response of isolated seminal vesicles to catecholamines and acetylcholine in the presence of prostaglandins. In *Nobel Symposium 2, Prostaglandins*, Bergström, S. and Samuelsson, B. (eds.), pp. 85–90 (Stockholm: Almqvist and Wiksell)

Euler, U. S. v. (1934). Zur Kenntnis der pharmakologischen Wirkungen von Nativsekreten und extrakten männlischer accessorischer Geschlechtsdrüsen. *Naunyn-Schmiedeberg's Arch. Pharmacol.*, **175**, 78

Euler, U. S. v. (1935). Über die specifische Blutdrucksenkende Substantz des menschlichen Prostata- und Samenblasensekretes. *Klin. Wschr.*, **14**, 1182

Euler, U. S. v. (1936). On the specific vaso-dilating and plain muscle stimulating substances from accessory genital glands in man and certain animals (prostaglandin and vesiglandin). *J. Physiol. (Lond.)*, **88**, 213

Euler, U. S. v. (1939). Weitere Untersuchungen über Prostaglandin, die physiologisch aktive Substantz gewisser Genitaldrüsen. *Skand. Arch. Physiol.*, **81**, 65

Euler, U. S. v. (1956). Noradrenaline: chemistry, physiology, pharmacology and clinical aspects. (Springfield: Thomas)

Euler, U. S. v. and Hedqvist, P. (1969). Inhibitory action of prostaglandins E_1 and E_2 on the neuromuscular transmission in the guinea-pig vas deferens. *Acta Physiol. Scand.*, **77**, 510

Fain, Jn., Psychoyos, S., Czernik, A. J., Frost, S. and Cash, W. D. (1973). Indomethacin, lipolysis and cyclic AMP accumulation in white fat cells. *Endocrinology*, **93**, 632

Ferreira, S. H., Herman, A. and Vane, J. R. (1972). Prostaglandin generation maintains the smooth muscle tone of the rabbit isolated jejunum. *Br. J. Pharmac.*, **44**, 328P

Ferreira, S. H. and Moncada, S. (1971). Inhibition of prostaglandin synthesis augments the effects of sympathetic nerve stimulation in the cat spleen. *Br. J. Pharmac.*, **43**, 419P

Ferreira, S. H., Moncada, S. and Vane, J. R. (1971). Indomethacin and aspirin abolish prostaglandin release from the spleen. *Nature (New Biology)*, **231**, 237

Ferreira, S. H., Moncada, S. and Vane, J. R. (1973). Some effects of inhibiting endogenous prostaglandin formation on the responses of the cat spleen. *Br. J. Pharmac.*, **47**, 48

Ferreira, S. H. and Vane, J. R. (1967). Prostaglandins: their disappearance from and release into the circulation. *Nature (Lond.)*, **216**, 868

Frame, M. H. and Hedqvist, P. (1974). Effects of prostaglandin E_2 on the sympathetic neuroeffector system of the rabbit kidney *in vitro* and *in situ*. *Acta Physiol. Scand.*, **91**, 25A

Frame, M. H. and Hedqvist, P. (1975). Evidence for prostaglandin mediated prejunctional control of renal vascular sympathetic tone. *Br. J. Pharmac.*, **54**, 189

Frame, M. H., Hedqvist, P. and Åström, A. (1974). Effect of prostaglandin E_2 on vascular responses of the rabbit kidney to nerve stimulation and noradrenaline, *in vitro* and *in situ*. *Life Sci.*, **15**, 239

Fredholm, B. B. and Hedqvist, P. (1973a). Increased release of noradrenaline from stimulated guinea-pig vas deferens after indomethacin treatment. *Acta Physiol. Scand.*, **87**, 570

Fredholm, B. B. and Hedqvist, P. (1973b). Role of pre- and post-junctional inhibition by prostaglandin E_2 of lipolysis induced by sympathetic nerve stimulation in dog subcutaneous adipose tissue *in situ*. *Br. J. Pharmac.*, **47**, 711

Fredholm, B. B. and Hedqvist, P. (1975a). Indomethacin and the role of prostaglandins in adipose tissue. *Biochem. Pharmacol.*, **24**, 61

Fredholm, B. B. and Hedqvist, P. (1975b). Indomethacin induced increase in noradrenaline turnover in some rat organs. *Br. J. Pharmac.*, **54**, 295

Fredholm, B. B. and Rosell, S. (1970). Effects of prostaglandin E_1 in canine subcutaneous adipose tissue *in situ*. *Acta Physiol. Scand.*, **80**, 450

Fuder, H. and Muscholl, E. (1974). The effect of methacholine on noradrenaline release from the rabbit heart perfused with indomethacin. *Naunyn-Schmiedeberg's Arch. Pharmacol.*, **285**, 127

Gilmore, N., Vane, J. R. and Wyllie, J. H. (1968). Prostaglandins released by the spleen. *Nature (Lond.)*, **218**, 1135

Graham, J. D. P. and Al Katib, H. (1967). Adrenolytic and sympatholytic properties of 2-halogenoalkylamines in the vas deferens of the guinea-pig. *Br. J. Pharmac.*, **31**, 42

Greenberg, R. (1974). The effects of indomethacin and eicosa-5,8,11,14-tetraynoic acid on the response of the rabbit portal vein to electrical stimulation. *Br. J. Pharmac.*, **52**, 61–68

Greenberg, S., Engelbrecht, J. A. and Wilson, W. R. (1974). Prostaglandin B_2-induced cutaneous vasoconstriction of the canine hind paw. *Circulation Res.*, **34**, 491

Greenberg, S., Howard, L. and Wilson, W. R. (1974). Comparative effects of prostaglandins A_2 and B_2 on vascular and airway resistances and adrenergic neurotransmission. *Can. J. Physiol. Pharmacol.*, **52**, 699

Gryglewski, R. J. and Korbut, R. (1973). Prostaglandin feedback mechanism limits vasoconstrictor action of norepinephrine. *Experentia*, **31**, 89

Gustafsson. L. and Hedqvist, P. (1975). Prostaglandin formation participates in the control of tone and contractility in the iris sphincter muscle. *Acta Physiol. Scand.*, **95**, 55A

Gustafsson, L., Hedqvist, P. and Lagercrantz, H. (1973). Prostaglandin mediated enhancement of effector response to cholinergic nerve stimulation. *Acta Physiol. Scand.*, **suppl. 396**, 106

Gustafsson, L., Hedqvist, P. and Lagercrantz, H. (1975). Potentiation by prostaglandins E_1, E_2, and $F_{2\alpha}$ of the contraction response to transmural stimulation in the bovine iris sphincter muscle. *Acta Physiol. Scand.*, **95**, 26

Hadhazy, P., Illes, P. and Knoll, J. (1973). The effects of PGE_1 on responses to cardiac vagus nerve stimulation and acetylcholine release. *Eur. J. Pharmac.*, **23**, 251

Hahn, R. A. and Patil, P. N. (1972). Salivation induced by prostaglandin $F_{2\alpha}$ and modification of the response by atropine and physostigmine. *Br. J. Pharmac.*, **44**, 527

Hahn, R. A. and Patil, P. N. (1974). Further observations on the interaction of prostaglandin $F_{2\alpha}$ with cholinergic mechanisms in canine salivary glands. *Eur. J. Pharmac.*, **25**, 279

Hamberg, M. (1969). Biosynthesis of prostaglandins in the renal medulla of rabbit. *FEBS Lett.*, **5**, 127

Hedqvist, P. (1968). Reduced effector response to nerve stimulation in the cat spleen after administration of prostaglandin E_1. *Acta Physiol. Scand.*, **74**, 7A

Hedqvist, P. (1970a). Control by prostaglandin E_2 of sympathetic neurotransmission in the spleen. *Life Sci.*, **9**, 269

Hedqvist, P. (1970b). Studies on the effect of prostaglandins E_1 and E_2 on the sympathetic neuromuscular transmission in some animal tissues. *Acta Physiol. Scand.*, **79, suppl. 345**, 1

Hedqvist, P. (1970c). Antagonism by calcium of the inhibitory action of prostaglandin E_2 on sympathetic neurotransmission in the cat spleen. *Acta Physiol. Scand.*, **80**, 269

Hedqvist, P. (1970d). Inhibition by prostaglandin E_1 of vascular response to sympathetic nerve stimulation *in vivo*. *Acta Physiol. Scand.*, **80**, 6A

Hedqvist, P. (1972a). Prostaglandin-induced inhibition of vascular tone and reactivity in the cat's hindleg *in vivo*. *Eur. J. Pharmac.*, **17**, 157

Hedqvist, P. (1972b). Prostaglandin-induced inhibition of neurotransmission in the isolated guinea-pig seminal vesicle. *Acta Physiol. Scand.*, **84**, 506

Hedqvist, P. (1973a). Aspects on prostaglandin and α-receptor mediated control of transmitter release from adrenergic nerves. In *Frontiers in Catecholamine Research*, Usdin, E. and Snyder, S. (eds.), pp. 583–587 (Oxford: Pergamon Press)

Hedqvist, P. (1973b). Prostaglandin mediated control of sympathetic neuroeffector transmission. *Adv. Biosci.*, **9**, 461

Hedqvist, P. (1974a). Prostaglandin action on noradrenaline release and mechanical responses in the stimulated guinea-pig vas deferens. *Acta Physiol. Scand.*, **90**, 86

Hedqvist, P. (1974b). Interaction between prostaglandins and calcium ions on noradrenaline release from the stimulated guinea pig vas deferens. *Acta Physiol. Scand.*, **90**, 153

Hedqvist, P. (1974c). Effect of prostaglandins and prostaglandin synthesis inhibitors on norepinephrine release from vascular tissue. In *Prostaglandin Synthetase Inhibitors*, Robinson, H. J. and Vane, J. R. (eds.), pp. 303–309 (New York: Raven Press)

Hedqvist, P. (1974d). Restriction of transmitter release from adrenergic nerves mediated by prostaglandins and α-adrenoreceptors. *Pol. J. Pharmacol. Pharm.*, **26**, 119

Hedqvist, P. and Brundin, J. (1969). Inhibition by prostaglandin E_1 of noradrenaline release and of effector response to nerve stimulation in the cat spleen. *Life Sci.*, **8**, 389

Hedqvist, P. and Euler, U. S. v. (1972a). Prostaglandin-induced neurotransmission failure in the field-stimulated, isolated vas deferens. *Neuropharmacology*, **11**, 177

Hedqvist, P. and Euler, U. S. v. (1972b). Prostaglandin controls neuromuscular transmission in guinea-pig vas deferens. *Nature (New Biology)*, **236**, 113

Hedqvist, P., Stjärne, L. and Wennmalm, Å. (1971). Facilitation of sympathetic neurotransmission in the cat spleen after inhibition of prostaglandin synthesis. *Acta Physiol. Scand.*, **83**, 430

Hedqvist, P. and Wennmalm, Å. (1971). Comparison of the effects of prostaglandins E_1, E_2 and $F_{2\alpha}$ on the sympathetically stimulated rabbit heart. *Acta Physiol. Scand.*, **83**, 156

Hedwall, P. R., Abdel-Sayed, W. A., Mark, A. L. and Abboud, F. M. (1971). Vascular responses to prostaglandin E_1 in gracilis muscle and hindpaw of the dog. *Am. J. Physiol.*, **221**, 42

Herbaczynska-Cedro, K. and Vane, J. R. (1973). Contribution of intrarenal generation of prostaglandin to autoregulation of renal blood flow in the dog. *Circulation Res.*, **33**, 428

Herbaczynska-Cedro, K. and Vane, J. R. (1974). Prostaglandins as mediators of reactive hyperaemia in kidney. *Nature (Lond.)*, **247**, 402

Holmes, S. W., Horton, E. W. and Main, I. H. M. (1963). The effect of prostaglandin E_1 on responses of smooth muscle to catecholamines, angiotensin and vasopressin. *Br. J. Pharmac.*, **21**, 538

Horton, E. W. (1965). Biological activities of pure prostaglandins. *Experientia*, **21**, 113

Horton, E. W. and Main, I. H. M. (1967). Identification of prostaglandins in central nervous tissues of the cat and chicken. *Br. J. Pharmac.*, **30**, 582

Hoszowska, A. and Panczenko, B. (1974). Effects of inhibition of prostaglandin biosynthesis on noradrenaline release from isolated perfused spleen of the cat. *Pol. J. Pharmacol. Pharm.*, **26**, 137

Hubbard, J. I. (1970). Mechanism of transmitter release. *Progr. Biophys. Mol. Biol.*, **21**, 33

Hubbard, J. I. and Schmidt, R. F. (1963). An electrophysiological investigation of mammalian motor nerve terminals. *J. Physiol. (Lond.)*, **166**, 145

Hubbard, J. I. and Willis, W. D. (1962a). Hyperpolarization of mammalian motor nerve terminals. *J. Physiol. (Lond.)*, **163**, 115

Hubbard, J. I. and Willis, W. D. (1962b). Reduction of transmitter output by depolarization *Nature (Lond.)*, **193**, 1294

Ichikawa, S. and Yamada, J. (1962). Biological actions of free and albumin-bound arachidonic acid. *Am. J. Physiol.*, **203**, 681

Illes, P., Vizi, E. S. and Knoll, J. (1974). Adrenergic neuro-effector junctions sensitive and insensitive to the effect of PGE_1. *Pol. J. Pharmacol. Pharm.*, **26**, 127

Johnson, D. G., Thoa, N. B., Weinshilboum, R., Axelrod, J. and Kopin, I. J. (1971). Enhanced release of dopamine-β-hydroxylase from sympathetic nerves by calcium and phenoxybenzamine and its reversal by prostaglandins. *Proc. Nat. Acad. Sci. (USA)*, **68**, 2227

Jones, R. L. (1972). Properties of a new prostaglandin. *Br. J. Pharmac.*, **45**, 144P

Junstad, M. and Wennmalm, Å. (1972). Increased renal excretion of noradrenaline in rats after treatment with the prostaglandin synthesis inhibitor indomethacin. *Acta Physiol. Scand.*, **85**, 573

Junstad, M. and Wennmalm, Å. (1973). On the release of prostaglandin E_2 from the rabbit heart following infusion of noradrenaline. *Acta Physiol. Scand.*, **87**, 573

Junstad, M. and Wennmalm, Å. (1974). Release of prostaglandin from the rabbit isolated heart following vagal nerve stimulation or acetylcholine infusion. *Br. J. Pharmac.*, **52** 357

Kadlec, O., Masek, K. and Seferna, I. (1974). A modulating role of prostaglandins in contractions of the guinea-pig ileum. *Br. J. Pharmac.*, **51**, 565

Kadowitz, P. J., George, W. J., Joiner, P. D. and Hyman, A. L. (1973). Effect of prostaglandins E_1 and $F_{2\alpha}$ on adrenergic responses in the pulmonary circulation. *Adv. Biosci.*, **9**, 501

Kadowitz, P. J., Sweet, C. S. and Brody, M. J. (1971a). Blockade of adrenergic vasoconstrictor responses in the dog by prostaglandins E_1 and A_1. *J. Pharmac. Exp. Ther.*, **179**, 563

Kadowitz, P. J., Sweet, C. S. and Brody, M. J. (1971b). Differential effects of prostaglandins E_1, E_2, $F_{1\alpha}$ and $F_{2\alpha}$ on adrenergic vasoconstriction in the dog hindpaw. *J. Pharmac. Exp. Ther.*, **177**, 641

Kadowitz, P. J., Sweet, C. S. and Brody, M. J. (1971c). Potentiation of adrenergic venomotor responses by angiotensin, prostaglandin $F_{2\alpha}$ and cocaine. *J. Pharmac. Exp. Ther.*, **176**, 167

Kadowitz, P. J., Sweet, C. S. and Brody, M. J. (1972). Effect of prostaglandins on adrenergic neurotransmission to vascular smooth muscle. In *Prostaglandins in Cellular Biology*, Ramwell, P. W. and Pharriss, B. B. (eds.), pp. 479–511 (New York: Plenum Press)

Kaplan, H. R., Greca, G. J., Sherman, G. P. and Buckley, J. P. (1969). Central and reflexogenic cardiovascular actions of prostaglandin E_1. *Int. J. Neuropharmac.*, **8**, 15

Karim, S. M. M., Hillier, K. and Devlin, J. (1968). Distribution of prostaglandins E_1, E_2, F_1 and $F_{2\alpha}$ in some animal tissues. *J. Pharm. Pharmac.*, **20**, 749

Karim, S. M. M. and Somers, K. (1972). Cardiovascular and renal actions of prostaglandins. In *The Prostaglandins, Progress in Research*, Karim S. M. M. (ed.), pp. 165–203 (Oxford: MTP)

Kayaalp, S. O. and McIsaac, R. J. (1968). Absence of effects of prostaglandins E_1 and E_2 on ganglionic transmission. *Eur. J. Pharmac.*, **4**, 283

Kecskemeti, V., Kelemen, K. and Knoll, J. (1973). Effect of prostaglandin E_1 on the transmembrane potentials of the mammalian heart. *Adv. Biosci.*, **9**, 373

Kecskemeti, V., Kelemen, K. and Knoll, J. (1974). Microelectrophysiological analysis of the cardiac effect of prostaglandin E_2. *Pol. J. Pharmacol. Pharm.*, **26**, 171

Kopin, I. J., Breese, G. R., Krauss, K. R. and Weise, V. K. (1968) Selective release of newly synthetized norepinephrine from the cat spleen during sympathetic nerve stimulation. *J. Pharmac. Exp. Ther.*, **161**, 271

Larsson, C. and Änggård, E. (1973a), Regional differences in the formation and metabolism of prostaglandins in the rabbit kidney. *Eur. J. Pharmac.*, **21**, 30

Larsson, C. and Änggård, E. (1973b). Arachidonic acid lowers and indomethacin increases the blood pressure of the rabbit. *J. Pharm. Pharmac.*, **25**, 653

Larsson, C. and Änggård, E. (1974). Increased juxtamedullary blood flow on stimulation of intrarenal prostaglandin biosynthesis. *Eur. J. Pharmac.*, **25**, 326

Leduc, J. (1961). Catecholamine production and release in exposure and acclimation to cold. *Acta Physiol. Scand.*, **53, supp.** 183

Lee, J. B., Crowshaw, K., Takman, B. H., Attrep, K. and Gougoutas, J. Z. (1967). The identification of prostaglandins E_2, $F_{2\alpha}$ and A_2 from rabbit kidney medulla. *Biochem. J.*, **105**, 1251

Lonigro, A. J., Terragno, N. A., Malik, K. U. and McGiff, J. C. (1973). Differential inhibition by prostaglandins of the renal actions of pressor stimuli. *Prostaglandins*, **3**, 595

Mantegazza, P. and Naimzada, M. K. (1965). Attivita della prostaglandia E_1 sul preparato nervo ipogastrico-deferente di varie specie animali. *Atti Accad. Med. Lomb.*, **20**, 58

Mayer, H. E., Abboud, F. M., Schmid, P. G. and Mark, A. L. (1970). Release of norepinephrine by prostaglandin E_1. *Clin. Res.*, **18**, 594

McGiff, J. G., Crowshaw, K., Terragno, N. A. and Lonigro, A. J. (1970). Renal prostaglandins: possible regulators of the renal actions of pressor hormones. *Nature (Lond.)*, **227**, 1255

McGiff, J. C. and Itskowitz, H. D. (1973). Prostaglandins and the kidney. *Circulation Res.*, **33**, 479

Messina, E. J., Weiner, R. and Kaley, G. (1974). Microcirculatory effects of prostaglandins E_1, E_2 and A_1 in the rat mesentery and cremaster muscle. *Microvascular Res.*, **8**, 77

Miele, E. (1969). Lack of effect of prostaglandin E_1 and $F_{1\alpha}$ on adreno-medullary catecholamine secretion evoked by various agents. In *Prostaglandins, Peptides and Amines*, Mantegazza, P. and Horton, E. W. (eds.), pp. 85–93 (London and New York: Academic Press)

Miledi, R. and Slater, C. R. (1966). The action of calcium on neuronal synapses in the squid. *J. Physiol. (Lond.)*, **184**, 473

Minkes, M. S., Douglas, J. R. and Needleman, P. (1973). Prostaglandin-release by the isolated perfused rabbit heart. *Prostaglandins*, **3**, 439

Naimzada, M. K. (1969a). Effect of some naturally-occurring prostaglandins (PGE_1, PGE_2, PGA_1 and $PGF_{1\alpha}$) on the hypogastric nerve vas deferens and seminal vesicle preparations of the guinea-pig. *Chimica Ther.*, **4**, 34

Naimzada, M. K. (1969b). Effects of some naturally occurring prostaglandins on the isolated hypogastric nerve seminal vesicle preparation of the guinea pig. *Life Sci.*, **8**, 49

Nakano, J. (1973). Cardiovascular actions. In *The Prostaglandins, Vol. I*, Ramwell, P. W. (ed.), pp. 239–316 (New York and London: Plenum Press)

Nakano, J. and McCurdy, R. (1967). Cardiovascular effects of prostaglandin E_1. *J. Pharmac. Exp. Ther.*, **156**, 538

Needleman, P., Douglas, J. R. Jnr., Jalsetik, B., Stocklein, P. B. and Johnson, E. M. Jr. (1974). Release of renal prostaglandin by catecholamines: relationship to renal endocrine function. *J. Pharmac. Exp. Ther.*, **188**, 453

Park, M. K., Dyer, D. C. and Vincenzi, F. F. (1973). Prostaglandin E_2 and its antagonists: effects on autonomic transmission in the isolated sino-atrial node. *Prostaglandins*, **4**, 717

Persson, N. Å. and Hedqvist, P. (1973). Reduced intestinal muscular response to adrenergic nerve stimulation after the administration of prostaglandins, *Acta Physiol. Scand*, **108**, suppl. 396

Posner, J. (1973). Prostaglandin E_2 and the bovine sphincter pupillae. *Br. J. Pharmac.*, **49**, 415

Radmanovic, B. (1968). Prostaglandins in perfusate of the rat small intestine after vagal stimulation. *Jugoslav. Physiol. Pharmac. Acta*, **4**, 123

Robert, A. (1968). Antisecretory property of prostaglandins. In *Prostaglandin Symp.*, *Worcester Found. Exp. Biol.*, Ramwell, P. W. and Shaw, J. E. (eds.), pp. 47–54 (New York: Interscience)

Robinson, B. F., Collier, J. G., Karim, S. M. M. and Somers, K. (1973). Effect of prostaglandins A_1, A_2, B_1, E_2 and $F_{2\alpha}$ on forearm arterial bed and superficial hand veins of man. *Clin. Sci.*, **44**, 367

Sanner, J. (1971). Prostaglandin inhibition with a dibenzoxazepine hydrazide derivative and morphine. *Ann. N.Y. Acad. Sci.*, **180**, 396

Shaw, J. E. and Ramwell, P. W. (1968). Inhibition of gastric secretion in rats by prostaglandin E_1. In *Prostaglandin Symp. Worcester Found. Exp. Biol.*, Ramwell, P. W. and Shaw, J. E. (eds.), pp. 55–66 (New York: Interscience).

Simpson, L. L. (1968). The role of calcium in neurohumoral and neurohormonal extrusion processes. *J. Pharm. Pharmac.*, **20**, 889

Simpson, L. L. (1974). The effect of chemical sympathectomy on vascular responses in spontaneously hypertensive rats. *Neuropharmacology*, **13**, 895

Sjöstrand, N. (1972). A note on the dual effect of prostaglandin E_1 on the motor responses of the guinea-pig vas deferens to nerve stimulation. *Experientia*, **28**, 431

Sjöstrand, N. and Swedin, G. (1968). Potentiation by smooth muscle stimulants of the hypogastric nerve–vas deferens preparation from normal and castrated guinea-pigs. *Acta Physiol. Scand.*, **74**, 472

Sjöstrand, N. and Swedin, G. (1970). Potentiation by various smooth muscle stimulants of an isolated sympathetic nerve–seminal vesicle preparation from the guinea-pig. *Acta Physiol. Scand.*, **80**, 172

Sjöstrand, N. and Swedin, G. (1974). On the mechanism of the enhancement by smooth muscle stimulants of the motor responses of the guinea-pig vas deferens to nerve stimulation. *Acta Physiol. Scand.*, **90**, 513

Steinberg, D., Vaughan, M., Nestel, P. J. and Bergström, S. (1963). Effects of prostaglandin E opposing those of catecholamines on blood pressure and on triglyceride breakdown in adipose tissue. *Biochem. Pharmac.*, **12**, 764

Stjärne, L. (1972a). Enhancement by indomethacin of cold-induced hypersecretion of noradrenaline in the rat *in vivo* by suppression of PGE mediated feed-back control? *Acta Physiol. Scand.*, **86**, 388

Stjärne, L. (1972b). Prostaglandin E restricting noradrenaline secretion–neural in origin. *Acta Physiol. Scand.*, **86**, 574

Stjärne, L. (1973a). Prostaglandin- versus α-adrenoceptor-mediated control of sympathetic neurotransmitter secretion in guinea-pig isolated vas deferens. *Eur. J. Pharmac.*, **22**, 233

Stjärne, L. (1973b). Frequency dependence of dual negative feed-back control of secretion sympathetic neurotransmitter in guinea-pig vas deferens. *Br. J. Pharmac.*, **49**, 358

Stjärne, L. (1973c). Inhibitory effect of prostaglandin E_2 on noradrenaline secretion from sympathetic nerves as a function of external calcium. *Prostaglandins*, **3**, 105

Stjärne, L. (1973d). Kinetics of secretion of sympathetic neurotransmitter as a function of external calcium: mechanism of inhibitory effect of prostaglandin E. *Acta Physiol. Scand.*, **87**, 428

Stjärne, L. (1973e). Lack of correlation between profiles of transmitter efflux and of muscular contraction in response to nerve stimulation in isolated guinea-pig vas deferens. *Acta Physiol. Scand.*, **88**, 137

Stjärne, L. and Gripe, K. (1973). Prostaglandin-dependent and independent feedback control of noradrenaline secretion in vasoconstrictor nerves of normotensive human subjects. *Naunyn-Schmiedeberg's Arch. Pharmac.*, **280**, 441

Stjärne, L. and Wennmalm, Å. (1971). Preferential secretion of newly formed noradrenaline in the perfused rabbit heart. *Acta Physiol. Scand.*, **80**, 428

Strong, C. G. and Chandler, J. T. (1972). Interactions of prostaglandin E_1 and catecholamines in isolated vascular smooth muscle. In *Prostaglandins in cellular biology*, Ramwell, P. W. and Pharriss, B. B. (eds.), pp. 369–383 (New York and London: Plenum Press)

Swedin, G. (1971a). Studies on neurotransmission mechanisms in the rat and guinea-pig vas deferens. *Acta Physiol. Scand.*, **369**, (suppl.), 1

Swedin, G. (1971b). Endogenous inhibition of the mechanical response of the isolated rat and guinea-pig vas deferens to pre- and postganglionic nerve stimulation. *Acta Physiol. Scand.*, **83**, 473

Taira, N. and Satoh, S. (1973). Prostaglandin $F_{2\alpha}$ as a potent excitant of the parasympathetic postganglionic neurons of the dog salivary gland. *Life Sci.*, **13**, 501

Taylor, G. S. and Einhorn, V. F. (1972). The effect of prostaglandins on junction potentials in the mouse vas deferens. *Eur. J. Pharmac.*, **20**, 40

Tobian, L. and Viets, J. (1970). Potentiation of *in vitro* norepinephrine vasoconstriction with prostaglandin E_1. *Fed. Proc.*, **29**, 387

Vane, J. R. (1971). Inhibition of prostaglandin synthesis as a mechanism of action for aspirin-like drugs. *Nature (New Biology)*, **231**, 232

Vergroeson, A. J., De Boer, J. and Gottenbos, J. J. (1967). Effects of prostaglandins on perfused isolated rat hearts. In *Nobel Symposium 2, Prostaglandins*, Bergström, S. and Samuelsson, B. (eds.), pp. 211–218 (Stockholm: Almqvist and Wiksell)

Weiner, R. and Kaley, G. (1969). Influence of prostaglandin E_1 on the terminal vascular bed. *Am. J. Physiol.*, **217**, 563

Wennmalm, Å. (1971). Studies on mechanisms controlling the secretion of neurotransmitters in the rabbit heart. *Acta Physiol. Scand.*, suppl. **365**, 1

Wennmalm, Å. and Hedqvist, P. (1971). Inhibition by prostaglandin E_1 of parasympathetic neurotransmission in the rabbit heart. *Life Sci.*, **10**, 465

Wennmalm, Å., Chanh, P. H. and Junstad, M. (1974). Hypoxia causes prostaglandin release from perfused rabbit heart. *Acta Physiol. Scand.*, **91**, 133

3
Prostaglandins and the Eye

KENNETH E. EAKINS

3.1 INTRODUCTION 63

3.2 BIOSYNTHESIS OF PROSTAGLANDINS IN OCULAR TISSUES 64

3.3 ACTIONS OF PROSTAGLANDINS ON INTRAOCULAR PRESSURE 65

3.4 ACTIONS OF PROSTAGLANDINS ON AQUEOUS HUMOUR DYNAMICS 67

3.5 APPEARANCE OF PROSTAGLANDINS IN THE AQUEOUS HUMOUR 69
3.5.1 *In experimental animals* 69
3.5.2 *In patients with open angle glaucoma* 70
3.5.3 *In patients with ocular inflammation* 71

3.6 REMOVAL OF PROSTAGLANDINS FROM INTRAOCULAR FLUIDS 71

3.7 OTHER ACTIONS OF PROSTAGLANDINS ON OCULAR TISSUES 71

3.8 DRUGS WHICH INHIBIT THE ACTIONS/SYNTHESIS OF PROSTAGLANDINS
AND THE EYE 73
3.8.1 *Prostaglandin antagonists* 73
3.8.2 *Inhibitors of prostaglandin biosynthesis* 75

3.9 CONCLUSIONS 78

REFERENCES 78

3.1 INTRODUCTION

Interest in the ocular effects of prostaglandins began in the 1950's with the discovery by Ambache (1955, 1957) of 'IRIN', an ether-soluble smooth muscle stimulating agent in extracts of iris tissue. Ocular tissues were among the first from which prostaglandins were extracted and identified and the actions of prostaglandins on the eye have been the subject of many investigations. Prostaglandins have been implicated in certain inflammatory eye diseases and this, in turn, has led to studies on the ocular actions of substances that inhibit the action and/or synthesis of prostaglandins.

The purpose of this chapter is to review the ocular actions of prostaglandins and to consider the possibility of physiological or pathological roles for these substances in the eye. In addition, the potential use of inhibitors of prostaglandin synthesis or action in the treatment of eye disease will be assessed.

3.2 BIOSYNTHESIS OF PROSTAGLANDINS IN OCULAR TISSUES

A long chain unsaturated hydroxy-fatty acid with smooth muscle stimulating properties, which he called IRIN, was found by Ambache (1955, 1957) in extracts of rabbit iris. Prostaglandins of both the E- and F-type were subsequently identified as components of IRIN extracted from sheep, cat and rabbit irides (Änggård and Samuelsson, 1964; Ambache and Brummer, 1968). Van Dorp and co-workers (1967) reported that the isolated pig iris can synthesize PGE_1 and $PGF_{2\alpha}$ from dihomo-γ-linolenic acid in the presence of glutathione and hydroquinone. In the lens and retina, however, the conversion of the fatty acid to prostaglandins was negligible. It was also shown in this study that the ocular tissues of the pig contain predominantly arachidonic acid with negligible amounts of all-cis-8,11,14-eicosatrienoic acid. These tissues would therefore produce PGE_2 and $PGF_{2\alpha}$ rather than PGE_1 and $PGF_{1\alpha}$. Later studies (Eakins et al., 1972a; Cole and Unger, 1973) confirmed the original observation (Ambache and Brummer, 1968) that only a PGE_2 and a $PGF_{2\alpha}$-like material could be found in extracts of normal rabbit iris. In a wide-ranging study, a moderate conversion of substrate (dihomo-γ-linolenic acid) to prostaglandin was demonstrated in the rabbit iris (Christ and Van Dorp, 1972). Higher yields (20% or higher) were found only in sheep vesicular glands, rabbit renal medulla and frog bladder. A comparison

Table 3.1   Prostaglandin biosynthesis from added substrate by various rabbit tissues *in vitro*

| | PG-like activity (ng/mg protein)* | | |
	Zero-time	20 min	Increase in activity‡
Spleen	18.9 ± 3.3 (9)	56 ± 10.5 (9)	38 ± 10 (9)
Kidney (medulla)	69 ± 12 (7)	648 ± 10 (7)	578.5 ± 96 (7)
Anterior uvea†	60 ± 5 (15)	179 ± 14 (15)	117 ± 11 (15)
Conjunctiva	39 ± 7 (5)	244 ± 34 (5)	205 ± 28 (5)
Cornea	15 ± 6 (5)	30.5 ± 5 (5)	15 ± 1 (5)
Retina	18 ± 3 (6)	32 ± 5 (6)	14 ± 2 (6)

* ng prostaglandin-like activity assayed as prostaglandin E_2 generated by microsomes in incubation fluid containing 10 μg/ml arachidonic acid. Numbers in parentheses refer to the number of separate microsomal fractions from pooled tissue samples used for each determination. Results expressed as mean ± SE mean
† Iris and ciliary body
‡ Calculated from individual differences between zero time and 20 min samples (From Bhattacherjee and Eakins, 1974)

of prostaglandin synthetase activity for different rabbit tissues is shown in Table 3.1. Bhattacherjee and Eakins (1974) compared prostaglandin bio-synthesis from added substrate (arachidonic acid) by microsomal fractions of various rabbit tissues *in vitro*. In the ocular tissues, prostaglandin bio-synthesis was not limited to the iris, since conjunctival tissue was able to generate even higher quantities of prostaglandin-like activity than the iris. Some activity was also found in the cornea and retina.

3.3 ACTIONS OF PROSTAGLANDINS ON INTRAOCULAR PRESSURE

The ocular actions of the prostaglandins themselves were first studied in the rabbit by Waitzman and King (1967). Intracameral injections of E-type prostaglandins were found to produce a miosis associated with a sustained rise in intraocular pressure (IOP). This increase in IOP was accompanied by only small changes in the protein content of the aqueous humour leading the authors to conclude that prostaglandins raise IOP mainly by altering the metabolic processes which normally control the secretion of aqueous humour. This conclusion was challenged by Beitch and Eakins (1969) in a later study on the rabbit eye. Prostaglandins of both the E- and F-type were found to produce the miosis and raised IOP, which, however, was found to be closely associated with large increases in the protein levels of aqueous humour and marked ocular vasodilatation. As little as 5 ng PGE_2 injected into the anterior chamber was found to produce a significant increase in the protein content of the aqueous humour. It was therefore concluded that local ocular vaso-dilatation together with an increase in the permeability of the blood–aqueous barrier were the principal mechanisms by which prostaglandins raised IOP. These observations were confirmed and extended by Starr (1971 a, b) who showed that prostaglandins, particularly PGE_1, can raise IOP even when given by intravenous injection. Chiang and Thomas (1972a) confirmed the observation that prostaglandins particularly of the E-type, given by intra-venous injection, raise IOP in the rabbit. Some species differences are apparent in the effect of intravenous prostaglandins on IOP. Although IOP is raised in the dog (Nakano *et al.*, 1973) intravenous prostaglandins did not raise IOP in the monkey (Kelly and Starr, 1971) and neither PGE_2 nor $PGF_{2\alpha}$ given by intravenous infusion were found to raise IOP in man (Hillier and Embrey, 1972).

In contrast to the intravenous route of administration, the eyes of all species studied have responded to intracameral injections of prostaglandins in a manner qualitatively similar to the rabbit with pupillary miosis, a sustained increase in IOP and increased aqueous humour protein levels (Table 3.2). Thus the cat eye has been found to respond to intracameral injections of PGE_1 and $PGF_{2\alpha}$ (Eakins, 1970) and the cynomolgus monkey to prostaglandins of both the E- and F-type (Kelly and Starr, 1971). In the monkey E-type prostaglandins were approximately 10 times more effective than those of the F-type. It should be noted that Kelly and Starr could not detect an effect of the prostaglandins on pupil diameter in the monkey. However, a later study (Casey, 1974a) confirmed the apparent lack of miotic

Table 3.2 Actions of prostaglandins on the eye

Route of administration	Species	Prostaglandin	Rise in intraocular pressure	Aqueous protein	Pupillary constriction	Reference
Intracameral	Rabbit	E_1; E_2	+	±	+	Waitzman and King, 1967
	Rabbit	E_1; E_2; $F_{2\alpha}$	+	+	+	Beitch and Eakins, 1969
	Rabbit	E_1; E_2	+	ND	−	Starr, 1971a
	Cat	E_2; $F_{2\alpha}$	+	+	+	Eakins, 1970
	Monkey	E_1; E_2; $F_{1\alpha}$; $F_{2\alpha}$	+	+	−	Kelly and Starr, 1971
	Monkey	E_2	ND	ND	±	Casey, 1974a
Topical	Rabbit	E_1; E_2; $F_{2\alpha}$	+	+	+	Bethel and Eakins, 1972
	Rabbit	E_1	+	+	ND	Kass, Podos, Moses and Becker, 1972
	Monkey	E_2	ND	ND	±	Casey, 1974b
Intravenous	Rabbit	E_1	+	ND	−	Starr, 1971a
	Rabbit	E_1; E_2	+	+	+	Chiang and Thomas, 1972a, b
	Rabbit	A_1; A_2; E_1	+	+	ND	Chiang, 1974
	Dog	E_1; E_2; A_2	+	ND	ND	Nakano et al., 1973
		$F_{2\alpha}$	−	ND	ND	
	Monkey	E_1; E_2; A_1; A_2	−	−	−	Kelly and Starr, 1971
	Man	E_2; $F_{2\alpha}$	−	ND	ND	Hillier and Embrey, 1972

+ = effect   − = no effect   ND = not determined

effect of PGE_2 in the normal rhesus monkey, but demonstrated a prosta-glandin-induced miosis in the atropinized monkey which had a fully dilated pupil prior to the administration of either topical or intracameral prosta-glandin E_2.

Topical applications of PGE_2 and $PGF_{2\alpha}$ (Bethel and Eakins, 1972) and PGE_1 (Kass et al., 1972) have been shown to produce their characteristic effects on the rabbit eye, and recently Casey (1974b) has reported that topically applied prostaglandin E_2 produces a similar rise in IOP accom-panied by increased protein levels in the aqueous humour in the monkey.

When prostaglandins are administered topically or intracamerally to one eye, the rise in IOP in the eye may be followed by a smaller rise in the contralateral eye. This phenomenon was first observed by Beitch and Eakins (1969) and subsequently by others (Kass et al., 1972; Chiang and Thomas, 1972a, b). Chiang and Thomas (1972b) found that this consensual response was not prevented by intracranial transection of the optic nerve, the oculomotor nerve or the trigeminal nerve or by topical pretreatment with prostaglandin antagonists such as polyphloretin phosphate or SC-19220. Topical pretreatment of the contralateral eye with epinephrine was found to block the consensual response. The precise mechanism of the response remains to be elucidated.

Tachyphylaxis to repeated administration of prostaglandins has been observed with the IOP response (Beitch and Eakins, 1969; Starr, 1971b) and the blood flow response (Starr, 1971a) in the rabbit eye, and with the IOP response in the cat (Eakins, 1970) and monkey (Kelly and Starr, 1971). The reason for this effect is not fully understood. The observations that the IOP in the rabbit became refractory to repeated mechanical stimula-tion of the iris (Duke-Elder and Duke-Elder, 1931) and that protein may interfere with the action of irin on the hamster colon (Ambache, 1959) led Beitch and Eakins (1969) to suggest that the presence of plasma proteins in the aqueous humour (resulting from the breakdown of the blood–aqueous barrier) may inhibit the action of intracamerally administered prostaglandins.

3.4 ACTIONS OF PROSTAGLANDINS ON AQUEOUS HUMOUR DYNAMICS

Under normal conditions, the production of inflow of aqueous humour is balanced by a continual escape of fluid from the anterior chamber of the eye by means of specialized outflow channels. Any sustained increase in IOP must, therefore, be explained in terms of either an increased production of aqueous humour or a decreased outflow of the fluid from the eye.

First, let us consider the production of aqueous humour. Recent evidence underscores the importance of changes in vascular permeability as being mainly responsible for the raised IOP produced by prostaglandins. Although prostaglandins have been found to increase short circuit current in isolated ciliary processes, the concentrations required (10^{-5} M for PGE_1 and PGE_2) are substantially higher than any levels which could reasonably be expected to be present in aqueous humour (Cole and Nagasubramanian, 1973). Essentially, the same conclusions were reached by Green (1973) in his experiments using the isolated rabbit ciliary body. Stimulation of active transport was seen only with high concentrations of the prostaglandins (PGE_1, PGE_2, $PGF_{2\alpha}$), whereas smaller concentrations increased the passive permeability of the preparation. It was concluded that these results argued strongly against any significant effect of prostaglandins on a metabolically dependent inflow process.

Using fluorescein angiography, Whitelocke and Eakins (1973a) were able to demonstrate directly that topical application of either PGE_1 or PGE_2 (and to a lesser extent, $PGF_{2\alpha}$) produced vasodilatation and a marked increase in permeability to fluorescein (Figure 3.1). Two autoradiographic studies, one *in vitro* (Ehinger, 1973) and one *in vivo* (Bhattacherjee, 1974) using [^{3}H]PGE_1 indicate that the radioactivity appeared to be located mainly in the stroma of the ciliary body. Neufeld and Sears (1973) have proposed that the site of action of PGE_2 may be on the tight junctions of the non-pigmented epithelial cells of the ciliary body.

Turning now to the effect of prostaglandins on the outflow of aqueous humour from the eye, the results from several laboratories suggest that prostaglandins of the E-type have little or no effect on the true facility of outflow of aqueous humour through the drainage channels in the angle of the rabbit eye (Waitzman and King, 1967; Masuda, 1972). Other workers have reported a rise in the total outflow of aqueous humour from the rabbit

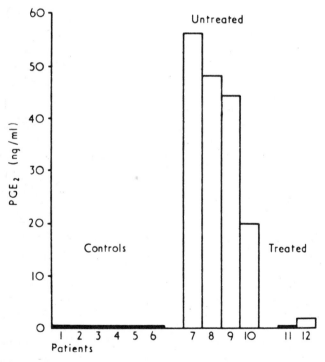

Figure 3.1   Prostaglandin-like activity (ng/ml assayed as PGE_2) in extracts of aqueous humour from control subjects and patients with treated and untreated acute anterior uveitis. (From Eakins *et al.*, 1972b)

eye (Kass *et al.*, 1972), following administration of PGE_1. Total outflow facility includes the component termed 'pseudofacility' which is defined as the suppressibility of aqueous humour production resulting from an increase in IOP. Thus, prostaglandins may only be increasing this pseudofacility without actually affecting true facility. A similar situation may exist in the monkey eye (Casey, 1974b).

3.5 APPEARANCE OF PROSTAGLANDINS IN AQUEOUS HUMOUR

3.5.1 In experimental animals

The observation (Ambache *et al.*, 1965) that irin was released into the aqueous humour of the rabbit eye in response to trauma was important in view of the suggestion (Ambache, 1961) that irin may play a role in certain pathological conditions such as injury and inflammation. The appearance of irin in perfusates of the anterior chamber occurred after various forms of mechanical trauma such as irritation of the iris, collapse of the anterior chamber and movement of the lens. A later report indicated the presence of a prostaglandin-like material (called oculo-tensin) in the aqueous humour of the cat eye which could increase intraocular pressure (Hakim, 1970).

When severe experimental uveitis was induced in rabbits using a single injection of bovine serum albumin (BSA) into the vitreous body, large amounts of PG-like activity (45–150 ng/ml) were found in the aqueous humour of the inflamed eyes (Eakins *et al.*, 1972a). Thin-layer and paper chromatography coupled with bioassay showed the material to be mainly PGE_1-like with only a little PGE_2-like activity. This finding was unexpected since only PGE_2 and $PGF_{2\alpha}$ had previously been found in iris extracts and again in this study, the authors could not detect PGE_1-like activity in iris extracts from normal or inflamed eyes. One clue to the source of the PGE_1-like material found in the aqueous humour 9–15 days after intravitreal BSA came from the work of Higgs and Youlten (1972). These authors showed that during phagocytosis rabbit polymorphonuclear leucocytes produce a PGE-like material which is now thought to be PGE_1 (Higgs and Youlten, personal communication.) It is therefore possible that the PGE_1-like material in aqueous humour comes from these white blood cells which are known to enter the anterior chamber of the eye during inflammation.

Miller *et al.* (1973) studied the release of prostaglandins into the aqueous humour of the rabbit eye during the relatively mild inflammation that follows paracentesis. Following the initial paracentesis (removal of aqueous humour from the anterior chamber) the secondary aqueous humour that had reformed some 1.5 h later had increased levels of protein and PG-like activity when compared to the primary (normal) fluid. There were some interesting differences between these results and the results obtained after BSA. Although in both cases ocular vasodilatation and increased vascular permeability were observed, no white blood cells could be observed in the aqueous humour after paracentesis in contrast to the large numbers of white blood cells in the aqueous humour following BSA. In addition, lower levels of PG-like activity (4–16 ng/ml) were found in the aqueous humour after paracentesis as opposed to the much higher levels (45–150 ng/ml) found after BSA. Furthermore, the PG-like material found after paracentesis was mainly PGE_2-like, in contrast to the PGE_1-like material found in the BSA experiments. These results lend some support to the hypothesis that the invading white blood cells are an important source of the PGE_1-like material observed during uveitis induced with BSA.

Mechanical stimulation of the iris of the rabbit was later found to produce levels of PG-like activity in the aqueous humour similar to those found after paracentesis (Cole and Unger, 1973). An alternative form of mechanical injury of the rabbit eye, namely, laser burn of the iris, also produces a rise in IOP associated with increased levels of PG-like activity in the aqueous humour (Perkins et al., 1973). In their study on the role of prostaglandins in the ocular response to trauma, Cole and Unger (1973) observed that although stimulation of the trigeminal nerve and intracameral injections of formaldehyde in the rabbit produced the usual ocular hypertension and miosis, these effects were not accompanied by any increase in PG-like activity in the aqueous humour. These results suggest that prostaglandins may not be involved in mediating all forms of ocular trauma. This subject will be dealt with in more detail when we consider the ocular effects of substances that block the actions and synthesis of prostaglandins.

3.5.2 In patients with glaucoma

Wyllie and Wyllie (1971) described slightly elevated levels of prostaglandin-like activity in aqueous humour taken from patients with open angle glaucoma. These results led the authors to suggest that prostaglandins (particularly PGE_1) may play some part in the aetiology of this disease. In contrast, Podos et al. (1972), using radioimmunoassay procedures, could not detect any significant difference in the levels of PGE_1 in aqueous humour samples from normal and glaucomatous eyes. Recently, Chiang (1974) has proposed that raised plasma levels of prostaglandins may play a role in the development of the increased IOP seen in glaucoma. This proposal is based on two findings, first that intravenous infusions of prostaglandins (particularly PGA_1, PGA_2 and PGE_1) raised IOP in the rabbit eye. Second, that plasma prostaglandin levels (measured by bioassay) were higher in patients with open angle glaucoma (3.25 ± 0.8 ng/ml in 6 patients) and narrow angle glaucoma (2.47 ± 0.08 ng/ml in 4 patients) than in non-glaucomatous patients (1.05 ± 0.08 ng/ml in 4 patients). However, it should be borne in mind that these differences are very small and are based on a very limited number of patients so their significance is open to question. Furthermore, it has already been shown that there are species differences in the response of the IOP to intravenous prostaglandins. Thus, although the rabbit responds to intravenous prostaglandins with a rise in IOP, the monkey and man apparently do not. Finally, it is now generally accepted that open angle glaucoma is a disease characterized by an impaired outflow of aqueous humour from the eye and, as we have seen, prostaglandins (if they have any effect) tend to raise outflow facility. It is, therefore, very difficult to see how prostaglandins can fit into this picture. In conclusion, there is little, if any, firm evidence that prostaglandins play a part in raising IOP in open angle glaucoma, a condition that does not involve any inflammatory process.

3.5.3 In patients with ocular inflammation

Using extraction methods coupled with bioassay, substantial amounts of PG-like activity (20–56 ng/ml assayed as PGE_2) were found in aqueous humour samples taken from patients with untreated acute anterior uveitis (Eakins *et al.*, 1972b). Little or no activity was found in the aqueous humour of control patients with cataract, or uveitis patients that had been treated with topical steroids (Figure 3.1). In contrast to the predominantly E-type PG-like activity found in rabbit aqueous humour, alkaline hydrolysis of the samples from the inflamed human eye indicated the presence of both E- and F-type prostaglandins. The authors concluded that prostaglandins may contribute to many of the clinial signs of anterior uveitis. These findings were substantially confirmed by Masuda *et al.* (1973). In this study radioimmunoassay was used to show elevated levels of E- and F-type prostaglandins in aqueous humour samples taken from patients with glaucomatocyclytic crises and Behcet's disease, both conditions which involve ocular inflammation.

3.6 REMOVAL OF PROSTAGLANDINS FROM INTRAOCULAR FLUIDS

It has recently been observed that supernatant fractions of rabbit ocular tissues (ciliary body/iris, conjunctiva, and lens) metabolize $[^3H]$-PGE_1 very slowly when compared to the rapid metabolism of ^3H-PGE_1 obtained with similar preparations of kidney and lung (Eakins *et al.*, 1974). Thus under standard conditions of temperature, pH and substrate concentration the ocular tissues showed little PG-dehydrogenase activity. However, evidence has recently been presented by Bito and co-workers which indicates that an absorptive transport mechanism may function in the normal eye to remove prostaglandins from the intraocular fluids. ^3H-PGE_1 injected into the vitreous body of the rabbit eye was found to be eliminated very rapidly from the eye with a half-time of 3 h as compared to 15 h for an inert substance of similar molecular weight, in this case, $[^{14}C]$ sucrose (Bito and Salvador, 1972). In contrast to $[^{14}C]$ sucrose, at no time following its intravitreal injection was $[^3H]$-PGE_1 detected in the aqueous humour. This rapid elimination of $[^3H]$-PGE_1 from the intraocular fluids is apparently due to an active transport of prostaglandin across the ciliary processes since it was shown that this tissue can actively accumulate ^3H-activity when incubated with $[^3H]$-PGE_1 *in vitro* (Bito, 1972a, b). Most of the accumulated ^3H remains associated with the original prostaglandin (Bito and Baroody, 1974). This absorptive transport across the blood–aqueous barrier (from aqueous to blood) appears to be analogous to the mediated transport of prostaglandins across the blood–cerebrospinal fluid barrier reported by Bito and Davson (1974). A similar prostaglandin transport system may be operative across the synovial membrane (Bito, 1973) and the blood–placental barrier of certain species (Bito, 1972a). Ehinger (1973) has confirmed the observation that prostaglandins are taken up by the rabbit iris/ciliary body preparation much more effectively than into several other tissues such as retina, cornea, heart and liver and concluded from autoradiographic studies that prostaglandins are transferred from the intraocular fluids to the stroma of the ciliary processes from where they enter the blood stream.

It has recently been observed that in experimental uveitis induced with BSA, the prostaglandin transport mechanism no longer functions (Bito, 1973), and this inhibition has been found to persist for a 20–week period (Bito, 1974). Irreversible blockade of this absorptive transport process in some forms of uveitis may account for the recurrent nature of this disease, since in the absence of a mechanism for the transfer of prostaglandins from the intraocular fluids to blood, any local irritation which normally would result in only slight prostaglandin accumulation within the eye, would now result in markedly elevated prostaglandin levels and render the eye extremely vulnerable to inflammatory stimuli.

3.7 OTHER ACTIONS OF PROSTAGLANDINS ON OCULAR TISSUES

Waitzman *et al.* (1972) have reported a reduced uptake of galactose by rat lenses incubated in media containing either prostaglandins E_1 or $F_{1\alpha}$. However, very high concentrations (10^{-3} M) of either prostaglandin were required to show an effect. Paterson and Eck (1973) studied the influence of prostaglandins on cation movements in incubated rabbit lenses. At 10^{-3} M, PGE_1, PGE_2 or $PGF_{2\alpha}$ but not $PGF_{1\alpha}$ increased Na^+ but decreased the K^+ content. Reduced rubidium-86 uptake was also observed in these lenses. However, at 10^{-4} M prostaglandins E_1, E_2 and $F_{2\alpha}$ appeared to stimulate the lens cation transport mechanism and enhance the uptake of rubidium-86. Lenses subjected to reduced calcium levels in the incubation medium were found to survive better in the presence of a 10^{-4} M concentration of these prostaglandins. The high concentrations of prostaglandins required to produce these effects suggest that the lens epithelium, like the corneal endothelium (Dikstein, 1973), is relatively insensitive to the prostaglandins.

The first indication of a possible physiological role for prostaglandins in the eye came from the studies of Posner (1973). The isolated bovine sphincter pupillae incubated in Krebs' solution were found to release a biologically active substance tentatively identified as PGE_2. This prostaglandin-like activity did not appear to be of neural origin or to result from tissue degeneration but seemed to be related to the tone of the sphincter muscle. Output increased as tone was acquired and fell when various procedures were used to reduce tone. The results of these experiments did not support any direct interaction of prostaglandins with adrenergic or cholinergic nerves or their receptors. It was suggested that the possible role of prostaglandins could be complementary to the autonomic nervous system and that PGE_2 may be continually synthesized by the smooth muscle cells and contribute to the acquisition and maintenance of tone in the bovine sphincter pupillae.

3.8 DRUGS THAT INHIBIT THE ACTIONS AND SYNTHESIS OF PROSTAGLANDINS IN THE EYE

The apparent importance of prostaglandins in certain forms of ocular inflammation suggests that drugs that inhibit either the actions or synthesis of prostaglandins may prove useful as ocular anti-inflammatory agents. Non-steroidal anti-inflammatory agents are needed in ophthalmology since there are serious problems associated with the use of anti-inflammatory steroids in the eye. Complications associated with the ophthalmic use of corticosteroids include inhibition of wound healing, and breakdown of connective tissue with subsequent facilitation of bacterial and viral infections. It is also well-documented that some patients respond to steroids with an increase in intraocular pressure accompanied by a reduction in visual function which, if recognized early enough, is reversed by cessation of treatment.

3.8.1 Prostaglandin antagonists and the eye

In vivo experiments

Cole (1961) first demonstrated that intra-arterial infusions of polyphloretin phosphate (PPP) in the rabbit prevented the increase in intraocular pressure and lowered the increased protein levels in aqueous humour, seen after either paracentesis or topical administration of mustine hydrochloride. Polyphloretin was thought to prevent the increased capillary permeability normally associated with ocular trauma. Close-arterial infusions of PPP were then found to prevent both the rise in intraocular pressure and the increased aqueous humour protein levels produced by intracameral injections of PGE_2 in the rabbit eye (Beitch and Eakins, 1969). Further studies showed that PPP could selectively antagonize contractions produced by both E- and F-type prostaglandins on certain isolated smooth muscle preparations (Eakins *et al.*, 1970; Mathe *et al.*, 1971; Bennett and Posner, 1971). This activity of PPP was related only to the low molecular weight polymers (Eakins, 1970). Further *in vivo* experiments on the eye, mainly in the rabbit, have been reported. Starr (1971b) showed that both intra-arterial infusions and intravitreal injections of PPP inhibited the rise in intraocular pressure produced by PGE. In this study, a second prolonged depressor effect of PGE_1 on intraocular pressure was observed after pretreatment with PPP, suggesting a dual action of PGE_1 on rabbit IOP. It is interestng to note here that Cole (1961) had observed that PPP converted the rise in IOP following irritation of the rabbit eye with mustine to a fall in IOP. However, intracameral injections of 1mg PPP into the monkey eye had virtually no effect on the rise in intraocular pressure produced by various prostaglandins. It is possible that this 1 mg dose may have been too small to produce inhibitory effects.

Further studies on the rabbit eye suggested that PPP may not penetrate into intraocular fluids very well following topical application to the surface of the cornea. Bethel and Eakins (1972) observed that topical instillation of 10 mg PPP into the rabbit eye inhibited the rise in IOP produced by topical $PGF_{2\alpha}$, but only slightly reduced the response to formaldehyde and had no effect on the response to topical PGE_2. In contrast, subconjunctival administration of this dose of PPP abolished or markedly reduced the rise in IOP produced by all three substances. Subconjunctival injections of the low molecular weight fraction of PPP also inhibited the rise in IOP produced by PGE_2, $PGF_{2\alpha}$ and formaldehyde. The high molecular weight fraction, as expected, was inactive against PGE_2 and $PGF_{2\alpha}$ but, unexpectedly, it inhibited the rise in IOP produced by formaldehyde, possibly as a result of known anti-hyaluronidase activity.

Chiang and Thomas (1972b) studied the actions of prostaglandin antagonists against the consensual response in the rabbit eye produced by intracameral injection of PGE_1 into the contralateral eye. This consensual response was inhibited by PPP given by close-arterial infusion. However, intravitreal or topical administration of either PPP or 7-oxa-13-prostynoic acid and SC-19220 either did not abolish or markedly enhanced the consensual response. It should be noted that the doses of PPP used in this study (0.1 ml 2% PPP topically and 200 μg PPP into the vitreous humour 24 h prior to the experiment) are very much lower than those used in previous experiments, which may account for these paradoxical results.

Other *in vivo* experiments in the rabbit, using fluorescein angiography, confirmed that subconjunctival injections of PPP antagonized the rise in IOP, together with the increased capillary permeability and vasodilatation of the iris blood vessels produced by PGE_1, E_2 and $F_{2\alpha}$ (Whitelocke and Eakins, 1973a, 1973b; Whitelocke *et al.*, 1973). In contrast to the active low molecular weight fraction of PPP, both the high molecular weight fraction and the analogue, diphloretin phosphate, were inactive as prostaglandin antagonists on the rabbit eye under the same experimental conditions.

Paterson and Pfister (1973) demonstrated an ocular hypertensive response to alkali burns in the monkey eye. Application of small volumes of 2 M NaOH to the cornea of anaesthetized monkeys resulted in a biphasic rise in IOP; a transient initial rapid increase which quickly subsided to be followed by a more sustained rise in pressure. The first rise was thought to be due to alkali-induced shrinkage of the outer coat of the eye. Subconjunctival injections of 10 mg PPP significantly reduced the secondary rise in IOP which is thought to be mediated in part by prostaglandins. These authors (Paterson and Pfister, 1974) later showed increased levels of PG-like activity in the aqueous humour of the rabbit which were associated with the sustained elevation of IOP after the alkali burn.

In vitro experiments

Using an Ussing-type chamber, prostaglandins of the E- and F-type were found to stimulate short circuit current in isolated preparations of rabbit ciliary tissue, the E-type prostaglandins being more effective than the F-type.

The responses obtained with PGE_1 and PGE_2 were antagonized by low molecular weight fractions of PPP (10 mg/ml in the bathing solution). Under the same conditions, the high molecular weight fraction of PPP was without effect (Cole and Nagasubramanian, 1973). In similar experiments, Gréen (1973) showed that PGE_1, PGE_2 and $PGF_{2\alpha}$ increased active transport and flow conductivity in isolated preparations of rabbit ciliary tissue. Pretreatment of the tissues with PPP (50, 100 and 200 μg/ml) successfully antagonized the responses produced by the prostaglandins. However, PPP was not effective in reducing an established response to the prostaglandin. Beitch et al. (1973) observed that both PPP and diphloretin phosphate antagonized the stimulation of chloride transport in the frog corneal epithelium produced by 10^{-5} M PGE_1.

Finally, it has recently been reported (Zink et al., 1973) that intraperitoneal injections of 250 mg/kg imidazole can antagonize the rise in IOP produced by topical application of 5 μg PGE_1 or PGE_2 to the rabbit eye. Imidazole is known to stimulate phosphodiesterase and the authors speculate that the actions of prostaglandins E_1 and E_2 on IOP may involve cyclic AMP.

3.8.2 Inhibitors of prostaglandin biosynthesis

In 1971 the so-called 'aspirin-like' drugs were shown to inhibit the synthesis of prostaglandins in several tissues (Vane, 1971; Ferreira et al., 1971; Smith and Willis, 1971). This discovery was of profound importance; first, it led to a clear hypothesis to account for the various therapeutic actions of the aspirin-like drugs; second, many other drugs which were prostaglandin synthetase inhibitors were immediately available to study the biosynthesis of prostaglandins, their function in vivo and their importance in the pathogenesis of certain disease states.

Studies on the ocular actions of aspirin and indomethacin

The effects of aspirin were studied on ocular trauma produced by either paracentesis or laser irradiation of the iris in the rabbit eye (Neufeld et al., 1972). In these experiments, the trauma was associated with a marked increase in protein levels in the aqueous humour, and this was greatly reduced in aspirin-treated animals (600 mg p.r.). The authors suggested that the greater stability of the blood–aqueous barrier, following pretreatment with aspirin, was due to local inhibition of prostaglandin biosynthesis. It was of further interest that aspirin did not prevent the rise in aqueous humour protein levels in response to nitrogen mustard, indicating that the ocular response produced by various irritants may be provoked by different chemical mediators.

In a later study (Miller et al., 1973) pretreatment of rabbits with aspirin (200 mg/kg p.r.) 1 h before initial paracentesis, was found to substantially inhibit the appearance of PG-like material, and partially prevent (60–70%) the increase in protein in the secondary aqueous humour. Furthermore, the generation of PG-like activity from arachidonic acid in microsomal fractions of anterior uvea taken from these animals, was markedly depressed in the aspirin-treated group. These results were thought to support the concept that the ocular anti-inflammatory actions of aspirin against paracentesis were, in fact, mediated via the prostaglandin system. The lack of effect of aspirin in the nitrogen mustard experiments indicates that the mechanism of action of this irritant does not involve the prostaglandin system. To further study this possibility, Cole and Unger (1974) examined the IOP, pupil response and prostaglandin levels in aqueous humour, following mechanical and chemical irritation and intercranial stimulation of the trigeminal nerve. Although the pattern of response was similar to all three stimuli, only mechanical stimulation of the iris increased PG-like activity in the aqueous humour and only in this case was the response blocked by pre-treatment with indomethacin. The authors suggested that chemical irritation (in this case intracameral injections of formaldehyde) and trigeminal nerve stimulation produce their effects by a mechanism which does not involve the prostaglandin system. An alternative form of mechanical stimulation, laser burn of the iris, also produced similar responses from the IOP and iris together with raised levels of PG-like activity in the aqueous humour. Indomethacin, given systematically, blocked the rise in IOP and the appearance of PG-like activity in the aqueous humour (Perkins et al., 1973).

This apparent difference between mechanical and chemical irritation of the eye and their involvement with the prostaglandin system may not be so clear however. Paterson and Pfister (1973) have shown that chemical irritation produced by topical sodium hydroxide on the rabbit eye is accompanied by an increase in PG-like activity in the aqueous humour. The effects produced by sodium hydroxide were abolished by pretreatment of the animals with either aspirin (200 mg/kg i.p.) or indomethacin (50 mg/kg i.p.).

This apparent discrepancy may be explained by the presence of an initial, sharp transient rise in IOP following the application of 2N sodium hydroxide to the rabbit cornea. This is followed by a secondary, sustained increase in pressure. The initial rise in pressure may be sufficient to activate the prostaglandin system and there is evidence to support this proposal. First of all, application of nitrogen mustard to the rabbit cornea does not produce the initial rise in IOP, there is no release of prostaglandins into the aqueous humour and the high levels of protein in the aqueous humour occur even in animals pretreated with aspirin (Jampol et al., 1974). Secondly, ocular compression has been shown to cause a secondary rise in IOP which can be prevented by pretreatment with aspirin or indomethacin (Ostbaum and Podos, 1974). Finally, it has been observed (Neufeld et al., 1973) that pretreatment with indomethacin (12.5 mg/kg i.p. three times at 8 h intervals) prevented the hyperaemia of the iris and conjunctiva normally associated with postganglionic sympathetic denervation of the rabbit eye. The mydriasis associated with local degeneration of sympathetic nerves was also antagonized by indomethacin. It was proposed that these effects were mediated by prostaglandins whose synthesis and release is dependent upon the release of norepinephrine from the degenerating nerve terminals. It was also suggested that some instances of epinephrine-induced hyperaemia seen in patients with glaucoma undergoing treatment with this catecholamine may be related to increased prostaglandin synthesis.

In vitro *studies on the inhibition of ocular prostaglandin biosynthesis*

Bhattacherjee and Eakins (1974) compared the sensitivity of the prostaglandin synthetase systems derived from microsomal fractions of rabbit ocular tissues with other tissues such as the kidney medulla and spleen, to inhibition by indomethacin. Generation of prostaglandin-like activity by the microsomal fractions from added arachidonic acid was studied by the method of Flower *et al.*, (1972). Under these arbitrarily chosen conditions, indomethacin was most potent in the spleen, then in decreasing order in the kidney medulla, conjunctiva, anterior uvea and retina. These results suggested a differential sensitivity to inhibition of the various prostaglandin synthetase systems. However, later studies carried out under optimal conditions for each enzyme (Ku *et al.*, 1976) did not support this conclusion. One season for this discrepancy may have been that the hydroquinone which was used as a cofactor in the original method, has been found to inhibit prostaglandin synthetase itself and may have modified the response to indomethacin.

In a further study (Bhattacherjee and Eakins, 1974), the potency of various compounds as inhibitors of prostaglandin biosynthesis in microsomal preparations of ocular tissues were compared under standard conditions of temperature, pH, substrate concentration and time. The non-acidic anti-inflammatory agent, indoxole was approximately 100 times more potent than indomethacin on the anterior uvea and 25 times more potent on the conjunctiva. Pirprofen (SU-21524) was also more potent than indomethacin on the ocular tissues. Other compounds such as naproxen, phenylbutazone and oxyphenbutazone were all essentially equiactive with indomethacin on the anterior uvea, whereas indomethacin was more potent than either phenylbutazone or oxyphenbutazone on the conjunctiva. Aspirin, paracetamol and dexamethasone had little or no activity in these experiments. Variations in the relative potencies of aspirin and indomethacin have been noted previously: in dog spleen preparations, aspirin was approximately 100 times less active than indomethacin (Flower *et al.*, 1972) and in bovine seminal vesicles (Flower *et al.*, 1973) aspirin was some 225 times less effective. Therefore, considering the lower absolute potency of indomethacin found in these experiments (using a relatively high concentration of arachidonic acid) the lack of effect of aspirin is not surprising. In a later study (Ku *et al.*, 1976), using much lower substrate concentrations, aspirin was found to be approximately 1000 times less active than indomethacin on the iris.

In vivo *studies on the inhibition of the ocular effects of arachidonic acid*

Topical application of arachidonic acid to eyes of rabbits and monkeys was found to raise IOP. Pretreatment with indomethacin (50 mg/kg i.p.) prevented the rise in IOP produced by arachidonic acid but failed to inhibit the rise in pressure produced by topical PGE_2 (Podos *et al.*, 1973a). The authors suggested that indomethacin inhibited prostaglandin production from arachidonic acid in the eye. In a more detailed study the authors (Podos *et al.*, 1973b) showed that in the rabbit and monkey eyes either topical arachidonic acid (0.1–20%) or in the case of the rabbit experiments, intravenous arachidonic acid (10–20 mg per animal) produced a dose-dependent rise in IOP associated with increased levels of protein in the aqueous humour. Both these effects were prevented by pretreatment with either indomethacin (10 mg/kg i.p.) or aspirin (600 mg i.p. per animal). Under these conditions low levels of prostaglandins were detected in the aqueous humour (1 ng/ml) following the instillation of arachidonic acid (Jaffe *et al.*, 1973). In a later study using the rabbit (Bhattacherjee and Eakins, 1975) topical administration of sodium arachidonate was found to increase IOP, constrict the pupil and increase both the protein and prostaglandin content of aqueous humour. Arachidonic acid itself (dissolved in arachis oil – was less effective than the sodium salt, although addition of polysorbate mono-oleate to the vehicle greatly increased the effects produced by arachidonic acid. The increased activity observed with these modifications of the original method was reflected in the higher level of PG-like activity, 16 ng/ml, found in the aqueous humour as opposed to the 1 ng/ml reported previously by Jaffe *et al.* (1973). Pretreatment with topically applied non-steroidal anti-inflammatory agents prevented the ocular effects of sodium arachidonate, indomethacin being 2–4 times as potent as either indoxole or pirprofen. The steroid dexamethasone was without effect in these experiments.

3.9 CONCLUSIONS

There are a number of pathological conditions involving increased permeability of the blood–aqueous barrier with consequent inflammatory damage to the eye. It is likely that prostaglandins are involved in some, but not all, of these clinical situations. These may include secondary glaucomas, inflammation produced by trauma (including surgery) inflammation of immunogenic origin and certain chemical irritants.

The finding that prostaglandins may be important in certain forms of ocular inflammation has paved the way for a fresh approach to the development of new compounds for use as ocular anti-inflammatory agents. This would include the use of prostaglandin synthetase inhibitors which can be used topically on the eye. This form of administration should minimize some of the more unpleasant side-effects sometimes associated with these compounds. We can also expect the development of new drugs which will block the actions of prostaglandins already present in ocular tissues and fluids. Some compounds will act by a combination of the actions described above. Finally, compounds that can protect or restore the normal mechanisms responsible for the facilitated removal of prostaglandins from the intraocular fluids may be of potential benefit in the treatment of ocular inflammation.

References

Ambache, N. (1955). Irin, a smooth muscle contracting substance present in rabbit iris. *J. Physiol. (Lond.)*, **129**, 65P
Ambache, N. (1957). Properties of irin, a physiological constituent of the rabbit iris. *J. Physiol. (Lond.)*, **135**, 114

Ambache, N. (1959). Further studies on the preparation, purification and nature of irin J. Physiol. (Lond.), **146**, 255

Ambache, N. (1961). Prolonged erythema produced by chromatographically pure irin. J. Physiol. (Lond.), **160**, 3P

Ambache, N., Kavanagh, L. and Whiting, J. (1965). Effect of mechanical stimulation on rabbit's eyes: release of active substance in anterior chamber perfusates. J. Physiol. (Lond.), **176**, 378

Ambache, N. and Brummer, H. C. (1968). A simple chemical procedure for distinguishing E from F prostaglandins, with application to tissue extracts. Br. J. Pharmac., **33**, 162

Änggård, E. and Samuelsson, B. (1964). Smooth muscle stimulating lipids in sheep iris. The identification of prostaglandin $F_{2\alpha}$. Prostaglandins and related factors 21. Biochem. Pharmacol., **13**, 281

Beitch, B. R. and Eakins, K. E. (1969). The effects of prostaglandins on the intraocular pressure of the rabbit. Br. J. Pharmac., **37**, 158

Beitch, B. R., Beitch, I. and Zadunaisky, J. A. (1973). Chloride transport activation by prostaglandins in the frog cornea. Fed. Proc., **32** (3), 245, Abs.

Bennett, A. and Posner, J. (1971). Studies on prostaglandin antagonists. Br. J. Pharmac., **42**, 584

Bethel, R. A. and Eakins, K. E. (1972). The mechanism of the antagonism of experimentally induced ocular hypertension by polyphloretin phosphate. Exp. Eye Res., **13**, 83

Bhattacherjee, P. (1974). Autoradiographic localization of intravitreally- or intracamerally-injected [^{3}H] prostaglandins. Exp. Eye Res., **18**, 181

Bhattacherjee, P. and Eakins, K. E. (1974). Inhibition of the prostaglandin synthetase systems in ocular tissues by indomethacin. Br. J. Pharmac., **50**, 227

Bhattacherjee, P. and Eakins, K. E. (1975). Inhibition of the ocular effects of sodium arachidonate by anti-inflammatory compounds. Prostaglandins, (submitted for publ.)

Bito, L. Z. (1972a). Accumulation and apparent active transport of prostaglandins by some rabbit tissues in vitro. J. Physiol. (Lond.), **221**, 371

Bito, L. Z. (1927b). Comparative study of concentrative prostaglandin accumulation by various tissues of mammals and marine vertebrates and invertebrates. Comp. Biochem. Physiol., **43A**, 65

Bito, L. (1973). Inhibition of uveal protaglandin transport in experimental uveitis. In Prostaglandins and Cyclic AMP, Kahn, R. H. and Lands, W. E. M. (eds.), pp. 213–214 (New York and London: Academic Press, Inc.)

Bito, L. Z. (1974). The effects of experimental uveitis on anterior uveal prostaglandin transport and aqueous humor composition. Invest. Ophthal., **13/12**, 959

Bito, L. Z. and Salvador, E. V. (1972). Intraocular fluid dynamics. III. The site and mechanism of prostaglandin transfer across the blood intraocular fluid barriers. Exp. Eye Res., **14**, 233

Bito, L. Z. and Baroody, R. (1974). Concentrative accumulation of ^{3}H prostaglandins by some rabbit tissues in vitro: the chemical nature of the accumulated ^{3}H-labelled substances. Prostaglandins, **7** (2), 131

Bito, L. Z. and Davson, H. (1974). Carrier-mediated removal of prostaglandins from cerebrospinal fluid. J. Physiol. (Lond.), **236**, 39P

Casey, W. J. (1974a). The effect of prostaglandin E_2 on the rhesus monkey pupil. Prostaglandins, **6**, 243

Casey, W. J. (1974b). Prostaglandin E_2 and aqueous humor dynamics in the rhesus monkey eye. In press

Chiang, T. S. and Thomas, R. P. (1972a). Ocular hypertension following intravenous infusion by prostaglandin E_1. Arch. Ophthal., **88**, 418

Chiang, T. S. and Thomas, R. P. (1972b). Consensual ocular hypertensive response to prostaglandin E_2. Invest. Ophthal., **11** (3), 845

Chiang, T. S. (1974). Effects of intravenous infusions of histamine, 5-hydroxytryptamine, bradykinin and prostaglandins on intraocular pressure. Archs. int. Pharmacodyn. Ther., **207**, 131

Christ, E. J. and Van Dorp, D. A. (1972). Comparative aspects of prostaglandin biosynthesis in animal tissues. Biochim. Biophys. Acta, **270**, 537

Cole, D. F. (1961). Prevention of experimental ocular hypertension with polyphloretin phosphate. Brit. J. Ophthal., **46**, 291

Cole, D. F. and Nagasubramanian, S. (1973). Substances affecting active transport across the ciliary epithelium and their possible role in determining intraocular pressure. *Exp. Eye Res.*, **16**, 251

Cole, D. F. and Unger, W. G. (1973). Prostaglandins as mediators of the responses of the eye to trauma. *Exp. Eye Res.*, **17**, 357

Cole, D. F. and Unger, W. G. (1974). The role of prostaglandins in ocular response to trauma. *J. Physiol. (Lond.)*, **236**, 18P

Dikstein, S. (1973). Discussion after paper by C. A. Paterson and B. A. Eck. *Exp. Eye Res.*, **15**, 767

Duke-Elder, P. M., and Duke-Elder, W. S. (1931). The vascular responses of the eye. *Proc. R. Soc. B*, **109**, 19

Eakins, K. E. (1970). Increased intraocular pressure produced by prostaglandins E_1 and E_2 in the cat eye. *Exp. Eye Res.*, **10**, 87

Eakins, K. E., Karim, S. M. M. and Miller, J. D. (1970). Antagonisms of some smooth muscle actions of prostaglandins by polyphloretin phosphate. *Br. J. Pharmac.*, **39**, 556

Eakins, K. E., Whitelocke, R. A. F., Perkins, E. S., Bennett, A. and Unger, W. G. (1972a). Release of a prostaglandin in ocular inflammation. *Nature (Lond.)*, **239**, 248

Eakins, K. E., Whitelocke, R. A. F., Bennett, A. and Martenet, A. C. (1972b). Prostaglandin-like activity in ocular inflammation. *Br. Med. J.*, **3**, 452

Eakins, K. E., Atwal, M. and Bhattacherjee, P. (1974). Inactivation of prostaglandin E_1 by ocular tissues *in vitro*. *Exp. Eye Res*. In press

Ehinger, B. (1973). Localization of the uptake of prostaglandin E_1 in the eye. *Exp. Eye Res.*, **17**, 43

Ferreira, S. H., Moncada, S. and Vane, J. R. (1971). Indomethacin and aspirin abolish prostaglandin release from the spleen. *Nature (New Biology)*, **231**, 237

Flower, R. J., Cheung, H. S. and Cushman, D. W. (1973). Quantitative determination of prostaglandins and malondialdehyde formed by the arachidonate oxygenase (prostaglandin synthetase) system of bovine seminal vesicle. *Prostaglandins*, **4**, 325

Flower, R., Gryglewski, R., Herbacrynska-Cedro, K. and Vane, J. R. (1972). Effects of anti-inflammatory drugs on prostaglandin biosynthesis. *Nature (New Biology)*, **238**, 104

Gréen, K. (1973). Permeability properties of the ciliary epithelium in response to prostaglandins. *Invest. Ophthal.*, **12**, 752

Hakim, S. A. E. (1970). Ciliary-iris hormone regulates eye tension. *J. All-India Ophthal. Soc.*, **18**, 143

Higgs, G. A. and Youlten, L. J. F. (1972). Prostaglandin production by rabbit peritoneal polymorphonuclear leukocytes *in vitro*. *Br. J. Pharmac.*, **44**, 330P

Higgs, G. A. and Youlten, L. J. F. Personal communication

Hillier, K. and Embrey, M. P. (1972). High dose intravenous administration of prostaglandin E_2 and $F_{2\alpha}$ for the termination of mid-trimester pregnancies. *J. Obstet. Gynecol. Br. Commonwealth*, **79**, 14

Jaffe, E. B. M., Podos, S. M. and Becker, B. (1973). Indomethacin blocks arachidonic acid-associated elevation of aqueous humor prostaglandin E. *Invest. Ophthal.*, **12 (8)**, 621

Jampol, L. M., Neufeld, A. H. and Sears, M. L. (1974). Innervation and the ocular irritative response. Presented at the Spring Meeting of the Association for Research in Vision and Ophthalmology (ARVO), Sarasota, Fla.

Kass, M. A., Podos, S. M., Moses, R. A. and Becker, B. (1972). Prostaglandin E_2 and aqueous humor dynamics. *Invest. Ophthal.*, **11**, 1022

Kelly, R. G. M. and Starr, M. (1971). Effects of prostaglandins and a prostaglandin antagonist on intraocular pressure and protein in the monkey eye. *Can. J. Ophthal.*, **6**, 205

Ku, E. C. and Eakins, K. E. Unpublished observations

Ku, E. C., Signor, C. and Eakins, K. E. (1966). Anti-inflammatory agents and inhibition of ocular prostaglandin synthetase. In *Advances in Prostaglandin and Thromboxane Research*, **vol. 2**, Samuelsson, B. and Paoletti, R. (eds.), (New York: Raven Press). In the press

Masuda, K. (1972). Prostaglandins—their effect on the inflow and outflow of the aqueous humor in rabbits. *Nippon Ganka Gakkai Zasshi*, **76**, 664

Masuda, K., Izawa, Y. and Mishima, S. (1973). Prostaglandins and uveitis: a preliminary report. *Jap. J. Ophthal.*, **17**, 166

Mathe, A. A., Strandberg, K. and Astrom, A. (1971). Blockade by polyphloretin phosphate of the prostaglandin $F_{2\alpha}$ action on isolated human bronchi. *Nature (New Biology)*, **230**, 215

Miller, J. D., Eakins, K. E. and Atwal, M. (1973). Release of prostaglandin E_2-like activity into the aqueous humor of the rabbit following paracentesis. Presented at the Spring Meeting of the Association for Research in Vision and Ophthalmology (ARVO), Sarasota, Fla.

Nakano, J., Chang, A. C. K. and Fischer, R. G. (1973). Effects of prostaglandins E_1, E_2, A_2 and $F_{2\alpha}$ on canine carotid arterial blood flow, cerebrospinal fluid and ocular pressure. *J. Neurosurgery*, **38**, 32

Neufeld, A. H., Jampol, L. M. and Sears, M. L. (1972). Aspirin prevents disruption of the blood aqueous barrier in the rabbit eye. *Nature (Lond.)*, **238**, 158

Neufeld, A. H. and Sears, M. L. (1973). The site of action of prostaglandin E_2 on the disruption of the blood–aqueous barrier in the rabbit eye. *Exp. Eye Res.*, **17**, 445

Neufeld, A. H., Chavis, R. M. and Sears, M. L. (1973). Degeneration release of norepinephrine causes transient ocular hyperemia mediated by prostaglandins. *Invest. Ophthal.*, **12 (3)**, 167

Ostbaum, S. A. and Podos, S. M. (1974). Ocular compression and non-steroidal antiinflammatory agents. Presented at the Spring Meeting of the Association for Research in Vision and Ophthalmology (ARVO), Sarasota, Fla.

Paterson, C. A. and Eck, B. A. (1973). Influence of prostaglandins on the cation movement in the lens. *Exp. Eye Res.*, **15**, 767

Paterson, C. and Pfister, R. R. (1974). Prostaglandin-like activity in the aqueous humor following alkali burns. In press

Paterson, C. and Pfister, R. R. (1973). Ocular hypertensive response to alkali burns in the monkey. *Exp. Eye Res.*, **17**, 449

Perkins, E. S., Unger, W. G. and Bass, M. (1973). The role of prostaglandin in the ocular responses to laser irradiation of the iris. *Exp. Eye Res.*, **17**, 394

Podos, S. M., Jaffe, B. M. and Becker, B. (1972). Prostaglandins and glaucoma. *Br. Med. J.*, **4**, 232

Podos, S. M., Becker, B. and Kass, M. A. (1973a). Indomethacin blocks arachidonic acid-induced elevation of intraocular pressure. *Prostaglandins*, **3**, 7

Podos, S. M., Becker, B. and Kass, M. A. (1973b). Prostaglandin synthesis, inhibition and intraocular pressure. *Invest. Ophthal.*, **12 (6)**, 426

Posner, J. (1973). Prostaglandin E_2 and the bovine sphincter pupillae. *Br. J. Pharmac.*, **49**, 415

Smith, J. B. and Willis, A. L. (1971). Aspirin selectively inhibits prostaglandin production in human platelets. *Nature (New Biology)*, **231**, 235

Starr, M. (1971a). Effects of prostaglandin on blood flow in the rabbit eye. *Exp. Eye Res.*, **11**, 161

Starr, M. (1971b). Further studies on the effect of prostaglandin on intraocular pressure in the rabbit. *Exp. Eye Res.*, **11**, 170

Van Dorp, D. A., Jouvenaz, G. H. and Strujik, C. B. (1967). The biosynthesis of prostaglandin in pig eye iris. *Biochim. Biophys. Acta*, **137**, 396

Vane, J. R. (1971). Inhibition of prostaglandin synthesis as a mechanism of action for aspirin-like drugs. *Nature (New Biology)*, **231**, 232

Waitzman, M. B. and King, C. D. (1967). Prostaglandin influences on intraocular pressure and pupil size. *Am. J. Physiol.*, **212**, 329

Waitzman, M. B., Kuck, J. R. Jr., and Woods, W. D. (1972). Effect of prostaglandins (PGs) on galactose uptake by lenses and on adenylate cyclase of isolated lens cells. *Fed. Proc.*, **31**, 385

Whitelocke, R. A. F. and Eakins, K. E. (1973a). Vascular changes in the anterior uvea of the rabbit produced by prostaglandins. *Arch. Ophthal.*, **89**, 495

Whitelocke, R. A. F. and Eakins, K. E. (1973b). A comparison of some derivatives of phloretin as prostaglandin antagonists. *Exp. Eye Res.*, **17**, 395

Whitelocke, R. A. F., Eakins, K. E. and Bennett, A. (1973). Acute anterior uveitis and prostaglandins. *Proc. Roy. Soc. Med.*, **66, (5)** 429

Wyllie, A. M. and Wyllie, J. H. (1971). Prostaglandins and glaucoma. *Br. Med. J.*, **3**, 615

Zink, H. A., Podos, S. M. and Becker, B. (1973). Inhibition by imidazole of the increase in intraocular pressure induced by topical prostaglandin E. *Nature (New Biology)*, **245**, 21

4
Prostaglandins and the Respiratory System

ALEXANDER P. SMITH

4.1 INTRODUCTION   83

4.2 THE EFFECTS OF PROSTAGLANDINS ON BRONCHIAL MUSCLE TONE   84
    4.2.1 *A-series prostaglandins*   84
    4.2.2 *B-series prostaglandins*   85
    4.2.3 *E-series prostaglandins*   85
    4.2.4 *F-series prostaglandins*   88

4.3 EFFECTS OF PROSTAGLANDINS ON THE PULMONARY CIRCULATION   89

4.4 EFFECTS OF PROSTAGLANDINS ON VENTILATION   90

4.5 EFFECTS OF PROSTAGLANDIN ANTAGONISTS AND SYNTHESIS
    INHIBITORS ON BRONCHIAL MUSCLE TONE   90

4.6 METABOLISM OF PROSTAGLANDINS BY THE LUNGS   91

4.7 RELEASE OF PROSTAGLANDINS FROM THE LUNGS   95

4.8 PROSTAGLANDINS AND LUNG DISEASE   96
    4.8.1 *Asthma*   96
    4.8.2 *Pulmonary embolization*   97
    4.8.3 *Miscellaneous*   97

4.9 CONCLUSION   98
    REFERENCES   98

4.1 INTRODUCTION

Since the discovery of the prostaglandins in pulmonary tissues (Änggård, 1965; Karim *et al.*, 1967), and the description of their effects upon bronchial muscle (see Smith, 1972 for references) research has been directed towards the identification of their role in the physiology and pathology of the lungs, and the development of synthetic analogues of possible therapeutic value. Although neither of these objectives has yet been attained, the effects of the two naturally occurring prostaglandins in the lung, PGE_2 and $PGF_{2\alpha}$, have been fully described, and there has been much discussion as to the importance of these two substances in the pathogenesis of asthma. It has also become apparent that the lungs are involved in the metabolism of prostaglandins. However, although prostaglandins are used in gynaecological practice, little is known about the pharmacokinetics of these substances by the human lung, or about the biological activity of the metabolites that are formed. Marked differences exist between the regional distribution of PGE_2 and $PGF_{2\alpha}$ in cadaveric lung parenchyma and bronchial tissue (Karim *et al.*, 1967). This could be of physiological importance in view of the differences in the action of these two prostaglandins. Although lungs are known to release prostaglandins under a variety of different conditions, little is known about the factors which lead to *in vivo* synthesis of one or the other from their parent lipid, arachidonic acid. The effects of prostaglandins on bronchial muscle tone, and their metabolism and release by the lungs are therefore convenient headings for the detailed consideration of relationships between prostaglandins and the lungs.

4.2 THE EFFECTS OF PROSTAGLANDINS ON BRONCHIAL MUSCLE TONE

One of the most striking effects of prostaglandins is their ability to influence the tone of smooth muscle. Their effects on bronchial muscle vary, depending upon the prostaglandin used, its route of administration, and the species in which the experiment is conducted. Prostaglandins of the E- and F-series have been the most closely studied, but some information is also available concerning the A and B series prostaglandins.

4.2.1 A-series prostaglandins

The effects of PGA_1 on the cat and the guinea pig tracheal chain preparations were investigated by Horton and Jones (1969) who found that it inhibited the contractile effects of acetylcholine, but was less effective (by a factor of about 30) than PGE_2. In the anaesthetized dog, and the cat, however, intravenous PGA_1 and PGA_2 increased airway resistance and reduced lung compliance (Ballantyne *et al.*, 1973; Hirose and Said, 1971) indicating the occurrence of bronchoconstriction of both small and large airways. Prostaglandin A_2 was twice as potent as PGA_1. Increased tone caused by intravenous infusion of metacholine was further increased by the prostaglandins which also caused changes in blood pressure. In man the synthetic analogue 15-epi-PGA_2 increased airways resistance (inhaled dose of 200 μg) suggesting that it had a weak bronchoconstrictor effect (Smith, 1974b). In general it seems that the A-series prostaglandins have a weak stimulatory effect upon bronchial muscle tone.

4.2.2 B-series prostaglandins

Greenberg *et al.* (1973) reported that prostaglandin B_2 produced dose-dependent increases in airway resistance in anaesthetized dogs. Prostaglandin A_2 did not share this effect. Brookes and Marshall (1974) studied the changes in tidal volume and respiratory rate to various prostaglandins and their analogues in anaesthetized rabbits. These authors found that none of the PGs tested (including PGB_1, PGB_2, PGA_1, PGA_2) produced any significant changes in the tidal volume. The increases in respiratory rate elicited by these prostaglandins were smaller than those produced by $PGF_{2\alpha}$ or PGE_2 (exact potency difference not given).

Karim, Ganesan and Lo (1975) have studied the effects of B-series prostaglandins on guinea pig, cat and human respiratory tract smooth muscle *in vitro*. Like prostaglandins of the E series, PGB_1 and PGB_2 inhibit acetylcholine- and carbachol-induced contractions of cat tracheal muscle preparations *in vitro* but are about 50 times less potent than PGE_2. On isolated preparations of human tracheal and bronchial muscle and guinea pig tracheal chain both PGB_1 and PGB_2 are more potent stimulants than $PGF_{2\alpha}$.

4.2.3 E-series prostaglandins

E-series prostaglandins have been shown to be mainly inhibitory on bronchial muscle tone. Main (1964) investigated the effects of PGE_1, PGE_2 and PGE_3 on isolated tracheal muscle tone from several species and found that all three inhibited contractions due to histamine, acetylcholine and other agonists. He also found that a fall in lung inflation pressure (suggesting bronchodilatation) occurred in anaesthetized animals during PGE_1 infusion. In the cat, however, PGE_1 caused an increase in the inflation pressure, a finding of some interest in view of the effects of intravenous PGE_2 in man. Large *et al.* (1969) confirmed the bronchodilator effect of PGE_1 in the guinea pig, and found it to be 100 times more potent than isoprenaline when given by aerosol. Although bronchodilatation still occurred during intravenous administration, the potency of the prostaglandin was reduced. Rosenthale and his colleagues 1968, 1970, 1971) found that PGE_1 and PGE_2 were of similar bronchodilator potency to each other in a number of species, but were about 30 times more potent than isoprenaline when delivered by aerosol in the cat. The dog was less responsive to the prostaglandins than to isoprenaline, and the rhesus monkey was equally sensitive to the prostaglandins and isoprenaline. The bronchodilator effects of PGE_1 and PGE_2 were unaffected by β-adrenergic blockade, ganglionic blockade or destruction of the nervous system. The duration of their effect was dose related lasting up to 20 min with higher doses. Rosenthale *et al.* (1971) also found that the potency of the two prostaglandins was markedly reduced by intravenous administration, although bronchoconstriction was not observed. Systemic effects in the form of hypotension and changes in pulse rate were common when the drugs were given parenterally. Isoprenaline was a more potent drug than either prostaglandin under these conditions.

Both PGE_1 and PGE_2 relax human bronchial muscle *in vitro* (Sweatman and Collier, 1968) the effect being independent of adrenergic or cholinergic nerve activity. Furthermore, when inhaled as aerosols (55 μg) by normal subjects both prostaglandins produced a small (10–20%) increase in specific airways conductance (SGaw, a measurement of airways resistance) which was similar to the effect of inhalation of isoprenaline (550 μg). Asthmatics however were more sensitive to the effects of inhaled PGE_1 (55 μg) or PGE_2 (55 μg) (Cuthbert, 1969, 1971; Herxheimer and Roetscher, 1971; Smith and Cuthbert, 1973). Changes in measurements of airways resistance of the order of 30–40% reached their maximum after 10–20 min and lasted for 30–50 min. There was no significant difference between the effects of PGE_1, PGE_2 and

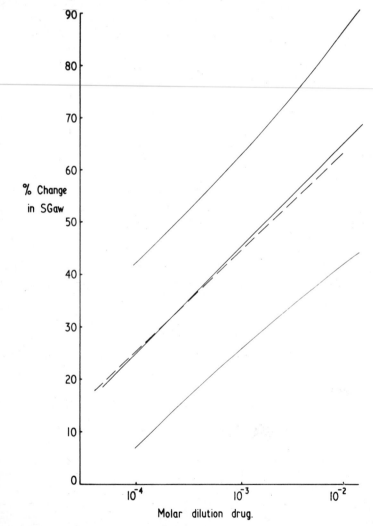

Figure 4.1   Dose related effects of inhaled PGE_2 (solid line) and isoprenaline (broken line) on specific airway conductance in 6 asthmatic patients with their confidence limits

isoprenaline under double-blind conditions, and no systemic side effects were noted after inhalation of these doses. Log molar dose/response regression lines for PGE_2 and isoprenaline indicate that they are of similar potency in man when given by aerosol (Figure 4.1). Two of the asthmatics taking part in the dose/response experiments developed systemic hypotension, headache and nausea, when doses of approximately 500 μg were inhaled. These side-effects disappeared after 10–15 min. All subjects, both normal and asthmatic, experienced bronchial and pharyngeal soreness after the inhalation of the free acids of either PGE_1 or PGE_2. Triethanolamine salts which were used subsequently also proved to be irritating when inhaled.

Occasionally PGE_1 or PGE_2 inhalation may cause bronchoconstriction (Cuthbert, 1969; Mathé et al., 1973) and an example of this phenomenon is shown in Figure 4.2. The effect was not prevented or reversed by inhalation of atropine methonitrate (in a dose sufficient to cause an increase in SGaw), prior to the experiment. The bronchodilator effect of isoprenaline was not affected by atropine. Their irritant effects and the risk of bronchoconstriction make the naturally occurring E-series prostaglandins unsuitable for clinical

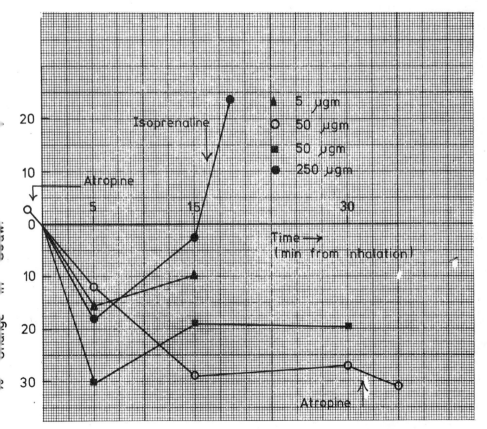

Figure 4.2 Idiosyncratic bronchoconstrictor effect of inhaled PGE_2 in one patient. The effect was not inhibited by inhalation of atropine methonitrate (1 mg)

use despite their lack of systemic side effects, and their potency, at low dosage. Neither 15(S) 15-methyl-PGE$_2$ (200 μg) nor 8-iso-PGE$_1$ (100 μg) were irritant to inhale, but in a limited study in 6 normal and 6 asthmatic subjects neither were effective bronchodilators in the doses used (Smith, 1974b). The recovery from histamine-induced bronchospasms in normal subjects was accelerated by 15-methyl-PGE$_2$ indicating a weak bronchodilator effect but clearly it lacks the potency on the bronchus which it exhibits on other organs (Karim *et al.*, 1973).

Prostaglandin E$_2$ when given intravenously to man loses its bronchodilator potency, and can cause bronchoconstriction. Five out of 7 women undergoing therapeutic termination of pregnancy experienced a minor but significant increase in lung resistance (airway interruptor valve method) during the course of PGE$_2$ infusion (5–100 μg/min) (Smith, 1973). Four out of ten asthmatic patients (Smith, 1974a) with proven reversibility of airway obstruction responded to intravenous PGE$_2$ with a reduction in forced expired volume in 1 s (FEV$_1$). A minor degree of bronchodilatation did occur in 4 of the asthmatic subjects, the mean change ($\pm$ SEM) being 0.2 ± 0.1 but one patient developed bronchoconstriction when the infusion was stopped. Systemic side effects (nausea, headache, hypotension) occurred in the patients who developed bronchoconstriction during PGE$_2$ infusion and in 3 of them treatment had to be terminated.

The occurrence of adverse effects during the infusion could not be correlated with age, sex, stage of pregnancy, smoking habits, diagnosis, or past medical history of allergic diseases. The reduction in the bronchodilator potency of PGE$_2$ when given intravenously may be due to its metabolism during its passage through the lungs. The bronchoconstriction and some of the systemic effects could be attributed to its metabolites. Intravenous PGE$_2$ should not therefore be given to patients with asthma without careful observation, and perhaps other routes of administration should also be avoided, as occasional attacks of asthma have been reported in patients receiving the drug via the extra-amniotic route (Frazer and Brash, 1974).

4.2.4 F-series prostaglandins

Although Änggård and Bergström (1963) showed that PGF$_{2\alpha}$ increased lung resistance in the cat, they were reluctant to attribute the response to bronchoconstriction as it failed to have any effect upon cat trachea *in vitro*. Main (1964) reported weak inhibition of cat tracheal tone by PGF$_{2\alpha}$ and Berry and Collier (1964) demonstrated a bronchoconstrictor effect of PGF$_{2\alpha}$ in the guinea pig. Later, Sweatman and Collier (1968) found that PGF$_{2\alpha}$ also contracted human bronchus *in vitro*, and that this effect was antagonized by PGE$_2$ and non-steroid anti-inflammatory drugs such as aspirin and the fenamates, but not by atropine or antihistamines (Collier and Sweatman, 1968). They concluded that PGF$_{2\alpha}$ was a constrictor agent acting upon the muscle itself rather than through any known pharmacological pathway.

PGF$_{2\alpha}$ is a potent bronchoconstrictor agent in man; normal volunteers inhaling it develop dose-related changes in specific airways conductance, and experience cough and sometimes wheezing (Hedqvist *et al.*, 1971; Smith and

Cuthbert, 1972; Mathe *et al.*, 1973, 1975; Smith *et al.*, 1975). The effect of $PGF_{2\alpha}$ was not inhibited by atropine methonitrate (in doses sufficient to cause bronchodilatation), disodium cromoglycate or flufenamic acid, but was reversed by inhalation of PGE_2 or isoprenaline (Smith and Cuthbert, 1972; Smith *et al.*, 1975). Asthmatics show very wide variation in sensitivity to inhaled $PGF_{2\alpha}$ but in general are much more sensitive to its action than are normal subjects, estimates ranging from about 8000 times (Mathé *et al.*, 1973) to about 200 times (Smith *et al.*, 1975) more than normal subjects. The difference in the reports of their increased sensitivity is probably due to individual variation between patients and the methods used to obtain the figures, but there is no doubt that asthmatics are much more sensitive to $PGF_{2\alpha}$ than are normal subjects. Like other prostaglandins which are active upon the bronchus, $PGF_{2\alpha}$ is irritating to inhale, and as asthmatics are more sensitive to the effects of inhalation of such irritants (Simonsson *et al.*, 1967), it is possible that their greatly increased sensitivity to $PGF_{2\alpha}$ is due to a combination of its pharmacological effects and reflex bronchoconstriction (Mathé *et al.*, 1975). Although atropine did not prevent $PGF_{2\alpha}$ induced bronchoconstriction in normal subjects, Alanko and Poppius (1973) found that the anticholinergic drug SC-1000 reduced its effect in patients with asthma, confirming that at least some of the bronchoconstriction was reflex in origin.

Prostaglandin $F_{2\alpha}$ retains its bronchoconstrictor effects when given intravenously. Fishburne and his colleagues (1972) reported the case of a patient receiving $PGF_{2\alpha}$ for the termination of pregnancy, who developed an attack of asthma; and subsequently measured ventilatory capacity by a number of volumetric methods in a group of 11 healthy pregnant women receiving $PGF_{2\alpha}$ infusions. Significant and dose-related changes occurred in FEV_1, vital capacity and other indices indicating that bronchoconstriction had occurred. Smith (1973) measuring lung resistance in a similar group of women also found dose-related changes which he attributed to bronchospasm. The effect is not confined to pregnant women as it also occurs in normal male volunteers (Smith *et al.*, 1975).

Prostaglandin $F_{2\beta}$ is a stereoisomer of $PGF_{2\alpha}$ which has been shown by Rosenthale *et al.* (1973) to possess inhibitory effects upon cholinergic bronchial muscle tone in the guinea pig and cat. Although it was about 100 times less potent than PGE_1 or PGE_2, it antagonized the bronchoconstrictor effect of $PGF_{2\alpha}$ and was effective by the intravenous route. Svanborg *et al.* (1973) reported that it gave rise to a modest increase in airways conductance when given by aerosol to asthmatics but quoted no specific figures.

4.3 EFFECTS OF PROSTAGLANDINS ON THE PULMONARY CIRCULATION

Prostaglandins are active upon pulmonary vascular smooth muscle. Prostaglandin A_1 and E_1 infusions in the anaesthetized dog resulted in reduction in pulmonary artery pressure (Nakano, 1968; Nakano and Cole, 1969). In the calf, PGE_1 and PGE_2 increased pulmonary artery pressure but in excised calf lungs these two prostaglandins produced a fall in vascular resistance (Lewis and Eyre, 1972). In man PGE_1 reduced pulmonary artery pressure

(Carlson *et al.*, 1969). Prostaglandin $F_{2\alpha}$ infusion produced a pressor response in the pulmonary artery of the dog (DuCharme and Weeks, 1967; Nakano and Cole, 1969) and in the calf (Lewis and Eyre, 1972). If it is injected into the portal vein, $PGF_{2\alpha}$ causes reduction in pulmonary resistance, possibly the result of an inhibitory metabolite (Cole and Nakano, 1968).

4.4 EFFECTS OF PROSTAGLANDINS ON VENTILATION

In general, systemic prostaglandins increase respiratory frequency and tidal volume. This effect occurs in the dog (Said, 1968; Hirose and Said, 1971), guinea pig (McQueen, 1973) and in man (Carlson *et al.*, 1969). The stimulatory effects are not inhibited by polyphloretin phosphate (PPP) (McQueen, 1973).

4.5 EFFECTS OF PROSTAGLANDIN ANTAGONISTS AND SYNTHESIS INHIBITORS ON BRONCHIAL MUSCLE TONE

Man and some animals possess intrinsic bronchial tone which varies in response to non-specific physical stimuli. Although it is recognized that a component of this tone *in vivo* is due to the cholinergic nervous system, it is possible that endogenous prostaglandin synthesis may contribute to it. Evidence in favour of this idea has been produced by Farmer *et al.* (1974), Lambley and Smith (1975), and Dunlop and Smith (1975). *In vitro* preparations of guinea pig trachea and human bronchial spiral strips exhibit a resting tone which is depressed by indomethacin or tetraynoic acid in doses which do not alter their response to $PGF_{2\alpha}$. Similar slow relaxation of tone occurs when the prostaglandin antagonists PPP or SC-19220 are added to the preparations in doses shown to inhibit the effects of $PGF_{2\alpha}$ suggesting that resting tone may be due to local prostaglandin synthesis particularly $PGF_{2\alpha}$ (Lambley and Smith, 1975). Conversely arachidonic acid causes contraction of the *in vitro* preparations which is progressively inhibited by indomethacin and SC-19220. Although prostaglandins were not directly assayed in any of these experiments, it seems likely that the resting tone and the subsequent changes were due to changes in their synthesis or due to inhibition of their effects. Whether these results justify the conclusion that prostaglandins affect physiological airway tone is open to question. No change in peak flow rate (a test of ventilatory performance) was found in 6 asthmatic patients receiving indomethacin 200 mg daily, a dose reported to inhibit endogenous prostaglandin synthesis (Samuelsson, 1973), and none experienced symptomatic improvement in a double-blind controlled trial of the drug in asthma (Smith, 1975). Prostaglandins are known to be released as a result of tissue damage and manipulation (see Section 4.6) and it may be that although resting *in vitro* bronchial tone is due to prostaglandin synthesis, it has not been shown to be the case *in vivo*, and the results of these studies should be evaluated with this in mind.

4.6 METABOLISM OF PROSTAGLANDINS BY THE LUNGS

The lung has a variety of metabolic functions in addition to its primary role as an organ of gas exchange (Bakhle and Vane, 1974), which include the metabolism and biosynthesis of prostaglandins. The cells which are responsible for these metabolic activities have not yet been fully identified but the removal of circulating substances from venous blood and their metabolism is thought to be conducted by pulmonary vascular endothelial cells (Smith and Ryan, 1970).

Labelled PGE_2 introduced into the high speed supernatant of guinea pig or swine lung homogenate was rapidly converted into two metabolites, 15-keto-dihydro-PGE_2 and dihydro-PGE_2 (Änggård and Samuelsson, 1967). The rate of metabolism of $PGF_{2\alpha}$ was slower. Metabolism of prostaglandins during passage through the pulmonary vascular bed was first demonstrated by Ferreira and Vane (1967) who showed that about 90% of PGE_1, PGE_2 and $PGF_{2\alpha}$ was removed by one passage through guinea pig lungs and McGiff et al. (1969) confirmed this finding in the dog lung. A-series prostaglandins are not so rapidly destroyed by passage through the lungs (McGiff et al., 1969; Piper et al., 1970) as those of the E-series or of the F-series. Large doses of aspirin reduces removal of prostaglandin by the lung (Jackson et al., 1973). Metabolism of prostaglandins has been directly demonstrated in several species, and in others, including man, indirect evidence exists, based upon reduction in pharmacological activity of the drugs when given intravenously (Carlson and Orö, 1966; Smith, 1974a) that such metabolism also occurs. Metabolites of $PGF_{2\alpha}$ (15-keto dihydro $PGF_{2\alpha}$ and dihydro $PGF_{2\alpha}$) occur in venous blood during $PGF_{2\alpha}$ infusion in women (Beguin et al., 1972). Measurement of $PGF_{2\alpha}$ by radioimmunoassay in pulmonary venous blood and aortic blood during $PGF_{2\alpha}$ infusion reveals reduction in the blood concentrations of this prostaglandin after passage through the lungs (Piper, P. J., Smith, A. P., Robinson, C., Jose, P., Neiderhauser, U., unpublished data).

Two enzyme systems exist in the lungs which are responsible for prostaglandin metabolism; 15-hydroxy prostaglandin dehydrogenase (PGDH) which converts PG to 15-keto PG; and 13, 14 prostaglandin reductase which converts 15-keto PG to 15-keto dihydro PG (Samuelsson, et al., 1971). Another enzyme, a β-oxidase, may also contribute to prostaglandin metabolism (Nakano and Morsy, 1971). There appears to be some species variation in the routes of prostaglandin metabolism, but in general it appears that the initial and rate limiting steps are due to PGDH. Prostaglandins E_1 and E_2 are the best substrates for this enzyme, PGE_3 and F-series prostaglandins are about 60% as effective, and A-series prostaglandins are but poor substrates (Änggård and Samuelsson, 1967). Metabolism of prostaglandins is thought to be associated with reduction in their biological activity (Piper et al., 1970; Änggård and Samuelsson, 1967), but Beguin et al. (1972) suggest that further reduction of 15-keto dihydro $PGF_{2\alpha}$ with formation of a 15-S hydroxyl group (as in dihydro $PGF_{2\alpha}$) could result in increased biological activity, and might be responsible for some of the effects hitherto attributed to the parent prostaglandin. Dawson et al. (1974) have shown

Table 4.1 Summary of the effects of prostaglandins on lung tissues

Prostaglandins	Species	Route	Effect on muscle in		Effect on ventilation	References
			Airways	Blood vessels		
A₁	Cat, Guinea pig	in vitro	Relaxation	—	—	Horton and Jones (1969)
	Guinea pig	i.v.	Relaxation	—	—	Dessy et al. (1973)
	Cat	i.v.	Contraction	—	—	Ballantyne et al. (1973)
	Dog	i.v.	Contraction	—	Stimulation	Hirose and Said (1971)
A₂	Guinea pig	i.v.	Relaxation	—	—	Rosenthale et al. (1973)
	Cat	i.v.	Contraction	—	—	Ballantyne et al. (1973)
15-epi A₂	Man	Aerosol	Contraction	—	—	Smith (1974b)
B₁ and B₂	Man	in vitro	Contraction	—	—	Karim et al. (1975)
D₂	Man	in vitro	Contraction	—	—	Dawson et al. (1974)
E₁	Cat, Monkey, Rabbit	in vitro	Relaxation	—	—	Main (1964)
	Guinea pig	Aerosol/i.v.	Relaxation	—	—	Large et al. (1969)
	Cat	i.v.	Contraction	—	—	Main (1964)
	Dog	i.v.	No effect	Relaxation	Stimulation	Hirose and Said (1971)
	Dog	i.v.	—	Relaxation	—	Nakano and Cole (1969)
	Man	i.v.	—	Relaxation	Stimulation	Carlson et al. (1969)
	Man	in vitro	Relaxation	—	—	Sweatman and Collier (1968)
	Man	Aerosol	Relaxation	—	—	Cuthbert (1969)
	Man	Aerosol	Relaxation	—	—	Herxheimer and Roetscher (1971)

Compound	Species	Route	Effect			Reference
E₂	Cat	in vitro	Relaxation	—	—	Main (1964)
	Guinea pig	in vitro	Relaxation/Contraction	—	—	Lambley and Smith (1975)
	Guinea pig, Dog, Cat, Monkey	Aerosol/i.v.	Relaxation	—	—	Rosenthale et al. (1968, 1970, 1971)
	Man	Aerosol	Relaxation	—	—	Cuthbert (1971)
	Man	i.v.	Relaxation/Contraction/no effect	—	—	Smith (1973, 1974a)
	Man	Extra-amniotic	?Contraction	—	—	Fraser and Brash (1974)
Dihydro-E₁	Guinea pig	i.v.	Relaxation	—	—	Rosenthale et al. (1973)
8-iso E₁	Man	Aerosol	No effect	—	—	Smith (1974b)
15-methyl E₂	Man	Aerosol	No effect	—	—	Smith (1974b)
F₁α	Cat	in vitro	Relaxation	—	—	Main (1964)
F₂α	Cat	i.v.	Contraction	—	—	Änggård and Bergström (1963)
	Dog	i.v.	—	Contraction	? Stimulation	DuCharme and Weeks (1967); Hirose and Said (1971); Nakano and Cole (1969)
	Man	in vitro	Contraction	—	—	Sweatman and Collier (1968)
	Man	Aerosol	Contraction	—	—	Mathé et al. (1973)
	Man	i.v.	Contraction	—	—	Fishburne et al. (1972)
F₂β	Guinea pig, Cat	Aerosol/i.v.	Relaxation	—	—	Rosenthale et al. (1973)
	Man	Aerosol	Relaxation	—	—	Svanborg et al. (1973)

Table 4.2   Stimuli leading to release of prostaglandins from lung tissues

Stimulus	Source of lung	Prostaglandin	Reference
Anaphylaxis	Rat	$E_1, E_2, F_{2\alpha}$	Piper and Vane, 1969
	Guinea pig	$E_1, E_2, F_{2\alpha}$	Piper and Vane, 1971
	Man	$E_2, F_{2\alpha}$	Piper and Walker, 1973
Chemicals			
Arachidonic acid	}		{ Palmer, Piper and
Dihomo-γ-linoleic	} Guinea pig	E-series	{ Vane, 1973
acid	}		{ Vargaftig and Dao, 1971
Acetylcholine	Rat		
	Dog		
	Cat		
Histamine	Rat		
	Dog		Alabaster and Bakhle,
	Cat	Uncharacterized	1970
	Guinea pig	prostaglandin	Bakhle and Smith,
β-phenylethylamine	Cat		1972
Tryptamine	Rat		
5-hydroxytryptamine	Dog		
Tyramine	Dog		
	Cat		
Overinflation	Guinea pig	E_2	Berry, Edmunds and Wyllie, 1971
	Dog	E-series	Said, Kitamura and Vreim, 1972
Embolization			
Prosparol	Guinea pig	E_2	Lindsey and Wyllie,
Sephadex	Guinea pig	E_2	1970
Latex spheres	Guinea pig		
Iron dextran	Guinea pig	Uncharacterized	Palmer, Piper and
Air	Guinea pig	prostaglandin	Vane, 1973
Mechanical			
Stroking	Guinea pig	E-series	Piper and Vane, 1971
Stirring	Man	$E_2, F_{2\alpha}$	Piper and Walker, 1973
Hypoxia	Cat	E-series	Said et al., 1975
	Dog	E-series	Weir et al., 1975

that the $PGF_{2\alpha}$ metabolite, 15-keto $PGF_{2\alpha}$ has more potent contractile effects on human bronchus *in vitro* than its parent $PGF_{2\alpha}$. As the latter prostaglandin is known to be released during anaphylaxis it is possible that its metabolites may be acting as bronchoconstrictor substances in addition to parent $PGF_{2\alpha}$ released with other humoral mediators of the response. The activity of PGDH may be reduced by PPP in doses less than those which inhibit the effects of $PGF_{2\alpha}$ (Crutchley and Piper, 1974).

In addition to the metabolism of prostaglandins, the lungs, under a variety of conditions, synthesize PGE_2 and $PGF_{2\alpha}$ from their common precursor, arachidonic acid (Änggård and Samuelsson, 1967), more $PGF_{2\alpha}$ being formed than PGE_2. The factors that determine the rate of prostaglandin biosynthesis and the type of prostaglandin synthesized are unknown, but are thought to be related to the presence of glutathione (Lands et al., 1971) and hydroquinone (Nugteren et al., 1966). The synthesis is inhibited by non-steroidal anti-inflammatory drugs such as aspirin or indomethacin (Vane,

1971), and the long chain fatty acid 5,8,11,14-eicosatetraynoic acid (tetraynoic acid) (Downing *et al.*, 1970).

The removal of prostaglandins by the lungs is consistent with the hypothesis that they act as venous hormones, but their ability to synthesize prostaglandins, and the wide variety of stimuli leading to prostaglandin release by the lungs would suggest that the object of the enzyme systems described is primarily to remove prostaglandins that are released locally.

4.7 RELEASE OF PROSTAGLANDINS FROM THE LUNGS

Although the biochemical factors leading to prostaglandin synthesis are not well understood, release of prostaglandins by lung tissue may be initiated by a wide variety of stimuli which may conveniently be divided into: anaphylaxis, chemical agents and physical stimuli, some of which may be interrelated.

Sensitized lungs from both man and experimental animals, and human bronchial spirals *in vitro*, release a mixture of smooth muscle active substances including histamine, SRS-A, prostaglandins and prostaglandin metabolites when they are exposed to antigen (Piper and Vane, 1969; Piper and Walker, 1973; Mathé and Levine, 1973; Dunlop and Smith, 1975). The form of allergic sensitivity seems to be unimportant, as it occurs when the tissues are sensitized with either IgE or IgG antibodies. E-series prostaglandins appear in excess of the F-series in a ratio of about 6:1 (Mathé and Levine, 1973) when guinea pig lungs are antigenically shocked. Since then Mathé *et al.* (1975) and Ruff *et al.* (1975) have shown that sensitized guinea pig lungs synthesize more $PGF_{2\alpha}$ than PGE_2, but the source of these prostaglandins and their contribution to the allergic response is doubtful. The relationship between the appearance of histamine following antigen exposure and the release of prostaglandins would suggest that the latter is a secondary phenomenon occurring either as a direct effect of histamine, or the resultant of smooth muscle contraction. Prostaglandins are known to be released as a result of histamine- or acetylcholine-induced muscle contraction in guinea pig trachea (Orehek *et al.*, 1973) but not from human bronchus when it contracts in response to acetylcholine (Dunlop and Smith, 1975). Furthermore, the inhibition of $PGF_{2\alpha}$ synthesis in human bronchus *in vitro* by indomethacin is associated with a reduction in antigen challenge-induced contractions. Further evidence in favour of the involvement of prostaglandins in allergic bronchospasm was the demonstration that PPP, which inhibits bronchoconstriction due to $PGF_{2\alpha}$ in the guinea pig and the cat (Mathé *et al.*, 1972) also reduced the effects of anaphylaxis (Strandberg, *et al.*, 1972).

Another explanation for the appearance of E-series prostaglandins during anaphylaxis would invoke one of the autoregulatory hypotheses concerning the biological role of the prostaglandins. Thus E-series prostaglandins, which are predominantly bronchodilator in effect, may be released in an attempt to restore normal bronchial tone. Histamine release from challenged sensitized leucocytes or human lung tissue is inhibited by PGE_1 or PGE_2, probably through their effect upon adenylate cyclase resulting in elevation of cell cyclic AMP (Lichtenstein *et al.*, 1972; Tauber *et al.*, 1973). Thus PGE_2 released during anaphylaxis could act as a feedback mechanism designed to restore cell levels of cyclic AMP to the pre-challenge state. Inhibition of prostaglandin synthesis in sensitized tissues might therefore be expected to potentiate the effect of antigen challenge, but this has not been observed. Release of prostaglandins from sensitized lung and bronchial tissues is inhibited by indomethacin (Piper and Walker, 1973; Dunlop and Smith, 1975) or by disodium cromoglycate, but in the latter case, only when the release of SRS-A and histamine is almost completely suppressed (Piper and Walker, 1973). Catecholamines also reduce the release of histamine and prostaglandins from sensitized guinea pig lungs on challenge with antigen (Mathé and Levine, 1973) and in this preparation too inhibition of prostaglandin synthesis and release occurred in parallel with inhibition of histamine release. On balance the evidence favours the hypothesis that prostaglandins released during anaphylaxis are a secondary phenomenon due to either distortion of cells during exocytosis of histamine granules or muscle contraction or the effect of histamine itself, rather than primary bronchoconstrictor mediators of anaphylaxis. It would appear however that they participate to some extent in the bronchospasm that occurs.

In addition to anaphylaxis, other physical stimuli cause the release of prostaglandins from whole or chopped lung tissue. Squeezing, stroking or stirring lung tissue (Piper and Vane, 1971; Piper and Walker, 1973) cause release of prostaglandins and other smooth muscle active substances. Their release by stirring is reduced by indomethacin but not by disodium cromoglycate (Piper and Walker, 1973). Ventilation of excised perfused dog lung also causes release of PGE_2 (Berry et al., 1971) and prostaglandin-like activity has been noted in anaesthetized dogs during artificial ventilation in response to increasing tidal volumes (Vane, quoted by Bakhle and Vane, 1974). Another stimulus leading to prostaglandin release from the lungs is pulmonary embolization and it is suggested that the release of PGE_2 might contribute to the circulatory effects of pulmonary embolization (Lindsey and Wyllie, 1970). The implications of some of these factors are discussed in Section 4.8.

4.8 PROSTAGLANDINS AND LUNG DISEASE

4.8.1 Asthma

The potent effects of PGE_2 and $PGF_{2\alpha}$ on the tone of bronchial muscle and their release during anaphylaxis have led to the suggestion that they could be involved in the pathogenesis of bronchial asthma. The levels of $PGF_{2\alpha}$ in the serum of asthmatic patients are reported to be about twice the levels found in the serum of non-allergic subjects (Okazaki et al., 1974) and increased amounts of prostaglandin metabolites have been reported in serum (15-keto, 13, 14 dihydro $PGF_{2\alpha}$, Gréen et al., 1974) and in urine (5α, 7α, dihydroxy-11-keto tetranor, prostane-1, 16-dioic acid (Svanborg et al., 1973) from allergic asthmatic patients and guinea pigs undergoing inhalation antigen challenge testing.

Passively sensitized human bronchus in vitro releases $PGF_{2\alpha}$ during antigen challenge-induced contraction, which is reduced by 20–30% by indomethacin or PPP (Dunlop and Smith, 1975). It would appear therefore that at least *in vitro* $PGF_{2\alpha}$ does contribute to the allergic response of the human bronchus. Indomethacin in doses which reduced the metabolites of $PGF_{2\alpha}$ in the urine also reduced the bronchoconstrictor effect of antigen challenge (Svanborg *et al.*, 1973), but another study has failed to confirm this finding (Smith, 1975) when doses which inhibit endogenous prostaglandin synthesis (200 mg orally for one week) (Samuelsson, 1973) were given prior to challenge. Technical differences may account for the variation in these results but small amounts of $PGF_{2\alpha}$ produced by residual synthesis could affect airway muscle which is known to be extremely sensitive to its action. A similar experiment, in which exercise asthma was induced before and after indomethacin therapy also failed to show any inhibitory effect of the drug. Furthermore, although $PGF_{2\alpha}$ metabolites were excreted in the urine of antigen challenged sensitized guinea pigs, suppression of $PGF_{2\alpha}$ synthesis by indomethacin failed to prevent the effects of anaphylaxis (Strandberg and Hamberg, 1974). $PGF_{2\alpha}$ is released by both lung and bronchial muscle during anaphylaxis in animals and in man and it is possible that it does contribute to the bronchospasm that occurs, particularly in view of its extremely potent effect on the bronchi. However, the failure of indomethacin to exert a protective effect in patients with asthma would suggest that the presence of $PGF_{2\alpha}$ is secondary and unlikely to be of the same importance as the other mediators of the allergic response such as histamine and SRS-A in the pathogenesis of asthma.

4.8.2 Pulmonary embolization

Following pulmonary embolization, or occlusion of the pulmonary arteries by other means, bronchoconstriction occurs in the affected areas of lung (Severinghaus *et al.*, 1961; Clarke *et al.*, 1970). This effect is independent of the nervous system (Nisell, 1950) and could therefore be due to release of pharmacological agents such as prostaglandins (Lindsey and Wyllie, 1970). Nakano and McLoy (1973) showed that bronchoconstriction in the dog, which occurred as a result of pulmonary embolization with barium sulphate, was inhibited by indomethacin in doses which did not inhibit the bronchoconstrictor effect of $PGF_{2\alpha}$. Although they did not measure prostaglandin release the results of their experiments suggest that prevention of bronchospasm was due to inhibition of prostaglandin synthesis. It should be noted, however, that barium sulphate particles probably act as nuclei for platelet aggregation (Bø *et al.*, 1974) and prostaglandins released during this process could cause local effects on smooth muscle. Some of the systemic manifestations of pulmonary emboli and the associated bronchoconstriction could, however, be caused by release of vasoactive substances from the lungs.

4.8.3 Miscellaneous

Prostaglandin release has been reported in other conditions, for example during the development of pulmonary edema, during hypoxic breathing

(Said, 1973) and during ventilation of the lungs (Berry *et al.*, 1970) especially in the presence of a metabolic alkalosis (Said *et al.*, 1972) but the significance of prostaglandins during these events is not known. Vasoconstriction caused by hypoxia in the cat lung (Said *et al.*, 1975) is partially inhibited by aspirin or indomethacin, which also reduced the associated release of prostaglandin-like material. The authors suggest that prostaglandins may act as local autoregulatory agents. Weir *et al.* (1975) have reported the release of an inhibitory prostaglandin from lungs during hypoxia-induced pulmonary vasoconstriction. Although not conclusive, the data suggest that prostaglandins may modulate pulmonary vascular tone in response to changes in alveolar gas tensions.

4.9 CONCLUSION

Prostaglandins are a group of substances with potent effects upon bronchial and pulmonary vascular smooth muscle, and the lungs have evolved enzyme systems for their removal. Although a definite role for prostaglandins in the lung has yet to be defined it seems likely that they act as autoregulatory agents, being rapidly synthesized and then destroyed in response to as yet unknown physiological requirements. Prostaglandins are released in asthma, but their role is probably secondary and may be related to physiological attempts to restore the bronchi to a more normal state. Prostaglandins may be involved in the maintenance of normal bronchial tone and thereby adjust local ventilation perfusion ratios in the lungs but the use of E-series prostaglandins for the treatment of patients with asthma has proved disappointing, because of their irritant effect when given by inhalation and their loss of potency when given intravenously. Possibly the 15-methyl ester of PGE_2 would be more effective on the bronchus by the intravenous route, but to date prostaglandin analogues have proved less active upon the bronchus than the naturally occurring compounds, when given by aerosol. Prostaglandins may play a part in the pathology of other lung diseases in particular pulmonary embolization and pulmonary edema particularly in relation to the bronchospasm that occurs in these conditions but further research is needed before a definite conclusion may be reached regarding the importance of prostaglandins in the pathogenesis of lung diseases.

References

Alabaster, V. A. and Bakhle, Y. S. (1970). The release of biologically active substances from isolated lungs by 5-hydroxytryptamine and tryptamine. *Br. J. Pharmacol.*, **40**, 582P

Alanko, K. and Poppius, H. (1973). Anticholinergic blocking of prostaglandin-induced bronchoconstriction. *Br. Med. J.*, **1**, 294

Änggård, E. (1965). The isolation and determination of prostaglandins in the lungs of sheep, guinea pig, monkey and man. *Biochem. Pharmacol.*, **14**, 1507

Änggård, E. and Bergström, S. (1963). Biological effects of an unsaturated trihydroxy acid ($PGF_{2\alpha}$) from normal swine lung. *Acta Physiol. Scand.*, **58**, 1

Änggård, E. and Samuelsson, B. (1967). The metabolism of prostaglandins in lung tissue. In *Prostaglandins (Proc. Nobel Symposium 2)*, Bergström, S. and Samuelsson, B.(eds.), pp. 97–105 (Stockholm: Almqvist and Wiksell)

Bakhle, Y. S. and Smith, T. W. (1972). Release of spasmogenic substances induced by vaso-active amines from isolated lungs. *Br. J. Pharmac.*, **46**, 543P

Bakhle, Y. S. and Vane, J. R. (1974). Pharmacokinetic function of the pulmonary circulation. *Physiol. Rev.*, **54**, 1007

Ballantyne, A., Jones, R. L. and Ungar, A. (1973). The actions of prostaglandins A_1 and A_2 on airway resistance and compliance in the cat. *Br. J. Pharmac.*, **47**, 630P

Beguin, F., Bygdeman, M., Gréen, K., Samuelsson, B., Toppozada, M. and Wiqvist, N. (1972). Analysis of prostaglandin $F_{2\alpha}$ and metabolites in blood during constant intravenous infusion of prostaglandin $F_{2\alpha}$ in the human female. *Acta Physiol. Scand.*, **86**, 430

Berry, P. A. and Collier, H. O. J. (1964). Bronchoconstrictor action and antagonism of a slow reacting substance from anaphylaxis of guinea-pig isolated lung. *Br. J. Pharmac.*, **23**, 201

Berry, E. M., Edmonds, J. F. and Wyllie, J. H. (1971). Release of prostaglandin E_2 and unidentified factors from ventilated lungs. *Br. J. Surg.*, **58**, 189

Bø, G., Hognestad, J. and Vooge, J. (1974). The role of blood platelets in pulmonary response to micro-embolisation with barium sulphate. *Acta Physiol. Scand.*, **90**, 244

Brookes, G. and Marshall, R. C. (1974). The effects of some prostaglandins on respiration in the rabbit. *J. Pharm. Pharmacol.*, **26**, 80

Carlson, L. A. and Orö, L. (1966). Effect of prostaglandin E_1 on blood pressure and heart rate in the dog. *Acta Physiol. Scand.*, **67**, 89

Carlson, L. A., Ekelund, L. G. and Orö, L. (1969). Circulatory and respiratory effects of different doses of PGE_1 in man. *Acta Physiol. Scand.*, **75**, 161

Clarke, S. W., Graf, P. D. and Nadel, J. (1970). *In vivo* visualisation of small airway constriction after pulmonary microembolization in cats and dogs. *J. Appl. Physiol.*, **29**, 646

Cole, B. and Nakano, J. (1968). Effects of $PGF_{2\alpha}$ on the systemic venous return and splanchnic circulation. *Pharmacologist*, **2**, 175

Collier, H. O. J. and Sweatman, W. J. F. (1968). Antagonism by fenamates of prostaglandin $F_{2\alpha}$ and of slow reacting substance on human bronchial muscle. *Nature (Lond.)*, **219**, 864

Crutchley, D. J. and Piper, P. J. (1974). Prostaglandin inactivation in guinea pig lung and its inhibition. *Br. J. Pharmac.*, **52**, 197

Cuthbert, M. F. (1969). Effect on airway resistance of prostaglandin E_1 given by aerosol to healthy and asthmatic volunteers. *Br. Med. J.*, **4**, 723

Cuthbert, M. F. (1971). Bronchodilator activity of aerosols of prostaglandin E_1 and E_2 in asthmatic subjects. *Proc. Roy. Soc. Med.*, **64**, 15

Dawson, W., Lewis, R. L., McMahon, R. E. and Sweatman, W. J. F. (1974). Potent bronchoconstrictor activity of 15-keto prostaglandin $F_{2\alpha}$. *Nature (Lond.)*, **250**, 331

Dessy, F., Maleux, M. R. and Cognioul, A. (1973). Bronchospasmolytic activity of some prostaglandins in the guinea pig. *Archs. int. Pharmacodyn. Ther.*, **206**, 368

Downing, D. T., Ahern, D. G. and Bachta, M. (1970). Enzyme inhibition by acetylenic compounds. *Biochem. Biophys. Res. Comm.*, **40**, 218

DuCharme, D. W. and Weeks, J. R. (1967). Cardiovascular pharmacology of prostaglandin $F_{2\alpha}$, a unique pressor agent. In *Prostaglandins (Proc. Nobel Symposium 2)*, Bergström, S. and Samuelsson, B. (eds.), pp. 173–181 (Stockholm: Almqvist and Wiksell)

Dunlop, L. S. and Smith, A. P. (1975). Reduction of antigen induced contraction of sensitised human bronchus *in vitro* by substances which inhibit the synthesis and effects of prostaglandin $F_{2\alpha}$. *Br. J. Pharmac.*, **541**, 495

Farmer, J. B., Farrar, D. G. and Wilson, J. (1974). Antagonism of tone and prostaglandin mediated responses in a tracheal preparation by indomethacin and SC–19220. *Br. J. Pharmac.*, **52**, 559

Ferreira, S. H. and Vane, J. R. (1967). Prostaglandins: their disappearance from and release into the circulation. *Nature (Lond.)*, **216**, 868

Fishburne, J. I., Brenner, W. E., Braaksma, J. T. and Hendricks, C. H. (1972). Bronchospasm complicating intravenous prostaglandin $F_{2\alpha}$ for therapeutic abortion. *Obstet. Gynecol.*, **39**, 892

Fishburne, J. I., Brenner, W. E., Braaksma, J. T., Staurovsky, L. G., Mueller, R. A., Hoffer, J. L. and Hendricks, C. H. (1972). Cardiovascular and respiratory responses to intravenous infusion of prostaglandin $F_{2\alpha}$ in the pregnant woman. *Am. J. Obstet. Gynecol.*, **114**, 765

Frazer, I. S. and Brash, J. H. (1974). Comparison of extra- and intra-amniotic prostaglandins for therapeutic abortion. *Obstet. Gynecol.*, **43**, 97

Gréen, K., Hedqvist, P. and Svanborg, N. (1974). Increased plasma levels of 15-keto, 13,14 dihydro $PGF_{2\alpha}$ after allergen provoked asthma in man. *Lancet*, **ii**, 1419

Greenberg, S., Howard, L. and Wilson, W. R. (1973). Comparative effects of prostaglandins A_2 and B_2 on vascular and airway resistances and adrenergic neurotransmission. *Can. J. Physiol. Pharmacol.*, **52**, 699

Hedqvist, P., Holmgren, A. and Mathé, A. A. (1971). Effect of prostaglandin $F_{2\alpha}$ on airway resistance in man. *Acta Physiol. Scand.*, **82**, 29a

Herxheimer, H. and Roetscher, I. (1971). Effects of prostaglandin E_1 on lung function in bronchial asthma. *Eur. J. Clin. Pharmacol.*, **3**, 123

Hirose, T. and Said, S. I. (1971). Respiratory effects of prostaglandins A_1, E_1 and $F_{2\alpha}$. *Clin. Res.*, **19**, 512

Horton, E. W. and Jones, R. L. (1969). Prostaglandins A_1, A_2 and 19-hydroxy A_1; their action on smooth muscle and their inactivation on passage through the pulmonary or hepatic portal vascular beds. *Br. J. Pharmac.*, **37**, 705

Jackson, H. R., Hall, R. C., Hodge, R. L., Gibson, E. L., Katic, F. P. and Stevens, M. (1973). The effect of aspirin on the pulmonary extraction of $PGF_{2\alpha}$ and cardiovascular response to $PGF_{2\alpha}$. *Aust. J. Exp. Biol. Med. Sci.*, **51**, 837

Karim, S. M. M., Sandler, M. and Williams, E. D. (1967). Distribution of prostaglandins in human tissues. *Br. J. Pharmac.*, **31**, 340

Karim, S. M. M., Sharma, S. D., Filshie, G. M., Salmon, J. A. and Ganesan, P. A. (1973). Termination of pregnancy with prostaglandin analogues. *Adv. Biosci.*, **9**, Bergström, S. (ed.), p 811–830 (Vieweg: Pergamon Press)

Karim, S. M. M., Adaikan, P. G. and Lo., P. Y. (1975). Effects of prostaglandins A_1, A_2, B_1 and B_2 on respiratory smooth muscle of guinea pig and man *in vitro*. Personal communication

Lambley, J. and Smith, A. P. (1975). The effects of arachidonic acid, indomethacin and SC–19220 on guinea pig tracheal tone. *Eur. J. Pharmacol.*, **30**, 148

Lands, W., Lee, R. and Smith, W. (1971). Factors regulating the biosynthesis of various prostaglandins. *Ann. N.Y. Acad. Sci.*, **180**, 107

Large, B. J., Leswell, P. F. and Maxwell, D. R. (1969). Bronchodilator activity of an aerosol of prostaglandin E_1 in experimental animals. *Nature (Lond.)*, **224**, 78

Lewis, A. J. and Eyre, P. (1972). Some cardiovascular and respiratory effects of prostaglandins E_1, E_2 and $F_{2\alpha}$ in the calf. *Prostaglandins*, **2**, 55

Lichtenstein, L. M., Gillespie, E., Bourne, H. R. and Henney, C. S. (1972). The effects of a series of prostaglandins on *in vitro* models of allergic response and cellular immunity. *Prostaglandins*, **2**, 519

Lindsey, H. E. and Wyllie, J. H. (1970). Release of prostaglandins from embolised lungs. *Br. J. Surg.*, **57**, 738

Main, I. H. M. (1964). The inhibitory actions of prostaglandins on respiratory smooth muscle. *Br. J. Pharmac.*, **22**, 511

Mathé, A. A., Hedqvist, P., Holmgren, A. and Svanborg, N. (1973). Bronchial hyperreactivity to prostaglandin $F_{2\alpha}$ and histamine in patients with asthma. *Br. Med. J.*, **1**, 193

Mathé, A. A. and Hedqvist, P. (1975). Effect of prostaglandins $F_{2\alpha}$ and E_2 on airway conductance in healthy subjects and asthmatic patients. *Am. Rev. Resp. Dis.*, **111**, 313

Mathé, A. A., Levine, L., Yen, S. S., Sohn, R. and Hedqvist, P. (1975). Release of prostaglandins and histamine from guinea pig lung. *Abstr. Int. Conf. Prostaglandins*, Florence, May 1975, p. 188

Mathé, A. A. and Levine, L. (1973). Release of prostaglandins and metabolites from guinea pig lung: inhibition by catecholamines. *Prostaglandins*, **4**, 877

Mathé, A. A., Strandberg, K. and Fredholm, B. (1972). Antagonism of prostaglandin $F_{2\alpha}$ induced bronchoconstriction and blood pressure changes by polyphloretin phosphate in the guinea pig and cat. *J. Pharm. Pharmacol.*, **24**, 378

McGiff, J. C., Terragno, N. A., Strand, J. C., Lee, J. B., Lonigro, A. J. and Ng, K. K. F. (1969). Selective passage of prostaglandins across the lung. *Nature (Lond.)*, **223**, 742

McQueen, D. S. (1973). The effects of prostaglandin E_2 and prostaglandin $F_{2\alpha}$ and polyphloretin phosphate on respiration and blood pressure in anaesthetised guinea-pigs. *Life Sci.*, **12**, 163

Nakano, J. (1968). Effect of prostaglandins E_1, A_1 and $F_{2\alpha}$ on cardiovascular dynamics in dogs. In *Prostaglandin Symposium of the Worcester Foundation for Experimental Biology*, Ramwell, P. W. and Shaw, J. E. (eds.), pp. 201–214 (New York: Interscience)

Nakano, J. and Cole, B. (1969). Effects of prostaglandins E_1 and $F_{2\alpha}$ on systemic, pulmonary and splanchnic circulations in dogs. *Am. J. Physiol.*, **217**, 222

Nakano, J. and McLoy, R. B. (1973). Effects of indomethacin on the pulmonary vascular and airway resistances responses to pulmonary microembolization. *Proc. Soc. Exp. Biol. Med.*, **143**, 218

Nakano, J. and Morsy, N. H. (1971). Beta-oxidation of prostaglandins E_1 and E_2 in rat lung and kidney homogenate. *Clin. Res.*, **19**, 142

Nisell, O. I. (1950). The actions of O_2 and CO_2 on the bronchioles and blood vessels of isolated perfused lungs. *Acta Physiol. Scand. Suppl.*, **21**, 73

Nugteren, D. H., Beerthuis, R. K. and Van Dorp, D. A. (1966). The enzymic conversion of all cis-8,11,14, eicosatrienoic acid into prostaglandin E_1. *Recl. Trav. Chim. Pays. Belg.*, **85**, 405

Okazaki, T., Vervloet, D., Attalah, A., Lee, J. and Arbesman, C. E. (1974). Prostaglandin synthesis and allergic reactions. *J. Allergy Clin. Immunol.*, **53**, 75

Orehek, J., Douglas, J. S., Lewis, A. J. and Bouhuys, A. (1973). Prostaglandin regulation of airway smooth muscle tone. *Nature New Biology*, **245**, 84

Palmer, M. A., Piper, P. J. and Vane, J. R. (1973). Release of rabbit aorta contracting substance (RCS) and prostaglandins induced by chemical or mechanical stimulation of guinea pig lung. *Br. J. Pharmac.*, **49**, 226

Piper, P. J. and Vane, J. R. (1969). Release of additional factors in anaphylaxis and its antagonism by anti-inflammatory drugs. *Nature (Lond.)*, **223**, 29

Piper, P. J. and Vane, J. R. (1971). The release of prostaglandins from lung and other tissues. *Ann. N.Y. Acad. Sci.*, **180**, 363

Piper, P. J., Vane, J. R. and Wyllie, J. A. (1970). Inactivation of prostaglandins by the lungs. *Nature (Lond.)*, **225**, 600

Piper, P. J. and Walker, J. L. (1973). The release of spasmogenic substances from human chopped lung tissue and its inhibition. *Br. J. Pharmac.*, **47**, 291

Rosenthale, M. E., Dervinis, A., Begany, A. J. and Lapidus, M. (1968). Bronchodilator activity of the prostaglandin E_2. *Pharmacologist*, **10**, 175

Rosenthale, M. E., Dervinis, A., Begany, A. J., Lapidus, M. and Gluckman, M. I. (1970). Bronchodilator activity of PGE_2 when administered by aerosol to three species. *Experientia*, **26**, 1119

Rosenthale, M. E., Dervinis, A. and Kassarich, J. (1971). Bronchodilator activity of the prostaglandins E_1 and E_2. *J. Pharmac. exp. Ther.*, **178**, 541

Rosenthale, M. E., Dervinis, A., Kassarich, J., Blumenthal, A. and Gluckman, M. I. (1973). Bronchodilating properties of the prostaglandin $F_{2\beta}$ in the guinea pig and cat. *Prostaglandins*, **3**, 767

Ruff, F., Dray, F., Santais, M. C., Allouche, G., Foussand, C. and Parrot, J. L. (1975). Determination of lung prostaglandins during induced anaphylactic shock. *Abstr. Int. Conf. Prostaglandins*, Florence, May 1975, p. 189

Said, S. I. (1968). Some respiratory effects of prostaglandins E_2 and $F_{2\alpha}$. In *Prostaglandin Symposium of the Worcester Foundation for Experimental Biology*, Ramwell, P. W. and Shaw, J. E. (eds.), pp. 267–277 (New York: Interscience)

Said, S. I., Kitamura, S. and Vreim, C. (1972). Prostaglandins: release from the lung during mechanical ventilation at large tidal volumes. *J. Clin. Invest.*, **51**, 83a

Said, S. I. (1973). The lung in relation to vasoactive hormones. *Fed. Proc.*, **32**, 1972

Said, S. I., Hova, N. and Yoshida, T. (1975). Hypoxic pulmonary vasoconstriction in cats; modification by indomethacin and aspirin. *Fed. Proc.*, **34**, 1229

Samuelsson, B. (1973). Quantitative aspects of prostaglandin synthesis in man. *Adv. Biosci.*, **9**, Bergström, S. (ed.), pp. 7–14 (Vieweg: Pergamon Press)

Samuelsson, B., Granström, E., Gréen, K. and Hamberg, M. (1971). Metabolism of prostaglandins. *Ann. N.Y. Acad. Sci.*, **180**, 138

Severinghaus, J. W., Swenson, E. W., Finley, T. N., Lategola, M. T. and Williams, J. (1961). Unilateral hypoventilation in dogs produced by occluding one pulmonary artery. *J. Appl. Physiol.*, **16**, 53

Simonsson, B. G., Jacobs, F. M. and Nadel, J. A. (1967). Role of autonomic nervous system and the cough reflex in the increased responsiveness of airways in patients with obstructive airways disease. *J. Clin. Invest.*, **46**, 1812

Smith, A. P. (1973). The effects of intravenous infusion of graded doses of prostaglandins $F_{2\alpha}$ and E_2 on lung resistance in patients undergoing termination of pregnancy. *Clin. Sci.*, **44**, 17

Smith, A. P. and Cuthbert, M. F. (1972). Antagonistic action of aerosols of prostaglandins $F_{2\alpha}$ and E_2 on bronchial muscle tone in man. *Br. Med. J.*, **2**, 212

Smith, A. P. (1974a). A comparison of the effects of prostaglandin E_2 and salbutamol by intravenous infusion on the airways obstruction of patients with asthma. *Br. J. Clin. Pharmac.*, **1**, 399

Smith, A. P. (1974b). Effects of three prostaglandin analogues on airway tone in asthmatics and normal subjects. *Int. Res. Commun. System*, **2**, 1457

Smith, A. P. (1975). Effect of indomethacin in asthma, evidence against a role for prostaglandins in its pathogenesis. *Br. J. Clin. Pharmac.*, **2**, 307

Smith, A. P. and Cuthbert, M. F. (1973). The effects of inhaled prostaglandins on bronchial tone in man. *Adv. Biosci.*, **9**, Bergström, S. (ed.) pp. 213–217 (Vieweg: Pergamon Press)

Smith, A. P., Cuthbert, M. F. and Dunlop, L. S. (1975). The effects of prostaglandins E_1, E_2, $F_{2\alpha}$ on airway resistance in normal and asthmatic subjects. *Clin. Sci.*, **48**, 421

Smith, U. and Ryan, J. W. (1970). An electron microscopic study of the vascular endothelium as a site for bradykinin and adenosine-5-triphosphate inactivation in rat lung. *Adv. Exp. Biol. Med.*, **8**, 249

Strandberg, K. and Hamberg, M. (1974). Increased excretion of 5α, 7α-dihydro-11-keto tetranor prostanoic acid in anaphylaxis in the guinea-pig. *Prostaglandins*, **6**, 159

Strandberg, K., Mathé, A. A. and Fredholm, B. (1972). Protective effect of polyphloretin phosphate in anaphylaxis in the guinea-pig. *Life Sci.*, **11**, 701

Svanborg, N., Hamberg, M. and Hedqvist, P. (1973). Aspects of prostaglandin action in asthma. *Acta Physiol. Scand.*, **Suppl. 396**, 22

Sweatman, W. J. F. and Collier, H. O. J. (1968). Effect of prostaglandins on human bronchial muscle. *Nature (Lond.)*, **217**, 69

Tauber, A. I., Kaliner, M., Stechschulte, D. J. and Austen, K. F. (1973). Immunologic release of histamine and slow reacting substance of anaphylaxis from human lungs. V. Effects of prostaglandins on release of histamine. *J. Immunol.*, **111**, 27

Vane, J. R. (1971). Inhibition of prostaglandin synthesis as a mechanism of action for aspirin-like drugs. *Nature New Biology*, **231**, 232

Vargraftig, B. B. and Dao, Hai W. (1971). Release of vasoactive substances from guinea-pig lungs by slow reacting substance C and arachidonic acid. *Pharmacology*, **6**, 99

Weir, E. K., McMurtry, I. F., Tucker, A., Reeves, J. T. and Grover, R. F. (1975). Inhibition of prostaglandin synthesis or blockade of prostaglandin action increases the pulmonary pressor response to hypoxia. *Abst. Inf. Conf. Prostaglandins*, Florence, May 1975, p. 128

5

Cardiovascular Actions of Prostaglandins

KAFAIT U. MALIK and JOHN C. McGIFF

5.1 INTRODUCTION   104

5.2 ANIMAL STUDIES   104
   5.2.1 *Blood pressure*   104
      5.2.1.1 E Prostaglandins and their derivatives   104
      5.2.1.2 A Prostaglandins and their derivatives   109
      5.2.1.3 F Prostaglandins and their derivatives   113
   5.2.2 *Cardiac output*   117
   5.2.3 *Inotropic effects*   118
   5.2.4 *Chronotropic effects*   121
   5.2.5 *Coronary circulation*   124
   5.2.6 *Myocardial metabolism*   126
   5.2.7 *Pulmonary circulation*   127
   5.2.8 *Splanchnic circulation*   129
      5.2.8.1 Gastric circulation   129
      5.2.8.2 Mesenteric circulation   129
      5.2.8.3 Pancreatic circulation   130
      5.2.8.4 Splenic circulation   130
      5.2.8.5 Hepatic and portal circulation   132
   5.2.9 *Forearm, hindlimb and cutaneous circulation*   133
   5.2.10 *Carotid circulation*   136
   5.2.11 *Cerebral circulation*   137
   5.2.12 *Female and male reproductive organs circulation*   139
   5.2.13 *Isolated vascular smooth muscle*   141
   5.2.14 *Cardiovascular reactivity to other vasoactive substances*   144
   5.2.15 *Prostaglandins in hypertension*   153
   5.2.16 *Cardiovascular neurotransmission*   156
      5.2.16.1 Adrenergic neuromuscular transmission   156
      5.2.16.2 Cholinergic neuromuscular transmission   169

5.3 HUMAN STUDIES   170
    5.3.1   E Prostaglandins   170
    5.3.2   A Prostaglandins   175
    5.3.3   F Prostaglandins   182

In the previous edition, this chapter was written by Prof. S. M. M. Karim and Prof. K. Somers. We have attempted to retain most of the content of the previous chapter. The section on animal studies has been rewritten and expanded whereas the section on human studies has been revised to include the results of some recent studies.

5.1 INTRODUCTION

Goldblatt (1933, 1935) and Euler (1935) independently observed that extracts of human seminal plasma and of the vesicular gland of sheep produced a fall in blood pressure and stimulated a variety of smooth muscle organs. Further studies by Euler (1936) showed that the biological activity of vesicular extract was due to lipid-soluble material with acidic properties which he named prostaglandin. In 1957, Bergström and Sjövall succeeded in isolating two active compounds in crystalline forms from sheep vesicular gland and designated them prostaglandins E and F. Since then, prostaglandins have been isolated from various tissues, their structure characterized and their cardio-vascular actions examined in many different animal species. From these studies it has become evident that there are marked qualitative as well as quantitative differences in the responses of various species as well as between various prostaglandins.

5.2 ANIMAL STUDIES

5.2.1 Blood pressure

5.2.1.1 E prostaglandins and their derivatives

Prostaglandins of the E series (PGE_1, PGE_2, and PGE_3) lower arterial blood pressure in all animal species thus far studied. These include dog (Steinberg et al., 1963; Berti et al., 1964; Bergström et al., 1964; Carlson and Orö, 1966; Nakano and McCurdy, 1967; Maxwell, 1967; Glaviano and Masters, 1968; Hollenberg et al., 1968; Weeks et al., 1969; Wendt and Baum, 1972), cat (Berti et al., 1964; Kannegiesser and Lee, 1971; Wendt and Baum, 1972; Koss et al., 1973), rabbit (Bergström and Euler, 1963; Horton and Main, 1963), rat (Weeks and Wingerson, 1964; DuCharme and Weeks, 1967; Weeks et al., 1969), mouse (Weeks, 1969), chick (Horton and Main, 1967), monkey (Welch et al., 1974) and calf (Lewis and Eyre, 1972). In most of these species the dose of PGE_1 or PGE_2 required to lower arterial blood pressure ranged from 0.1 to 10 μg/kg. The action of PGE_1, PGE_2 and PGE_3 on arterial blood pressure was qualitatively similar. However, the activity of these agents varied in different animal species. Thus, the threshold dose of

PGE_1 required to lower arterial blood pressure after intravenous administration, was 180 ng/kg per min in cats, 440 ng/kg per min in dogs and 1 μg/kg per min in rabbits (Horton and Jones, 1969). Prostaglandins E_1 and E_2 were equipotent in most animal species. However, in rat and dog, Weeks et al. (1969) found PGE_2 to be somewhat more active in lowering blood pressure than PGE_1. The cardiovascular effects of E PGs were dependent upon the route of administration. Thus, intra-aortic injections produced more pronounced changes than single intravenous injections. Also, injections of PGE_1 into the thoracic aorta produced a greater vasodepressor effect than injections into the lower abdominal aorta (Bergström et al., 1964; Carlson and Orö, 1966). In the cat and dog, 2 μg/kg of PGE_2 was a depressor when given as a single intravenous injection. However, when injected intra-muscularly, 0.1 mg/kg, PGE_2 had no effect on the cardiovascular system in the cat and dog (cf. Karim and Somers, 1972). Rapid single injection of 50 μg PGE_2 resulted in tachycardia and a fall in the arterial blood pressure. In man, a slow intravenous infusion of as much as 6 mg PGE_2 per hour had no effect on the cardiovascular system (Karim et al., 1969, 1971; Karim, Hillier, Somers and Trussell, 1971). The above differences are explained by rapid uptake and/or metabolism of E prostaglandins by the lungs and liver as well as rapid diffusion from the blood (Änggård and Samuelsson, 1964; Ferreira and Vane, 1967; Hansson and Samuelsson, 1965; Horton and Jones, 1969; McGiff et al., 1969).

The fall in arterial blood pressure produced by E prostaglandins is most probably due to a decrease in total peripheral resistance as a result of their direct vasodilator action on resistance vessels. The increase in cardiac output in dogs and rats (Lee et al., 1965; Nakano and McCurdy, 1967; Weeks et al., 1969; Weeks and Wingerson, 1964) associated with the hypotensive effect of PGE_1 is presumably due to decreased peripheral resistance resulting in increased venous return and reflex increase in heart rate. Close arterial injections of PGE_1 have also been shown to decrease the resistance in carotid, femoral, brachial, coronary and renal vascular beds of the dog (Nakano and McCurdy, 1967) and the hindlimb vasculature of the cat (Holmes et al., 1963; Horton and Jones, 1969) and the rabbit (Beck et al., 1966). Euler (1939) observed that, in the cat, seminal fluid extracts did not decrease arterial blood pressure after the animal was eviscerated. Clamping of the abdominal aorta also abolished the vasodepressor action of seminal fluid extracts. Euler (1939) noticed a rise in portal vein pressure and blanching of the liver with the crude extract. These observations suggest that vasoconstriction in the portal circulation may be of importance for the systemic hypotensive effect of prostaglandins.

The hypotensive effect of E prostaglandins is also independent of peripheral autonomic mechanisms. Both Goldblatt (1935) and Euler (1936) found that atropine did not modify the depressor effect of crude seminal prostaglandins in anaesthetized cats and rabbits. Bergström et al. (1959) reported that the depressor action of PGE_1 was not prevented by doses of atropine and antihistaminics sufficient to block acetylcholine and histamine-induced vasodepression, respectively. Prostaglandin-induced fall in blood pressure was not abolished by vagotomy or after the administration of various anaesthetics (Giles et al., 1969), or by β-adrenergic blockade (Carlson and Orö, 1966;

Berti *et al.*, 1964; Nakano and McCurdy, 1967). Ganglionic blocking agents also did not modify cardiovascular responses to PGE_1 (Carlson, 1967; Carlson and Orö, 1966; DuCharme and Weeks, 1967; Lee *et al.*, 1966). Carlson and Orö (1966) found that PGE_1 decreased arterial blood pressure in reserpine pretreated animals which was confirmed by DuCharme and Weeks (1967). From these studies it was concluded that vasodilatation and the associated fall in arterial blood pressure produced by E prostaglandins was not mediated through cholinergic mechanism, release of histamine, stimulation of β-adrenergic receptors or through blockade of α-adrenergic receptors. Although E prostaglandins reduce sympathetic activity by decreasing the output of the adrenergic transmitter (cf. Hedqvist, 1973; cf. Brody and Kadowitz, 1974), their vasodilator effects and vasodepression seemed to be independent of these mechanisms (Bergström *et al.*, 1964; Steinberg *et al.*, 1963). In agreement with this conclusion was the observation that catecholamines, angiotensin II or vasopressin still increased blood pressure in dogs receiving infusions of PGE_1, PGE_2 or PGE_3 (Holmes *et al.*, 1963;

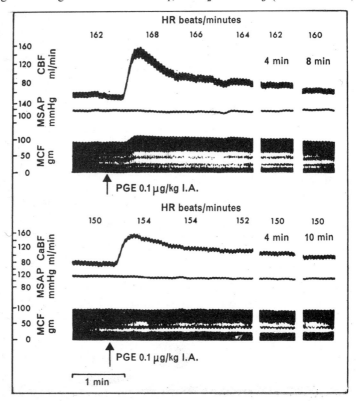

Figure 5.1 Upper tracing. Effects of intra-arterial injection of 0.1 μg/kg of PGE_1 into the anterior descending branch of the left coronary artery on heart rate (HR), coronary arterial blood flow (CBF), mean systemic arterial pressure (MSAP) and myocardial contractile force (MCF) in a dog. Lower tracing: Effects of the intra-arterial administration of 0.1 μg/kg of PGE_1 on heart rate, the right common carotid arterial blood flow (Ca BF), mean systemic arterial pressure and myocardial contractile force of a dog. Reproduced from Nakano and McCurdy (1967), by courtesy of *J. Pharmac. Exp. Ther.*

Nakano and McCurdy, 1967) and that ganglionic stimulation by electrical or chemical means caused a rise in blood pressure in dogs during infusion of PGE_1 (Carlson and Orö, 1966). Similarly, when blood pressure was raised by norepinephrine infusion, simultaneous administration of PGE_1, PGE_2 or PGE_3 caused a fall in blood pressure in the dog, rabbit, cat or rat (Steinberg *et al.*, 1963; Bergström *et al.*, 1964; Holmes *et al.*, 1963). Moreover, after intravenous infusion of PGE_1 to the rat, the pressor response to angiotensin II was decreased but that to norepinephrine remained unaltered (Türker *et al.*, 1968).

The possibility that prostaglandins may have cardiovascular effects which are mediated by the central nervous system was suggested by Kaplan *et al.* (1969). In cross-circulation experiments in dogs they sectioned the buffer nerves and found that the cardiovascular response to cranial arterial infusions of PGE_1 was abolished by the administration of a ganglionic blocking drug, hexamethonium. Lavery *et al.* (1969, 1970) studied the role of the central nervous system in the cardiovascular effects of PGE_1 in the intact anaesthetized dog. These authors showed that PGE_1, in doses which had no effect when given intravenously, produced tachycardia when injected into the vertebral artery. The mechanism of action is not certain. Carlson and Orö (1966) reported that infusion of PGE_1 into the common carotid artery of the dog increased the systemic arterial blood pressure which could be abolished or reversed by ganglionic blocking drugs. This suggests stimulation of sympathetic vasoconstrictor activity through an effect of PGE_1 on the carotid sinus or on the central nervous system. However, Nakano and McCurdy (1967) did not observe such systemic effects after intracarotid injection in anaesthetized dogs (Figures 5.1 and 5.2).

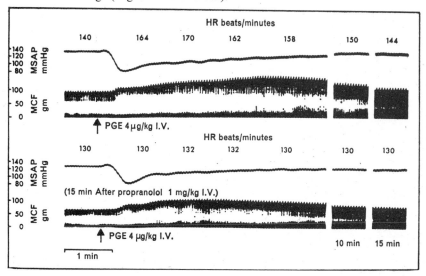

Figure 5.2   Effects of the intravenous administration of 4 μg/kg of PGE_1 on heart rate (HR), mean systemic arterial pressure (MSAP) and myocardial contractile force (MCF) before (upper tracing) and after (lower tracing) the intravenous administration of 1 mg/kg of propranolol in a vagotomized dog. Reproduced from Nakano and McCurdy (1967), by courtesy of *J. Pharmac. Exp. Ther.*

Prostaglandin E_2-methyl ester and 15-methyl prostaglandin E_2-methyl ester

Intravenous administration of PGE_2 methyl ester (PGE_2ME) and 15-methyl PGE_2 methyl ester (PGE_2-15S), 0.032 to 3.2 $\mu g/kg$, in anaesthetized dogs, produced a similar dose-dependent decrease in arterial blood pressure (Weeks *et al.*, 1973). Prostaglandin E_2ME produced a dose related increase in cardiac output and decreased total peripheral resistance, while left ventricular dp/dt and cardiac rate remained essentially unchanged. The effects of PGE_2-15S on these cardiac parameters were similar to PGE_2ME up to a dose of 0.32 $\mu g/kg$ but at doses of 1.0 and 3.2 $\mu g/kg$ it produced a sharp decrease in cardiac output, left ventricular dp/dt and increased total peripheral resistance. On the basis of these results it was concluded that the hypotensive effect of PGE_2ME was due to a decrease in total peripheral resistance presumably due to a direct peripheral vasodilator action of the compound. The increase in cardiac output caused by PGE_2ME could be secondary to the decrease in total peripheral resistance since myocardial contractile force was not altered by this agent as indicated by minimal changes in left ventricular dp/dt. The hypotensive effect of PGE_2-15S at low doses was primarily due to peripheral vasodilatation whereas, that of larger doses was attributed to a fall

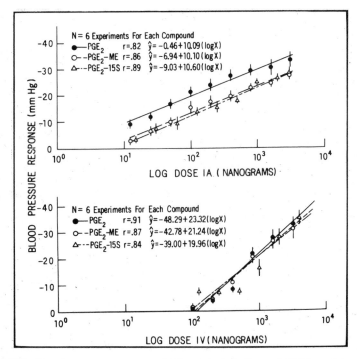

Figure 5.3 Vasodepressor responses of the rat to injections of PGE_2 and its methyl ester analogues given i.a. and i.v. Each symbol indicates the mean and SEM for six observations in six rats. The equation and correlation coefficient (*r*) of the regression line for each compound are shown. Reproduced from Strand, Miller and McGiff (1974), by courtesy of *Eur. J. Pharmacol.*

in cardiac rate and left ventricular dp/dt. PGE$_2$ME and PGE$_2$-15S have also been reported to cause a fall in arterial blood pressure in the rat (Weeks *et al.*, 1973; Strand *et al.*, 1974). Intravenous administration of these agents produced a similar degree of fall in arterial blood pressure as that produced by PGE$_2$, whereas, to produce a similar degree of fall in blood pressure by intra-aortic administration, the doses of PGE$_2$, PGE$_2$ME and PGE$_2$-15S were 29, 6 and 5 times less, respectively, than those required by the intravenous route (Figure 5.3). The difference in the degree of reduction in blood pressure between i.v. and i.a. administration produced by these agents was attributed to pulmonary inactivation. The degree of pulmonary inactivation of analogues (approximately 80%) was substantially less than that of natural PGE$_2$ (97%). Additional evidence for less pulmonary inactivation of the analogues than of PGE$_2$ was suggested by the observation that on i.v. administration, PGE$_2$ and its analogues were equipotent in their hypotensive activity whereas on intra-aortic administration the hypotensive effect of PGE$_2$ME and PGE$_2$-15S which did not differ from each other were 4 to 5 times less potent than PGE$_2$ (Strand *et al.*, 1974). (See also Chapter 11.)

Dihydro-PGE$_1$, 15-keto-PGE$_1$ and 15-epimer-PGE$_1$

Intravenous administration of dihydro-PGE$_1$ and 15-keto-PGE$_1$ in the dog, produced a fall in arterial blood pressure to a greater degree than PGE$_1$ (Nakano, 1971). The increase in myocardial contractility produced by dihydro PGE$_1$ was similar to PGE$_1$, whereas 15-keto-PGE$_1$ was less active than PGE$_1$ for this action. Nakano (1973) studied the effects of the 15-epimer PGE$_1$ (15R-PGE$_1$) in anaesthetized dogs and did not observe any significant effect on heart rate, arterial blood pressure or myocardial contractile force.

5.2.1.2 A prostaglandins and their derivatives

Prostaglandins of the A series are derived from E prostaglandins by dehydration which results in a marked decrease in potency on smooth muscle of the gastrointestinal, respiratory and reproductive tracts, but an increase in the reactivity of cardiovascular smooth muscle (Bygdeman *et al.*, 1966; Lee *et al.*, 1965; Pike *et al.*, 1967; Bygdeman and Hamberg, 1967; Weeks *et al.*, 1969). Prostaglandins A$_1$, A$_2$ and their 19-hydroxy derivatives are present in human seminal plasma (Hamberg and Samuelsson, 1966). Prostaglandin A$_2$ was recovered from purified extracts of the rabbit, rat and dog renal medulla (Lee *et al.*, 1967; Daniels *et al.*, 1967; Crowshaw *et al.*, 1970; Papanicolaou *et al.*, 1974). Cardiovascular effects of A prostaglandins are qualitatively similar to E prostaglandins. Prostaglandins A$_1$ and A$_2$ have a potent blood pressure lowering effect in both conscious and anaesthetized dogs and rats (Lee *et al.*, 1965; Bergström *et al.*, 1967; Nakano, 1968a, b; Horton and Jones, 1969; Pike *et al.*, 1967; Weeks, 1969; Higgins *et al.*, 1970, 1972; Higgins *et al.*, 1971; Barner *et al.*, 1972; Greenberg *et al.*, 1974), anaesthetized cats (Horton and Jones, 1969; Kannegiesser and Lee, 1971) and rabbits (Horton and Jones,

1969). Like E prostaglandins, the activity of A prostaglandins varies in different animal species. For example, threshold doses of PGA_1 required to lower blood pressure were 0.37 $\mu g/kg$ in dogs; 0.045 $\mu g/kg$ in cats and 6.3 $\mu g/kg$ in rabbits; of PGA_2 were 0.08 $\mu g/kg$ in cats and 0.11 $\mu g/kg$ in dogs (Horton and Jones, 1969). Prostaglandins A_1 and A_2 have been reported to be equipotent in rats and dogs (Weeks et al., 1969) but they are more potent in lowering blood pressure than either PGE_1 or PGE_2 in most animal species when given by the intravenous route. This includes dogs (Bergström, 1967a; Lee, 1968; Nakano, 1968a, b; Horton and Jones, 1969; Weeks et al., 1969) rabbits (Euler, 1936), cats (Horton and Jones, 1969), guinea pigs (Änggård, 1966), rats (Weeks et al., 1969) and man (Christlieb et al., 1969). Differences in the magnitude of fall in blood pressure produced by PGA_1 have also been observed in anaesthetized and unanaesthetized animals. Higgins et al. (1971) found that PGE_1 decreased arterial blood pressure and increased cardiac output to a greater extent in the conscious dog than either PGA_1 or PGE_1 in the anaesthetized dog. Kannegiesser and Lee (1971) showed that PGE_1 and PGE_2 were more potent than PGA_1 or PGA_2 on intra-aortic administration to the cat as compared to intravenous administration. This difference is due to the fact that intravenous injection necessitates passage through the lungs which selectively inactivates E prostaglandins but not A prostaglandins which pass freely across the pulmonary circulation (Ferreira and Vane, 1967; McGiff et al., 1969). The inability of the pulmonary circulation to inactivate A prostaglandins is most likely due to their lesser specificity for 15-hydroxy-prostaglandin dehydrogenase than those of the E series (Nakano et al., 1969).

Like E prostaglandins, the hypotensive effect of A prostaglandins is most likely due to marked dilatation of the peripheral vasculature resulting in a decrease in total peripheral resistance (Nakano, 1968a, b; Horton and Jones, 1969; Weeks et al., 1969). The fall in arterial blood pressure produced by A prostaglandins is not due to changes in heart rate or myocardial contractile force since these functions are increased reflexly by PGA_1. Thus, after β-adrenergic blockade with propranolol, the increase in heart rate produced by PGA_1 was greatly diminished (Higgins et al., 1971). Moreover, after β-adrenergic and cholinergic receptor blockade or when heart rate was kept constant by electrical pacing, PGA_1 resulted in a fall in arterial blood pressure comparable to that seen before autonomic blockade and in unpaced hearts (Higgins et al., 1971). The increase in myocardial contractile force produced by PGA_1 was markedly diminished when indirect effects of PGA_1 were precisely controlled (Higgins et al., 1972). Thus, when alterations of reflex sympathetic activity, afterload and tachycardia were prevented by β-adrenergic blockade, inflation of an intra-aortic balloon catheter and electrical pacing of the atrium, respectively, resulted in insignificant changes in response to PGA_1 in the parameters of contractile force in the conscious dog (Higgins et al., 1972). These observations taken together with failure of PGA_1 to alter the contractile force of isolated dog and cat atria (Su et al., 1973) and of the rabbit heart (Lee et al., 1965) and the inability of the ganglionic blocking agent, pentolinium, to abolish the hypotensive effect of PGA_1 and PGA_2 (Kannegiesser and Lee, 1971) suggest that the fall in arterial blood pressure produced by A prostaglandins is due to a decrease in peripheral resistance as a result of their direct vasodilator actions. To determine whether the site of action of PGA_2 as a blood pressure lowering agent is central or peripheral, Lee *et al.* (1966) injected 50 µg PGA_2 into the femoral, carotid, mesenteric and renal arteries of anaesthetized dogs. Femoral blood flow increased from 50 ml/min to 140 ml/min. Similar increases in blood flow were observed in all other regional vascular beds. There was also a significant fall in mean arterial blood pressure. At the time of maximum vasodepression, cardiac output increased so that there was a decrease in calculated peripheral resistance (Figure 5.4). Thus the hypotensive effect of A prostaglandins is primarily due to vasodilatation. The fall in arterial blood pressure produced by PGA_1 and PGA_2 in the anaesthetized cat was found by Kannegiesser and Lee (1971) to be gradual with a relatively slow return to pre-injection levels. Jones (1972a) observed that the fall in arterial blood pressure in this species produced by PGA_1 (100 ng/kg) was biphasic; the initial fall reached a maximum 15 s after injection followed by a prolonged and more pronounced fall with a maximum

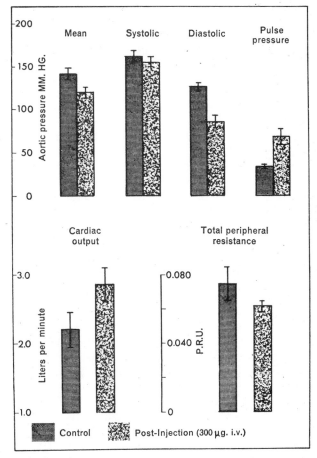

Figure 5.4   Cardiovascular effects of intravenous injection of 300 µg PGA_2 in the dog (average of eight experiments). Reproduced from Lee, Covino, Takman and Smith (1965), by courtesy of *Circulation Res.*

at 85 s. On the basis of these observations it has been concluded that the peripheral arteriolar dilatation produced by A prostaglandins occurred, at least in part, by an indirect mechanism (Kannegiesser and Lee, 1971) probably through their conversion by prostaglandin isomerase in the plasma, to C prostaglandins, which have a 3-fold greater depressor activity than the precursor (Jones, 1972a).

19-hydroxy-PGA$_1$ and 15-epimer-PGA$_2$

19-hydroxy-PGA$_1$, like PGA$_1$ decreased blood pressure in dogs, cats and rabbits. Horton and Jones (1969) have shown that in the cat where 0.045 μg/kg was the threshold dose of PGA$_1$ needed to lower mean arterial blood pressure, the threshold dose of 19-hydroxy-PGA$_1$ was 0.25 μg/kg. Nakano (1969) found that 15-epimer-PGA$_2$ (15-R-PGA$_2$) a stereoisomer of PGA$_2$, isolated from a sea animal, gorgonian *Plexaura homomalla*, was devoid of any effect on systemic arterial pressure, heart rate and myocardial contractile force in anaesthetized dogs when administered intravenously in doses of 2.25–256 μg/kg. In contrast, 0.25–4.0 μg/kg of PGE$_2$ and PGA$_2$ decreased mean systemic arterial pressure and increased heart rate and myocardial contractile force. Thus, it appears that stereochemical modification at C-15 renders PGA$_2$ inactive.

Prostaglandin C$_1$, PGC$_2$, PGB$_1$, PGB$_2$ and 19-hydroxy-PGB$_1$

Prostaglandins of the B and C series are formed from A prostaglandins by the action of a prostaglandin isomerase which has been shown to be present in the plasma of a number of animal species (Jones, 1972b; Jones *et al.*, 1972; Jones and Cammock, 1973). Jones (1972a) compared the effect of PGE$_1$, PGA$_1$, PGB$_1$ and PGC$_1$ on the blood pressure of anaesthetized cats after a rapid injection into the thoracic aorta. By comparing the fall in blood pressure 15 s after injection, estimates of their potencies relative to PGE$_1$ (= 100), were PGA$_1$ (16), PGB$_1$ (0.9) and PGC$_1$ (44). Similarly, PGA$_2$, PGB$_2$ and PGC$_2$ were found to possess 16, 1.2 and 47% of the activity of PGE$_2$. The fall in blood pressure produced by PGC$_2$ in the anaesthetized cat was associated with a fall in left ventricular and diastolic pressure (LVEDP) and dp/dt max. The effect on dp/dt max was absent when the heart was paced and LVEDP and mean arterial pressure kept constant (Jones *et al.*, 1974). These observations indicate that the fall in arterial blood pressure produced by PGC$_2$ is primarily due to a decrease in peripheral resistance. The fall in LVEDP, in conjunction with a fall in cardiac output, could be due to reduced venous return as a result of pooling of blood in the portal circulation (as shown by Euler (1939) with crude PG) or to relaxation of capacitance vessels. In contrast, PGC$_2$ in dog as in cat, although producing a fall in mean arterial pressure, increased dp/dt max in spite of the fact that LVEDP and mean arterial blood pressure were held constant (Jones *et al.*, 1974). These observations indicate that PGC$_2$ may have a direct inotropic action. Prostaglandin, B$_1$, PGB$_2$ and 19-hydroxy-PGB$_1$ have also been reported to produce a fall in arterial blood pressure in the anaesthetized dog (Greenberg *et al.*, 1973) and cat (Horton and Jones, 1969). In the dog, PGB_1 was less potent in decreasing blood pressure than PGB_2. However, PGB_1 was a more potent depressant of left ventricular pressure than PGB_2. Prostaglandin B_1 and PGB_2 also decreased the heart rate in the dog, PGB_1 being less potent than PGB_2 (Greenberg *et al.*, 1973). These agents constricted the perfused hindlimb and hindpaw vasculature (Greenberg, *et al.*, 1973).

5.2.1.3 F prostaglandins and their derivatives

The cardiovascular effects of F prostaglandins are complicated by qualitative species variations. Thus, $PGF_{1\alpha}$ or $PGF_{2\alpha}$ are depressor in the rabbit (Änggård and Bergström, 1963; Bergström and Euler, 1963; Horton and Main, 1963, 1965b; Levy and Lindner, 1971) and cat (Änggård and Bergström, 1963; Koss *et al.*, 1973; Villanueva *et al.*, 1972; Mathé *et al.*, 1972) and pressor in rat, dog (DuCharme and Weeks, 1967; DuCharme *et al.*, 1968; Nakano and McCurdy, 1968; Nakano and Cole, 1969; White and Pennink, 1972) guinea pig (Mathé *et al.*, 1972; McQueen, 1973) spinal chick (Horton and Main, 1967) calf (Lewis and Eyre, 1972) baboon and monkey (Karim, personal communication) and man (Karim, Hillier *et al.*, 1971; Karim, Somers and Hillier, 1971). In the anaesthetized chick (Horton and Main, 1967) the response may be pressor, depressor or biphasic.

The mechanism of cardiovascular effects of F prostaglandins in various animal species is still unclear. In the cat, where $PGF_{2\alpha}$ is depressor, intra-arterial injection into the vasculature of different muscles produced vaso-dilatation (Änggård and Bergström, 1963; Horton and Main, 1965a). Moreover, it increased pulmonary resistance (Änggård and Bergström, 1963). On the basis of these observations it was suggested that the hypotensive effect of $PGF_{2\alpha}$ in the cat might be due to an increase in pulmonary vascular resistance and cardiac slowing and to some extent by its direct vasodilator action on muscle blood vessels (Änggård and Bergström, 1963). Koss and Nakano (1973) found that intra-arterial administration of $PGF_{2\alpha}$ in the perfused hindlimb of the cat produced vasodilatation which was highly variable from animal to animal and was more transient than the overall systemic response. They observed that in addition to direct vasodilator action, several other cardiovascular effects of $PGF_{2\alpha}$ contributed in a larger measure to its vasodepressor action and the extent of their contribution varied from animal to animal. Thus, in some experiments, the fall in blood pressure was related mainly to a decrease in cardiac output which occurred concomitantly with the increase in pulmonary arterial resistance. In other cases, vagal activation seemed to play a predominant role in the depressor response and also contributed to the slow recovery phase. In contrast, in rabbit, $PGF_{2\alpha}$ failed to increase right ventricular pressure after intravenous administration as it did in the cat (Änggård and Bergström, 1963). Moreover, polyphloretin phosphate (PPP) which antagonized the hypotensive action of $PGF_{2\alpha}$ in the cat (Villanueva *et al.*, 1972; Mathé *et al.*, 1972) failed to abolish the depressor effect of $PGF_{2\alpha}$ in the rabbit (Levy and Lindner, 1971). In the rabbit, meclofenamic acid selectively blocked the hypotensive effect of

$PGF_{2\alpha}$ (Levy and Lindner, 1971). These observations indicate that the hypotensive effect of $PGF_{2\alpha}$ in the cat and rabbit may be mediated by a somewhat different mechanism. The hypotensive effect of $PGF_{2\alpha}$ in these species, does not appear to be due to its central actions. Thus, Koss *et al.* (1973) demonstrated that injections of up to 3 μg/kg of $PGF_{2\alpha}$, directly into the vertebral artery did not produce any cardiovascular effects as reported in the dog (Lavery *et al.*, 1969, 1970).

The mechanism of the pressor action of F prostaglandins in rat and dog has been studied by several investigators. DuCharme and Weeks (1967) showed that the pressor activity of $PGF_{2\alpha}$ in the rat was not mediated by an alteration of sympathetic vasoconstrictor activity since the effect persists after administration of a ganglionic blocking agent or pretreatment of the animals with reserpine. In experiments on the perfused hindlimb of the dog it was observed that $PGF_{2\alpha}$ constricted veins rather than arterioles (DuCharme and Weeks, 1967; DuCharme *et al.*, 1968). Prostaglandin $F_{2\alpha}$ therefore, by constricting the veins, could increase the venous return and consequently increase the cardiac output. DuCharme *et al.* (1968) have shown that in unanaesthetized dogs intravenously administered $PGF_{2\alpha}$ increased cardiac output and mean systemic arterial blood pressure without altering peripheral resistance (Figure 5.5). Using a right-heart-bypass preparation, these authors concluded that the pressor action of $PGF_{2\alpha}$ was primarily due to venoconstriction leading to an increase in cardiac output. Nakano and McCurdy (1968) and Nakano and Cole (1969) also demonstrated that $PGF_{2\alpha}$ increases arterial blood pressure in dogs but their observations suggest a different

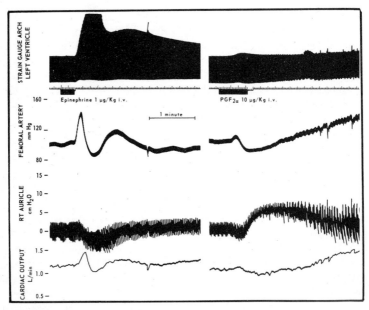

Figure 5.5   Effect of epinephrine and $PGF_{2\alpha}$ on myocardial contractility, mean arterial blood pressure, right auricular pressure and cardiac output of an anaesthetized dog. Reproduced from DuCharme, Weeks and Montgomery (1968), by courtesy of *J. Pharmac. Exp. Ther.*

mechanism of action. They found that $PGF_{2\alpha}$ increased cardiac output and total and regional vascular resistance. The increase in cardiac output produced by $PGF_{2\alpha}$ was suggested to be primarily due to increased myocardial contractility and not secondary to increased venous return (Nakano and Cole, 1969). The increase in myocardial contractile force and cardiac output in the absence of a change in systemic arterial pressure by $PGF_{1\alpha}$ has been shown in the dog heart–lung preparation by Katori et al. (1970). Emerson et al. (1971) observed that when cardiac inflow was adjusted continually to match venous return, a continuous 5 min intra-arterial infusion of $PGF_{2\alpha}$ in anaesthetized dogs caused a transient increase in venous return whereas, total peripheral resistance and systemic arterial blood pressure remained elevated throughout the infusion of this agent. The transient increase in venous return occurring at the onset of $PGF_{2\alpha}$ infusion was accompanied by an increase in heart rate and myocardial contractile force. From these studies it appears that the transient constriction of capacitance vessels was followed by the delayed constriction of various resistance blood vessels. Prostaglandin $F_{2\alpha}$ has been shown to cause constriction of both venous (DuCharme et al., 1968; Greenberg and Sparks, 1969; Mark et al., 1971) as well as various peripheral arterial vessels (Nakano, 1968a, b; Greenberg and Sparks, 1969; Hodgman et al., 1970; Powell and Brody, 1973; Csépli and Erdelyi, 1973).

The cardiovascular changes produced by the central actions of $PGF_{2\alpha}$ were studied by Lavery et al. (1970) and Lavery et al. (1971). They found that infusions of $PGF_{1\alpha}$ (4–360 ng/kg per min) and $PGF_{2\alpha}$ (4–64 ng/kg per min) into the vertebral artery of the anaesthetized dog increased blood pressure, heart rate and cardiac output. There was also a fall in central venous pressure but no change in total peripheral resistance. The same doses infused intravenously or into the internal carotid artery did not have any effect on any of the above cardiovascular parameters. The reduction in central venous pressure contrasts with an increase in central venous pressure when $PGF_{2\alpha}$ was injected intravenously (DuCharme et al., 1968). The increase in arterial blood pressure and heart rate produced by intravertebral arterial injection of $PGF_{2\alpha}$ in greyhounds was not altered after β-adrenergic receptor blockade with propranolol or by cervical cord section at C4–6 (Lavery et al., 1971). Since tachycardia and the pressor responses were greatly reduced by vagotomy or atropine, it was concluded that the cardiovascular effects produced by intravertebral arterial infusion of $PGF_{2\alpha}$ is due to withdrawal of vagal tone to the heart. Lavery et al. (1971) also observed that the residual pressor response after vagotomy was abolished by subsequent sympathetic blockade with bethanidine or bretylium (Figure 5.6). Since these agents (but not propranolol or cervical cord section) also reduced both the tachycardia and the pressor response to $PGF_{2\alpha}$ in animals with intact vagi, it was concluded that bretylium and bethanidine probably interfere with central adrenergic pathways involved in the response to $PGF_{2\alpha}$. The increase in mean arterial blood pressure on intravertebral arterial infusion of $PGF_{2\alpha}$ (in doses devoid of any effect by intravenous or intracarotid administration) have also been reported in conscious dogs by Sweet et al. (1971). Since these authors failed to observe any changes in heart rate, they suggested that the central hypertensive effect of $PGF_{2\alpha}$ was mediated through activation of the sympathetic fibres to peripheral vessels as well as to the heart. No attempt was made to examine the central hypertensive effects of $PGF_{2\alpha}$ after adrenergic blockade. Although these studies indicate that in the dog $PGF_{2\alpha}$ may cause a rise in arterial blood pressure by a central mechanism, the work of DuCharme *et al.* (1968), Nakano and Cole (1969) and Emerson *et al.* (1971) suggests that the hypertensive effect of $PGF_{2\alpha}$ is primarily due to direct vascular and cardiac actions.

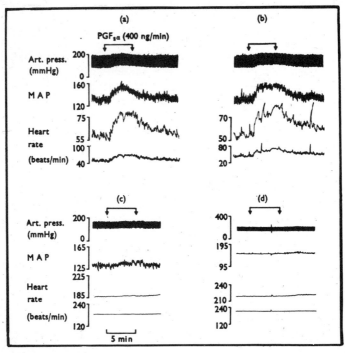

Figure 5.6   Effect of infusion of prostaglandin $F_{2\alpha}$ (400 ng/min for 5 min) into the vertebral artery in the chloralose-anaesthetized greyhound. Pulsatile arterial pressure (Art. press.), mean arterial pressure (MAP) and heart rate (at two different gain factors) are illustrated. The response in the intact dog (a) is shown and then the sequential effects of (b) propranolol, (c) vagotomy and (d) bethanidine. Reproduced from Lavery, Lowe and Scroop (1971), by courtesy of *Br. J. Pharmacol.*

Prostaglandin $F_{2\alpha}$ methyl ester and 15-methyl-$PGF_{2\alpha}$ methyl ester

Prostaglandin $F_{2\alpha}$ methyl ester ($PGF_{2\alpha}ME$) and 15-methyl-PGF_2 methyl ester ($PGF_{2\alpha}$-15S) produced a dose-related (0.032–3.2 $\mu g/kg$) rise in systemic and pulmonary arterial pressure in anaesthetized dogs (Weeks *et al.*, 1973). Although comparable pressor effects on both systemic and pulmonary arterial pressure were obtained by these agents, the effects of $PGF_{2\alpha}$-15S were more prolonged than $PGF_{2\alpha}ME$. Neither agent produced any significant effect on heart rate, cardiac output or myocardial contractile force. A rise in systemic and pulmonary arterial pressure by these agents was also observed in rats (Weeks *et al.*, 1973). Prostaglandin $F_{2\alpha}$-15S was somewhat less active at the higher dose, but a significant difference was obtained only at doses of 5.6 $\mu g/kg$. The mean duration of action ranged from about 1 min after the lowest dose to about 5 min at the highest dose for both compounds, but with large individual variations.

5.2.2 Cardiac output

Prostaglandins have been reported to increase, decrease, produce a biphasic effect or no effect on the cardiac output. Thus, PGE_1 increased cardiac output in rats (Weeks and Wingerson, 1964) and anaesthetized or unanaesthetized dogs (Lee et al., 1965; Nakano and McCurdy, 1967, 1968; Maxwell, 1967). Nakano and McCurdy (1967) found that PGE_1 produced a biphasic change in cardiac output followed by a transient return to the control value before a second greater and sustained increase in cardiac output occurred. Intra-coronary administration of PGE_1 and PGA_1 in anaesthetized dogs produced an increase followed by a more persistent fall in cardiac output (Nutter and Crumly, 1972). An increase in cardiac output has also been observed after the administration of PGA_1 (Nakano and McCurdy, 1968; Higgins et al., 1970, 1971, 1972, 1973) and $PGF_{2\alpha}$ (Nakano and McCurdy, 1968) in the dog. However, Murphy et al. (1970) and Rowe and Afonso (1974) failed to observe any effect of PGE_1 and PGA_1 and PGE_1 and PGE_2, respectively, on the cardiac output in the dog. Similarly, PGE_2 did not alter the cardiac output in the calf (Anderson et al., 1972) nor did $PGF_{2\alpha}$ in the pregnant woman (Fishburne et al., 1972). However, in cat (Koss et al., 1973) and cattle (Anderson et al., 1972) $PGF_{2\alpha}$ increased pulmonary arterial pressure and decreased cardiac output; whereas in dog it caused an unsustained decrease in cardiac output (Maxwell, 1969). These variable effects of prostaglandins on cardiac output may be related to their other cardiovascular actions. If a prostaglandin causes a decrease in venous compliance, then cardiac filling pressure will decrease which will result in a fall in cardiac output, whereas, if arterial pressure falls more and venous pressure is maintained, cardiac output would be increased. On the other hand, if there is constriction of veins, such as that produced by PGB_1 and $PGF_{2\alpha}$ (Robinson et al., 1973) then it will tend to raise venous return and increase cardiac output. Thus, the net effect of a prostaglandin on cardiac output will depend on the sum of its actions on myocardial contractility and heart rate as well as on the capacitance vessels and regional vascular resistance. Studies in anaesthetized and conscious animals have shown that increase in cardiac output caused by PGE_1 or PGA_1 was independent of reflexly-induced sympathetic stimulation of heart rate since it persisted after β-adrenergic receptor blockade (Nakano and McCurdy, 1968; Higgins et al., 1971). Katori et al. (1970) demonstrated that PGE_1 increased myocardial contractile force and cardiac output without causing any change in arterial blood pressure or heart rate in the dog heart–lung preparation. Therefore, increases in cardiac output produced by prostaglandins in some animal species, independent of sympathetic stimulation of heart rate, could result from decreased afterload consequent to generalized vasodilatation, tachycardia due to reflex withdrawal of vagal restraint and possibly a direct positive inotropic effect. Although the work of

Higgins *et al.* (1972) in conscious dogs indicates that the direct positive inotropic effect of PGA_1 plays a minor role in the increased cardiac output
produced by this agent, studies in anaesthetized animals indicate that
prostaglandins of the E, A or F series do exert a positive inotropic effect
(Nakano and McCurdy, 1967, 1968; Jones *et al.*, 1974) whereas studies in
isolated cardiac tissue, as will be discussed later in this chapter, are conflicting
and show species differences.

5.2.3 Inotropic effects

The inotropic effects of prostaglandins are qualitatively as well as quantitatively different and vary in different animal species. The intravenous
injection or infusion of PGE_1 or PGA_1 in anaesthetized dog (Nakano and
McCurdy, 1967, 1968; Nakano and Cole, 1969; Emerson *et al.*, 1971),
increased myocardial contractile force as the arterial blood pressure decreased. The intra-arterial injection of PGE_1 into the anterior descending
branch of the left coronary artery, in doses that did not affect systemic
blood pressure, produced a significant increase in myocardial contractility
as well as an increase in coronary blood flow (Figures 5.1 and 5.2). Nutter
and Crumly (1972) demonstrated that intracoronary administration of PGE_1
and PGA_1 in anaesthetized dog caused a sustained and significant increase in
isometric contractile force. The positive inotropic action was immediate in
onset, paralleled the duration of the coronary and systemic vasodilator effect
and occurred at all dose levels (0.1 to 12.5 µg). Moreover, the increase in
contractile force was also observed with doses having little effect on systemic
blood pressure. A similar but less pronounced inotropic effect of PGE_1 has
been reported in the dog (Hollenberg, *et al.*, 1968). The persistence of increased myocardial contractility produced by these agents after β-adrenergic
blockade (Nakano and McCurdy, 1967, 1968; Nutter and Crumly, 1972)
indicate that prostaglandins of the E and A series exert a direct positive
inotropic effect on the myocardium. This conclusion is in agreement with the
observations of Katori *et al.* (1970) that administration of PGE_1 into the left
atrium or intravenous injection of PGE_1 into the dog heart–lung preparation
increased myocardial contractility, coronary blood flow and cardiac output
without altering the heart rate and arterial blood pressure. When left ventricular end-diastolic pressure and mean arterial blood pressure were held
constant, PGE_2 and PGC_2, in the anaesthetized dog but not in the cat,
increased myocardial contractility (Jones *et al.*, 1974). However, in conscious
dogs Higgins *et al.* (1972) failed to demonstrate any significant increase in
myocardial contractile force with PGA_1 when alterations in the effect of
sympathetic activation on myocardium, afterload and heart rate were prevented. Since the major portion of the increase in myocardial contractility
produced by PGA_1 was blocked by β-adrenergic receptor blockade, it was
secondary to reflex sympathetic activation of the myocardium. In contrast,
Giles *et al.* (1969) found that intracoronary administration of PGE_1 decreased
heart rate, myocardial contractile force and systemic and pulmonary arterial
pressure but did not alter right ventricular pressure and contractile force.
Similarly, a decrease in myocardial contractile force and an associated fall in

systemic pressure and coronary flow by intrapulmonary administration of PGA_1 in the anaesthetized dog was reported by Barner *et al.* (1972). These discrepancies in the inotropic actions of E and A prostaglandins may be due to differences in doses and in the experimental procedures used by various investigators.

Variations in the inotropic actions of prostaglandins and differences among various animal species have also been observed in the isolated perfused heart and in strips of cardiac muscle. Euler (1936) found that a crude extract of prostaglandins was without inotropic effect on the isolated rabbit heart or on the cat heart–lung preparation. These observations were confirmed by using PGE_1 in the isolated rabbit heart (Berti *et al.*, 1965; Lee *et al.*, 1965) and cat heart (Berti *et al.*, 1965; Sunahara and Talesnik, 1974). Similarly, Lee *et al.* (1965) observed that PGA_2 was devoid of any significant inotropic effect on the isolated perfused rabbit heart. Prostaglandin E_1 and PGA_1 also failed to produce an inotropic effect on the isolated rabbit atria (preliminary observations, Nutter and Crumly, 1972), dog and cat atria (Su *et al.*, 1973) and PGE_2 on the human atrial appendage (Levy and Killebrew, 1971) and cultured chicken heart (Sperelakis and Lehmkuhl, 1965). However, on the isolated cat papillary muscle, PGE_1, markedly increased the tension (Türker *et al.*, 1971) whereas on dog papillary muscle only a slight increase in tension was observed at higher concentrations of PGE_1 (Antonaccio and Lucchesi, 1970). Wennmalm and Hedqvist (1970) also observed a slight increase in both rate and contractile force of the rabbit heart in response to PGE_1 and PGE_2. A positive inotropic effect of PGE_1 on the isolated electrically driven and isolated spontaneously beating rabbit atria have been reported by Tuttle and Skelly (1968) and Levy and Killebrew (1971). The amplitude of contraction of the isolated rat heart was only modestly increased (Berti *et al.*, 1965; Vergroesen *et al.*, 1967; Vergroesen and de Boer, 1968) whereas, that of spontaneously beating atria of normal and genetically hypertensive rats was increased markedly by PGE_1 and PGE_2, respectively (Levy, 1973a). Prostaglandin E_1 also increased the amplitude of contraction of the frog heart (Berti *et al.*, 1965; Klaus and Piccinini, 1967; Vergroesen and de Boer, 1968) and ventricular strips (Baysal and Vural, 1974) guinea pig heart (Berti *et al.*, 1965; Mantegazza, 1965; Sobel and Robison, 1969; Nutter and Crumly, 1972) and chicken heart (Horton and Main, 1967). Sabatini-Smith (1970) showed that PGE_1 and PGE_2 increased the amplitude of contraction of isolated guinea pig atria.

The intracoronary administration of $PGF_{2\alpha}$ in the anaesthetized dog did not cause any change in coronary arterial blood flow and myocardial contractile force (Nakano, 1968a, b). DuCharme *et al.* (1968) and Hollenberg *et al.* (1968) also failed to demonstrate any effect of $PGF_{2\alpha}$ and $PGF_{1\alpha}$, respectively, on myocardial contractile force. In contrast, Nutter and Crumly (1972) observed a small but consistent increase in canine isometric contractile force after intracoronary administration of $PGF_{2\alpha}$ in doses too small to elicit systemic and hence reflex effect on the heart. Nakano and McCurdy (1968), Nakano and Cole (1969) and Emerson *et al.* (1971) found a small increase in the myocardial contractile force in the anaesthetized dog after intravenous administration of this agent. Katori *et al.* (1970), in the dog heart–lung preparation, showed an increase in myocardial contractile force in response to large doses of $PGF_{1\alpha}$ (50 μg). Prostaglandin $F_{1\alpha}$ and $PGF_{1\beta}$ were also reported to have a positive inotropic effect on the isolated rat heart, $PGF_{1\beta}$ being less active than $PGF_{1\alpha}$ (Vergroesen et al., 1967). Prostaglandin $F_{1\alpha}$ did not affect the isolated guinea pig heart (Sobel and Robison, 1969) while $PGF_{2\alpha}$ produced a slight positive inotropic effect on isolated guinea pig atria (Nutter and Crumly, 1972) and had no effect on the isolated or cultured chicken heart (Horton and Main, 1967; Sperelakis and Lehmkuhl, 1965) and isolated cat and dog atria (Su et al., 1973).

The mechanism by which prostaglandins produce positive inotropic effects in some animal species appears to be a direct action on the myocardium. Although the inotropic action of PGE_1 on the isolated cat papillary muscle (Türker et al., 1971) has been reported to be mediated through an adrenergic mechanism, the majority of studies in intact and isolated heart indicate that the positive inotropic actions of prostaglandins are independent of adrenergic and cholinergic mechanisms. Thus, the positive inotropic action of prostaglandins, in vivo and in vitro, was not abolished by β-adrenergic blockade (Nakano and McCurdy, 1967, 1968; Nutter and Crumly, 1972; Berti et al., 1965; Mantegazza, 1965; Levy and Killebrew, 1971; Berti et al., 1967; Baysal and Vural, 1974), α-adrenergic blockade (Levy and Killebrew, 1971) reserpine pretreatment (Berti et al., 1965, 1967; Mantegazza, 1965; Levy and Killebrew, 1971), vagotomy (Nakano and McCurdy, 1968) or atropine (Levy and Killebrew, 1971). Although PGE_1 increased the sensitivity of isolated rabbit atria to ouabain (Tuttle and Skelly, 1968) the effect of PGE_1 in frog ventricular strips was not altered by ouabain, thereby suggesting that PGE_1-induced change may not be directly related to the sodium pump (Baysal and Vural, 1974). There are some studies (Sobel and Robison, 1969; Piccinini et al., 1969; Klein and Levey, 1971; Curnow and Nuttall, 1971) which indicate that the positive inotropic action of prostaglandins may be mediated by the adenylate cyclase–cyclic 3′, 5′-adenosine monophosphate system. The positive inotropic action of PGE_1 and $PGF_{1\alpha}$ was associated with an increased myocardial adenylate cyclase activity in the isolated guinea pig heart (Sobel and Robison, 1969) and PGE_1 increased intracellular cyclic 3′, 5′-adenosine monophosphate (cAMP) levels in the rat heart and activated phosphorylase (Piccinini et al., 1969; Curnow and Nuttall, 1971). In guinea pig heart homogenates, PGE and PGA but not PGF, compounds markedly increased the accumulation of cAMP (Klein and Levey, 1971). The accumulation of cAMP in particulate preparations of cat left ventricle was unaffected by PGE_2, PGA_1, PGA_2 and $PGF_{2\alpha}$ and only slight increases were observed with PGE_1 (Levey and Epstein, 1969a, b). Whether the positive inotropic effect of prostaglandins is mediated by the adenylate cyclase–cAMP system and whether the variable effects of prostaglandins on this myocardial enzyme system are a reflection of variable inotropic effects of prostaglandins in different animal species remain to be investigated. Considerable attention has been given to the effect of prostaglandins on cardiac membrane permeability to Ca^{2+} as a possible mechanism for the inotropic effect of these agents. The available data suggests a close relationship between the positive inotropic action of PGE_1 and increased ^{45}Ca uptake although total myocardial Ca^{2+} content did not increase (Klaus and Piccinini, 1967). Prostaglandins may produce their positive inotropic effect by enhancing the availability of free Ca^{2+} to the excitation–contraction coupling process (Piccinini *et al.*, 1969). This effect may result from a direct increase in cellular membrane permeability to Ca^{2+} (Klaus and Piccinini, 1967) or by enhancing the uptake of Ca^{2+} by the sarcoplasmic reticulum (Sabatini-Smith, 1970). Since PGE_1 produced a marked positive inotropic action in the K^+-intoxicated frog heart and restored the normal function in K^+-arrested heart it has been proposed that PGE_1 may act by antagonizing the effect of K^+ rather than facilitating Ca^{2+} uptake (Vergroesen and de Boer, 1968).

5.2.4 Chronotropic effects

Prostaglandins of the E and A series produced a marked increase in heart rate and a fall in systemic arterial pressure in anaesthetized or unanaesthetized dog (Steinberg *et al.*, 1964; Lee *et al.*, 1965; Carlson and Orö, 1966; Nakano and McCurdy, 1967, 1968; Bergström *et al.*, 1966, 1967; Maxwell, 1967; Emerson *et al.*, 1971; Higgins *et al.*, 1970, 1971, 1972; Wendt and Baum, 1972; Rowe and Afonso, 1974) cat (Koss *et al.*, 1973), calf (Anderson *et al.*, 1972; Lewis and Eyre, 1972) and man (Bergström *et al.*, 1959; Bergström *et al.*, 1965a, b). The chronotropic effect of E prostaglandins varied according to experimental conditions. Thus, in intact cats, intravenous injection of PGE_1 or PGE_2 produced no change or a slight reduction in heart rate, whereas in open-chest cats, no change or a slight increase occurred (Wendt and Baum, 1972). Suzuki *et al.* (1969) failed to observe any change in heart rate after intravenous administration despite a marked decrease in arterial blood pressure. Similarly, Nutter and Crumly (1972) did not find any change in the heart rate during the systemic hypotension accompanying the large doses of PGE_1 and PGA_1 which was suggested to result from the fluothane anaesthesia. Fluothane has been shown to alter baroreceptor reflexes (Skovsted *et al.*, 1969). On the other hand, Giles *et al.* (1969) found a decrease in heart rate by either intravenous or intracoronary infusion of PGE_1 whereas, intra-aortic infusion of PGE_1 increased the heart rate.

The increase in heart rate produced by PGE_1 in dogs was not abolished by bilateral cervical vagotomy (Nakano and McCurdy, 1967), by β-adrenergic blockade (Nakano and McCurdy 1967; Higgins *et al.*, 1971, 1972; Nutter and Crumly, 1970; Rowe and Afonso, 1974) or by reserpine pretreatment (Carlson and Orö, 1966). When alterations in β-adrenergic activation and afterload were prevented by propranolol and inflation of intra-aortic balloon catheter, respectively, administration of PGA_1 did not produce any significant change in heart rate of conscious dogs (Higgins *et al.*, 1972). Katori *et al.* (1970) showed that PGE_1 administered into the right atrium or by intravenous injection in the dog heart–lung preparation did not change the heart rate or arterial blood pressure. Moreover, direct injection of graded doses of PGE_1 into the sinus node artery did not produce any significant change in heart rate in the anaesthetized dog (Chiba *et al.*, 1972). From these observations it appears that the increase in heart rate is due to reflex sympathetic activation and/or stimulation of cardioaccelerator centres in the medulla rather than a direct intrinsic effect of prostaglandins on the myocardium. Lavery *et al.* (1970) studied the central mechanism for the cardiovascular effects of PGE_1 and PGA_1. They showed that infusion of PGE_1 (4–360 ng/kg per min) into the vertebral artery increased heart rate more than either intravenous or intracarotid administration of this agent. No significant effect on systemic arterial blood pressure was observed. Infusion of PGA_1 (0.1–9 μg/min) produced a small reduction in arterial blood pressure which was accompanied by an increase in heart rate. However, the magnitude of these effects was similar to that obtained by either intravenous or intracarotid routes of administration. Higgins *et al.* (1971) has shown that withdrawal of vagal activity also contributes to the tachycardia in response to PGA_1. Thus, after β-adrenergic blockade with propranolol, there was still an increase in heart rate averaging 39% in conscious dogs. Cardiac acceleration, produced by PGA_1, was totally abolished after combined β-adrenergic and cholinergic blockade thereby suggesting that tachycardia produced by PGA_1 is a summation of reflex activation of β-adrenergic receptors and withdrawal of vagal inhibition on the sino-atrial node. The failure of studies in anaesthetized animals after treatment with propranolol, reserpine and ganglionic blocking agents, (Nakano and McCurdy, 1967; Carlson and Orö, 1966) to demonstrate the contribution of vagal withdrawal to tachycardia produced by E and A prostaglandins could be due to the basic difference in the mechanism of the baroreceptor reflex-mediated tachycardia in conscious and anaesthetized animals. Thus, reductions in resting vagal tone occur in the anaesthetized state (Vatner *et al.*, 1971). In most of the above studies sodium pentobarbital was used as the anaesthetic agent. This agent has been reported to depress vagal activity (Brown and Hilton, 1956). This is supported by the observation that resting heart rates in excess of 140/min in anaesthetized dogs are frequently encountered; control rate in conscious dogs is about 72/min. (Higgins *et al.*, 1971).

Variable chronotropic effects of prostaglandins of the E and A series have also been reported on the isolated heart and various cardiac preparations from different animal species. Euler (1939) showed that crude extracts of prostaglandins did not affect the rate of the isolated rabbit heart or the cat heart–lung preparation. Prostaglandin E_1 also failed to alter the rate of the isolated heart of the rabbit (Berti *et al.*, 1965; Mantegazza, 1965), cat (Berti *et al.*, 1965; Mantegazza, 1965; Sunahara and Talesnik, 1974) and chicken (Horton and Main, 1967). However, PGE_1 increased contractile force and rate of isolated guinea pig and frog hearts (Mantegazza, 1965; Berti *et al.*, 1965) and frog ventricular strips (Baysal and Vural, 1974). In the isolated rat heart PGE_1 and PGE_2 produced either no effect or had variable chronotropic effects (Vergroesen *et al.*, 1967). However, Levy (1973a) found that PGE_2 increased the force of contraction and rate of spontaneously beating isolated atria of normal and genetically hypertensive rats. Although PGE_1 does not alter the rate of the cat heart (Berti *et al.*, 1965; Mantegazza, 1965; Sunahara and Talesnik, 1974), it increased the frequency of contraction of isolated cat atria but not that of dog atria (Su *et al.*, 1973). In the dog (Su *et al.*, 1973) and in rabbit atria (Nutter and Crumly, 1972), PGE_1 and PGA_1 were devoid of any chronotropic effect. Similar results have been obtained with PGE_2 in the isolated rabbit atria driven electrically or beating spontaneously (Levy and Killebrew, 1971) and with PGA_2 in the isolated chicken and rabbit heart (Lee *et al.*, 1965). Although cardiac tissues of various animal species respond differently to prostaglandins of the E and A series, the positive chronotropic effect observed in some isolated cardiac tissues may be due to a direct action on the myocardium. Thus, in the isolated guinea pig heart, PGE_1 consistently produced a positive chronotropic effect which was not blocked by pretreatment with either propranolol or reserpine (Mantegazza, 1965).

Chronotropic effects of F prostaglandins are qualitatively as well as quantitatively different in various animal species. Prostaglandin $F_{2\alpha}$, which produced a fall in arterial blood pressure of the anaesthetized cat resulted in a marked bradycardia after a delay of 10 to 30 s (Änggård and Bergström, 1963; Koss et al., 1973). Since the bradycardia produced by $PGF_{2\alpha}$ in these studies was abolished by vagotomy or atropine treatment, it appears to be reflex in origin. Hollenberg et al. (1968) on the other hand, did not find any effect of $PGF_{1\alpha}$ and $PGF_{2\alpha}$ after intracoronary infusion, on myocardial blood flow, heart rate or contractility, in the anaesthetized dog. However, DuCharme et al. (1968), Nakano and McCurdy (1968) and Nakano and Cole (1969) found that the intravenous injection or administration of $PGF_{2\alpha}$ into the left atrium of the anaesthetized dog increased mean arterial blood pressure and heart rate. The increase in heart rate produced by injection of $PGF_{2\alpha}$ into the left atrium was greater than after intravenous administration. Similarly, Emerson et al. (1971) observed a marked increase in heart rate after intravenous administration of $PGF_{2\alpha}$ in the anaesthetized dog. Lavery et al. (1970, 1971) reported that $PGF_{1\alpha}$ (9–60 μg/min) and $PGF_{2\alpha}$ (4–64 ng/kg per min), when given into the vertebral artery of anaesthetized dogs, produced a marked increase in heart rate and arterial blood pressure. The intravenous and intracarotid infusion of similar doses of these agents failed to produce any haemodynamic effect. Since tachycardia produced by $PGF_{2\alpha}$ was not affected by propranolol or cervical cord section but was abolished by vagotomy or atropine, it was concluded that the tachycardia, in response to $PGF_{2\alpha}$, is due to inhibition of vagal tone (Figure 5.6). Activation of adrenergic nerves probably contributed partly to intravertebrally-induced $PGF_{2\alpha}$ tachycardia because after vagotomy, a residual pressor response remained, which was abolished by subsequent adminstration of bethanidine or bretylium. However, in conscious dogs infusion of $PGF_{2\alpha}$ (4–40 ng/kg per min) into the vertebral artery raised arterial blood pressure without any significant increase in heart rate. Moreover, in anaesthetized cats, $PGF_{2\alpha}$, up to 3 μg/kg, injected into the left vertebral artery produced no demonstrable cardiovascular effect (Koss et al., 1973). From these observations it appears that the cardiovascular effects of $PGF_{2\alpha}$ depend upon the experimental conditions and the animal species. Prostaglandin $F_{2\alpha}$ does not seem to produce its chronotropic effects directly since infusion of $PGF_{2\alpha}$ into the canine sinus node artery was without a chronotropic effect (Chiba et al., 1972). Moreover, most of the in vitro studies have failed to demonstrate a chronotropic action of prostaglandins of the F series. Katori et al. (1970), in the dog heart–lung preparation, did not find any effect of $PGF_{1\alpha}$ on the heart rate. Similarly, Vergroesen et al. (1967) found $PGF_{1\alpha}$ and $PGF_{1\beta}$ to be ineffective in altering the rate of the isolated rat heart. $PGF_{2\alpha}$ was also demonstrated to be ineffective in altering the rate of the isolated rabbit or chicken heart (Lee et al., 1965; Horton and Main, 1967), had a weak positive chronotropic effect on guinea pig atria and no effect on rabbit (Nutter and Crumly, 1972) and dog atria (Su *et al.*, 1973) but produced a marked positive chronotropic effect on cat atria (Su *et al.*, 1973). The positive chronotropic effect of $PGF_{2\alpha}$ in the latter, exemplifies the significance of species differences.

5.2.5 Coronary circulation

Prostaglandins of the E and A series (E_1, E_2 or A_1) increased coronary blood flow and decreased coronary vascular resistance in anaesthetized and un-anaesthetized dogs (Nakano and McCurdy, 1967, 1968: Nakano, 1968a; Maxwell, 1967; Hollenberg *et al.*, 1968; Hedwall *et al.*, 1970; Bloor and Sobel, 1970; Higgins *et al.*, 1970, 1971; Nutter and Crumly, 1970, 1972; Glaviano and Masters, 1971; Rowe and Afonso, 1974). The degree of fall in coronary perfusion pressure, produced by intracoronary administration of PGE_1 in doses of 12.5 μg, was similar to that produced by 1.0 μg of intracoronary acetylcholine or by reactive hyperaemia (Nutter and Crumly, 1972). Although the systemic hypotensive effect of PGA_1 exceeded that produced by PGE_1, the coronary vasodilator effect of PGA_1 was much less than that caused by equivalent doses of PGE_1 (Nutter and Crumly, 1972). Moreover, PGE_1 and PGE_2 have been reported to be more potent coronary vasodilators than adenosine; exceeding the efficacy of adenosine by 5 to 10 times per unit of drug weight (Rowe and Afonso, 1974). The duration and magnitude of the coronary vasodilator action of PGE_1 have also been shown to be greater than those of the well-known coronary vasodilator, nitroglycerine (Nakano and McCurdy, 1968). Glaviano and Masters (1971) found that intracoronary administration of PGE_1 (0.5 μg/kg per min) increased the left circumflex coronary arterial flow within 1 min, but this declined progressively to control levels within 10 min despite continued infusion of PGE_1. Since coronary vascular resistance was not significantly altered, the decline in coronary flow during prolonged infusion of PGE_1 could be due to lowering of coronary perfusion pressure. In contrast to studies demonstrating increased coronary blood flow with E and A prostaglandins Barner *et al.* (1972) observed that administration of PGA_1 into the pulmonary artery (1–5 μg/kg) of the anaes-thetized dog decreased coronary blood flow progressively with increasing doses. The maximum fall in coronary flow occurred 30 to 60 s after infusion of PGA_1 and coincided with the maximal fall in arterial blood pressure. Since coronary vascular resistance declined in response to PGA_1, it was concluded that the decrease in coronary flow was due to a greater vasodilator effect of PGA_1 on other vascular beds, the net effect of which would be a fall in coronary blood flow.

Increased coronary blood flow and decreased coronary vascular resistance, produced by intracoronary administration of prostaglandins of the E and A series in the dog, has been shown to occur without any change in heart rate or systemic blood pressure (Nakano and McCurdy, 1967, 1968; Nakano, 1968a; Hollenberg *et al.*, 1968; Nutter and Crumly, 1970, 1972). In the dog heart–lung preparation, Katori *et al.* (1970) found that intravenous injection of PGE_1 or injection of $PGF_{1\alpha}$ into the left atrium markedly increased coronary blood flow, cardiac output and myocardial contractile force without altering the heart rate and arterial blood pressure. Although intravenous administration of E or A prostaglandins increased heart rate and systemic arterial pressure (Maxwell, 1967, Nakano, 1968a, b; Higgins et al., 1970, 1971; Bloor and Sobel, 1970) the increase in coronary blood flow appears to be independent of these changes. Thus, β-adrenergic blockade with propranolol and cholinergic blockade with atropine, failed to abolish the increase in coronary blood flow produced by prostaglandins of the E and A series (Nakano, 1968a; Hollenberg et al., 1968; Hedwall et al., 1970, Nutter and Crumly, 1972; Rowe and Afonso, 1974). Moreover, when heart rate was controlled by electrical stimulation at a rate above that produced by PGA_1 (180/min) and after β-receptor blockade alone or combined with blockade of cholinergic receptors with atropine, PGA_1 still produced a substantial increase in coronary blood flow and decreased coronary vascular resistance although less than that observed before autonomic blockade (Higgins et al., 1971). Although, under these conditions, arterial pressure was markedly decreased, PGA_1 still produced a 42% decrease in coronary resistance. Increased coronary oxygen tension occurred at the time of peak coronary blood flow. The observations of Nutter and Crumly (1972) that PGE_1 produced coronary vasodilatation in the absence of systemic circulatory effect, increased myocardial oxygen consumption or myocardial potassium release as well as in the fibrillating and hypocalcaemic arrested heart indicate that PGE_1 produces coronary vasodilatation by a direct effect on vascular smooth muscle.

Prostaglandins of the E and A series have also been reported to increase coronary blood flow in the isolated perfused heart of some animal species. Thus, PGE_1 enhanced coronary blood flow in the rat, cat and rabbit heart without any significant effect on the rate and myocardial contractile force (Mantegazza, 1965). In contrast, in the isolated guinea pig heart, PGE_1 increased coronary flow, heart rate and myocardial contractile force (Berti et al. 1965; Mantegazza, 1965). Similar observations were made by Wennmalm and Hedqvist (1970) in the isolated rabbit heart. Although Berti et al. (1965) failed to find any effect of PGE_1 on heart rate and coronary blood flow in the isolated rat heart, Vergroesen et al. (1967) demonstrated that PGE_1, PGE_2 or PGA_1 increased coronary blood flow and myocardial contractile force without any consistent effect on heart rate. Similarly, Willebrands and Tasseron (1968) showed that, in the isolated rat heart, PGE_1 increased coronary flow and contractile force. In the isolated guinea pig heart the increase in coronary flow produced by PGE_1 was not blocked by β-adrenergic blocking agents, propranolol or pronethalol, or by reserpine pretreatment (Berti et al., 1965; Mantegazza, 1965).

Prostaglandins of the F series did not appear to affect the coronary blood flow in intact animals. Thus, intracoronary administration of $PGF_{2\alpha}$ in the anaesthetized dog did not change coronary arterial blood flow or myocardial contractile force (Nakano, 1968a, b). These findings have been confirmed by Hollenberg et al. (1968) and Nutter and Crumly (1970, 1972) who did not find any effect of $PGF_{1\alpha}$ and $PGF_{1\alpha}$ and $PGF_{2\alpha}$ respectively on myocardial blood flow, heart rate or contractility after intracoronary administration. Intravenous injection of $PGF_{2\alpha}$ also failed to affect the coronary vascular bed of the dog (Bloor and Sobel, 1970). In contrast, Maxwell (1969) observed a transient increase in coronary blood flow with $PGF_{2\alpha}$. Moreover, high doses of $PGF_{1\alpha}$ (50 µg/kg) increased coronary blood flow, myocardial contractile force and cardiac output without altering heart rate and arterial blood pressure in the isolated dog heart–lung preparation (Katori *et al.*, 1970). Vergroesen *et al.* (1967) found that in the isolated rat heart $PGF_{1\alpha}$ increased myocardial contractile force and that $PGF_{1\alpha}$ or $PGF_{1\beta}$ failed to alter coronary blood flow, whereas, Willebrands and Tasseron (1968) showed that $PGF_{1\alpha}$ increased both coronary blood flow and myocardial contractile force. The reason for this discrepancy is not known.

5.2.6 Myocardial metabolism

Prostaglandins, particularly those of the E series, have marked effects on lipid and carbohydrate metabolism, whereas those of the A series are essentially inactive and those of the F series have much weaker actions in this respect. Prostaglandin E_1 is the most potent inhibitor of basal lipolysis (Steinberg *et al.*, 1964; Carlson, 1965), lipolysis induced by catecholamines (Steinberg *et al.*, 1963) and sympathetic nerve stimulation (Berti and Usardi, 1964) and by a wide variety of hormones (Steinberg *et al.*, 1963, 1964; Mandel and Kuehl, 1967; Fain, 1967). This action of PGE_1, *in vivo*, was dose-dependent. Small doses stimulate and large doses inhibit lipolysis (Carlson, 1967). Intracoronary administration of PGE_1 (Maxwell, 1967) increased coronary flow and cardiac oxygen extraction in anaesthetized dogs. The rise in oxygen uptake and coronary blood flow was accompanied by decreased glucose and free fatty acid levels and increased lactate concentration in the coronary sinus blood. The concentration of pyruvate, on the other hand, was not altered. It was concluded that PGE_1 enhanced uptake of glucose and free fatty acids. However, Glaviano and Masters (1971) found that the intracoronary infusion of PGE_1 in anaesthetized dogs produced a fall in arterial levels and the myocardial extraction ratio of free fatty acids. This was found to be associated with increased arterial levels, myocardial extraction ratio and uptake of glucose. Cardiac muscle triglyceride fatty acids were increased. Moreover, PGE_1, when added to cardiac muscle homogenates of untreated control dogs, decreased lipolytic activity as determined by the levels of free fatty acids. These authors concluded that PGE_1 inhibited basal myocardial lipolysis. Since the levels of cyclic AMP in the left ventricular cardiac muscle subjected to intracoronary administration of PGE_1 were decreased by 83 % as compared to those in cardiac muscle from control dogs, it was postulated that the antilipolytic effect of PGE_1 on myocardium is mediated by decreased myocardial cyclic AMP. However, this is in contrast to studies in other species. PGE_1 has been shown to increase cyclic AMP levels in rat heart (Curnow and Nuttall, 1971), enhance adenylate cyclase activity (Sobel and Robison, 1969) and activate phosphorylase activity in the guinea pig and rat heart (Piccinini *et al.*, 1969) respectively. In view of these observations, it appears that the antilipolytic action of PGE_1 involving cyclic AMP may have been species-dependent. A myocardial metabolic effect of PGE_1 was also demonstrated by Willebrands and Tasseron (1968) who found that PGE_1 and $PGF_{1\alpha}$ increased production of

$^{14}CO_2$ from [^{14}C]glucose and [^{14}C]palmitate when coronary blood flow, myocardial contractile force and myocardial oxygen consumption increased. Maxwell (1969) showed that $PGF_{2\alpha}$ increased coronary venous flow which was associated with decreased aortic flow but it did not alter myocardial oxygen consumption. Moreover, in contrast to the effects of PGE_1, $PGF_{2\alpha}$ did not produce a significant effect upon either arterial glucose, myocardial glucose or free fatty acid extraction, whereas it increased both lactate and pyruvate levels in arterial as well as in coronary sinus blood.

5.2.7 Pulmonary circulation

In 1959, Bergström and his colleagues made the observation in human subjects that intravenous injection of PGE_1 caused a small, transient decrease in pulmonary arterial pressure, probably due to a decrease in cardiac output. However, studies in anaesthetized dogs (Maxwell, 1967, 1969; Said, 1968; Giles et al., 1969) showed that PGE_1 or PGE_2 increased pulmonary arterial pressure and decreased pulmonary vascular resistance. An increase in pulmonary arterial pressure by PGE_1 or PGE_2 has also been reported in both anaesthetized (Lewis and Eyre, 1972) and unanaesthetized (Anderson et al., 1972) calves. A vasodilator effect of PGE_1, as indicated by decreased pulmonary arterial perfusion pressure, has also been demonstrated by Nakano and Cole (1969) and Nakano and Kessinger (1970) in anaesthetized dogs when either cardiac input or pulmonary blood flow was kept constant. Similarly, in the blood perfused lobar artery of the anaesthetized dog, administration of PGE_1 produced a decrease in mean pulmonary arterial pressure, lobar perfusion pressure and lobar venous pressure (Hyman, 1969). Since lobar blood flow was kept constant and there was no change in arterial pressure during intralobar infusion of PGE_1 the progressive decrease in the pressure gradient between the lobar artery and the small pulmonary lobar vein and left atrium was assumed to be due to active dilatation of lobar pulmonary veins and the blood vessels upstream to the venous segment, presumably the lobar arteries. Alpert et al. (1973) found that administration of PGE_1 into the right atrium of the anaesthetized dog did not alter the mean pulmonary arterial pressure but produced a significant increase in pulmonary blood volume and cardiac output thereby suggesting a mild active pulmonary vasodilatation. Prostaglandin E_2 had very little effect on the pulmonary circulation. A pulmonary vasodilator effect of PGE_1 or PGE_2 was reported in the isolated perfused lungs of rabbit (Hauge et al., 1967), cat (Hauge et al., 1967; Wendt and Baum, 1972), guinea pig (Okpako, 1972) and calf (Lewis and Eyre, 1972). The decrease in pulmonary vascular resistance produced by PGE_1 or PGE_2 was not abolished by propranolol or phentolamine (Hauge et al., 1967; Okpako, 1972) thereby suggesting that the vasodilator action of PGE_1 and PGE_2 was not mediated by stimulation of β-adrenergic receptors or blockade of α-adrenergic receptors. Prostaglandin E_1 has been shown to cause relaxation of helical strips of pulmonary lobar artery and vein of the dog in concentrations similar to those which produced pulmonary vasodilatation, in vivo (Kadowitz et al., 1973). Prostaglandins E_1 and E_2 relaxed pulmonary arterial and venous strips contracted by histamine,

5-HT or acetylcholine and also relaxed in high doses uncontracted vein and arterial strips (Lewis and Eyre, 1972). The effect of prostaglandins of the A series on the pulmonary circulation has not been as thoroughly investigated as those of the E series. Barner *et al.* (1972) showed that administration of PGA_1 into the pulmonary artery of anaesthetized dog produced a significant fall in pulmonary arterial pressure only after high doses (5 $\mu g/kg$) of PGA_1. Alpert *et al.* (1973) found that PGA_1 caused marked dilatation of the peripheral circulation but had little effect on the pulmonary circuit. Pulmonary blood volume, cardiac output and compliance index did not change significantly while mean pulmonary arterial pressure decreased, most probably due to passive shrinkage of the pulmonary vascular bed secondary to a shift of blood to the peripheral circulation.

In contrast to E and A prostaglandins, $PGF_{2\alpha}$ caused constriction of the pulmonary vascular bed and increased pulmonary arterial pressure. Thus, intravenous administration of $PGF_{2\alpha}$ increased pulmonary arterial pressure in the dog (Nakano and McCurdy, 1968; DuCharme *et al.*, 1968; Said, 1968; Kadowitz *et al.*, 1973; Hyman, 1969; Emerson *et al.*, 1971; Nakano, *et al.*, 1973; Alpert *et al.*, 1973), calf (Lewis and Eyre, 1972; Anderson *et al.*, 1972) and cat (Änggård and Bergström, 1963). The increase in pulmonary arterial pressure caused by $PGF_{2\alpha}$ has been shown to be secondary to constriction of pulmonary veins (DuCharme *et al.*, 1968; Said, 1968; Hyman, 1969). Hyman (1969) and Kadowitz *et al.* (1973) showed that in the anaesthetized dog, administration of $PGF_{2\alpha}$ into the pulmonary lobar artery caused an abrupt increase in lobar arterial pressure and a progressive increase in lobar venous pressure without alteration of pulmonary blood flow or right and left atrial pressures. Moreover, an abrupt increase in the pressure gradient, from the lobar artery to the small lobar vein was observed. On the basis of these observations it was concluded that $PGF_{2\alpha}$ increased pulmonary arterial pressure by a direct constrictor action on the lobar veins and arteries. Alpert *et al.* (1973) found that in the dog, $PGF_{2\alpha}$ increased mean pulmonary arterial pressure and pulmonary vascular resistance without altering pulmonary blood volume and total peripheral resistance, thereby suggesting an active pulmonary vasoconstriction. Similar results have been obtained by other investigators (Nakano and McCurdy, 1968; Nakano and Cole, 1969; Emerson *et al.*, 1971). $PGF_{2\alpha}$ also increased pulmonary vascular resistance in the isolated perfused guinea pig lung at threshold doses of 0.05 to 0.2 μg (Okpako, 1972). Since this effect of $PGF_{2\alpha}$ was not abolished by an antihistaminic agent, mepyramine, or an α-adrenergic blocking agent, phentolamine, it was concluded that the pulmonary vasoconstriction produced by $PGF_{2\alpha}$ was neither due to stimulation of histaminergic or adrenergic receptors nor to release of catecholamines but most probably to a direct effect. Prostaglandin $F_{2\alpha}$ caused contraction of helical strips of isolated pulmonary lobar arteries and veins (Kadowitz *et al.*, 1973). These observations indicate that the increased pulmonary arterial pressure is due to its direct action on the pulmonary vessels.

5.2.8 Splanchnic circulation

5.2.8.1 Gastric circulation

Intravenous administration of PGE_1 to the dog has been shown to reduce histamine or pentagastrin-induced gastric acid secretion and decrease the gastric mucosal blood flow (as determined by aminopyrine clearance) (Wilson and Levine, 1969, 1972; Jacobson, 1970). The inhibitory action of PGE_1 on histamine or pentagastrin-induced gastric secretion was not the result of decreased blood flow since the ratio of clearance to volume secretion did not change during inhibition of pentagastrin and rose significantly during inhibition of histamine-induced gastric acid secretion (Jabobson, 1970; Wilson and Levine, 1972). Similar observations have been made by Main and Whittle (1973a) with PGE_1, PGE_2, PGA_1 and PGA_2 in the rat. Although PGE_1 in the dog (Wilson and Levine, 1969, 1972) and PGE_1, PGE_2, PGA_1 and PGA_2 in the rat (Main and Whittle, 1973a) inhibited gastric secretion induced by histamine or pentagastrin and decreased gastric mucosal blood flow, they produced an initial increase in gastric mucosal blood flow (as indicated by increased clearance of aminopyrine and $[^{14}C]$aniline) when gastric secretion was inhibited. Moreover, PGE_1, PGE_2, PGA_1 and PGA_2 in the rat increased gastric mucosal blood flow under basal conditions, viz. in the absence of histamine or pentagastrin stimulation (Main and Whittle, 1973a). Since indomethacin, an inhibitor of prostaglandin synthesis (Vane, 1971) which increased pentagastrin stimulation secretion, reduced the mucosal blood flow without altering acid secretion (Main and Whittle, 1973b), prostaglandins may fulfil a role as mediators of functional vasodilatation in the gastric mucosa. In the anaesthetized dog, Nakano et al. (1971) perfused the stomach vasculature with arterial blood at a constant flow and administered PGE_1 and PGA_1 intravenously. They found that these agents decreased arterial blood pressure, gastric perfusion pressure and gastric vascular resistance, PGA_1 being more active than PGE_1. However, on intra-arterial administration, PGE_1 and PGA_1 produced qualitatively similar effects without altering mean arterial blood pressure or heart rate; PGE_1 was more active than PGA_1 by this route of administration.

5.2.8.2 Mesenteric circulation

Prostaglandins E_1, E_2, A_1 and A_2, when given by intra-arterial injection (Lee, 1968) or infusion of PGE_1 (Shehadeh et al., 1969) in the anaesthetized dog, increased mesenteric blood flow and decreased mesenteric vascular resistance. Similar results have been reported with intravenous administration of PGA_1 in conscious dogs (Higgins et al., 1970, 1973). Murphy et al. (1970) found that the intravenous infusion of large doses of PGA_1 in anaesthetized normotensive and hypertensive dogs decreased both mesenteric and renal blood flow. However, Higgins et al. (1973) observed that similar doses of PGA_1 (1.0 µg/kg) in conscious dogs produced a large increase in mesenteric blood flow and a small or no increase in renal blood flow. In fact, in some experiments a decrease in renal blood flow was observed while mesenteric blood flow was increased. Prostaglandin E_1 and PGA_1 in anaesthetized dogs also caused a marked increase in mesenteric blood flow without altering renal or femoral blood flow (Covino et al., 1968). Direct infusion of PGE_1 (0.1 μg/kg per min) into the mesenteric artery dilated the mesenteric vasculature, previously constricted by haemorrhagic shock and restored the blood flow nearly to prehaemorrhage values without altering systemic arterial pressure (Ulano et al., 1972). Moreover, in the rat, topical application of PGE_1 but not PGA_1, on the mesoappendix in vivo, has been shown to produce dilatation of mesenteric meta-arterioles and precapillary sphincters (Messina et al., 1974). From these studies one may conclude that prostaglandins E and A produce vasodilatation by a direct action on the mesenteric vasculature.

In contrast, $PGF_{2\alpha}$ was shown to decrease the resistance and blood flow in the superior mesenteric artery of the anaesthetized dog after intra-arterial administration (Lee, 1968). Shehadeh et al. (1969) however, observed variable effects on the mesenteric circulation after intra-arterial administration of $PGF_{2\alpha}$. Prostaglandin $F_{2\alpha}$ caused constriction of blood perfused colic veins in a dose-related manner; $PGF_{2\alpha}$ being less potent than norepinephrine (Mark et al., 1971). These constrictor effects of $PGF_{2\alpha}$ contribute to its hypertensive action in the dog (DuCharme and Weeks, 1967; Nakano and Cole, 1969).

5.2.8.3 Pancreatic circulation

The effects of prostaglandins on pancreatic circulation have not yet been thoroughly investigated. Saunders and Moser (1972a) reported that in the isolated perfused rat pancreas, PGE_2 (0.01–10 μg/ml) produced a dose-related decrease in vascular resistance, whereas $PGF_{2\alpha}$ had an opposite effect. Like $PGF_{2\alpha}$, PGB_1 and PGB_2 also increased vascular resistance in this preparation (Saunders and Moser, 1972b). Since the increase in perfusion pressure, produced by PGB_2 was only partially reduced by phentolamine, it was concluded that at least part of the pressor action of PGB_2 was not mediated by release of catecholamines from sympathetic fibres. In view of the presence of E and F prostaglandins in the bovine pancreas (Bergström, 1967b) and their potent vascular effects on the pancreatic blood vessels, Kaley and Weiner (1968) have proposed that prostaglandins serve as regulators of pancreatic blood flow.

5.2.8.4 Splenic circulation

The effect of prostaglandins on the splenic circulation was studied by Davies and Withrington (1968, 1969, 1971) using the blood perfused isolated spleen of the dog. They showed that PGE_1, 0.5 to 5 μg/min and PGE_2 0.5 to 4 μg/min increased splenic blood flow and reduced splenic vascular resistance. The magnitude of reduction in splenic vascular resistance, produced during infusion of PGE_1 was slightly less than that produced by acetylcholine.

Prostaglandin E_2 was considerably less effective than either of these agents (Figure 5.7). An increase in splenic volume accompanied the reduction in splenic vascular resistance during the infusion of PGE_1 and PGE_2. The volume increase, however, was always very much slower than changes in vascular resistance (Davies and Withrington, 1968). Prostaglandins A_1, A_2, $F_{1\alpha}$, and $F_{2\alpha}$, at rates of up to 4 μg/min, also reduced vascular resistance but none of these agents was more effective than PGE_1. Infusions of these agents were also accompanied by a slight increase in splenic volume (Davies and With-

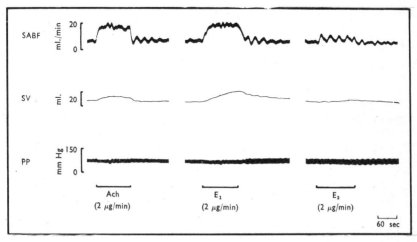

Figure 5.7 Dog (11.4 kg). Effect of close-arterial infusion of acetylcholine (Ach), prostaglandin E_1 (E_1) and prostaglandin E_2 (E_2) on splenic arterial blood flow (SABF) and spleen volume (SV) at constant perfusion pressure (PP). Reproduced from Davies and Withrington (1968), by courtesy of *Br. J. Pharmacol.*

rington, 1969). Although $PGF_{2\alpha}$ in lower concentrations (less than 10 μg/100 ml) produced a reduction in splenic vascular resistance, higher concentrations (greater than 100 μg/100 ml) caused an increase in splenic vascular resistance. The effect of PGE_1, PGE_2, PGA_1, PGA_2 and $PGF_{2\alpha}$ on the splenic vascular resistance was not abolished by propranolol, whereas, phenoxybenzamine did not block the effect of PGE_1, PGE_2, PGA_1, and $PGF_{1\alpha}$ but converted the vasodilator effect of PGA_2 and $PGF_{2\alpha}$ to vasoconstriction (Davies and Withrington, 1968, 1969). The mechanism of this latter effect of phenoxybenzamine on the vasodilator actions of PGA_2 and $PGF_{2\alpha}$ was not determined. The inability of phenoxybenzamine or propranolol to abolish the vasodilator effect of these agents suggested that their effect was not mediated by stimulation of either α- or β-adrenergic receptors. In view of the demonstration of their presence (Papanicolaou *et al.*, 1974) and release, in response to a wide variety of stimuli (Davies *et al.*, 1968; Gilmore *et al.*, 1968; Peskar and Hertting, 1973), and their marked effects on the splenic vasculature (Davies and Withrington, 1968, 1969, 1971) prostaglandins may play an important role in regulation of splenic blood flow and modulation of action of various vasoactive stimuli.

5.2.8.5 Hepatic and portal circulation

Prostaglandin E_1 (1 μg/ml), when given by intravenous injection into the anaesthetized dog, produced a transient increase in the hepatic arterial blood flow which was associated with a significant decrease in vascular resistance (Geumei *et al.*, 1973). This was accompanied by a fall in systemic arterial pressure. Injection of PGE_1 (0.1–10 μg) directly into the hepatic artery, increased hepatic arterial blood flow and reduced hepatic vascular resistance without altering systemic arterial pressure. Since the hepatic vascular response to PGE_1 was not abolished by denervation or by prior intravenous administration of propranolol, the increase in hepatic blood flow is most probably due to its direct vasodilator action on the hepatic vasculature.

Euler (1939) found that administration of seminal fluid extracts in the anaesthetized cat produced a rise in portal venous pressure, caused blanching of the liver and a fall in systemic arterial blood pressure. Nakano and Cole (1969) showed that intrafemoral or intraportal administration of PGE_1 (4 μg/kg) produced a biphasic change in portal venous pressure, i.e., an initial increase followed by a decrease. The initial rise in portal vein pressure was suggested to be due to reflex sympathetic stimulation, and the subsequent decrease due to direct vasodilator effects on portal venous vasculature. However, on intravenous injection, PGE_1 1 μg/kg, produced a decrease in mean systemic arterial pressure and blood flow in the portal vein which was accompanied by a rise in portal venous pressure with an insignificant change in its resistance (Geumei *et al.*, 1973). These effects were not altered by either denervation or by the administration of propranolol. Thus, the increase in portal venous blood flow is most likely secondary to the vasodilator effect of PGE_1 on the mesenteric vasculature (Covino *et al.*, 1968; Shehadeh *et al.*, 1969). In contrast, intraportal injection of PGE_1 was found to have no significant immediate or delayed effect on portal venous blood flow, mean portal venous pressure or mean systolic arterial pressure. However, portal venous blood flow and pressure were increased in a few experiments after intraportal injection of large doses of PGE_1 (10–30 μg) which were accompanied by a fall in systemic arterial pressure. The marked decrease in systemic arterial pressure, produced by femoral vein injection of PGE_1 (Nakano and Cole, 1969; Geumei *et al.*, 1973), in contrast to unchanged systemic blood pressure after administration of PGE_1 into the hepatic artery or into the portal vein, indicates substantial metabolism and inactivation of PGE_1 in the liver, probably by nonspecific β- and ω-oxidation (Samuelsson, 1970).

Prostaglandin $F_{2\alpha}$ when given via the femoral vein increased portal venous and systemic arterial pressure (Nakano and Cole, 1969). However, administration of $PGF_{2\alpha}$ into the portal vein increased portal vein pressure and decreased systemic, pulmonary arterial and right atrial pressure. The increase in the portal venous pressure produced by administration of $PGF_{2\alpha}$ into the portal vein, was more prolonged and greater than that produced by its intrafemoral route. From these observations it was concluded that $PGF_{2\alpha}$, when given into the portal veins, acts directly on the venous vasculature to decrease venous return, pulmonary arterial blood flow and pressure, atrial pressure and cardiac output and hence decreases systemic arterial pressure.

5.2.9 Forearm, hindlimb and cutaneous circulation

Prostaglandins were first demonstrated by Euler (1939) to produce a marked vasodilatation in the isolated perfused rabbit hindleg. Beck *et al.* (1966) using PGE_1 confirmed these observations. Prostaglandin E_1 or E_2 also increased blood flow and decreased vascular resistance in the limb of man (Bevegard and Orö, 1969; Robinson *et al.*, 1973), dog (Lee *et al.*, 1965; Lee, 1968; Nakano and McCurdy, 1967; Nakano, 1968a, b; Smith *et al.*, 1968; Greenberg and Sparks, 1969; Horton and Jones, 1969; Daugherty, 1971; Kadowitz, 1972; Conway and Hatton, 1973; Strand *et al.*, 1974), calf Anderson *et al.*, 1972), cat (Holmes *et al.*, 1963; Horton and Jones, 1969) and frog (Euler, 1936). In addition to relaxation of resistance vessels, PGE_1 or PGE_2 also caused dilatation of capacitance vessels in the hindleg of the dog (Greenberg and Sparks, 1969; Daugherty, 1971; Conway and Hatton, 1973). When compared with other vasodilator agents in the femoral bed of dog, PGE_1 on a molar basis, was found to be slightly more potent than isoprenaline, nitroglycerine, acetylcholine and histamine (Nakano and McCurdy, 1967; Lee *et al.*, 1965; Lee, 1968; Smith *et al.*, 1968) but less potent than bradykinin and eledoisin (Nakano, 1964, 1965a, b). Prostaglandin E_2 is either a less potent vasodilator (Conway and Hatton, 1973) or has the same potency as PGE_1 in the perfused hindleg (Kadowitz, 1972) but is about 6 times more potent than its methyl ester, PGE_2-methyl ester, in the femoral vascular bed of the dog (Strand *et al.*, 1974). Prostaglandin E_1 also caused dilatation in the isolated perfused gracilis muscle and hindpaw of the dog (Abdel-Sayed *et al.*, 1970; Hedwall *et al.*, 1971). Kadowitz *et al.* (1971a) found that PGE_1 produced a greater degree of vasodilatation in the in-nervated canine hindpaw than in the denervated preparation. Since glyceryl trinitrate, which does not interfere with sympathetic transmission, also produced a greater dilator effect in the innervated than in the denervated paw, it was suggested that the greater dilator effect of PGE_1 and glyceryl trinitrate in the innervated preparation may be due to a higher degree of vasoconstrictor tone (Hedwall *et al.*, 1971). Using the cross-perfusion circu-lation technique, Horton and Jones (1969) showed that intravenous adminis-tration of PGE_1 and PGA_1 in the recipient cat produced a fall in mean arterial blood pressure and increased heart rate and hindlimb perfusion pressure; whereas intra-arterial injection of these agents into the hindlimb decreased perfusion pressure. Vagotomy and denervation of the carotid sinus bodies in the recipient cat abolished the rise in hindlimb perfusion pressure and decreased the rise in heart rate without altering arterial blood pressure. They concluded that the rise in perfusion pressure and heart rate was due to reflex sympathetic activation as a result of a fall in arterial blood pressure, and that the vasodilator effect of PGE_1 and PGA_1 was due to their direct action on the hindlimb vasculature. The vasodilator action of PGE_1 in the forearm of man and in the hindlimb of the dog has been shown to be independent of either adrenergic, cholinergic or histaminergic mechanisms (Smith *et al.*, 1968; Bevegard and Orö, 1969).

Prostaglandins A_1 or A_2 have similar vasodilator actions as PGE_1 and PGE_2 in the fore and/or hindlimb of the dog (Lee *et al.*, 1965; Lee, 1968;

Nakano, 1968 a, b; Barner *et al.*, 1973) and man (Robinson *et al.*, 1973). Higgins *et al.* (1973) have shown that intravenous administration of PGA_1 in graded doses of 0.01 $\mu g/ml$, produced an increase in iliac blood flow and decreased iliac vascular resistance. Although PGA_1 was a less potent vasodilator than PGE_1 in the perfused hindlimb of the dog (Greenberg and Sparks, 1969), they were equipotent in the perfused canine hindpaw (Kadowitz *et al.*, 1971a). In the human forearm, PGA_1 was less potent than PGE_2 (Robinson *et al.*, 1973). Similarly, PGA_2 was a considerably less potent vasodilator than PGE_1 or PGE_2 in the dog hindlimb (Kadowitz, 1972). Moreover, the vasodilator action of PGA_2 in the hindlimb of dog was not maintained in spite of continuous infusion of this agent. Greenberg *et al.* (1974) found that small concentrations of PGA_2 produced a non-sustained dilatation of the innervated perfused hindpaw of the dog followed by a secondary increase in perfusion pressure. Higher concentrations, although producing a fall in systemic arterial pressure, caused vasoconstriction in the hindpaw. In denervated hindpaw, the magnitude of PGA_2-induced vasodilatation was increased and the vasoconstrictor effect was reduced, but not abolished, thereby suggesting that the constrictor effect of PGA_2 may be partly dependent upon tonic sympathetic activity. Since PGA_2 is converted to PGC_2 and subsequently to PGB_2 by prostaglandin isomerase (Jones, 1972b), the vasoconstrictor action of PGA_2 in the hindpaw of the dog has been postulated to be mediated through its conversion to PGB_2 which is about 6–7 times more potent a vasoconstrictor than PGA_2 (Greenberg *et al.*, 1974). Prostaglandin B_2, 50–1600 ng/kg per min, produced a dose-dependent vasoconstriction and a non-sustained vasodilatation after pretreatment with bretylium, phentolamine or reserpine, or after acute denervation in the canine hindpaw (Greenberg *et al.*, 1974a, b). Similarly, PGB_1 produced vasodilatation in small doses (50–200 ng/kg per min) whereas, higher doses (200–3200 ng/kg per min) caused vasoconstriction. Since acute denervation or pretreatment with bretylium, phentolamine or reserpine reduced but did not abolish the vasoconstrictor effect of PGB_1 and PGB_2, it was concluded that these agents act partly by releasing catecholamines from adrenergic nerves as well as by a direct action on the hindpaw vasculature (Greenberg *et al.*, 1974a, b). The vasodilator effects of PGB_1 and PGB_2 (after catecholamine depletion and adrenergic blockade) were not abolished by either cholinergic, histaminergic or β-adrenergic receptor blocking agents (Greenberg *et al.*, 1974b). Prostaglandin B_1 has also been reported to increase blood flow in the forearm of man and cause constriction of the superficial hand veins of man (Robinson *et al.*, 1973).

Prostaglandin $F_{2\alpha}$ increased vascular resistance in the brachial and femoral arteries of the dog (Greenberg and Sparks, 1969; Nakano, 1968a, b). Mean arterial blood pressure, myocardial contractile force and heart rate were not altered. Since the vasoconstrictor effect of $PGF_{2\alpha}$ was not blocked by phenoxybenzamine or methysergide, it was concluded that $PGF_{2\alpha}$ acts by a direct effect on the vessels (Nakano, 1968a, b). Intrapulmonary injection of $PGF_{2\alpha}$ 100 μg, produced a transient decrease or no change in the femoral arterial pressure of the calf (Anderson *et al.*, 1972). Prostaglandin $F_{2\alpha}$ in man, when administered in small doses into the brachial artery, caused a transient fall in forearm flow, whereas, high doses produced an increase in forearm flow

(Robinson *et al.*, 1973). DuCharme *et al.* (1968) found that $PGF_{2\alpha}$ in the perfused hindleg of the dog, had little effect on femoral arterial and small arterial pressure but produced a marked increase in pressure of the small veins. Blockade of tonic sympathetic discharge to the limb vasculature, produced by sectioning the sympathetic chain between the third and fourth lumbar ganglia or by treatment with hexamethonium or phenoxybenzamine, abolished the vasoconstrictor activity of $PGF_{2\alpha}$, whereas stimulation of the lumbar sympathetic trunk, distal to the point of section, resulted in restoration of $PGF_{2\alpha}$ induced vasoconstrictor activity. Since the removal or replacement of tonic sympathetic activity had no effect on the pressor activity of epinephrine, it was concluded that the sympathetic nervous system may contribute to the venoconstrictor effect of $PGF_{2\alpha}$. Hodgman *et al.* (1970) demonstrated that, in the forelimb of the dog, $PGF_{2\alpha}$ decreased skin blood flow but not muscle blood flow, and increased forelimb vascular resistance progressively. It was concluded that $PGF_{2\alpha}$ increased venous vascular resistance alone or to a greater degree than arteriolar resistance. Although Kadowitz *et al.* (1971b) failed to observe any effect on the perfused canine saphenous vein, Mark *et al.* (1971) found marked constriction. Since the venoconstrictor effect of $PGF_{2\alpha}$ in this preparation was not blocked by phentolamine, reserpine, hexamethonium or sectioning of the sympathetic chain, it appears that the constrictor effect of this agent was due to an effect independent of autonomic nervous activity. Prostaglandin $F_{2\alpha}$ also caused constriction of the superficial hand veins of man (Robinson *et al.*, 1973). In contrast, Kadowitz *et al.* (1971c, 1972) did not observe any effect of either $PGF_{1\alpha}$ or $PGF_{2\alpha}$ on the innervated, as well as denervated, perfused hindpaw of dog. From these studies it can be concluded that $PGF_{2\alpha}$ was a more potent constrictor of veins than arteries.

Effect of PGs of the E and F series on skin vessels

Prostaglandin E_1 is a potent vasodilator in guinea pig and human skin (Solomon *et al.*, 1968). Thus, intradermal injection of PGE_1 produced a small weal and an area of redness due to its potent vasodilator action. In rabbit skin, PGE_1, 100 μg, had very little effect but higher doses, 250 μg, produced erythema. Similar observations were made by Juhlin and Michaelsson (1969) and Jørgensen and Søndergaard (1973). The intradermal injection of as little as 1 ng was enough to produce erythema in normal skin. With higher doses the erythema was more intense, persisted for several hours and was more pronounced in patients with chronic urticaria. Prostaglandin E_1-induced erythema was not abolished by α-adrenergic blocking agents, dibenzyline, atropine, histamine depletion or antihistaminics; whereas it was reduced by β-adrenergic blockade, lidocaine and fluocinolone acetonide cream (Juhlin and Michaelsson, 1969). The mechanism of this inhibition of PGE_1-induced erythema is not known. Since an inhibitor of kallikrein, Trasylol, reduced the effect of high but not low doses of PGE_1-induced erythema, it would appear that kinins are involved in this effect of PGE_1. In contrast, Solomon *et al.* (1968) failed to demonstrate the inhibitory effect of lidocaine on the cutaneous response to PGE_1. Epinephrine and norepinephrine abolished the

PGE_1-induced erythema (Solomon *et al.*, 1968; Juhlin and Michaelsson, 1969), probably due to their constrictor effect opposing the dilator action of PGE_1. Prostaglandin E_1 was also shown to increase vascular permeability in guinea pig and rat skin (Weiner and Kaley, 1969). Crunkhorn and Willis (1969) made similar observations in human and rat skin. Although PGE_1 or PGE_2-induced erythema was not abolished by histamine depletion or antihistaminics (Juhlin and Michaelsson, 1969), the increased vascular permeability produced by PGE_2 was blocked by antihistaminics (Crunkhorn and Willis, 1969) thereby suggesting that other factors are also involved in the erythema produced by prostaglandins. In view of enhanced cutaneous vascular permeability and erythema produced by PGE_1 or PGE_2, and the demonstration that prostaglandins are synthesized in the skin (Änggård and Jonsson, 1972), it was concluded that prostaglandins may play a role in the inflammatory response.

Although prostaglandins of the E series cause vasodilatation of skin vessels *in vivo*, PGE_2 *in vitro* has been reported to produce contraction of the cutaneous arterial smooth muscle strips of both dog and man (Goldyne and Winkelmann, 1973). Thus, PGE_2 produced contraction of the dog paw, back and ear vessels, and human breast and finger vessels. The percentage of blood vessels contracting in response to PGE_2 was variable. Moreover, PGE_2 did not cause relaxation of the vessels even when actively contracted by KCl or epinephrine. In fact, PGE_2 raised the tension level of a catecholamine or KCl-induced contraction. The opposite effect of PGE_2 on skin vessels, *in vitro* and *in vivo*, is probably due to differences in the calibre of vessels. With *in vitro* techniques, larger calibre vessels were used, which may, by the nature of regional differentiation, respond differently from smaller, terminal arterioles and capillaries. Moreover, *in vivo*, prostaglandins may also involve other substances which influence the final response of a given vascular bed.

In contrast to the ability of prostaglandins E_1 and E_2 to produce marked erythema in human skin, $PGF_{1\alpha}$ and $PGF_{2\alpha}$ caused erythema of considerably lesser degree and neither produced erythematous streak nor hyperalgesia which resulted from the intradermal injection of PGE_1 or PGE_2 (Juhlin and Michaelsson, 1969). The intradermal injection of $PGF_{2\alpha}$ also did not affect rabbit and guinea pig skin (Solomon *et al.*, 1968). Moreover, $PGF_{1\alpha}$ and $PGF_{2\alpha}$ did not alter the vascular permeability in man and rat (Crunkhorn and Willis, 1969). However, $PGF_{2\alpha}$, but not PGE_1, antagonized the increased vascular permeability to plasma protein caused by bradykinin, histamine, serotonin or lymph node permeability factor in rats (Willoughby, 1968). Similarly, $PGF_{2\alpha}$ inhibited the increased vascular permeability in thermal injury and the early phase of chemical injury in rats, whereas PGE_1 was ineffective.

5.2.10 Carotid circulation

Prostaglandins of the E and A series (E_1, E_2, A_1 or A_2), when given intra-arterially to the anaesthetized dog increased carotid arterial blood flow without altering the systemic arterial blood pressure, heart rate or myocardial contractile force (Nakano and McCurdy, 1967; Nakano, 1968a, b; Lee,

1968; Nakano *et al.*, 1973). Intravenous administration of PGE_1, PGE_2 and PGA_2 was also found to increase carotid arterial blood flow, intraocular pressure and heart rate as systemic arterial pressure and carotid arterial resistance decreased. However, intravenous injection of PGA_1 decreased internal carotid flow, as mean arterial blood pressure decreased; vascular resistance remained unchanged (Barner *et al.*, 1973). In anaesthetized monkeys, Welch *et al.* (1974) showed that the intracarotid infusion of PGE_1 (1 μg/kg per min) produced an immediate increase in external carotid flow which was maintained in spite of a fall in mean systemic arterial blood pressure. The external carotid resistance was significantly decreased. Low doses of PGE_1 (200 ng/kg per min) increased external carotid flow without altering systemic mean arterial pressure. Internal carotid flow was decreased as was cerebral perfusion pressure. Since the percentage decrease in blood flow was greater than the percentage decrease in cerebral perfusion pressure, cerebrovascular resistance was increased. When the external carotid artery was ligated and internal carotid flow alone was measured, after applying pressure packs and a tourniquet to the orbits and extracranial structures to prevent collateral flow to the extracranial tissues, PGE_1 produced no significant change in blood flow despite a slight decrease in cerebral perfusion pressure. Since PGE_1, in doses which decreased internal carotid flow, impaired autoregulation, it was concluded that PGE_1, by dilating the external carotid vascular bed and imparing cerebral autoregulation, may cause the redistribution of, or 'steal', blood away from the internal carotid system.

Prostaglandins of the F series ($PGF_{2\alpha}$) decreased carotid arterial blood flow and increased carotid vascular resistance (Lee, 1968; Nakano *et al.*, 1973). White *et al.* (1971) showed that administration of $PGF_{2\alpha}$ (10 μg/kg per min) into the internal carotid artery increased internal carotid pressure and cerebrovascular tone in the anaesthetized monkey. External carotid pressure and femoral arterial pressure were either unchanged or decreased. Since the effect of $PGF_{2\alpha}$ was not altered by either methysergide or phenoxybenzamine, which blocked the increase in internal carotid perfusion pressure produced by 5-HT and norepinephrine respectively, it was concluded that $PGF_{2\alpha}$ does not produce its constrictor effect on the internal carotid artery by the stimulation of serotoninergic or adrenergic receptors. During increased internal carotid pressure produced by $PGF_{2\alpha}$, the pH of the blood, pCO_2 and pO_2 were not altered. Similar effects of $PGF_{2\alpha}$ on the external and internal carotid arterial beds have been reported in the monkey (Welch *et al.*, 1974).

5.2.11 Cerebral circulation

Prostaglandin E_1 on intravenous administration in anaesthetized dog caused a marked increase of blood flow in the internal carotid artery and a slight increase in external carotid arterial blood flow (Katsuki *et al.*, 1969). Denton *et al.* (1972), using a standard perfusion pressure technique, showed that intracarotid infusion of PGE_1 (0.1–1 μg/kg per min) in the dog caused vasodilatation and decreased cerebrovascular tone which was related to the dose of this agent and was independent of the fall in systemic arterial blood pressure. In monkeys, PGE_1 even in higher doses (1 μg/kg per min), which produced a marked fall in systemic arterial blood pressure, failed to produce any appreciable change in cerebrovascular tone. Prostaglandin A_1 produced a simultaneous fall of similar magnitude in cerebrovascular resistance and systemic arterial blood pressure. However, in the baboon, PGE_1 increased cerebral blood flow (Pelofsky et al., 1972). In humans, PGE_1 produced only a modest change in cerebral blood flow and did not alter the intracerebral spasm following subarachnoid haemorrhage (Steiner et al., 1972). Welch et al. (1974), using a photomicrographic technique, showed that topical application of PGE_1 caused marked dilatation of pial arteries and the vessels close to the artery of application. In contrast to these studies, Yamamoto et al. (1971–1972, 1972) using fluorescein micrography and ^{133}Xe clearance techniques and by measurement of the diameter of the exposed epicerebral vessels, showed that intracarotid infusion of PGE_1 reduced regional cerebral blood flow with significant vasoconstriction in small epicerebral arteries. The blood flow in the ipsilateral carotid system was reduced and the collateral flow from the vertebrobasilar system increased. The discrepancy between these results and those of other investigators (Denton et al., 1972) may be due to differences in their experimental techniques and to the anatomic variability of the blood supply from the carotid system to cerebral arteries in dogs (Daniel et al., 1952–54; Echlin, 1968).

Prostaglandin $F_{2\alpha}$ increased cerebrovascular tone in dogs and monkeys (Denton et al., 1972). Similarly, Yamamoto et al. (1971–72, 1972) found that intracarotid infusion of $PGF_{2\alpha}$ reduced regional cerebral blood flow and caused selective vasoconstriction of small epicerebral arteries. In the anaesthetized baboon, Pickard (1973) observed that the intracarotid infusion of $PGF_{2\alpha}$ reduced cerebral blood flow and increased cerebrovascular resistance which was associated with a significant reduction in cerebral oxygen consumption. Since there was no dissociation between the effects on cerebral oxygen consumption and cerebral blood flow by varying either the dose of $PGF_{2\alpha}$ or pCO_2, it was concluded that the ability of $PGF_{2\alpha}$ to constrict cerebral vessels is primarily due to its action on cerebral oxygen consumption and not on cerebrovascular smooth muscle. However, in view of the demonstration that $PGF_{2\alpha}$ produced cerebrovascular constriction without altering blood pH, pCO_2 or pO_2 in the dog (White et al., 1971) and that carbon dioxide produced cerebrovascular changes primarily by acting on centres in the brain stem (Shalit et al., 1968), it would appear that $PGF_{2\alpha}$ produces its constrictor effect by acting directly on the cerebral vessels. Moreover, Welch et al. (1974) have demonstrated that topical application of $PGF_{1\alpha}$ in the anaesthetized cat produced a slight vasoconstriction, whereas $PGF_{2\alpha}$, applied in similar quantities, produced vasoconstriction that was more profound and prolonged than $PGF_{1\alpha}$. Neither $PGF_{1\alpha}$ nor $PGF_{2\alpha}$ altered the diameter of the pial veins. In view of these observations and the release of prostaglandins from the cerebral cortex by direct and evoked nerve stimulation in the cat (Ramwell and Shaw, 1966), it is possible that prostaglandins may play a part in the regulation of cerebral circulation. Moreover, $PGF_{2\alpha}$, but not PGE_1, injected into the chiasmatic cisterna increased the incidence of cerebral vasospasm; it has been suggested that endogenous $PGF_{2\alpha}$ may be involved in the pathogenesis of cerebral vasospasm (Pennink et al., 1972). Although the work of

Torre *et al.* (1974) indicates that there is no correlation between the concentration of $PGF_{2\alpha}$ in the cerebrospinal fluid and the appearance of cerebral vasospasm in patients with subarachnoid haemorrhage, further work with antagonists and inhibitors of the synthesis of prostaglandins is required to assess their role in cerebral vasospasm.

5.2.12 Female and male reproductive organs circulation

In 1934 Euler found that seminal fluid extract constricted the perfused human placenta. Hillier and Karim (1968) reported that the effect of prostaglandins on the umbilical cord vessels depended upon the gestation age. Prostaglandins E_2, $F_{1\alpha}$ and $F_{2\alpha}$ produced contraction of circular and longitudinal muscle strips obtained at 34–42 weeks of gestation. On the other hand, PGE_1 caused relaxation of these vessels although higher doses often produced contraction. In contrast, these prostaglandins did not produce any effect on the umbilical vessels obtained during early pregnancy. Park *et al.* (1972) have shown that human umbilical vessels obtained at normal delivery showed contraction in response to PGE_1, PGE_2, $PGF_{1\alpha}$ and $PGF_{2\alpha}$. Pharriss *et al.* (1970) have demonstrated that $PGF_{2\alpha}$ caused constriction of utero-ovarian veins and decreased the blood flow in rats, rabbits and dogs. Based on these observations it was proposed that $PGF_{2\alpha}$, but its direct vasoconstrictor action on the utero-ovarian vein may produce a contraceptive or abortifacient effect. Clark *et al.* (1973) found that in the blood-perfused canine uterine vasculature PGE_1, 1 μg/min, reduced the uterine perfusion pressure and potentiated the vasoconstrictor responses to norepinephrine. Uterine vasoconstriction produced by sympathetic nerve stimulation was inhibited by PGE_1 at low frequencies and potentiated at higher frequencies of stimulation. Prostaglandin $F_{2\alpha}$ on the other hand, failed to alter the vascular resistance but potentiated the vasoconstrictor responses to both adrenergic stimuli. In contrast, in the late stage pregnant dogs neither PGE_1 nor $PGF_{2\alpha}$ altered vascular resistance. The failure of exogenous prostaglandins to alter the uterine vascular resistance in late pregnancy does not appear to be due to enhanced synthesis of prostaglandins by the uteroplacental complex (Terragno *et al.*, 1974; Venuto *et al.*, 1975). Terragno *et al.* (1974) showed that in late pregnancy in dogs after the inhibition of prostaglandin synthesis with indomethacin, intra-aortic administration of PGE_2 at rates as high as 3000 ng/min failed to increase the uterine blood flow which was depressed by indomethacin. Since the administration of arachidonic acid, a precursor of PGE_2, increased uterine blood flow when given before but not after indomethacin, they concluded that the failure of exogenous PGE_2 to alter the uterine blood flow was not due to enhanced levels of endogenous prostaglandins but probably due to increased degradation or relative inaccessibility of exogenous PGE_2 to its site of action. Enhanced prostaglandin synthesis in the uteroplacental complex during late pregnancy, however, could be an important determinant of increased uterine blood flow in pregnancy (Metcalfe *et al.*, 1959) and decreased uterine vascular reactivity to vasoactive agents such as norepinephrine and angiotensin (Ladner *et al.*, 1970; Ferris *et al.*, 1972). Venuto *et al.* (1975) using radioimmunoassay have shown that in the late pregnant bilaterally nephrectomized rabbit the level of PGE-like substance in the uterine venous blood was 172.4 ng/ml, whereas arterial levels of 'PGE' were 2.1 ng/ml. After the administration of either meclofenamate or indomethacin, arterial blood pressure was increased and uteroplacental blood flow reduced. This was accompanied by reduced levels of 'PGE' in uterine venous blood, whereas the arterial blood levels of 'PGE' were decreased to 1 ng/ml. On the other hand, in the male and non-pregnant female rabbit arterial levels of 'PGE' were shown to be 0.37 ng/ml. Dr. Terragno (personal communication) in preliminary experiments, has found the levels of PGE-like substance in rabbit uterine venous blood to be 0.45 ng/ml. After indomethacin treatment, however, these levels were reduced to less than 100 pg/ml of blood (as measured by bioassay). Terragno et $al.$ (1974), in late pregnant dogs, found that the concentration of 'PGE' in the uterine venous blood was 0.38 ng/ml which was reduced to 0.03 ng/ml after administration of indomethacin. Moreover, they showed that angiotensin II, which increased uterine blood flow in late pregnant dogs, elevated uterine venous blood levels of 'PGE'. After administration of indomethacin, angiotensin II neither released 'PGE' nor increased uterine blood flow despite increased mean arterial blood pressure (Terragno et $al.$, 1974). Similar observations have been made in the pregnant monkey (Franklin et $al.$, 1974). These observations suggest that local synthesis of prostaglandins by the uteroplacental complex could play an important role in the well-known adaptive increase in uteroplacental blood flow and decrease uterine vascular responsiveness to various vasoactive agents during pregnancy. The capacity of PGE_2 to oppose the vasoconstrictor action of pressor hormones has been demonstrated in the kidney (Lonigro et $al.$, 1973). The ameliorating effect of pregnancy on both experimental (Page, 1947) and essential hypertension (Chesley and Annitto, 1947) may reside partially in the capacity of uteroplacental complex to synthesize one or more substances with antihypertensive actions such as PGE_2. In contrast, decreased synthesis of prostaglandins could result in toxaemia of pregnancy and increased responsiveness to vasoconstrictor stimuli such as norepinephrine and angiotensin II (Talledo et $al.$, 1968; Gant et $al.$, 1973).

Although prostaglandins were first discovered in male accessory gland tissues and seminal plasma (Goldblatt, 1933; Euler 1935) there has been very little work done on their action on the male reproductive circulation. Free and Jaffe (1972) have studied the effect of PGE_1, PGE_2 and $PGF_{2\alpha}$ on blood flow in the testes of conscious rats. Administration of PGE_1, PGE_2 and $PGF_{2\alpha}$ into the testicular artery increased venous pressure and reduced blood flow to the testis. Prostaglandin $F_{2\alpha}$ was shown to be the most potent venoconstrictor, while PGE_1 produced the greatest reduction in testicular blood flow. Einer-Jensen and Soofi (1974) using ^{133}Xenon clearance showed that intratesticular injection of $PGF_{2\alpha}$, 10 μg, decreased testicular blood flow. In view of testicular synthesis of prostaglandins of the E and F series (Carpenter et $al.$, 1971) and the demonstration of rapid metabolism of PGE_1 by the rat testis (Nakano and Prancan, 1971), it is possible that prostaglandins play a role in the regulation of testicular blood flow.

5.2.13 Isolated vascular smooth muscle

The effect of prostaglandins on isolated vascular smooth muscle, *in vitro*, varies according to the animal species, the vascular tissue under study, the existing tone of the tissue and the concentration of prostaglandins used in the study. Thus, Khairallah *et al.* (1967) found that PGE_1 constricted isolated rabbit aortic and cat carotid arterial strips, the response being almost linearly related to the dose of this agent. Crude extract containing PGE_2-217 (PGA_2) caused contraction of isolated rabbit aortic strips, but purified medullin did not alter the tone of these strips when they were partially contracted with norepinephrine or angiotensin II. Strong and Bohr (1967) showed that PGE_1, PGE_2 and PGA_1 contracted isolated resting rabbit aortic and dog coronary arterial strips and enhanced the contraction of these strips produced by angiotensin II and KCl. However, these agents were found to produce a biphasic effect on small isolated skeletal, mesenteric and renal arterial strips of the dog. Small concentrations of PGE_1, PGE_2, PGA_1 and $PGF_{1\alpha}$ caused relaxation whereas higher concentrations of these agents produced contraction. A comparison of the effect of PGE_1, PGE_2, PGA_1 and $PGF_{1\alpha}$ on canine mesenteric arteries revealed the following order of potency in producing contraction: $PGA_1 > PGE_2 > PGE_1 > PGF_{1\alpha}$, and for relaxation: $PGA_1 > PGE_1 = PGE_2 = PGF_{1\alpha}$. The relaxation of this preparation produced by small concentrations of PGE_1 was not blocked by β-adrenergic and cholinergic blocking agents. Similarly, the contractile effect of PGE_1, on the rabbit aortic and cat carotid arterial strips of animals pretreated with reserpine was not abolished (Khairallah *et al.*, 1967). Moreover, the contraction of canine mesenteric arterial strips, produced by PGE_1, was not blocked by α-adrenergic, histaminergic or serotoninergic blocking agents (Strong and Bohr, 1967). These observations indicate that the paradoxical effects of low and high doses of PGE_1 were not mediated through autonomic, serotoninergic or histaminergic receptors, but rather due to a direct effect of this agent on the vascular smooth muscle. Khairallah *et al.* (1967) have proposed that the contractile effect of PGE_1 on the vascular smooth muscle is due to depolarization of the cell membrane. In contrast, in the rabbit perfused ear, Al Tai and Graham (1972) showed that PGE_1 and $PGF_{2\alpha}$ produced constriction which was abolished by phentolamine, reserpine pretreatment or by denervation thereby suggesting that the constrictor effect of these agents was due to the liberation of norepinephrine from sympathetic fibres. The constrictor effect of PGE_1, PGE_2, PGA_2 and $PGF_{2\alpha}$ on the rat and $PGF_{2\alpha}$ on the rabbit renal blood vessels (Figure 5.8) was not altered by chemical sympathectomy with 6-hydroxydopamine or by phentolamine, thereby indicating that the effect of these agents is independent of adrenergic mechanisms. Similarly, PGE_2, PGB_1, PGB_2 and $PGF_{2\alpha}$ caused constriction of isolated perfused rat pancreatic arteries (Saunders and Moser, 1972a, b). In isolated superfused canine mesenteric arteries and veins, tibial arteries and dorsal metatarsal veins, PGE_1 and PGE_2 caused relaxation, whereas PGA_2 and PGB_2 produced contraction; $PGF_{2\alpha}$, however, was ineffective in altering the tone of these vessels (Greenberg and Long, 1973; Greenberg *et al.*, 1973a, b; Greenberg, Kadowitz, Diecke and Long, 1973). Kadar and Sunahara (1967, 1969) found that in the isolated mesenteric arterial strips, PGE_1 caused relaxation whereas $PGF_{1\alpha}$ and $PGF_{2\alpha}$ produced contraction. Moreover, PGE_1 inhibited the spontaneous contraction of the canine isolated superior mesenteric vein and $PGF_{1\alpha}$ and $PGF_{2\alpha}$ enhanced the spontaneous contraction of these strips. The effect of these agents on venous strips was not abolished by pretreatment with atropine, phenoxybenzamine, propranolol or tetrodotoxin. These observations also indicate that prostaglandins exert a direct effect on vascular smooth muscle. The dilator and constrictor effects of prostaglandins of the E and F series, respectively, have also been shown in other vascular preparations. Thus, PGE_1 caused relaxation whereas $PGF_{2\alpha}$ produced contraction of isolated helical strips of canine pulmonary artery and vein (Kadowitz *et al.*, 1973). Similarly, in the rabbit perfused renal blood vessels, PGE_1, PGE_2 and PGA_2 produced dilatation while $PGF_{2\alpha}$ caused constriction (Figure 5.8).

Prostaglandins also exert a potent action on umbilical blood vessels and the ductus arteriosus. Hillier and Karim (1968) showed that PGE_2, $PGF_{1\alpha}$ and $PGF_{2\alpha}$ produced contraction of human umbilical vessels, whereas PGE_1 caused relaxation. However, a mixture of four prostaglandins in proportion to that found in the umbilical cord produced contraction of the umbilical arteries and veins. (Karim, 1967). Prostaglandin $F_{2\alpha}$ was the most potent on umbilical arteries, whereas PGE_2 and $PGF_{2\alpha}$ were equipotent but more potent than PGE_1 or $PGF_{1\alpha}$ on umbilical veins (Park *et al.*, 1973). More recently prostaglandins A_2 and B_2 have been shown to be several times

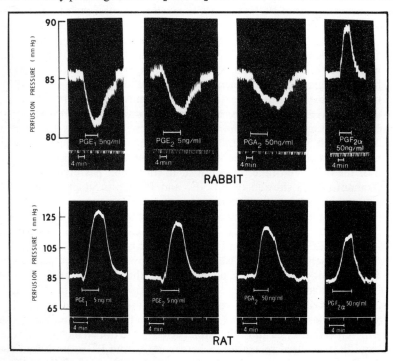

Figure 5.8   Effect of prostaglandins PG E_1, E_2, A_2 and $F_{2\alpha}$ on the basal pressure in isolated perfused rabbit (upper panel) and rat (lower panel) kidney. Reproduced from Malik and McGiff (1975), by courtesy of *Circulation Res.*

more potent than PGE_2 and $PGF_{2\alpha}$ in constricting human umbilical blood vessels (Adaikan and Karim, 1974). Serotonin was found to be 100 times more potent than prostaglandin for its contractile action on umbilical vessels. Coceani and Olley (1973) observed that PGE_1 and PGE_2 markedly relaxed anoxic isolated strips of lamb ductus arteriosus, whereas they had little effect on the tissues after exposure to oxygen. Further PGE_1 and PGE_2 were less active on the anoxic tissue depolarized by excess K^+. On the other hand, $PGF_{2\alpha}$ caused contraction of the ductus under anaerobic as well as aerobic conditions (Elliott and Starling, 1972). The response of the ductus to oxygen and $PGF_{2\alpha}$ was found to develop similarly with respect to fetal age. Moreover, the contraction of the vessels by oxygen did not occur in the presence of 7-oxa-13-prostynoic acid, an antagonist of prostaglandins, thereby indicating that exposure to oxygen may result in liberation of prostaglandins which in turn leads to closure of the ductus arteriosus at birth.

From the aforementioned studies it is apparent that the effect of prostaglandins on the isolated vascular smooth muscle is complex and varies in different vascular beds ranging from contraction to dilatation, biphasic response or no effect. The mechanism by which prostaglandins produce these variable effects may be related to alterations in permeability of cell membrane to various cations, such as Na^+ or Ca^{2+}, or binding or release of intracellular Ca^{2+}. The contractile effects of various prostaglandins on vascular smooth muscle has been shown to be antagonized by an inhibitor of cell membrane Na^+-K^+-ATPase, ouabain (Sunahara and Kadar, 1968). Moreover, there was a parallel relationship between the excitatory and inhibitory effects of Ca^{2+} and prostaglandins on smooth muscle. Thus, prostaglandins E_1 and A_1 increased the contractile frequency of the rat portal vein whereas they decreased it in the dog ureter (Strong and Bohr, 1967). On the basis of these observations these authors postulated that the opposite effect of prostaglandins, relaxation in small concentrations and contraction in higher concentrations, could be due to their effect on Ca^{2+}. Prostaglandins in low concentrations may have potentiated intracellular binding of Ca^{2+}, thus causing relaxation of contractile proteins, and in higher concentrations progressively decreased cell membrane stability, also by decreasing ionic Ca^{2+}, finally resulting in depolarization and contraction. However, the demonstration that the contractile effect of PGE_1 on rabbit aortic strip, previously depolarized by 100 mM K_2SO_4, though reduced, was not abolished, indicates that the contraction of vascular smooth muscle by PGE_1 may be mediated at least in part, by a mechanism other than membrane depolarization (Chandler and Strong, 1972) such as, pharmacological coupling (Somlyo and Somlyo, 1968a) or non-electric activation of the vascular smooth muscle (Bohr and Uchida, 1968). This latter mechanism might release Ca^{2+} from intracellular stores (Johansson et al., 1967) which would inactivate the troponin–tropomyosin ATP-ase inhibitory system (Ebashi and Ebashi, 1964). Prostaglandins may also interact directly with the contractile elements or affect cellular metabolism to alter vascular smooth muscle tone. Finally, prostaglandins could physically bind with Ca^{2+} ion and, in this way, alter membrane permeability since PGE_1 has been shown to act as a calcium ionophore (Kirtland and Baum, 1972).

5.2.14 Cardiovascular reactivity to other vasoactive substances

Prostaglandins of the E, A and F series modify the cardiovascular actions of a number of vasoactive substances. These include catecholamines, serotonin, histamine, angiotensin II and vasopressin. The direction of modification, viz. inhibition or potentiation, varies with the type of prostaglandin, its concentration, the vascular tissue and the animal species. Bergström et al. (1964, 1965a, 1966) demonstrated that PGE_1, PGE_2 and PGE_3 reduced the vasodepressor effect of norepinephrine in the dog. Similar observations were made by Steinberg et al. (1964), Steinberg and Pittman (1966) and Carlson and Orö (1966). Prostaglandin E_1 and E_2 have also been shown to reduce the pressor actions of catecholamines in rabbit (Holmes et al., 1963), rat (Somova, 1972) and man (Bergström et al., 1965a; Carlson et al., 1968, 1969). In contrast, $PGF_{1\alpha}$ did not alter the effect of catecholamines (Bergström et al., 1964). During the intravenous infusion of PGE_1, the administration of norepinephrine or stimulation of sympathetic ganglia with dimethylphenyl-piperazinium (DMPP) increased arterial blood pressure suggesting that the antagonism between PGE_1 and catecholamines is the result of summation of two opposite effects, viz vasoconstriction induced by catecholamines and a vasodilatation induced by PGE_1 (Bergström, et al., 1964, 1965a; Carlson et al., 1968, 1969). The inhibitory effect of PGE_1 on the pressor response to angiotensin II, but not to norepinephrine, was shown to occur in the anaesthetized rat (Türker et al., 1968). However, Somova (1972) showed that PGE_1 and PGE_2 inhibited the hypertensive effect of angiotensin II and vasopressin, as well as catecholamines. A similar, but much smaller inhibitory effect of papaverine and reserpine on the pressor responses to these agents was observed. Moreover, the inhibitory effect of PGE_1 and PGE_2 on the pressor response to angiotensin II, vasopressin and catecholamines was either markedly diminished or disappeared after ganglionic blockade and vagotomy. These observations indicate that the nervous component may participate in the pressor action of these agents. The inhibitory effect of PGE_1 and PGE_2 on the pressor actions of angiotensin II, vasopressin and catecholamines does not appear to involve a central mechanism since it was also demonstrable in spinal cats (Somova, 1972). Prostaglandin E_1 has also been reported to antagonize the pressor effect of angiotensin II and vasopressin in the rabbit (Holmes et al., 1963) and in conscious rats (Weeks and Wingerson, 1964). The interaction of prostaglandins and various vasoactive substances also occurs locally in the heart, spleen, kidney, aorta, mesenteric vessels and fore- and hindlimb vessels.

The effect of prostaglandins on the cardiac responses to catecholamines was small and inconsistent. Thus, Hedqvist and Wennmalm (1971) observed that the effect of PGE_1 and PGE_2 on the mechanical response of isolated perfused rabbit heart to norepinephrine was small and varied from slight inhibition to weak potentiation. The response to sympathetic nerve stimulation on the other hand, was inhibited by PGE_1 and PGE_2 due to diminished release of the neurotransmitter. Since many agents which inhibit adrenergic nervous activity by acting presynaptically (B-TM10, a bretylium-like substance, guanethidine and 6-hydroxydopamine) or postsynaptically (propranolol) are known to inhibit ouabain-induced arrhythmias (Roberts *et al.*, 1963; Dohadwalla *et al.*, 1969), prostaglandins have also been studied for their action against cardiac arrhythmias produced by various agents. Thus, PGE_1 has been reported to suppress arrhythmia produced by coronary occlusion in the dog (Zijlstra *et al.*, 1972) and to increase the doses of ouabain required to produce premature ventricular complexes, ventricular tachycardia and death in the cat (Kelliher and Glenn, 1973). Similar observations have been made with PGE_2 (Mest *et al.*, 1973). Since PGE_1 and PGE_2 have no depressant effect or β-adrenergic receptor blocking action on the heart (cf. Weeks, 1972), their ability to antagonize ouabain-induced arrhythmias could be, at least in part, due to their inhibitory effect on release of the adrenergic transmitter (Hedqvist, 1970a). Ouabain has been shown to increase release of catecholamines from the heart; this effect was associated with the development of arrhythmias (Ciofalo and Treece, 1973). However, $PGF_{2\alpha}$ which did not inhibit release of the adrenergic transmitter from the isolated rabbit heart (Hedqvist and Wennmalm, 1971), suppressed $CaCl_2$ and aconitine-induced arrhythmias in rats, $BaCl_2$-induced arrhythmias in rabbits and ouabain-induced arrhythmias in cats (Forster *et al.*, 1973). Similarly, PGA_2 and $PGF_{2\alpha}$ inhibited aconitine-induced tachycardia in isolated rabbit heart (Tanz, 1974). Therefore, it would appear that the ability of prostaglandins to suppress cardiac arrhythmias, induced by various types of agents, may also involve other mechanisms such as the changes in the permeability of the cell membrane and their effect on intracellular metabolism of different cations.

Prostaglandins of the E and A series, as mentioned earlier, not only produced coronary vasodilatation due to their direct action on the vascular smooth muscle but have also been shown to antagonize the coronary vasodilator effects of catecholamines. Thus, Talesnik and Sunahara (1973) and Sunahara and Talesnik (1974) showed that PGE_1, in the isolated perfused rat and cat heart respectively, in doses which were devoid of a direct vasodilator effect, antagonized the metabolically-induced coronary vasodilatation (MCD) in response to norepinephrine and Ca^{2+}. Prostaglandin E_1 did not antagonize the other cardiostimulatory effects of norepinephrine or Ca^{2+}. Moreover, β-adrenergic blocking agents, propranolol or pronethalol, abolished both the norepinephrine-induced cardiac activity and the consequent MCD but not the cardiac hyperactivity and MCD due to Ca^{2+} or the inhibitory effect of PGE_1 on MCD in response to Ca^{2+}. Since, (1) the inhibitors of prostaglandin synthesis, aspirin and indomethacin (Vane, 1971) potentiated the MCD in response to norepinephrine or Ca^{2+}, but not the cardiac hyperactivity produced by these agents (Figure 5.9), and (2) the infusion of PGE_2 (10 μg/litre) markedly inhibited the indomethacin-potentiated MCD in response to norepinephrine or Ca^{2+} without altering the cardiac hyperactivity produced by these substances, it has been proposed that endogenous prostaglandins may play a role as modulators of the MCD in response to catecholamines or Ca^{2+} (Sunahara and Talesnik, 1974; Talesnik and Sunahara, 1973). The mechanism by which PGE_1 produces this modulatory action may be mediated through the adenylate cyclase cyclic AMP system. The increased MCD response to cardiac hyperactivity (Sen *et al.*, 1972) has been shown to be correlated to cyclic AMP levels and the

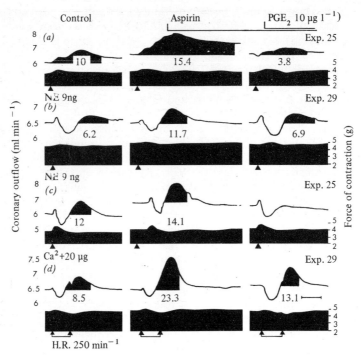

Figure 5.9 Effects of aspirin before and during PGE₂ infusion on MCD responses. The calibrations on the left refer to coronary outflow, the hatched portion represents the area measured for MCD responses and the numbers within the hatching denote % change from control level. The right hand calibration represents the force of heart contractions. Doses of norepinephrine (NE) and calcium chloride (Ca²⁺) were given (▲). Tachycardia (250 beats/min) was applied during the interval (↑ ↑). Reproduced from Talesnik and Sunahara (1973), by courtesy of *Nature*

prostaglandin-induced inhibition of MCD is associated with diminished cyclic AMP production (Sunahara *et al.*, 1972). On the basis of these observations it has been concluded that cardiac hyperactivity, in response to norepinephrine or Ca^{2+}, may lead to activation of adenylate cyclase which could be the triggering mechanism for the regulation of coronary vascular smooth muscle tone. Thus, if cyclic AMP levels were reduced as a result of inhibition of adenylate cyclase by E prostaglandins, cardiac hyperactivity would be followed by a reduced MCD response. In contrast, if cyclic AMP levels were increased by the administration of phosphodiesterase inhibitors (Sunahara *et al.*, 1972; Sen *et al.*, 1972) or by inhibitors of prostaglandin synthesis, MCD would be potentiated and the levels of cyclic AMP increased. Thus, prostaglandins, probably by regulating the activity of adenylate cyclase, modulated MCD in response to catecholamines and various other agents.

Prostaglandins also affected the splenic vascular and capsular smooth muscle responses to various vasoactive agents. Davies and Withrington (1968, 1969, 1971) found that close-arterial infusion of PGE₁, in the blood-perfused dog spleen did not alter the vasoconstrictor responses to epinephrine, norepinephrine, angiotensin II or sympathetic nerve stimulation. Similarly,

PGE_2 did not alter the effects of epinephrine or norepinephrine. The splenic capsular smooth muscle responses to catecholamines and angiotensin II were also unaltered by PGE_1, PGE_2 and PGA_2, whereas, a slight potentiation with PGA_1 and $PGF_{2\alpha}$ was observed. Hedqvist (1969, 1970b) and Hedqvist and Brundin (1969) showed that in the cat spleen the mechanical responses to sympathetic nerve stimulation and to norepinephrine were inhibited by PGE_1, while with PGE_2 the capsular response was largely unaffected and the vascular response was biphasic, i.e., inhibition in the presence of low concentrations and potentiation with high doses. On the basis of these observations, Hedqvist (1969) suggested that PGE_2, released during splenic contraction, may have a homeostatic function, reducing both the amount of norepinephrine released from sympathetic nerves and its effects on the smooth muscle. Ferreira *et al.* (1971) showed that administration of an inhibitor of prostaglandin synthesis, indomethacin, caused augmentation of the effect of epinephrine infusions in the dog spleen. Similarly, in the cat spleen, augmentation of the responses to norepinephrine, angiotensin II and nerve stimulation was observed after the administration of indomethacin (Figure 5.10). These

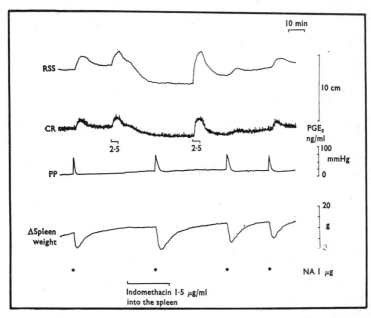

Figure 5.10 Inhibition of prostaglandin synthesis increases the effects of norepinephrine injections. Indomethacin (1.5 $\mu g/ml$) was infused into the splenic outflow except when applied to the spleen. The upper two tracings show the contractions of a rat stomach strip (RSS) and a chick rectum (CR) to prostaglandin (PG) infusions and release of prostaglandin by norepinephrine injections. The lower two tracings show the splenic perfusion pressure (PP) (mm Hg) and change in spleen weight (g). The infusion of indomethacin (1.5 $\mu g/ml$) into the spleen caused (a) relaxation of the assay tissues together with an increase in the sensitivity to calibrating infusions of prostaglandin E_2 (b) increased perfusion pressure and augmentation of the effects of norepinephrine injections (NA) (c) abolition of prostaglandin output induced by norepinephrine injections (experiment 12). Time 10 min; vertical scales 10 cm, 100 mm Hg and 20 g. Reproduced from Ferreira, Moncada and Vane (1973), by courtesy of *Br. J. Pharmacol.*

observations support the hypothesis that antagonism by endogenous prostaglandins of the effect of norepinephrine on smooth muscle may be an important homeostatic mechanism in addition to reduction in norepinephrine release.

Prostaglandins, particularly those of the E series, also play an important role in the modification of renal vascular reactivity to various vasoactive substances such as catecholamines and angiotensin. Lonigro *et al.* (1973) have shown that the infusion of PGE_2 antagonized the vasoconstrictor and antidiuretic actions of angiotensin II and norepinephrine when it was infused into the renal artery, at rates which established concentrations of approximately 0.5 ng PGE_2/ml of blood, comparable to those of a PGE-like substance reported in venous effluent of the kidney during escape from the renal effects of pressor hormones. Prostaglandin A_2, in concentrations 5 times greater than those of PGE_2, produced similar effects on the vasoconstrictor responses to angiotensin II and norepinephrine, whereas $PGF_{2\alpha}$ in concentrations up to 1000 ng/min was found to be ineffective. In the isolated perfused rabbit kidney, PGE_2 (Frame *et al.*, 1974) and PGE_1, PGE_2 and PGA_2 (Malik and McGiff, 1975) in higher concentrations, produced a fall in perfusion pressure and antagonized the vasoconstrictor responses to norepinephrine. In contrast, $PGF_{2\alpha}$ produced vasoconstriction and augmented the pressor effects of this agent (Malik and McGiff, 1975). In view of 1) the release of a PGE-like substance from the kidney in response to angiotensin II (McGiff *et al.*, 1970; Aiken and Vane, 1973; Needleman *et al.*, 1973; Gagnon *et al.*, 1974) renal ischaemia (McGiff *et al.*, 1970; Sweet *et al.*, 1972) and adrenergic stimuli (Dunham and Zimmerman, 1970; McGiff *et al.*, 1972; Davis and Horton, 1972) and (2) the demonstration that inhibition of prostaglandin synthesis enhances the renal vasoconstrictor action of angiotensin II and norepinephrine associated with failure of the pressor hormones to release prostaglandins intrarenally (Aiken and Vane, 1973), it has been proposed that prostaglandins of the E series, elaborated by the kidney in response to constrictor stimuli, play an important role in modulating the effect of vasopressor stimuli (McGiff and Iskoviz, 1973). However, this modulatory role of prostaglandins is species-dependent. In the isolated perfused rat kidney where prostaglandins of the E, A and F series produced constriction and enhanced the effect of the adrenergic stimuli, these agents may be prohypertensive (Malik and McGiff, 1975).

The interaction of prostaglandins and catecholamines as well as other vasoactive substances, also occurred in mesenteric blood vessels. Viguera and Sunahara (1969) found that the intravenous administration of PGE_1, at rates which did not produce vasodilatation, inhibited the vasoconstrictor effect of norepinephrine but not that of angiotensin II applied topically on the mesocaecal arteries. The norepinephrine-induced vasoconstriction was inhibited for a prolonged period of time after PGE_1 infusion had been terminated and the systemic arterial blood pressure had recovered to normal levels. In contrast, PGE_1 did not alter the vasoconstrictor responses to norepinephrine and angiotensin II in the cremaster muscle. However, Kaley and Weiner (1968), Weiner and Kaley (1969) and Messina *et al.* (1974) showed that PGE_1, in an anaesthetized rat, antagonized the constrictor effect of epinephrine, norepinephrine, angiotensin II and vasopressin applied topically on mesenteric and cremasteric blood vessels. The discrepancy between these results and those of Viguera and Sunahara (1969) could be due to the high doses used by these authors, for Messina et al. (1974) found that PGE_1 in the cremaster muscle did not affect the arteriolar response to the high doses of vasopressor agents but did inhibit the vasoconstrictor effects of low doses of angiotensin II, catecholamines and vasopressin. The constrictor effect of serotonin or the dilator effect of histamine or bradykinin was not altered by PGE_1 in the mesenteric and cremasteric blood vessels. Prostaglandin A_1 did not alter the responses to these vasopressor agents on the mesenteric and cremasteric blood vessels. The inhibitory effect of PGE_1 on the vascular responsiveness to vasoactive agents, was also demonstrated after the vasodilator effect of PGE_1 had subsided. Moreover, PGE_1 despite its greater vasodilator action in the cremasteric than in the mesenteric vessels, failed to antagonize the vasoconstrictor response to high doses of vasoactive agents in cremaster muscle whereas, in mesenteric vessels, it antagonized the constrictor responses to high doses of vasopressor agents. In the isolated perfused rabbit kidney, PGE_1 was also shown to inhibit the vasoconstrictor responses to injected norepinephrine (Malik and McGiff, 1975). In contrast, in the isolated perfused rat mesenteric arteries, PGE_1, PGE_2, PGA_2 and $PGF_{2\alpha}$ potentiated the vasoconstrictor responses to injected norepinephrine (Malik and McGiff, 1974). Similar observations were made by Tobian and Viets (1970) with PGE_1 in this preparation. These authors proposed that the inhibitory action of PGE_1 on the vasoconstrictor response to norepinephrine *in vivo* was probably due to its interaction with one or more humoral substances which are absent *in vitro*. Kadar and Sunahara (1969) found that the norepinephrine-induced contractions of the isolated canine mesenteric artery and vein strip preparations were inhibited by PGE_1 and enhanced by $PGF_{1\alpha}$ and $PGF_{2\alpha}$ (Figure 5.11). However, Greenberg and Long (1973), Greenberg et al. (1973b) and Greenberg, Kadowitz et al. (1973) found that the contractile response of the isolated superfused canine mesenteric arteries and veins, tibial arteries and dorsal metatarsal veins was enhanced by PGE_1, PGE_2, PGA_2 and $PGF_{2\alpha}$. The augmentation in the contractile response of these vascular strips to vasoactive agents was independent of changes in the vascular tone. Prostaglandins E_1 and E_2 reduced the vascular tone whereas PGA_2 raised the basal tone. Moreover, the increase in resting tension, produced by PGA_2 returned to control levels within 15 min of removal of PGA_2 from the perfusion fluid, whereas the response to each of the agonists was still enhanced 1 h after removal of PGA_2 from the medium. Prostaglandin $F_{2\alpha}$, on the other hand, did not alter the vascular tone.

Prostaglandins of the E, A and F series also affected the vascular reactivity to various vasoactive agents in the fore- and hindlimb vascular beds. Bevegard and Orö (1969) showed that the vasodilator action of PGE_1 was abolished by the simultaneous infusion of norepinephrine. In the human superficial hand veins, PGE_2, PGA_1 and PGA_2 antagonized the vasoconstrictor effect of norepinephrine and serotonin (Robinson et al., 1973). However, in the dog perfused forelimb, Daughtery et al. (1968) failed to find any effect of PGE_1 on the vasoconstrictor responses to epinephrine, norepinephrine or angiotensin II. In contrast, Holmes et al. (1963) showed that in the perfused hindlimb of the cat, PGE_1 reduced the vasoconstrictor responses to intra-arterial

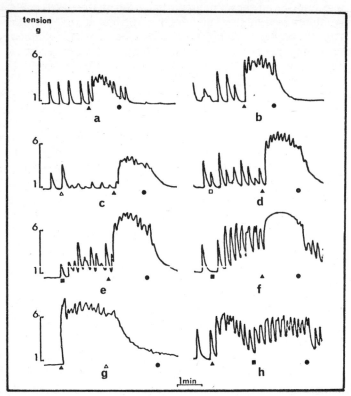

Figure 5.11   The influence of PGE$_1$, PGF$_{1\alpha}$ and PGF$_{2\alpha}$ on the norepinephrine-induced contractions in the isolated vein. ▲ norepinephrine; △ PGE$_1$; □ PGF$_{1\alpha}$; ■ PGF$_{2\alpha}$; ● wash. (a) norepinephrine, 24 ng/ml; norepinephrine, 50 ng/ml; (c) PGE$_1$, 100 ng/ml + norepinephrine, 50 ng/ml; (d) PGF$_{1\alpha}$, 100 ng/ml + norepinephrine, 50 ng/ml; (e) PGF$_{2\alpha}$, 25 ng/ml + norepinephrine, 50 ng/ml; (f) PGF$_{2\alpha}$, 50 ng/ml + norepinephrine, 25 ng/ml; (g) norepinephrine, 50 ng/ml + PGE$_1$, 200 ng/ml; (h) norepinephrine, 25 ng/ml + PGF$_{2\alpha}$, 50 ng/ml. Reproduced from Kadar and Sunahara (1969), by courtesy of *Can. J. Physiol. Pharmacol.*

injections of epinephrine, norepinephrine and angiotensin II. Similar antagonism to the vasoconstrictor response to sympathetic nerve stimulation and injected norepinephrine by PGE$_1$ and PGE$_2$ was observed in the cat hindleg (Hedqvist, 1972). He found that the low doses of PGE$_1$ produced a small and inconsistent effect varying from slight reduction to weak potentiation, while higher concentrations consistently caused small inhibition of the response to norepinephrine. Prostaglandin E$_2$ inhibited the responses to norepinephrine only in high concentrations. In dog hindlimb, PGE$_1$, PGE$_2$ and PGA$_2$ produced vasodilatation and reduced the vasoconstrictor responses to norepinephrine, angiotensin II and sympathetic nerve stimulation (Kadowitz, 1972). However, there was no relationship between the vasodilator and inhibitory effect of prostaglandins on the vascular responses to the vasoactive agents. Prostaglandin E$_1$ and E$_2$ were equipotent as vasodilators; however, PGE$_1$ was much more potent than PGE$_2$ in inhibiting the vasoconstrictor responses to nerve stimulation, norepinephrine and angiotensin II. Similarly, PGA_2 and PGE_2 had almost similar inhibitory effects on the vasoconstrictor response to these agents, while PGE_2 was more potent than PGA_2 as a vasodilator. In the perfused canine hindpaw and gracilis muscle, PGE_1 inhibited the vascular responses to sympathetic nerve stimulation, epinephrine, norepinephrine, angiotensin II or serotonin (Hedwall et al., 1971; Kadowitz et al., 1971c). The threshold concentration of PGE_1 which produced vasodilatation was lower in the vascular bed of the gracilis muscle than in that of the skin of the hindpaw (Hedwall et al., 1971), yet inhibition of vascular response to vasoconstrictor stimuli was more pronounced and longer lasting in the skin than in the skeletal muscle. Based on these observations, it was concluded that the inhibitory effect of PGE_1 on the vasoconstrictor responses to these agents was independent of the vasodilator actions of PGE_1. Moreover, the interaction of PGE_1 with vasoconstrictor stimuli was specific, since the reduction in the responsiveness to vasoconstrictor interventions produced by PGE_1 could not be duplicated by the infusion of the vasodilator agent, glyceryl trinitrate. Zimmerman et al. (1973) found that the infusion of a low dose of PGE_2 (110 ng/min) depressed the vasoconstrictor responses to both norepinephrine and nerve stimulation. Since the inhibitors of prostaglandin synthesis, indomethacin and eicosatetraynoic acid, potentiated the vasoconstrictor responses to adrenergic stimuli, it was suggested that prostaglandins of the E series, synthesized in the cutaneous vasculature, may play an important role in the modulation of vascular reactivity to adrenergic stimuli. In contrast, Mayer et al., (1970) showed that, in the isolated perfused hindpaw, the intra-arterial injection of PGE_1 (5 μg) augmented the vasoconstrictor response to nerve stimulation and reduced the response to norepinephrine. However, a large dose of PGE_1 (0.35 μg/min) reduced the vasoconstrictor responses to both adrenergic stimuli. Kadowitz et al. (1971c), on the other hand, found that PGE_2, 1 μg/min, did not alter the vasoconstrictor responses to sympathetic nerve stimulation, norepinephrine or angiotensin II in the canine hindpaw. However, high concentrations of PGE_2, 2 μg/min, potentiated the response to nerve stimulation without altering that to norepinephrine. Prostaglandin A_2, on the other hand, failed to alter the vasoconstrictor responses of the perfused canine hindpaw to tyramine and norepinephrine but potentiated the vasoconstrictor responses to sympathetic nerve stimulation, presumably due to enhanced release of the adrenergic transmitter (Greenberg et al., 1974). Since PGB_1 and PGB_2, which are formed from PGA_2 by the action of a prostaglandin isomerase (Jones, 1972b), produced similar actions on the vasoconstrictor response to nerve stimulation, tyramine and norepinephrine, it was concluded that the effect of PGA_2 is mediated by its conversion within the vascular tissue to PGB_2 (Greenberg, Howard and Wilson, 1974; Greenberg et al., 1974). Prostaglandin $F_{1\alpha}$ and $F_{2\alpha}$ augmented the vascular response of canine hindpaw to sympathetic nerve stimulation without altering the vascular resistance (Kadowitz et al., 1971c, 1972). Since $PGF_{1\alpha}$ decreased and $PGF_{2\alpha}$ produced no effect on the vasoconstrictor response to norepinephrine, these authors concluded that prostaglandins of the F series act presynaptically and facilitate adrenergic transmission. Prostaglandin $F_{2\alpha}$ was also shown to exert a similar action on the canine perfused saphenous vein (Kadowitz et al., 1971b).

The interaction of prostaglandins and various vasoactive agents has also been shown to occur in the isolated aorta and other vascular preparations. Khairallah *et al.* (1967) showed that the contractile effect of angiotensin II, serotonin and vasopressin, but not that of norepinephrine, was enhanced by subcontractile doses of PGE_1 (0.1–1.0 ng/ml). Augmentation of the contractile effect of vasopressin by PGE_1 was dependent on the catecholamine stores since it did not occur in norepinephrine depleted preparations and it was restored when norepinephrine stores were replenished by the infusion of this agent. On the other hand, potentiation by PGE_1 of the contractile response of aortic strips to serotonin and angiotensin II was independent of norepinephrine stores. Since subcontractile amounts of PGE_1 reduced the threshold voltage of vacular smooth muscle, it was concluded that augmentation of the contractile response to serotonin and angiotensin II by PGE_1 could be due to hypopolarization of the cell membrane. Strong and Bohr (1967) also showed that PGE_1, PGE_2, PGA_1 and $PGF_{2\alpha}$ enhanced the contractile effect of angiotensin II and KCl on the rabbit aortic strip. Lee *et al.* (1965) however, failed to demonstrate an effect of PGA_2 on the contractile response of the vascular smooth muscle to norepinephrine or angiotensin II. The antagonism between PGE_2 and papaverine on the isolated rabbit aortic strips has been demonstrated by Levy (1973b). Papaverine was shown to cause a concentration-dependent inhibition of PGE_2-induced contraction which was enhanced in zero Ca^{2+} and was unaltered by low K^+. The antagonistic effect of papaverine was not due to its phosphodiesterase inhibitory activity (Kukovetz and Pöch, 1970) since imidazole, which is known to stimulate phosphodiesterase activity in various tissues (Robison *et al.*, 1971), did not antagonize the effect of PGE_2 but rather potentiated it. Further dibutyryl cyclic AMP pretreatment did not greatly alter the effect of papaverine. From these observations it was postulated that papaverine antagonized the contractile effect of PGE_2 presumably by its action on Ca^{2+} and Ca^{2+}–contraction coupling mechanism, rather than by directly affecting the intracellular cyclic AMP levels. The interaction of PGE_1 and $PGF_{2\alpha}$ and norepinephrine and vasopressin in the perfused vessels of the rabbit ear and of PGE_1 and PGE_2 and norepinephrine in the rabbit central ear artery has been demonstrated by Al Tai and Graham (1972) and Kalsner (1974) respectively. Prostaglandin E_1 and E_2 reduced the vasoconstrictor responses to injected norepinephrine in the central ear artery, whereas in the rabbit perfused ear vessels the addition of norepinephrine or vasopressin to the Krebs' solution increased perfusion pressure which had been reduced by the simultaneous administration of either PGE_1 or $PGF_{2\alpha}$. The dilator effect was not affected by hyoscine or propranolol. Since treatments which elevate cyclic AMP levels in tissues such as perfusion with theophylline with added ATP, ADP, 3′,5′-AMP or pretreatment of animals with stilbestrol, antagonized the dilator effect of PGE_1 and/or $PGF_{2\alpha}$ on the norepinephrine-induced constriction of ear vessels, it was proposed that prostaglandins may produce this effect by regulating the activity of the adenylate cyclase–phosphodiesterase system.

From the aforementioned studies it is quite apparent that the antagonistic action of prostaglandins on the vascular responsiveness to various agents is independent of their direct dilator or constrictor actions on vascular smooth muscle. Moreover, the effect of a prostaglandin on the vascular reactivity to a vasoactive agent depends upon the vascular bed, the animal species and the concentration of prostaglandin as well as of the agonist used. The mechanism by which prostaglandins inhibit or potentiate the vascular responses to a wide variety of vasoactive agents has not yet been clearly elucidated. Studies thus far carried out have related the effect of prostaglandins, on the response of vascular tissues to vasoactive agents, to changes in the permeability of the cell membrane to Ca^{2+} (Clegg et al., 1966) and alterations in intracellular Ca^{2+} binding or release (Strong and Bohr, 1967). Khairallah et al. (1967) have postulated that subthreshold doses of PGE_1 may enhance the vascular responsiveness to other vasoactive agents by causing hypopolarization of the cell membrane. Greenberg and Long (1973) and Greenberg et al. (1973a, b) and Greenberg, Kadowitz et al. (1973), who have shown potentiation of the vascular tissues to norepinephrine, KCl and $BaCl_2$ by PGE_1, PGE_2, PGA_2 and $PGF_{2\alpha}$ and have measured the uptake and efflux of total ^{45}Ca in the tissues during some of these interventions, have suggested that prostaglandins of the E and F series produce their effect by modifying the membrane permeability to Ca^{2+} ions, whereas PGA_2 decreased the binding of Ca^{2+} to intracellular sites. However, in view of (1) preferential synthesis of prostaglandins of the E series in bovine mesenteric arteries and prostaglandins of the F series in veins under the action of vasoactive agents, such as bradykinin, (Terragno et al., 1975) and (2) conversion of PGE to PGF in various tissues (Leslie and Levine, 1973; Lee and Levine, 1974a) it is suggested that patterns of prostaglandin synthesis and interconversion of the primary prostaglandins also play an important role in the modification of vascular reactivity to vasoactive substances.

5.2.15 Prostaglandins in hypertension

Prostaglandins, particularly those of the E and A series which are synthesized in response to vasoactive stimuli in various organs, including kidney, and have potent antihypertensive actions, have led to the hypothesis that essential hypertension probably results from an inadequate amount of vasodepressor prostaglandins (Lee, 1969, McGiff and Iskovitz, 1973). Recently, Colina et al. (1975) have shown that the administration of indomethacin, in doses of 10–20 mg/kg per day for 17 days in unanaesthetized rabbits, caused a significant, progressive increase in blood pressure as compared to control animals. This was associated with a significant reduction in the urinary excretion of 'PGE' from 0.56 to 0.05 μg/day. Moreover, they showed that the conversion of radiolabelled arachidonic acid to prostaglandins of the E and F series by renomedullary homogenates was reduced by 75% in indomethacin-treated rabbits. From these studies they concluded that continuous synthesis of prostaglandins in renal and perhaps in extrarenal tissues may be an important factor in the maintenance of normal blood pressure. This conclusion is in agreement with the observations of Larsson and Änggård (1973) who showed that intravenous infusion of a precursor of prostaglandins, arachidonic acid, in anaesthetized rabbits caused a dose dependent fall in systemic arterial blood pressure. However, after the administration of an inhibitor of prostaglandin synthesis, indomethacin, this effect of arachidonic acid was abolished and the systemic arterial blood pressure was increased above control levels. Similarly, administration of arachidonic acid has been shown to cause a profound fall in systemic arterial blood pressure and increased heart rate in spontaneously hypertensive rats (SHR) (Cohen et al., 1973). This effect was also observed in animals receiving either PGE_1 or PGE_2. Since the administration of the anti-inflammatory agents, indomethacin, aspirin and phenylbutazone, produced a significant inhibition of the arachidonic acid-induced changes in arterial blood pressure but not that produced by PGE_1 or PGE_2, the effect of arachidonic acid was presumably mediated by its conversion to PGs. In contrast, in rats made hypertensive by unilateral nephrectomy and administration of desoxycorticosterone acetate (DOCA) and high salt diet, arachidonic acid, 200 mg/kg given by gastric intubation simultaneously with DOCA injection or after the onset of hypertension, aggravated the rise in blood pressure (Laborit and Valette, 1974). The discrepancy between these results and those of the former workers is probably due to a difference in the model of hypertension used. Moreover, Laborit and Valette (1974) did not study the effect of exogenous prostaglandins and inhibitors of prostaglandin synthesis on the arachidonic acid induced rise in blood pressure in their model of hypertension. Therefore, it is difficult to say if the effect of arachidonic acid on blood pressure in their experiments was mediated by its conversion to prostaglandins or by some other mechanism.

Somova and Dochev (1971) studied the effect of PGE_1 in renal hypertensive Wistar rats and found that chronic, daily intraperitoneal administration of this agent normalized the blood pressure within 2 weeks of treatment. In contrast, Wendling and DuCharme (1974), using the same route of administration (PGE_1, 15 μg/kg per day) in Sprague-Dawley rats made hypertensive by bilateral renal artery constriction or by unilateral renal artery constriction and contralateral nephrectomy, failed to confirm these observations. They also did not find any effect of PGE_1 in the SHR under similar experimental conditions. The discrepancy between these results and those of Somova and Dochev (1971) is probably due to differences in the strain of rats used by these workers. Moreover, PGE_1 is removed from blood on a single passage across the lung (Ferreira and Vane, 1967; McGiff et al., 1969) and the intraperitoneal route of administration used by these workers could result in very small but different arterial blood levels of PGE_1 which may or may not be sufficient to produce a change in blood pressure. Leach et al. (1973) studied the effect of PGA_2 and PGE_2 in anaesthetized spontaneously hypertensive rats (SHR) and found that intravenous injection of PGA_2 and PGE_2 caused a prolonged fall in systemic arterial blood pressure. This prolonged fall in blood pressure was evident only when prostaglandins were administered according to a rigid dose and time schedule in SHR but not in normotensive rats. Since the delayed fall in systemic arterial blood pressure in SHR was abolished by cutting the vagi or after efferent vagal blockade, they concluded that the prolonged fall in arterial blood pressure produced by PGA_2 and PGE_2, was mediated through stimulation of the vagus. In contrast, Simpson (1974) found that PGE_2 produced a fall in systemic arterial blood pressure in the normotensive rat as well as in SHR but the degree of fall in arterial blood pressure was greater in spontaneously hypertensive rats than in three different strains of normotensive rats. Moreover, the vasodepressor effect of PGE_2 was shown to be related to the degree of rise in blood pressure in SHR, viz., the higher the pressure, the greater the effect of PGE_2. When the development of high blood pressure in SHR was prevented by the oral administration of hydralazine or guanethidine the increased responsiveness to PGE_2 did not occur. Similarly, when established hypertension in SHR was reversed by administration of these agents, increased responsiveness to PGE_2 was lost. The increased responsiveness of SHR to PGE_2 appears to be specific since, other vasodilator agents acetylcholine and isoprenaline produced similar falls in arterial blood pressure in normotensive and SHR. Spontaneously hypertensive rats have also been shown to have enhanced responsiveness to the vasopressor and other cardiovascular effects of $PGF_{2\alpha}$. Thus, Ellis and Hutchins (1974) showed that $PGF_{2\alpha}$ increased systemic arterial blood pressure and pulse pressure and caused constriction of cremaster muscle arterioles to a greater degree in SHR than in normotensive rats. Although spontaneously hypertensive rats showed a greater responsiveness to the vasodilator effects of PGE_2 and vasopressor effects of $PGF_{2\alpha}$, the effect of prostaglandins on the isolated vascular preparations of these animals showed qualitative as well as quantitative differences. Thus, PGE_2 and its precursor, arachidonic acid, produced a greater increase in perfusion pressure in the isolated kidney of SHR than in the kidney of normotensive rats (Armstrong et al., 1975). The increase in perfusion pressure produced by arachidonic acid was abolished by indomethacin, an inhibitor of prostaglandin synthesis (Vane, 1971). The vasoconstrictor effect of angiotensin II was also found to be greater in SHR. Since the greater release of prostaglandins from the kidney of SHR caused by angiotensin II was prevented by indomethacin, it was concluded that renal prostaglandins could contribute to the elevated blood pressure of SHR. Levy (1973a) showed that PGE_2 increased the contractile force and beat of isolated atria of the SHR to a similar degree as in normotensive rats. Further, the basal rate of beat of the atria of SHR and normotensive rat was similar. In contrast, the effect of prostaglandins on the isolated aortic strips from SHR was found to be variable (Levy, 1973c). Thus, PGE_2 and $PGF_{2\alpha}$ produced significantly less contractile effect on the aortic strips isolated from SHR than those from normotensive rats. Prostaglandin A_1, on the other hand, produced a similar degree of contraction of aortic strips from SHR and normotensive rats; whereas PGE_1 produced greater contraction of aortic strips of SHR than of normotensive rats. Similarly, the ability of papaverine to reduce the contractile effect of PGE_2, $PGF_{2\alpha}$ and PGA_1 on the isolated aortic strip of SHR was found to be reduced (Levy, 1974). Thus, the concentration of papaverine required to produce 50% inhibition of the contractile response of isolated aortic strips to PGA_1, $PGF_{2\alpha}$ and PGE_2 was increased to 2.8, 5.1 and 6.2 fold, respectively, in SHR compared to normal rats. In contrast, inhibition of the contractile effect of norepinephrine and KCl on aortic strips of SHR was not significantly different from those of normal animals. Since papaverine is a powerful inhibitor of phosphodiesterase activity and enhanced intracellular levels of cyclic AMP may cause vascular smooth muscle relaxation (Pöch and Kukovetz, 1972), the decreased ability of papaverine to antagonize the contract ileresponse to prostaglandins could be due to enhanced phosphodiesterase activity in the isolated aorta of SHR (Amer, 1973) and possibly a difference in PG-induced Ca^{2+} translocation (Carsten, 1972) in the aorta of SHR compared to that of normotensive animals.

5.2.16 Cardiovascular neurotransmission

5.2.16.1 Adrenergic neuromuscular junction

The adrenergic nervous system plays an important role in the maintenance of vascular tone. Although the activity of the adrenergic nervous system is ultimately controlled by the central nervous system, it is greatly susceptible to modulation by various vasoactive hormones such as angiotensins and prostaglandins. In addition to their direct effect on the cardiovascular system prostaglandins also affect adrenergic transmission in cardiovascular tissues. Recent studies have shown that there are not only quantitative and qualitative differences between the action of prostaglandins on the adrenergic neuromuscular junction but their actions differ in various animal species and vary with the concentration of the agent used. The activity of prostaglandins at the adrenergic neuromuscular junction and their role as mediators of a feedback control of neurotransmission has been the subject of several recent reviews (Hedqvist, 1973; Horton, 1973; Brody and Kadowitz, 1974). (See also Chapter 2.)

Of the various types of prostaglandins synthesized in cardiovascular tissues in response to various stimuli, (cf. Ramwell and Shaw, 1970; cf. Horton, 1973; cf. Hedqvist, 1973; cf. Crowshaw and McGiff, 1973), those of the E series appear to be the most likely physiological modulators of adrenergic transmission (Hedqvist, 1973). The proposed role of prostaglandins of the E series as modulators of adrenergic transmission is supported by the following:

(1) the ability of E prostaglandins to modify the response of adrenergic tissues to sympathetic nerve stimulation and to administered norepinephrine. Alterations in the response of various tissues produced by prostaglandins was associated with changes in the output of the adrenergic transmitter

(2) stimulation of adrenergic nerves as well as administration of norepinephrine enhanced release of PGE-like substances as a result of activation of their synthesis in cardiovascular tissues. This enhanced output of prostaglandins in response to adrenergic stimuli was abolished after the administration of inhibitors of prostaglandin synthesis

(3) inhibition of prostaglandin synthesis modified the response of adrenergic tissues to sympathetic nerve stimulation in a direction opposite to that produced by exogenous prostaglandins, especially PGE compounds. These alterations in the response to sympathetic nerve stimulation were usually associated with changes in the output of adrenergic transmitter

(4) finally, adrenergic tissues contain the enzymes for the synthesis, interconversion and degradation of prostaglandins.

Although other prostaglandins (PGA, PGF) also affect the adrenergic neuromuscular junction they have not yet been thoroughly investigated for their role in sympathetic transmission. Most of the available evidence indicates that PGA and PGF compounds are less likely modulators of adrenergic transmission. They are synthesized in cardiovascular tissues in relatively small amounts as compared to prostaglandins of the E series (Karim, 1967, Karim, Sandler and Williams, 1967; Karim, Hillier and Devlin, 1968; cf. Horton, 1973; cf. Crowshaw and McGiff, 1973; Papanicalaou *et al.*, 1974). Moreover, inhibitors of prostaglandin synthesis in many adrenergic tissues produce effects expected to result from inhibition of the synthesis of endogenous prostaglandins of the E and not those of the F series. Similarly, the involvement of A prostaglandins as physiological modulators of adrenergic transmission is uncertain in view of the lack of conclusive evidence supporting their natural occurrence in tissues such as the kidney (cf. Crowshaw and McGiff, 1973). However, when one considers the presence of enzymes (Lee and Levine, 1974a; Lee *et al.*, 1975) capable of converting one type of prostaglandin to another type of prostaglandin such as E to F it becomes evident that the effect of endogenous prostaglandins on the modulation of adrenergic transmission will finally depend on the type of prostaglandin synthesized as well as the rate of synthesis. Moreover, these factors may also determine the direction of modulation, viz., facilitation or inhibition of adrenergic transmission.

Effect of prostaglandins on the response of cardiovascular tissues to sympathetic nerve stimulation and administered catecholamines

E Prostaglandins: Prostaglandins E_1 and E_2 have been shown to reduce the vasoconstrictor responses to sympathetic nerve stimulation and catecholamines in the spleen of the cat (Hedqvist, 1969; Hedqvist, 1970b; Hedqvist and Brundin, 1969), kidney of the dog (Lonigro *et al.*, 1973) and the rabbit (Frame *et al.*, 1974; Malik and McGiff, 1975), hindlimb of the cat (Holmes *et al.*, 1963; Hedqvist, 1972) and the dog (Kadowitz, 1972), the dog paw (Hedwall *et al.*, 1971; Kadowitz *et al.*, 1971a, c), the rabbit portal vein (Greenberg, 1974) and mesenteric arteries (Malik and McGiff, 1974), the isolated heart (Hedqvist *et al.*, 1971; Hedqvist and Wennmalm, 1971) as well as reduce the chronotropic responses of the rabbit sino-atrial node (Park *et al.*, 1973) and guinea pig atria (Illés *et al.*, 1973) to sympathetic nerve stimulation at low frequencies. The degree of inhibition produced by PGE_1 and PGE_2 of the responses of several of these tissues to sympathetic nerve stimulation was greater than the response to administered norepinephrine. Moreover, doses too low to alter the response of adrenergic tissues to norepinephrine, inhibited that to sympathetic nerve stimulation. Thus, in the hindpaw of the dog, PGE_1 tended to inhibit the pressor response to nerve stimulation to a greater degree than to norepinephrine (Kadowitz *et al.*, 1971a). In the isolated perfused rabbit kidney, infusion of PGE_1 and PGE_2 in doses (0.1 ng/ml) which failed to alter the basal perfusion pressure and the vasoconstrictor responses to injected norepinephrine, markedly inhibited the equiconstrictor response to sympathetic nerve stimulation (Figure 5.12). Similar results have been obtained in the cat hindlimb (Hedqvist, 1972) rabbit heart (Hedqvist and Wennmalm, 1971) and rabbit portal vein (Greenberg,

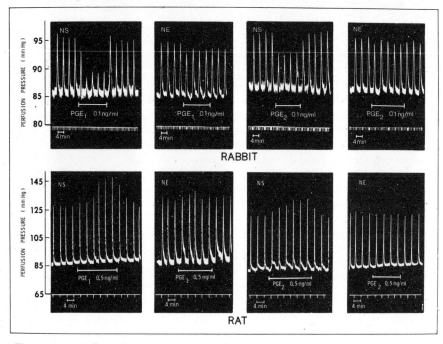

Figure 5.12 Effect of PGE_1 and PGE_2 on the vasoconstrictor responses of isolated perfused rabbit (upper panel) and rat (lower panel) kidney to sympathetic nerve stimulation (NS) and to equiconstrictor responses to injected norepinephrine (NE). Sympathetic nerves to the renal vessels were stimulated for 22 s at 4 min intervals. NE (50–75 ng) was injected directly into the arterial cannula at 4 min intervals. Reproduced from Malik and McGiff (1975), by courtesy of *Circulation Res.*

1974). These observations indicate that PGE_1 and PGE_2, in addition to their postsynaptic actions may also act on the presynaptic sites of the adrenergic neuromuscular junction. Thus, in the isolated, saline perfused cat spleen, Hedqvist (1970b) found that the reduction in responses to sympathetic nerve stimulation following administration of PGE_2 was associated with decreased output of the adrenergic transmitter. On increasing the doses of PGE_2 (6×10^{-8} to 6×10^{-6} M), its inhibitory effect on the release of norepinephrine evoked by nerve stimulation was progressively increased and closely paralleled the reduction in the vasoconstrictor responses with regard to onset, intensity and recovery (Figure 5.13). Similar observations were made in the isolated rabbit heart (Hedqvist and Wennmalm, 1971). Administration of PGE_1 and PGE_2 progressively and reversibly inhibited the mechanical responses of this organ associated with reduced output of the adrenergic transmitter to sympathetic nerve stimulation. In human arteries and veins PGE_2 inhibited the output of preloaded radiolabelled norepinephrine in response to sympathetic nerve stimulation (Stjärne and Gripe, 1973).

The inhibitory effect of prostaglandins on the release of the adrenergic transmitter has been shown not to be due to increased inactivation of liberated norepinephrine by either metabolic degradation or increased neuronal

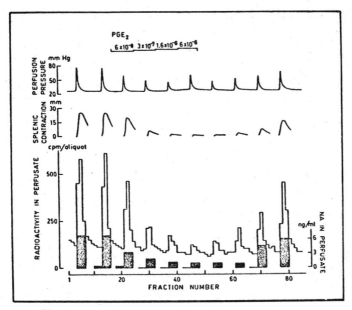

Figure 5.13 Isolated perfused cat spleen loaded with ^{3}H-DL-NA. Lower panel: outflow of radioactivity and of fluorimetrically determined NA from the spleen, resting and in response to supramaximal nerve stimulations (NS) 200 pulses at 10 s. Upper panel: perfusion pressure and splenic contraction responses to NS. Effect of increasing doses of PGE$_2$ (molar concentrations). Reproduced from Hedqvist (1970), by courtesy of *Acta Physiol. Scand.*

re-uptake. Thus, in the cat spleen previously loaded with radioactive norepinephrine, PGE$_1$ and PGE$_2$ were found to cause a simultaneous, closely parallel and reversible reduction of the efflux of total radioactive material and of fluorimetrically determined norepinephrine in response to nerve stimulation (Hedqvist and Brundin, 1969; Hedqvist, 1970b). Moreover, PGE$_2$ did not alter the removal of tritium-labelled norepinephrine infused into the spleen (Hedqvist, 1970b). Nor was the inhibitory effect of PGE$_1$ or PGE$_2$ on the output of adrenergic transmitter evoked by nerve stimulation the result of decreased norepinephrine synthesis since prostaglandins did not alter the biosynthesis of norepinephrine from tyrosine in isolated bovine splenic nerves (Hedqvist, 1973). Moreover, an inhibitory effect of PGE$_1$ and PGE$_2$ directly on the nerve granules is unlikely. Thus, PGE$_2$ in doses which reduced the release of norepinephrine produced by sympathetic nerve stimulation did not alter the tyramine-induced release of the adrenergic transmitter (Hedqvist, 1970c). The inhibitory effect of prostaglandins on the release of the adrenergic transmitter has also been shown to be independent of the negative feedback mechanism mediated through stimulation of presynaptic α-adrenoceptors (Stjärne, 1973). These observations taken together with the failure of PGE compounds to alter the basal efflux of norepinephrine, in the isolated rabbit heart (Hedqvist *et al.*, 1970), strongly suggest that PGE compounds inhibit outflow of norepinephrine from adrenergic nerves indirectly by interfering with some of the steps in the release mechanism triggered by nerve impulses. The release of norepinephrine from sympathetic fibres by nerve impulses requires Ca^{2+} (Huković and Muscholl, 1962), and the output of the adrenergic transmitter as well as the response of an organ to sympathetic nerve stimulation is related to the concentration of Ca^{2+} in the medium (Kirpekar and Misu, 1967; Burn and Gibbons, 1964; Malik and McGiff, 1972). On the basis of these observations it has been proposed that, upon the arrival of a nerve action potential, depolarization causes entry of Ca^{2+} into the nerve terminal which, in some still unknown way, activates the process of release of the neurotransmitter (cf. Rubin, 1970; cf. Hubbard, 1970). In view of the demonstration of: (a) the close interrelationship between the concentration of Ca^{2+} and the direct actions of prostaglandins in some tissues (Bygdeman, 1964; Mantegazza, 1965; Mantegazza and Naimzada, 1965; Clegg et al., 1966; Fassina and Contessa, 1967; Emmons et al., 1967; Fassina et al., 1969) and (b) the ability of increased Ca^{2+} concentrations to counteract the inhibitory action of PGE_2, and restore to normal the output of norepinephrine in response to nerve stimulation (Hedqvist, 1970c); it has been postulated that PGE compounds may inhibit release of the adrenergic transmitter by decreasing the potential of the nerve terminal membrane possibly by increasing Na^+ permeability, and thereby, upon arrival of a nerve action potential, reduce the influx of Ca^{2+} or charged Ca^{2+} complex required for release of the adrenergic transmitter. Alternatively, prostaglandins may exert a direct action on the membrane bound Ca^{2+}, and in this way reduce the influx of Ca^{2+} to further nerve impulses (Hedqvist, 1973).

Although prostaglandins of the E series, in general, inhibit the response of cardiovascular tissues to sympathetic nerve stimulation or administered norepinephrine, they have also been shown to be either ineffective or to potentiate the response of some vascular tissues to adrenergic stimuli in various animal species. Thus, in the dog spleen (Davies and Withrington, 1968, 1969), PGE_1 and PGE_2 did not affect the vasoconstrictor responses to sympathetic nerve stimulation or to norepinephrine. Prostaglandin E_1 augmented the response to norepinephrine in the isolated rabbit aortic strip (Strong and Chandler, 1972), PGE_1 (Mayer et al., 1970) and PGE_2, in higher concentrations (Kadowitz et al., 1971c) to sympathetic nerve stimulation in the dog paw vasculature, PGE_1 to norepinephrine and, at higher frequencies, to sympathetic nerve stimulation in the dog uterine vasculature (Clark et al., 1973) and PGE_1 and PGE_2 to sympathetic nerve stimulation and injected norepinephrine in the rat mesenteric arteries (Malik and McGiff, 1974) and kidney (Malik and McGiff 1975). Since, in these vascular tissues PGE_1 or E_2 potentiated the vasoconstrictor response to sympathetic nerve stimulation when the response to norepinephrine was either unaltered (Kadowitz et al., 1971c) or decreased (Mayer et al., 1970) or potentiated to a lesser degree than the response to nerve stimulation (Figure 5.12), it appears that E prostaglandins enhanced release of the adrenergic transmitter in these tissues. These observations were supported by the demonstration that PGE_1 increased the output of adrenergic transmitter in response to sympathetic nerve stimulation from the dog spleen (Blakely et al., 1969). Although the mechanism by which E prostaglandins facilitate adrenergic transmission in some vascular tissues remains to be investigated, they may produce this effect by enhancing the availability of Ca^{2+} for the release process of the adrenergic transmitter in a way similar to that proposed for their direct actions on the excitation–contraction coupling process in vascular smooth muscle (Clegg et al., 1966). Thus, it would appear that E prostaglandins may either inhibit or facilitate adrenergic transmission by decreasing or increasing the availability of Ca^{2+} for the release process of the neurotransmitter, respectively, depending upon the vascular tissue and animal species.

A prostaglandins: The effects of A prostaglandins on adrenergic neurotransmission has not been as extensively studied as those of E prostaglandins. Like the latter, prostaglandins of the A series have been shown to inhibit the response of various vascular tissues to sympathetic nerve stimulation and administered catecholamines. Prostaglandins A_1 and A_2 reduced the vasoconstrictor response of perfused dog paw and hindlimb vasculature (Kadowitz et al., 1971a; Kadowitz, 1972). In the perfused dog paw, PGA_1 was 100 times less potent than PGE_1 in depressing the vasoconstrictor responses to adrenergic stimuli. Renal vasoconstriction produced by sympathetic nerve stimulation and norepinephrine was also antagonized by PGA_2 and PGE_2, PGA_2 being 5 times less potent than PGE_2 (Lonigro et al., 1973). Similar results were obtained in the isolated perfused rabbit kidney (Malik and McGiff, 1975). In this preparation, PGA_2 was 10–50 times less active than PGE_1 or PGE_2 in inhibiting the response to sympathetic nerve stimulation. Since the degree of reduction produced by PGA_2 in the vasoconstrictor response to sympathetic nerve stimulation was greater than that to injected norepinephrine, it was concluded that PGA_2 inhibited release of the adrenergic transmitter by its presynaptic actions. The mechanism by which A prostaglandins inhibit release of the adrenergic transmitter may be similar to that of E prostaglandins.

In addition to their inhibitory effect on adrenergic transmission A prostaglandins have also been shown to facilitate adrenergic transmission in various vascular beds of different animal species. Thus, in the blood-perfused spleen, they enhanced the splenic contraction to sympathetic nerve stimulation (Davies and Withrington, 1969). In the isolated perfused rat mesenteric (Malik and McGiff, 1974) and renal vasculature (Malik and McGiff, 1975) PGA_2 potentiated the vasoconstrictor responses to adrenergic nerve stimulation as well as to injected norepinephrine. Since augmentation of the rat renal vasoconstrictor response to sympathetic nerve stimulation also occurred in concentrations which did not alter the response to injected norepinephrine, it was concluded that PGA_2 enhanced release of the adrenergic transmitter in this preparation (Figure 5.12). In the canine perfused paw, PGA_2 in high doses enhanced the vasoconstrictor responses to sympathetic nerve stimulation (Greenberg et al., 1974). Since PGB_2, which is formed from PGA_2 under the action of prostaglandin isomerase (Jones, 1972b), produced similar results and is more active than PGA_2, it has been suggested that the facilitatory effect of PGA_2 on adrenergic transmission may be mediated by its conversion to a PGB in vascular smooth muscle (Greenberg et al., 1974).

F prostaglandins: Prostaglandins of the F series were either ineffective or exerted a facilitatory effect on the adrenergic neuromuscular junction in various cardiovascular tissues. Hedqvist and Wennmalm (1971) observed that in the isolated rabbit heart $PGF_{2\alpha}$ altered neither the chronotropic nor the inotropic effect, nor the release of the adrenergic transmitter produced by sympathetic nerve stimulation. The effect of exogenous norepinephrine also remained unchanged. Prostaglandin $F_{2\alpha}$ also failed to alter the effect of sympathetic nerve stimulation on the cat and dog heart (Brody and Kadowitz, 1974). However, in dog spleen, $PGF_{1\alpha}$ and $PGF_{2\alpha}$ enhanced the splenic contraction and the vascular smooth muscle response to sympathetic nerve stimulation as well as to administered catecholamines (Davies and Withrington, 1969, 1971). Prostaglandin $F_{2\alpha}$ produced similar effects in the canine perfused saphenous vein (Kadowitz et al., 1971b). In the perfused dog paw vasculature, both $PGF_{1\alpha}$ and $PGF_{2\alpha}$ enhanced the vasoconstrictor responses to sympathetic nerve stimulation whilst $PGF_{1\alpha}$ decreased the vasoconstrictor responses to injected norepinephrine, and $PGF_{2\alpha}$ neither altered the responses to noradrenaline nor tyramine. It was suggested that the F prostaglandins facilitated adrenergic transmission by enhancing release of the adrenergic transmitter (Kadowitz, 1971c, Kadowitz et al., 1972). Augmentation of the vasoconstrictor responses to sympathetic nerve stimulation and/or injected norepinephrine by $PGF_{2\alpha}$ has also been reported to occur in the perfused canine uterine vasculature (Clark et al., 1973), rat mesenteric arteries (Malik and McGiff, 1974), rabbit and rat kidneys (Malik and McGiff, 1975) and in the isolated superfused dog tibial artery (Brody and Kadowitz, 1974). Since, in some of these vascular tissues, such as the canine tibial artery (Brody and Kadowitz, 1974) and the rat and rabbit renal vasculature (Malik and McGiff, 1974, 1975), potentiation of the vasoconstrictor responses to sympathetic nerve stimulation occurred in concentrations which failed to alter the response to norepinephrine it was concluded that $PGF_{2\alpha}$ facilitated adrenergic transmission by enhancing release of the neurotransmitter. Facilitation of adrenergic transmission by $PGF_{2\alpha}$ was also shown to occur in vivo. Thus, intra-arterial administration of $PGF_{2\alpha}$ was shown to potentiate the reflex vasoconstrictor responses to both nicotine and carotid occlusion in the canine paw vasculature and skeletal muscle, but did not affect the systemic pressor responses or the vasoconstrictor responses to administered norepinephrine (Powell and Brody, 1973). The mechanism by which prostaglandins of the F series facilitated adrenergic transmission and enhanced the response of various vascular tissues to exogenous norepinephrine may be through increased availability of Ca^{2+} to the neurotransmitter release process and to the contractile process of vascular smooth muscle, respectively, since Ca^{2+} plays an important role in each process (cf. Rubin, 1970; cf. Somlyo and Somlyo, 1968b).

Prostaglandin release by adrenergic nerve stimulation and administered catecholamines

Part of the important evidence which supports the function of prostaglandins as modulators of adrenergic transmission was the demonstration that stimulation of adrenergic nerves or administration of catecholamines released prostaglandin-like substances from cardiovascular tissues such as spleen

(Davies *et al.*, 1968; Ferreira and Vane, 1967; Gilmore *et al.*, 1968; Ferreira *et al.*, 1973), heart (Hedqvist *et al.*, 1971; Wennmalm, 1971; Chanh and Carthery, 1973; Junstad and Wennmalm, 1973) and kidney (Dunham and Zimmerman, 1970; McGiff *et al.*, 1972; Davis and Horton, 1972). Since prostaglandins are not stored, their release from an organ in response to a stimulus denotes activation of their synthesis rather than release from any preformed source (cf. McGiff *et al.*, 1974). The major type of prostaglandin released from cardiovascular tissues in response to adrenergic stimuli was type E although small amounts of PGF were also detected. Thus, Davies *et al.* (1968) found that venous effluent collected from the perfused dog spleen during and immediately after splenic nerve stimulation contained several prostaglandin-like substances, whereas blood collected before stimulation contained no prostaglandin-like activity. Using gas chromatographic, mass spectrometric and parallel bioassay procedures, PGE_2 and $PGF_{2\alpha}$ were identified in the venous effluent obtained during sympathetic nerve stimulation (Horton, 1973). Similar results have been reported in the dog spleen (Ferreira and Vane, 1967; Gilmore *et al.*, 1968) and in the cat spleen (Hedqvist *et al.*, 1971; Ferriera *et al.*, 1973). Adrenergic nerve stimulation or administration of norepinephrine also released a smooth muscle stimulating material having the physicochemical characteristics of a PGE-like substance from the isolated rabbit heart (Wennmalm, 1971; Chanh and Carthery, 1973; Junstad and Wennmalm, 1973) and kidney of dog (Dunham and Zimmerman, 1970; McGiff *et al.*, 1972) and rabbit (Davis and Horton, 1972; Needleman *et al.*, 1974). In addition to the release of E prostaglandins from the rabbit kidney, smaller amounts of PGF compounds were identified in response to sympathetic nerve stimulation (Davis and Horton, 1972).

The release of prostaglandins from cardiovascular tissues evoked by adrenergic stimuli has been shown to be reduced or abolished after the administration of inhibitors of prostaglandin synthesis such as eicosatetraynoic acid (ETA) (Downing *et al.*, 1970) and aspirin-like drugs (Vane, 1971). Thus, in the isolated cat spleen (Hedqvist *et al.*, 1971; Ferreira *et al.*, 1973) and rabbit heart (Samuelsson and Wennmalm, 1971; Chanh *et al.*, 1972) administration of either ETA or indomethacin reduced the output of prostaglandins evoked by sympathetic nerve stimulation. Using indomethacin, similar results were obtained in the rabbit kidney (Davis and Horton, 1972). These observations indicate that adrenergic stimuli enhance prostaglandin synthesis in various cardiovascular tissues. The evidence for release and hence synthesis of prostaglandins during adrenergic nerve stimulation obtained in most of the above studies has been based on the detection of substances having the smooth muscle stimulating and physicochemical properties of prostaglandins. Further work is required for the quantitation and final identification of prostaglandin-like substances released from various cardiovascular tissues in response to adrenergic stimuli in different animal species. Moreover, the exact site and mechanism by which nerve impulses promote prostaglandin synthesis in adrenergic tissues remains to be investigated.

Most of the studies thus far carried out on adrenergic tissues indicate that release of prostaglandins is closely associated with the function of the effector cell membrane. For example, in the dog spleen denervation or α-adrenergic receptor blockade abolished the release of prostaglandins evoked by either sympathetic nerve stimulation or administration of epinephrine as well as abolishing splenic contractions. (Davies *et al.*, 1968; Gilmore *et al.*, 1968). However, release of prostaglandins from the spleen was also found to occur in response to the administration of colloid particles even in the absence of splenic contraction (Gilmore *et al.*, 1969) indicating that the latter was not a necessary condition for release of prostaglandins. Adrenergic denervation of the vas deferens (Hedqvist, 1973) did not abolish the efflux of prostaglandins in response to direct electrical stimulation of this organ. Similarly, in the isolated rabbit heart obtained from animals chemically sympathectomized by pretreatment with 6-hydroxydopamine the amount of prostaglandins released by the administration of norepinephrine was not different from that released from hearts of non-treated animals (Junstad and Wennmalm, 1973). Although prostaglandins have been detected in nervous tissue (Kataoka *et al.*, 1967; Karim *et al.*, 1968), the above evidence, when taken together with the release of prostaglandins from various tissues in response to non-adrenergic stimuli (Gilmore *et al.*, 1969; cf. Ramwell and Shaw, 1970; McGiff, Crowshaw *et al.*, 1970; McGiff, *et al.*, 1972; Needleman, Douglas *et al.*, 1974; Needleman, Minkes and Douglas, 1974) suggests that the effector cells are the major site for the synthesis of prostaglandins. The sympathetic transmitter, released from adrenergic neurons, acts on sites of the effector cells, and possibly, coupled with cyclic AMP formation, causes the activation of prostaglandin synthesis (Hedqvist, 1973). Since the release of prostaglandins produced by the administration of either catecholamines or sympathetic nerve stimulation from the rabbit kidney was blocked by phenoxybenzamine, Needleman, Douglas *et al.* (1974) proposed that the adrenergic-induced release of prostaglandins in the kidney is mediated through α-adrenergic receptor stimulation. However, Junstad and Wennmalm, (1973) failed to observe an alteration in the output of prostaglandins from the rabbit heart evoked by norephinephrine after the administration of either phentolamine, phenoxybenzamine or propranolol. The reason for the failure of α-adrenergic blocking agents in the latter and not in the rabbit kidney is unknown at present. Since prostaglandin release, mediated by non-adrenergic stimuli such as angiotensin II, was not abolished by either α- or β-adrenergic receptor blocking agents (Needleman, Douglas *et al.*, 1974), it would appear that the release was mediated by mechanisms independent of α- or β-adrenergic receptors. Catecholamines, released from nerve fibres or administered exogenously, and various non-adrenergic stimuli may promote prostaglandin synthesis by activation of a phospholipase-A_2 (Kunze and Vogt, 1971) which may be the regulating factor for the synthesis of prostaglandins. This enzyme would liberate precursor fatty acids from a phospholipid of the effector cell membranes and in this way provide substrate to the synthesis complex for conversion to prostaglandins.

Effect of inhibitors of prostaglandin synthesis on the response of cardiovascular tissues to adrenergic nerve stimulation and to administered catecholamines

If endogenous prostaglandins are involved in the modulation of adrenergic transmission, the inhibition of their biosynthesis would be expected to modify the response of cardiovascular tissues to sympathetic nerve stimulation in a direction opposite to that produced by the administration of exogenous prostaglandins. Thus, in the cat spleen where exogenous PGE_2 inhibited the vasoconstrictor response to nerve stimulation and diminished release of the adrenergic transmitter, administration of an inhibitor of prostaglandin synthesis, ETA (Downing et al., 1970) produced an opposite effect (Hedqvist et al., 1971). It increased the pressor response to sympathetic nerve stimulation, enhanced release of the adrenergic transmitter and abolished the output of previously detectable PGE-like activity. Anti-inflammatory agents such as indomethacin and aspirin which also inhibit prostaglandin synthesis (Vane, 1971), reduced prostaglandin release from the dog spleen and augmented the response of the effector cells to epinephrine (Ferreira et al., 1971). Similar results have been reported in the cat spleen (Ferreira et al., 1973). In these experiments the vasoconstrictor response to nerve stimulation was increased and the output of prostaglandins diminished. Moreover, the increase in perfusion pressure, in response to nerve stimulation, was abolished by the simultaneous infusion of PGE_2. In the rabbit kidney, administration of indomethacin reduced the output of prostaglandins (Davis and Horton, 1972) and enhanced the vasoconstrictor response to sympathetic nerve stimulation without altering the equiconstrictor response to injected norepinephrine (Figure 5.14). Inhibition of prostaglandin synthesis in the isolated rabbit heart with either ETA (Samuelsson and Wennmalm, 1971) or indomethacin (Chanh et al., 1972), reduced the output of PGE and enhanced release of the adrenergic transmitter in response to sympathetic nerve stimulation. Moreover, infusion of the perfusate or purified extract of the perfusate, obtained from the rabbit heart during adrenergic nerve stimulation, into a recipient heart, inhibited the outflow of norepinephrine from the recipient heart evoked by nerve stimulation (Wennmalm and Stjärne, 1971). However, when the recipient heart was infused with an extract of the perfusate obtained from the donor heart after pretreatment with ETA, it did not alter the outflow of norepinephrine produced by sympathetic nerve stimulation of the recipient heart. These observations indicated that the donor heart liberated prostaglandins in response to nerve stimulation which were responsible for reducing the outflow of norepinephrine (from the recipient heart) evoked by adrenergic nerve stimulation. In human arteries and veins administration of ETA also enhanced the output of preloaded radiolabelled norepinephrine in response to nerve stimulation (Stjärne and Gripe, 1973).

Inhibition of prostaglandin synthesis also affected responses of the various vascular beds to adrenergic nerve stimulation and/or to administered catecholamines. Thus, indomethacin or ETA potentiated the vasoconstrictor response of perfused dog paw vasculature to adrenergic nerve stimulation as well as to administered norepinephrine (Zimmerman et al., 1973). Potentiation of the vasoconstrictor response of the perfused rabbit ear artery to norepinephrine by aspirin (Jackson and Hall, 1973) and the contractile response of the rabbit portal vein to sympathetic nerve stimulation after the administration of either ETA or indomethacin have also been observed (Greenberg, 1974).

Endogenous as well as exogenous prostaglandins mediated inhibition of adrenergic transmission appeared to operate at lower, 'physiological' nerve

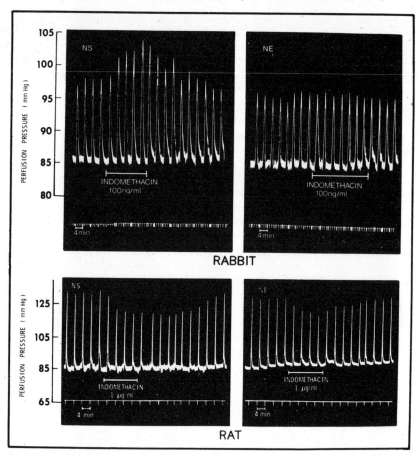

RABBIT

RAT

Figure 5.14 Effect of indomethacin on the vasoconstrictor responses of isolated perfused rabbit (upper panel) and rat (lower panel) kidneys to sympathetic nerve stimulation (NS) and to equiconstrictor responses to injected norepinephrine (NE). Reproduced from Malik and McGiff (1975), by courtesy of *Circulation Res.*

impulse frequencies (1–2 Hz) and not at higher frequencies of stimulation (8–10 Hz). Junstad and Wennmalm (1973) demonstrated that in the isolated rabbit heart, stimulation of sympathetic fibres released greater amounts of the adrenergic transmitter at 10 Hz than it did at 2 Hz. However, after administration of ETA, there was a significant increase in overflow of norepinephrine at 2 Hz, while at 10 Hz overflow of norepinephrine was not altered. Due to the fact that a 5 times higher frequency only approximately doubled the outflow of prostaglandins, it was neither correlated in a linear way to the stimulation frequency nor to the amount of sympathetic transmitter released. Since the chronotropic response of the heart to nerve stimulation was found to be inhibited by exogenous PGE$_2$ more markedly at 2 Hz than at 10 Hz, it was concluded that the failure of the endogenous prostaglandin 'brake' at the higher nerve impulse frequency was due to a decrease in sensitivity to prostaglandins of the mechanism governing transmitter release despite augmented release of prostaglandins at higher frequencies. In the rabbit portal vein the inhibitory effect of PGE_2 on the response to nerve stimulation has also been reported to be inversely related to the frequency of stimulation. Moreover, indomethacin and ETA, which potentiated the contractile response of this tissue to nerve stimulation at 1–2 Hz, failed to alter the responses to stimulation at 4–8 Hz (Greenberg, 1974). In the guinea pig isolated, field-stimulated atria, an inverse correlation was found between the number of pulses and sympathetic blockade by exogenous PGE_1 (Illés et al., 1973). Similarly, in the isolated rabbit sino-atrial node, the chronotropic response to sympathetic nerve stimulation was almost completely blocked at lower frequencies (2–5 Hz) while it had no effect at higher frequencies of stimulation (20–100 Hz) (Park et al., 1973).

In cardiovascular tissues, where inhibition of prostaglandins synthesis augmented the effects of adrenergic nerve stimulation or administered nor-epinephrine, enhancement of prostaglandin synthesis, achieved by administration of precursors of PGE_1 or PGE_2, di-homo-γ-linolenic acid and arachidonic acid respectively, produced an inhibitory effect. The inhibitory effect of PG precursors on adrenergic transmission was either reduced or abolished by the administration of prostaglandin synthetase inhibitors. Thus, in the isolated perfused rabbit kidney (Figure 5.15) infusion of arachidonic acid inhibited the vasoconstrictor response to sympathetic nerve stimulation which was abolished by the simultaneous infusion of indomethacin. Prostaglandin precursors, di-homo-γ-linolenic acid and arachidonic acid, also depressed the vasoconstrictor responses of the perfused dog paw vasculature to exogenous norepinephrine (Ryan and Zimmerman, 1974). This inhibitory effect of prostaglandin precursors was antagonized after the administration of prostaglandin synthetase inhibitors, ETA and indomethacin. Moreover, in these studies, α-linolenic acid, which is not a precursor of prostaglandins, failed to alter the vasoconstrictor responses to administered norepinephrine. These observations support the modulatory role of endogenous prostaglandins on adrenergic transmission.

Although in most cardiovascular tissues of different animal species, inhibitors of prostaglandin synthesis and prostaglandin precursors exert facilitatory and inhibitory effects respectively, at the adrenergic neuromuscular junction they have also been reported to produce opposite effects in some animal species. Thus, in the isolated perfused rat mesenteric (Malik and McGiff, 1974) and renal vasculature (Malik and McGiff, 1975) where exogenous prostaglandins E_1, E_2, A_2 and $F_{2\alpha}$ augmented the vasoconstrictor responses to sympathetic nerve stimulation, indomethacin and meclofenamate reduced the vasoconstrictor responses to nerve stimulation (Figure 5.15). Horrobin et al. (1974) have also made similar observations in rat mesenteric arteries with aspirin on the response to administered norepinephrine. The facilitatory effect of prostaglandins on adrenergic transmission was demonstrated by the observation that arachidonic acid, a precursor of PGE_2 and $PGF_{2\alpha}$, potentiated the vasoconstrictor response of the rat renal vasculature to adrenergic nerve stimulation. Since this potentiating effect was abolished by indomethacin, it was concluded that the facilitatory effect of arachidonic acid on adrenergic transmission was mediated by enhanced endogenous generation of prostaglandins in the rat kidney. These

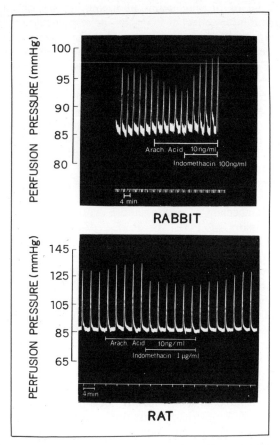

Figure 5.15 Effect of arachidonic acid on the vasoconstrictor responses to sympathetic nerve stimulation of the isolated perfused rabbit (upper panel) and rat (lower panel) kidney. Reproduced from Malik and McGiff (1975), by courtesy of *Circulation Res.*

results, when taken together with the facilitatory effects of exogenous prostaglandins on adrenergic transmission, strongly suggest that prostaglandins may not only effect a negative feedback control of neurotransmission but may also facilitate neurotransmission in various vascular beds of some species.

Synthesis, interconversion and degradation of prostaglandins in cardiovascular tissues

Prostaglandins, which are primarily tissue hormones, are not stored and thus their release from an organ in response to a stimulus denotes enhanced synthesis (cf. McGiff *et al.*, 1974). Christ and Van Dorp (1973) have systematically examined the activity of prostaglandin synthetase from a wide range of tissues. In mammalian tissue the biosynthetic capacity, as measured by the conversion of tritiated di-homo-γ-linolenic acid to PGE_1, of lung and kidney was 10–40% which was surpassed only by ox and sheep seminal vesicles. The spleen and aorta showed the lowest conversion (1% or less). Using radiolabelled arachidonic acid Hollander *et al.* (1974) also found a very low conversion in the rabbit aorta. Terragno *et al.* (1975) have shown that incubation with radiolabelled arachidonic acid resulted in formation of prostaglandin-like substances in mesenteric arteries and veins 210 ng/g and 186 ng/g respectively after one hour of incubation. An inhibitor of prostaglandin synthesis, meclofenamate, was found to decrease the rate of synthesis by 86% in arteries and 90% in veins. The enzyme responsible for prostaglandin synthesis which has been partially purified in a number of tissues (Samuelsson *et al.*, 1967) was found in the microsomal fraction. Limas and Cohen (1973) found that the microsomal fraction of canine myocardium (as determined by incubation with arachidonic acid) contained active prostaglandin synthetase, while the biosynthetic capacity of the supernatant was considerably less.

In addition to prostaglandin synthetase, enzymes responsible for interconversion and degradation of prostaglandins have also been demonstrated in various tissues. Thus, an enzyme, PGE 9-keto-reductase, which converts prostaglandins of the E series to those of the F series, has been demonstrated in various tissues of different animal species (Leslie and Levine, 1973; Lee and Levine, 1974a; Wagner *et al.*, 1975; Wong *et al.*, 1975).

Prostaglandins of the E and F series, synthesized in various organs and entering the circulation are rapidly metabolized on a single passage through the pulmonary circulation, whereas those of the A series survive passage across the lung and may function as circulating hormones (McGiff *et al.*, 1969). Metabolism of prostaglandins proceeds through oxidation of the 15-hydroxyl group by 15-hydroxy PG-dehydrogenase, reduction of the $^{13}\Delta$ double bond and ω- and β-oxidation of the side chains (Samuelsson *et al.*, 1971; Samuelsson, 1972). Although the lung was shown to be the major source of these enzymes (Änggård and Samuelsson, 1964, 1966) they have also been found in various other tissues, and partially purified and characterized (Nagasawa *et al.*, 1974; Schlegel *et al.*, 1974; Lee and Levine, 1974b; Lee *et al.*, 1975).

5.2.16.2 Cholinergic neuromuscular junction

Junstad and Wennmalm (1974) showed that the infusion of acetylcholine or vagal nerve stimulation at 5 Hz released 1.8–6.2 ng/min and 5.2–8.3 ng/min of a PGE-like substance from the isolated rabbit heart. Administration of atropine completely abolished not only the mechanical response but also the enhanced 'PGE' release produced by acetylcholine, thereby indicating that the release of 'PGE' by acetylcholine was associated with stimulation of muscarinic receptors. Wennmalm and Hedqvist (1971) found that PGE_1 inhibited the chronotropic response to stimulation of the vagus nerve but not to exogenous acetylcholine, thereby indicating a presynaptic action of PGE_1. On the basis of these observations, it was concluded that prostaglandins of the E series may control release of the cholinergic transmitter by a negative feedback mechanism analogous to that of the adrenergic transmitter.

However, Park *et al.* (1973) failed to find any inhibitory effect of PGE_2 on the chronotropic response to electrical stimulation of intranodal parasympathetic fibres at low frequencies of stimulation (2–20 Hz) and at higher frequency stimulation (50–100 Hz) a slight increase was observed. In the isolated guinea pig atria PGE_1 reduced the negative chronotropic responses to vagal stimulation as well as to exogenous acetylcholine, probably due to its postsynaptic actions (Hadházy *et al.*, 1973). The absence of a presynaptic action of PGE_1 at the cholinergic neuromuscular junction in this species was supported by the observation that PGE_1 did not alter the output of acetylcholine from the isolated ileum in response to parasympathetic nerve stimulation. Although an inhibitor of prostaglandin synthesis, indomethacin, reduced the output of prostaglandins (Botting and Salzmann, 1974) and decreased the response of the guinea pig ileum to transmural stimulation (Kaldec *et al.*, 1974), it failed to alter the output of acetylcholine in response to nerve stimulation (Botting and Salzmann, 1974). These observations indicate that the modulatory action of prostaglandins on cholinergic transmission may depend upon the tissue, the concentration of prostaglandins and the animal species as shown for adrenergic transmission. Moreover, the anticholinergic action of PGE_1 may be related to activation of the cyclic AMP system. Prostaglandin E_1 has been shown to elevate the cyclic AMP levels in the guinea pig heart (Sobel and Robison, 1969) while acetylcholine reduced cyclic AMP formation (Murad *et al.*, 1962).

5.3 HUMAN STUDIES

5.3.1 E prostaglandins

The first study of the effect of PGE_1 on the cardiovascular system in man was carried out by Bergström *et al.* (1959). Chemically-pure PGE_1 was infused in doses of 0.2–0.7 μg/kg per min in two healthy male subjects over periods of 4–10 min. Tachycardia, reddening of the face, headache and an oppressive feeling in the chest were some of the effects observed. A fall in systolic and diastolic pressure and an increase in heart rate occurred in both subjects (Figure 5.16). There was also a moderate decrease in cardiac output. Some of the above effects persisted for up to 15 min after discontinuing the infusion which lasted 4–10 min. In subsequent studies reported by Bergström *et al.* (1965a) PGE_1 was infused at a rate of 0.1–0.2 μg/kg per min into three healthy male subjects for 20 min. With these doses no consistent changes in arterial blood pressure occurred but the heart rate increased by 20 beats per minute. When PGE_1 was infused simultaneously with norepinephrine in two subjects, the increase in blood pressure produced by norepinephrine was less. Prostaglandin E_1 completely inhibited norepinephrine induced bradycardia. Even with the small rates of infusion of 0.1–0.2 μg/kg per min PGE_1, subjective side effects did occur. They included reddening of the face, abdominal cramps, pulsating headache in the temples, inability to fixate the eyes and visual symptoms which continued for about 20 min. In addition the arm into which PGE_1 was infused showed intense flushing and pronounced edema which developed within 10 min and lasted for over one hour. The inhibition

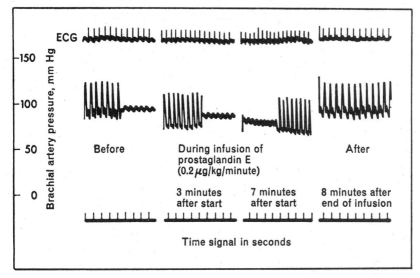

Figure 5.16 Effect of intravenous infusion of 0.2 μg/kg per min of PGE$_1$ on the cardiovascular system in a healthy young man. Reproduced from Bergström *et al.* (1959), by courtesy of *Acta Physiol. Scand.*

of the pressor effect of norepinephrine by PGE$_1$ has been thought to be due to a summation of opposite effects, i.e. physiological antagonism. The abolition of the bradycardia produced by norepinephrine was probably the result of the combined effect of PGE$_1$ in increasing the heart rate and reducing the pressor effect of norepinephrine.

Karim *et al.* (1969) infused PGE$_1$ in one male volunteer at the rate of 0.2 μg/kg per min for 30 min. This produced an increase in heart rate of 22 beats per minute; mean brachial arterial pressure was reduced by 11 mm Hg. The subject complained of pulsating headache and abdominal cramps 10 min after the start of the infusion (Figure 5.17).

When PGE$_1$ was infused in five women at the rate of 0.1 μg/kg per min to stimulate the uterus in an attempt to induce abortion, it produced a fall in blood pressure, tachycardia, flushing of the face and pulsating headache in three of the subjects. These effects, particularly the headache, were so severe that the infusion had to be discontinued in all three patients after 30 min, 2 h and 2½ h respectively. In the other two women no cardiovascular changes were produced. The infusion was continued for 10 and 15 h respectively. In all five subjects PGE$_1$ produced erythema in the arm in which the drug was infused (cf. Karim and Somers, 1972). Bygdeman *et al.* (1968) have also infused PGE$_1$ in doses of 0.01–0.15 μg/kg per min in eleven pregnant women to stimulate the uterus. The duration of infusion varied between 5 and 45 min and contrary to the findings reported above (Bergström *et al.*, 1965a; Karim *et al.*, 1969) there were no effects on the cardiovascular system in their patients. Embrey (1970) infused PGE$_1$ in two pregnant patients at the rate of 2–5 μg/min for up to 16½ h and encountered no cardiovascular effects. Carlson *et al.* (1969) reported the effects of different doses of PGE$_1$ in eight healthy male subjects in doses from 0.032 to 0.58 μg/kg per min. With doses

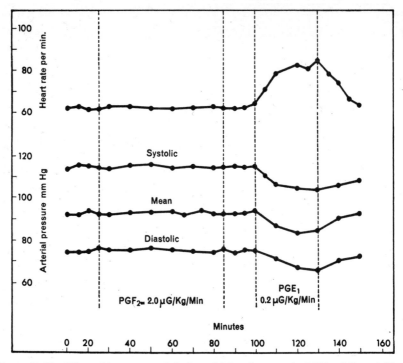

Figure 5.17 Effect of intravenous infusion of 2.0 μg/kg per min PGF$_{2\alpha}$ followed fifteen minutes later by 0.2 μg/kg per min PGE$_1$ on the arterial pressures and heart rate of a healthy fasting man. Reproduced from Karim, Somers and Hillier (1969), by courtesy of *Eur. J. Pharmacol.*

of 0.058–0.1 μg/kg per min the effects produced included an increase in heart rate, stroke volume and a decrease in peripheral resistance. At higher than 0.1 μg/kg per min infusion there was a further increase in heart rate and a decrease in arterial blood pressure. The increase in stroke volume was less but there was still an increase in cardiac output. The subjective side-effects were similar to those previously reported by Bergström, Duner *et al.* (1959). Since it was possible to produce an increase in heart rate with doses that have no effect on the blood pressure, Carlson *et al.* (1969) suggested that the increase in pulse rate was not due to baroreceptor reflex stimulation induced by a blood pressure fall but due to sympathetic nervous stimulation (Carlson and Orö, 1966), or due to a direct action on the heart. In contrast to the reduction in cardiac output reported by Bergström, Duner *et al.* (1959), Carlson *et al.* (1969) showed an increase in cardiac output with PGE$_1$ infusion. These discrepancies could be the result of different rates of infusion used by the two groups.

Flushing of the face with PGE$_1$ has been reported by all authors who have infused PGE$_1$ in man. The mechanism of action is not certain. Prostaglandin E$_1$ may have a direct vasodilator effect on the vessels of the skin, or the dilatation of cutaneous vessels by PGE$_1$ could be due to a release of other vasoactive substances. Flushing of the face during serotonin infusion has been previously reported (Carlson *et al.*, 1967). The pulsating headache and abdominal cramps likewise could result from a direct action of PGE_1 or from release of another vasoactive substance. However, it has been shown that PGE_1 does not release 5-hydroxytryptamine (Thompson and Angulo, 1968, 1969).

In nine healthy male volunteers, Bevegard and Orö (1969) studied the effects of PGE_1 on forearm blood flow by means of strain gauge plethysmography. Brachial artery infusion of as little as 0.01 ng/kg per min doubled blood flow, and with a 1 ng/kg per min infusion there was a ten-fold increase in blood flow. The PGE_1-induced vasodilatation was not blocked by atropine or propranolol (Figure 5.18).

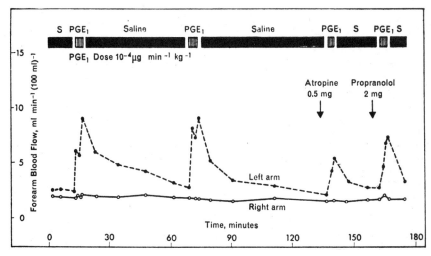

Figure 5.18 Effect of repeated infusions of PGE_1 into the brachial artery on forearm blood flow before and after local intra-arterial administration of 0.5 mg atropine and 2 mg propranolol. The unbroken line connects mean values of 3–6 blood flow determinations during 1–2 minute periods. Result of a typical experiment. Reproduced from Bevegard and Orö (1969), by courtesy of *Scand. J. Clin. Lab. Invest.*

Okada *et al.* (1974) showed that intravenous administration of PGE_1 (50 µg) had little effect on the blood pressure of healthy individuals except for a slight decrease in the diastolic blood pressure within 5 min. However, in cases of essential hypertension, the blood pressure was decreased immediately after administration of PGE_1. The antihypertensive effect of PGE_1 was also demonstrated in renal and renovascular hypertension and hypertension associated with Takayasu's arteritis, primary aldosteronism, phaeochromocytoma and anephric subjects having the Kimmelstiel–Wilson syndrome. The pattern of the blood pressure response to PGE_1 in all types of hypertension studied was almost similar. Flushing of the face was observed during and after the injection in one-third of the cases. A summary of the human cardiovascular effects of prostaglandins is given in Table 5.3.

Prostaglandin E_2 also increased heart rate and decreased arterial blood pressure but was less potent than PGE_1. Infusion of 0.8 µg/kg per min of PGE_2 was required to produce an increase in heart rate (comparable to that

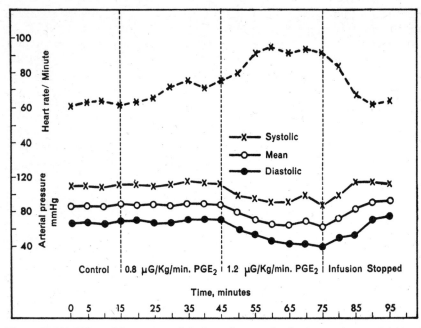

Figure 5.19 Effect of intravenous infusion of prostaglandin E_2 on the arterial blood pressure and heart rate in a healthy fasting female. Reproduced from Karim, Somers and Hillier (1971), by courtesy of *Cardiovasc. Res.*

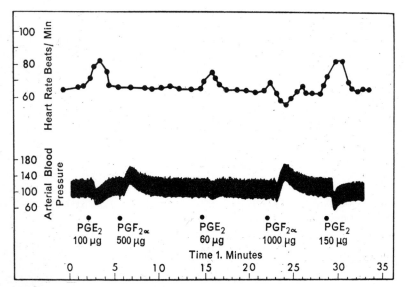

Figure 5.20 Effect of rapid single intravenous injections of prostaglandins E_2 and $F_{2\alpha}$ on the arterial blood pressure and heart rate in a healthy young male subject. Reproduced from Karim, Somers and Hillier (1971), by courtesy of *Cardiovasc. Res.*

produced by less than 0.1 μg/kg per min infusion of PGE_1) and there was no fall in blood pressure until an infusion rate of 1.2 ug/kg per min was reached (Figure 5.19). With rapid single intravenous injections of 60 μg, PGE_2 produced an increase in heart rate, while 100–150 μg produced a fall in arterial blood pressure lasting 3–7 min (Figure 5.20). Given intramuscularly or subcutaneously, the minimum dose of PGE_2 required to produce an effect on the cardiovascular system was 5 mg (Karim, Hillier et al., 1971). Prostaglandin E_2, given by mouth in a dose up to 5 mg, had no effect on the cardiovascular system (Karim, 1971). Similarly, intravaginal administration of 20 mg was without any effect on the cardiovascular system in pregnant women (Karim and Sharma, 1971). The above findings suggested that E prostaglandins are very rapidly metabolized or inactivated (Tables 5.1, 5.2, 5.3). Infusion of PGE_2 at the rate of 5–20 μg/min has been given by several investigators to produce abortion. In some cases, the infusion was continued for up to 48 h. However, even with such prolonged infusions, no effect on the cardiovascular system has been produced (Karim and Filshie, 1970; Embrey, 1970; Kaufman et al., 1971).

Robinson et al. (1973) showed that the administration of PGE_2, 0.5–12.8 ng/min into the brachial artery produced a dose-dependent increase in human forearm flow. Prostaglandin E_2 in doses of 10 to 100 ng/ml infused into the superficial relaxed hand veins did not produce any effect. However, PGE_2 caused a dose-dependent dilatation over the range of 10–1000 pg/ml of the veins preconstricted with either norepinephrine or 5-hydroxytryptamine. Infusion of PGE_2 at rates of 10 ng/min and 100 ng/min resulted in the appearance of a flare in the skin over the veins draining the infusion site. The flare lasted for up to 2 h and with small doses of 100 ng/min was accompanied by a burning sensation, especially when the veins were distended. Venous erythema leading to phlebitis of the arm has been observed after the administration of prostaglandin E_2 (Embrey, 1970; Kaufman et al., 1971).

5.3.2 A prostaglandins

Lee et al. (1965) studied the effect of PGA_2 on cardiovascular haemodynamics in a 25-year-old hypertensive subject. Eighteen seconds following a single intravenous injection of medullin (PGA_2, 50 μg) there was a fall in blood pressure from 185/116 to 160/95 mm Hg which reached a maximum 23 s after injection and returned to control levels 32 s after injection. The heart rate increased from 102 to a maximum of 114 beats/minute. This occurred after the maximal fall in blood pressure suggesting a tachycardia of reflex origin. The cardiac output increased from 8.4 to 9.5 l/min so that the calculated total peripheral resistance fell from 17.5 to 14.1 peripheral resistance units (Lee et al., 1965). With a prolonged infusion at a dose of 191 μg/min in the same subject, systolic blood pressure fell from a control of 186 to 180 mm Hg and diastolic from 114 to 106 mm Hg. With an increase in infusion rate to 382 μg/min the blood pressure fell to 165/97 mm Hg. With the fall in blood pressure there was an increase in heart rate from 92 to 114 beats/min and an increase in cardiac output from 8.4 to 10.5 l/min and a fall in the calculated total peripheral resistance from 17.5 to 12.5 units. There was also a marked

Table 5.1   Effect of intravenous infusion of prostaglandin E_2 on the mean arterial blood pressure and heart rate in three subjects

Subject No.	Control		Prostaglandin dose and duration of infusion	Maximum change		Prostaglandin dose and duration of infusion	Maximum change	
	BP	*HR*		*BP*	*HR*		*BP*	*HR*
1 (M)	88	62	PGE_2 infused at the rate of 0.8 μg/kg per min for 30 min	0	+12	PGE_2 infused at the rate of 1.2 μg/kg per min for 30 min	−20	+26
2 (M)	82	70	PGE_2 infused at the rate of 0.8 μg/kg per min for 30 min	−2	+10	PGE_2 infused at the rate of 1.2 μg/kg per min for 30 min	−18	+29
3 (F)	90	60	PGE_2 infused at the rate of 0.8 μg/kg per min for 30 min	0	+14	PGE_2 infused at the rate of 1.2 μg/kg per min for 30 min	−12	+42

BP = Mean arterial blood pressure mm Hg
HR = Heart rate per min
+ = Increase ⎫
− = Decrease ⎬ in HR or BP
0 = No change ⎭
M = Male
F = Female
$PGF_{2\alpha}$ infused at the rate of 4.0 μg/kg per min for 30 min in three subjects did not produce any changes in HR or BP
Reproduced from Karim, Somers and Hillier (1971), by permission of the publisher

Table 5.2 Effect of single intravenous injections of prostaglandins E$_2$ and F$_{2\alpha}$ on the mean arterial blood pressures and heart rate in six human subjects

Subject No.	Control BP	Control HR	PG and dose	Change BP	Change HR	Control BP	Control HR	PG and dose	Change BP	Change HR	Control BP	Control HR	PG and dose	Change BP	Change HR
1 (F)	90	60	PGE$_2$ 60 µg	0	+6	92	62	PGE$_2$ 100 µg	−10	+12	90	60	PGE$_2$ 150 µg	−24	+22
2 (F)	102	66	PGE$_2$ 60 µg	−2	0	102	66	PGE$_2$ 100 µg	−2	+13	100	66	PGE$_2$ 150 µg	−24	+18
3 (M)	82	70	PGE$_2$ 60 µg	+2	+10	84	70	PGE$_2$ 100 µg	−6	+22	86	72	PGE$_2$ 150 µg	−16	+28
4 (M)	90	62	PGF$_{2\alpha}$ 250 µg	0	−2	92	60	PGF$_{2\alpha}$ 500 µg	+12	−2	90	58	PGF$_{2\alpha}$ 1000 µg	+39	−6
5 (M)	84	63	PGF$_{2\alpha}$ 250 µg	−4	+2	82	64	PGF$_{2\alpha}$ 500 µg	+24	0	80	63	PGF$_{2\alpha}$ 1000 µg	+54	−9
6 (F)	92	68	PGF$_{2\alpha}$ 250 µg	−2	−2	92	72	PGF$_{2\alpha}$ 500 µg	+24	−4	94	70	PGF$_{2\alpha}$ 1000 µg	+34	−8

BP = Mean arterial pressure mm Hg
HR = Heart rate/min
+ = Increase ⎱
− = Decrease ⎰ in HR or BP
0 = No change
F = Female
M = Male
Reproduced from Karim, Somers and Hillier (1971), by permission of the publisher

Table 5.3 Summary of the actions of prostaglandins on the human cardiovascular system

Prostaglandin	Mode of administration	Dose	BP	HR	CO	Reference
PGE$_1$	i.v. Infusion	0.2–0.7 µg/kg per min	↓	↑	↑	Bergström, Duner et al. (1959)
	i.v. Infusion	0.2 µg/kg per min	↓			Bergström, Carlson et al. (1963)
	i.v. Infusion	0.058–0.1 µg/kg per min	↓	↑		Karim, Somers and Hillier (1969)
	i.v. Infusion	0.1–0.58 µg/kg per min	↓	↑	↓	Carlson, Ekelund and Orö (1969)
	i.v. Infusion	50 µg	↓		↓	Okada, Nukada, Yamauchi, Abe (1974)
	Brachial artery infusion	0.01–0.1 ng/kg per min	Increase in forearm blood flow			Bevegård and Orö (1969)
PGE$_2$	i.v. Infusion	0.8 µg/kg per min	↓	↑		Karim, Somers and Hillier (1971)
	i.v. Infusion	1.2 µg/kg per min	↓	↑		Karim, Hillier, Somers, Trussell (1971)
	i.v. Injections	60 µg		↑		
	i.v. Injections	100 µg	↓	↑		
	i.m. Injections	5 mg	↓	↑		
	s.c. Injections	5 mg	↓	↑		
	Vaginal	20 mg	No effect			cf. Karim and Somers (1972)
	Oral	5 mg	No effect			cf. Karim and Somers (1972)
	Brachial artery infusion	0.5–12.8 ng/min	Increase in forearm blood flow			Robinson, Collier, Karim and Somers (1973)
PGA$_1$	i.v. Infusion	0.22 µg/kg per min	↓	↑	↓	Lee et al. (1969)
	i.v. Infusion	0.48–1.32 µg/kg per min	↓	↑		Carr (1970)
	i.v. Infusion	1.2 µg/kg per min	↓	↑		Westura et al. (1970)
	i.v. Infusion	0.3–1.2 µg/kg per min	↓	↑		Christlieb et al. (1969)
	i.v. Infusion	0.03–5.0 µg/kg per min	↓	↑		Fichman (1969, 1970)
	i.v. Infusion	0.4 µg/kg per min	↓			Krakoff, Guia, Vlachakis, Stricker and Goldstein, (1973)
						Slotkoff (1974)
	i.v. Infusion	0.6–2.4 µg/kg body weight per min	↓			
	i.v. and i.a. Infusion	25–50 µg/min	Increased coronary, femoral and popliteal blood flow			Barner, Kaiser, Jellinek and Lee (1973)

	Route	Dose	Effect	Reference
PGA$_2$	Brachial artery infusion	0.1–10 μg/min	Increased forearm blood flow	Robinson, Collier, Karim and Somers (1973)
	i.v. Injection	50 μg	→ ↓ ←	Lee, Covino, Takman and Smith (1965)
	i.v. Infusion	191–382 μg/min	→ ↓ ←	Hornych, Safar, Papanicolaou, Meyer and Milliez (1973)
	i.v. Infusion	2–9 μg/kg per min	↑ ← ←	Karim (unpublished)
	Oral and vaginal	20 mg	→ ↑	Karim, Somers and Hillier (1969)
	i.v. Infusion	4 μg/kg per min	No effect	Fishburne, Brenner, Braaksma, Stavrorsky, Mueller, Hoffer and Hendricks (1972)
	i.v. Infusion	25–200 μg/min	No effect	
PGF$_{2\alpha}$	i.v. Injection	500 μg	← →	Karim, Somers and Hillier (1971)
	i.m. Injection	20 mg	No effect	Karim, Hillier, Somers and Trussell (1971)
	s.c. Injection	20 mg	No effect	cf. Karim and Somers (1972)
	Oral	50 mg	No effect	
	Vaginal	50 mg	No effect	cf. Karim and Somers (1972)
	Brachial artery infusion	0.4–2 μg/min	Transient reduction in forearm blood flow	Robinson, Collier, Karim, and Somers (1973)
		10 μg/min	Increased forearm blood flow	

↑ = Increase in blood pressure (BP); heart rate (HR); or cardiac output (CO)
↓ = Decrease in blood pressure (BP); heart rate (HR); or cardiac output (CO)
i.v. = Intravenous
i.m. = Intramuscular
s.c. = Subcutaneous

diuresis with PGA_2 infusion. In another study, Lee *et al.* (1969) infused PGA_1 in six patients with essential hypertension at the rate of 0.22 μg/kg per min for 1 h. Within 20 min urine flow and sodium excretion increased threefold; potassium excretion also increased. Subsequently the blood pressure fell from 185/104 to 150/90 mm Hg associated with a reduction in total peripheral resistance and blood volume. Carr (1970) studied the effect of PGA_1 in five patients with mild essential vascular hypertension. Prostaglandin was infused at the rate of 0.48 to 1.32 μg/kg per min. Infusion of PGA_1 decreased systolic, diastolic and mean blood pressure in all subjects. Westura *et al.* (1970) have reported their findings in six patients with essential hypertension infused with PGA_1. After the first 15 min control period, PGA_1 was infused at the rate of 1.0 μg/kg per min for 15 min followed by 2.0 μg/kg per min for a further 15 min. During the first period of infusion there was an initial rise in sodium excretion and urine flow. This was followed by a progressive fall in blood pressure and a drop in peripheral resistance. Stroke volume and cardiac index rose slightly and there was a reflex increase in the heart rate from an average of 72 beats to 96 beats per min. During the higher rate of infusion, there was a further small fall in the systolic blood pressure but the diastolic pressure was unaffected. The heart rate had continued to increase but the cardiac index decreased only slightly. No direct effect of PGA_1 was demonstrable on cardiac performance, e.g. the stroke volume was not significantly altered. The fall in blood pressure was accompanied by an increase in the cardiac output which seemed to be the result of a reflex tachycardia (Figure 5.21).

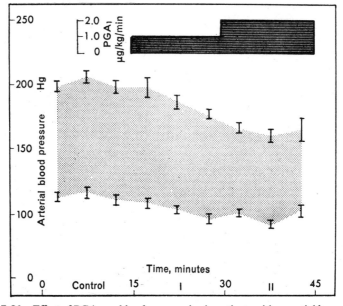

Figure 5.21   Effect of PGA_1 on blood pressure in six patients with essential hypertension. Mean of 12 to 18 determinations. Control period (15 min) and period I and period II (15 min each) during PGA_1 infusion (1 and 2 μg/kg per min intravenously, respectively) are subdivided into three consecutive five-minute intervals. Reproduced from Westura *et al.* (1970), by courtesy of *Circulation Res.*

Christlieb *et al.* (1969) reported the results of infusion of 0.3 to 1.2 μg/kg per min PGA$_1$ for 30–60 min. Blood pressure was lowered during the infusion but post-infusion rebound of the blood pressure was common and severe at times.

Fichman (1969, 1970) infused PGA$_1$ in a total of 35 normal hypertensive, hyponatremic, cirrhotic and anephric patients at rates varying from 0.03 to 5 μg/kg per min. The studies were carried out mainly to investigate the natriuretic actions of PGA$_1$. The greatest natriuretic effect was produced in cirrhotic patients with ascites (Table 5.3).

Krakoff *et al.* (1973) have shown that in 10 hypertensive subjects maintained on a constant diet containing 40 mEq of sodium and 80 mEq of potassium, the intravenous infusion of PGA$_1$, 0.4 μg/kg per min, caused a small but significant reduction in arterial blood pressure, and increased urine flow, renal plasma flow and sodium and potassium excretion. Plasma renin activity was not markedly altered. After sodium depletion with furosemide (80 mg/day for one week), PGA$_1$ infusion did not significantly alter the arterial blood pressure. Although urine flow, sodium excretion and renal plasma flow rose with PGA$_1$ infusion, the degree of increase in these parameters was less than that observed prior to furosemide administration. Moreover, in salt-depleted subjects a significant rise in plasma renin activity was observed during PGA$_1$ infusion. Based on these observations it was concluded that extracellular fluid volume depletion reduces the vasodilator response to PGA$_1$ and that the increase in plasma renin activity could partly account for the preservation of arterial blood pressure and the smaller increase in renal plasma flow.

Slotkoff (1974) infused PGA$_1$ into a woman with severe hypertension in congestive heart failure in doses of 0.6–2.4 μg/kg body weight per min. At low doses (0.6 μg) a marked diuresis occurred during the first 15 min with little change in blood pressure (210/110 mm Hg) or pulse rate. After 30 min when the infusion rate was increased fourfold the blood pressure fell from 210/110 mm Hg to 100/60 mm Hg within 2 min and within several hours of PGA$_1$ administration signs and symptoms of congestive heart failure were cleared.

Prostaglandin A$_1$ has also been shown to increase blood flow in several vascular beds of man. Barner *et al.* (1973) studied the effect of PGA$_1$ on 19 aortocoronary bypass grafts, five internal carotid arteries, eight aorto-femoral bypass grafts and seven femoral popliteal bypass grafts in man. They found that intra-arterial or intravenous administration of PGA$_1$ (25–50 μg) increased coronary, femoral and popliteal blood flow. Internal carotid flow did not increase after intravenous injection of PGA$_1$ but decreased as mean aortic pressure decreased and vascular resistance did not change. Robinson *et al.* (1973) showed that PGA$_1$ and PGA$_2$ infused into the brachial artery of man in doses varying from 0.1 to 10 μg/min produced a dose-dependent increase in forearm blood flow, PGA$_1$ being about 10 times more potent than PGA$_2$. In the superficial hand veins infusion of PGA$_1$ and PGA$_2$ in doses of 10–100 ng/min had no effect on the relaxed vein whereas when infused into veins preconstricted with either norepinephrine or 5-hydroxytryptamine both PGA$_1$ and PGA$_2$ produced a dose-dependent dilatation. These effects of PGA$_1$ and PGA$_2$ on both arteries and veins in man are qualitatively similar to the action of these agents in the dog (Nakano, 1968a, b; Greenberg and Sparks, 1969; Hyman, 1969; Hedwall et al., 1970; Mark et al., 1971; Emerson et al., 1971). Prostaglandin B_1 which is formed from PGA_1 by a prostaglandin isomerase (Jones, 1972b) also increased forearm blood flow in man at doses ranging from 2–10 $\mu g/min$ (Robinson et al., 1973). In contrast, PGB_1 in subconstrictor doses (2–32 ng/min) did not affect the veins preconstricted with norepinephrine whereas PGE_2 in doses 100 times greater than that required to overcome the constriction produced by norepinephrine caused dilatation of veins preconstricted with PGB_1 (500 ng/min). These observations suggest that PGB_1 has a differential effect on arteries and veins. In the dog hindpaw, PGB_1 has been reported to produce vasodilatation in small concentrations (50–200 ng/kg per min) whereas higher doses (200–3200 ng/kg per min) caused vasoconstriction (Greenberg, Howard et al., 1974).

Hornych et al. (1973) studied the effect of PGA_2 in 9 essential hypertensive patients and one patient with renovascular hypertension. They found that intravenous infusion of PGA_2 in doses (0.1–0.2 $\mu g/kg$ per min) which were devoid of hypotensive effects increased free water clearance and renal blood flow without producing other haemodynamic changes. The natriuretic effect was less pronounced than the diuretic actions thereby suggesting that PGA_2 is not a specific natriuretic agent. High doses of PGA_2, 2–9 $\mu g/kg$ per min caused a fall in systemic arterial blood pressure accompanied by an increase in cardiac output and decreased total peripheral resistance. The increased cardiac output was due to increased heart rate. Renal blood flow was increased in all patients except in one with renovascular hypertension. In this patient diuresis was not observed. Plasma renin activity was not altered during infusion of PGA_2 despite a large decrease in blood pressure. In contrast, in patients with renal artery stenosis, PGA_2 increased renin activity. Lee et al. (1971) have also reported an increase in renal venous renin in hypertensive patients after the administration of PGA_1 whereas Krakoff et al. (1973) found only a slight increase in plasma renin activity of hypertensive patients. At present no explanation is available for these contradictory results, although differences in sodium intake are probably contributory.

5.3.3 F prostaglandins

Karim et al. (1969) studied the cardiovascular effects of $PGF_{2\alpha}$ infusion in one female and five male volunteers. Continuous infusion of 0.01–2.0 $\mu g/kg$ per min $PGF_{2\alpha}$ for 60 min was without any effect on the systolic or diastolic blood pressure, heart rate or electrocardiogram (Figure 5.17). In another study, the same authors showed that up to 4 $\mu g/kg$ per min $PGF_{2\alpha}$ infusion for 60 min or 20 mg given intramuscularly or subcutaneously did not affect the blood pressure or heart rate in males and non-pregnant females (Karim et al., 1971; Karim, Hillier et al., 1971). However, with rapid single intravenous injections, 500 mg $PGF_{2\alpha}$ raised the arterial blood pressure (Figure 5.20). This effect was similar to that seen in the dog and rat (DuCharme and Weeks, 1967), but unlike that produced by $PGF_{2\alpha}$ in the cat and rabbit. As much as

50 mg $PGF_{2\alpha}$ given by mouth, rectally or per vaginam does not have any effect on the human cardiovascular system (Karim, 1971; Karim and Sharma, 1971) (Tables 5.1, 5.2 and 5.3). Infusions of $PGF_{2\alpha}$ up to 200 μg/min, have been given by many investigators to stimulate the human uterus in early pregnancy. In none of these studies has $PGF_{2\alpha}$ produced any apparent changes in the cardiovascular system (Karim and Filshie, 1970; Roth-Brandel et al., 1970; Embrey, 1970; Kaufman et al., 1971; Hendricks et al., 1971; Fishburne et al., 1972).

The mechanism of the pressor action of $PGF_{2\alpha}$ in man has so far not been studied. In the dog and the rat, $PGF_{2\alpha}$ is believed to raise the blood pressure due to selective venoconstriction (DuCharme and Weeks, 1967) and/or due to increased peripheral resistance (Nakano and McCurdy, 1968; Nakano and Cole, 1969). Robinson et al. (1973) have shown that infusion of $PGF_{2\alpha}$ into the brachial artery of man in higher doses, 10 μg/min increased the forearm blood flow, whereas lower doses (0.4 μg/min) caused a transient reduction in flow. In superficial hand veins infusion of $PGF_{2\alpha}$, 100–500 ng/min, caused a dose-dependent constriction of the vein. These observations also support the view that the rise in blood pressure produced by $PGF_{2\alpha}$ may be due to venoconstriction.

Acknowledgements

We wish to express our thanks to Miss Patricia Ryan, Mary Houde, Susan Ryan and Mrs. Sadžida Hamamdžić for their excellent assistance during the preparation of this manuscript.

This work was supported in part by research grants from U.S. Public Health Service (HL 17530-01 and HL 13624), American Heart Association (73692) and Wisconsin Heart Association.

References

Abdel-Sayed, W., Abboud, F. M., Hedwall, P. R. and Schmid, P. G. (1970). Vascular responses to prostaglandin E_1 (PGE_1) in muscular and cutaneous beds. *Circulation*, **42, Suppl. III,** 126

Adaikan, P. G. and Karim, S. M. M. (1974). Effect of prostaglandins A_1, A_2, B_1, B_2, E_2 and $F_{2\alpha}$ on human umbilical cord vessels. *Prostaglandins*, **8,** 411

Aiken, J. W. and Vane, J. R. (1973). Intrarenal prostaglandin release attenuates the renal vasoconstrictor activity of angiotensin. *J. Pharmac. exp. Ther.*, **184,** 678

Alpert, J. S., Haynes, F. W., Knutson, P. A., Dalen, J. E. and Dexter, L. (1973). Prostaglandins and the pulmonary circulation. *Prostaglandins*, **3,** 759

Al Tai, S. A. and Graham, J. D. P. (1972). The actions of prostaglandins E_1 and $F_{2\alpha}$ on the perfused vessels of the isolated rabbit ear. *Br. J. Pharmac.*, **44,** 699

Amer, M. S. (1973). Cyclic adenosine monophosphate and hypertension in rats. *Science*, **179,** 807

Anderson, F. L., Kralios, A. C., Tsagaris, T. J. and Kuida, H. (1972). Effects of prostaglandins $F_{2\alpha}$ and E_2 on the bovine circulation. *Proc. Soc. Exp. Biol. Med.*, **140,** 1049

Änggård, E. (1966). The biological activities of three metabolites of prostaglandin E_1. *Acta Physiol. Scand.*, **66,** 509

Änggård, E. and Bergström, S. (1963). Biological effects of an unsaturated trihydroxy acid ($PGF_{2\alpha}$) from normal swine lung. *Acta Physiol. Scand.*, **58,** 1

Änggård, E. and Jonsson, C. E. (1972). Formation of prostaglandins in the skin following a burn injury. In: *Prostaglandins in Cellular Biology*, Ramwell, P. W. and Pharriss, B. B. (eds.), pp. 269–291 (New York and London: Plenum Press Inc.)

Änggård, E. and Samuelsson, B. (1964). Metabolism of prostaglandin E_1 in guinea-pig lung: the structure of two metabolites. *J. Biol. Chem.*, **239**, 4097

Änggård, E. and Samuelsson, B. (1966). Purification and properties of a 15-hydroxyprostaglandin dehydrogenase from swine lung. *Ark. Kem.*, **25**, 293

Antonaccio, M. J. and Lucchesi, B. R. (1970). The interaction of glucagon and theophylline, PGE_1, isoproterenol, ouabain and $CaCl_2$ on the dog isolated papillary muscle. *Life Sci.*, **9**, 1081

Armstrong, J. M., McGiff, J. C. and Mullane, K. (1975). Renal prostaglandins (PGs): their possible prohypertensive action in rats. *Sixth International Congress of Pharmacol.*, *Helsinki, Finland*

Barner, H. B., Kaiser, G. C., Hahn, J. W., Jellinek, M., Amako, H., Lee, J. B. and Willman, V. L. (1972). Effects of prostaglandin A_1 on cardiovascular dynamics and myocardial metabolism. *J. Surg. Res.*, **12**, 168

Barner, H. B., Kaiser, G. C., Jellinek, M. and Lee, J. B. (1973). Effect of prostaglandin A_1 on several vascular beds in man. *Am. Heart J.*, **85**, 584

Baysal, F. and Vural, H. (1974). Effects of PGE_1 on the frog ventricular strip. *Experientia*, **30**, 71

Beck, L., Pollard, A. A., Kayaalp, S. O. and Weiner, L. M. (1966). Sustained dilatation elicited by sympathetic nerve stimulation. *Fed. Proc.*, **25**, 1596

Bergström, S. (1967a). Prostaglandins: members of a new hormonal system. *Science*, **157**, 382

Bergström, S. (1967b). Isolation, structure and action of the prostaglandins. In *Nobel Symposium Prostaglandins*, Bergström S., and Samuelsson, B. (eds.), pp. 21–30 (Stockholm: Almqvist and Wiksell)

Bergström, S., Carlson, L. A., Ekelund, L. G. and Orö, L. (1965a). Cardiovascular and metabolic response to infusions of prostaglandin E_1 and to simultaneous infusions of noradrenaline and prostaglandin E_1 in man. *Acta Physiol. Scand.*, **64**, 332

Bergström, S., Carlson, L. A., Ekelund, L. G. and Orö, L. (1965b). Effect of prostaglandin E_1 on blood pressure, heart rate and concentration of free fatty acids of plasma in man. *Proc. Soc. Exp. Biol. Med.*, **118**, 110

Bergström, S., Carlson, L. A. and Orö, L. (1964). Effect of prostaglandins on catecholamine-induced changes in the free fatty acids of plasma and in blood pressure in the dog. *Acta Physiol. Scand.*, **60**, 170

Bergström, S., Carlson, L. A. and Orö, L. (1966). Effect of different doses of prostaglandin E_1 on free fatty acids of plasma, blood glucose and heart rate in the non-anaesthetized dog. *Acta Physiol. Scand.*, **67**, 185

Bergström, S., Carlson, L. A. and Orö, L. (1967). A note on the cardiovascular and metabolic effects of prostaglandin A_1. *Life Sci.*, **6**, 449

Bergström, S., Duner, H., Euler, U.S.v., Pernow, B. and Sjövall, J. (1959). Observations on the effects of infusion of prostaglandin E in man. *Acta Physiol. Scand.*, **45**, 145

Bergström, S., Eliasson, R., Euler, U.S.v. and Sjövall, J. (1959). Some biological effects of two crystalline prostaglandin factors. *Acta Physiol. Scand.*, **45**, 133

Bergström, S. and Euler, U.S.v., (1963). The biological activity of prostaglandin E_1, E_2 and E_3. *Acta Physiol. Scand.*, **59**, 493

Bergström, S. and Sjövall, J. (1957). The isolation of prostaglandin. *Acta Chem. Scand.*, **11**, 1086

Berti, F., Borroni, V., Fumagalli, R., Marchi, P. and Zocche, G. P. (1964). Sullattivita pressoria della prostaglandina. *Atti Accad. Med. Lomb.*, **19**, 397

Berti, F., Lentati, R. and Usardi, M. M. (1965). The species specificity of prostaglandin E_1 effects on isolated heart. *Med. Pharmacol. Exp.*, **13**, 233

Berti, F., Naimzada, M. K., Lentati, R., Usardi, M. M., Mantegazza, P. and Paoletti, R. (1967). Relations between some *in vitro* and *in vivo* effects of prostaglandin E_1. *Progr. Biochem. Pharmacol.*, **3**, 110

Berti, F. and Usardi, M. M. (1964). Investigations on a new inhibitor of free fatty acid mobilization. *G. Arterioscler*, **2**, 261

Bevegard, S. and Orö, L. (1969). Effect of prostaglandin E_1 on forearm blood flow. *Scand. J. Clin. Lab. Invest.*, **23**, 347

Blakely, A. G. H., Brown, L., Dearnaley, D. P. and Woods, R. I. (1969). Perfusion of the spleen with blood containing prostaglandin E_1: Transmitter liberation and uptake. *Proc. Soc. London (Biol.)*, **174**, 281

Bloor, C. M. and Sobel, B. E. (1970). Enhanced coronary blood flow following prostaglandin infusion in the conscious dog. *Circulation*, **42, Suppl. III**, 123

Bohr, D. F. and Uchida, E. (1968). Activation of vascular smooth muscle. In *The pulmonary circulation and interstitial space*, Fisherman, A. P. and Hecht, H. H. (eds.). pp. 133–45 (University of Chicago Press)

Botting, J. H. and Salzmann, R. (1974). The effect of indomethacin on the release of prostaglandin E_2 and acetylcholine from guinea-pig isolated ileum at rest and during field stimulation. *Br. J. Pharmac.*, **50**, 119

Brody, M. J. and Kadowitz, P. J. (1974). Prostaglandins as modulators of the autonomic nervous system. *Fed. Proc.*, **33**, 48

Brown, R. V. and Hilton, J. G. (1956). The effectiveness of the baroreceptor reflexes under different anesthetics. *J. Pharmac. exp. Ther.*, **118**, 198

Burn, J. H. and Gibbons, W. R. (1964). The part played by calcium in determining the response to stimulation of sympathetic post-ganglionic fibres. *Br. J. Pharmac.*, **22**, 540–8

Bygdeman, M. (1964). The effect of different prostaglandins on the human myometrium *in vitro*. *Acta Physiol. Scand.*, **63, Suppl. 242**, 1

Bygdeman, M. and Hamberg, M. (1967). The effect of eight new prostaglandins on human myometrium. *Acta Physiol. Scand.*, **69**, 320

Bygdeman, M., Hamberg, M. and Samuelsson, B. (1966). The content of different prostaglandins in human seminal fluid and their threshold doses on the human myometrium. *Mem. Soc. Endocr.*, **14**, 49

Bygdeman, M., Kwon, S. U., Mukherjee, T. and Wiqvist, N. (1968). Effect of intravenous infusion of prostaglandin E_1 and E_2 on motility of the pregnant human uterus. *Am. J. Obstet. Gynecol.*, **102**, 317

Carlson, L. A. (1965). Inhibition of the mobilization of free fatty acids from adipose tissue. *Ann. N.Y. Acad. Sci.*, **131**, 119

Carlson, L. A. (1967). Metabolic and cardiovascular effects *in vivo* of prostaglandins. In *Nobel Symposium, Prostaglandins*, Bergström, S. and Samuelsson, B. (eds.), pp. 123–132 (Stockholm: Almqvist and Wiksell)

Carlson, L. A., Ekelund, L. G. and Orö, L. (1967). Metabolic and cardiovascular effects of serotonin. *Life Sci.*, **6**, 261

Carlson, L. A., Ekelund, L. G. and Orö, L. (1968). Clinical and metabolic effects of different doses of prostaglandin E_1 in man. *Acta Med. Scand.*, **183**, 423

Carlson, L. A., Ekelund, L. G. and Orö, L. (1969). Circulatory and respiratory effects of different doses of prostaglandin E_1 in man. *Acta Physiol. Scand.*, **75**, 161

Carlson, L. A. and Orö, L. (1966). Effect of prostaglandin E_1 on blood pressure and heart rate in the dog. *Acta Physiol. Scand.*, **67**, 89

Carpenter, M. P., Manning, L. and Wiseman, B. (1971). Prostaglandin synthesis in rat testis. *Fed. Proc.*, **30**, 1081 Abs

Carr, A. A. (1970). Hemodynamic and renal effects of a prostaglandin, PGA_1, in subjects with essential hypertension. *Am. J. Med. Sci.*, **259**, 21

Carsten, M. E. (1972). Prostaglandins' part in regulating uterine contraction by transport of calcium. *J. Reprod. Med.*, **9**, 277

Chandler, J. T. and Strong, C. G. (1972). The actions of prostaglandin E_1 on isolated rabbit aorta. *Archs. int. Pharmacodyn. Ther.*, **197**, 123

Chanh, P. H. and Carthery, M. C. N. (1973). Prostaglandin-releasing effect of exogenous noradrenaline in isolated rabbit heart. *Naturwess*, **60**, 482

Chanh, P. H., Junstad, M. and Wenmalm, A. (1972). Augmented noradrenaline release following nerve stimulation after inhibition of prostaglandin synthesis with indomethacin. *Acta Physiol. Scand.*, **86**, 563

Chesley, L. C. and Annitto, J. E. (1947). Pregnancy in the patient with hypertensive disease. *Am. J. Obstet. Gynec.*, **53**, 372

Chiba, S., Nakajima, T. and Nakano, J. (1972). Effect of prostaglandins E_1 and $F_{2\alpha}$ on heart rate by direct injection into the canine sinus node artery. *Jap. J. Pharmacol.* **22**, 734

Christ, E. J. and Van Dorp, D. A. (1973). Comparative aspects of prostaglandin biosynthesis in animal tissue. *Adv. Biosci.*, **9**, 35

Christlieb, A. R., Dobrzinsky, S. J., Lyons, C. J. and Hickler, R. B. (1969). Short term PGA$_1$ infusions in patients with essential hypertension. *Clin. Res.*, **17**, 234

Ciofalo, F. and Treece, G. (1973). Ouabain-induced myocardial catecholamine release: inhibition by propranolol. *Res. Commun. Chem. Path. Pharmac.*, **5**, 73

Clark, K. E., Ryan, M. J. and Brody, M. J. (1973). Effects of prostaglandins E$_1$ and F$_{2\alpha}$ on uterine hemodynamics and motility. *Adv. Biosci.*, **9**, 779

Clegg, P. C., Hall, W. J. and Pickles, V. R. (1966). The action of ketonic prostaglandins on the guinea-pig myometrium. *J. Physiol. (Lond.)*, **183**, 123

Coceani, F. and Olley, P. M. (1973). The response of the ductus arteriosus to prostaglandins. *Canad. J. Physiol. Pharmac.*, **51**, 220

Cohen, M., Sztokalo, J. and Hinsch, E. (1973). The antihypertensive action of arachidonic acid in the spontaneous hypertensive rat and its antagonism by anti-inflammatory agents. *Life Sci.*, **13**, 317

Colina, J. C., McGiff, J. C. and Nasjletti, A. (1975). Development of high blood pressure following inhibition of prostaglandin synthesis. *Fed. Proc.* (In press)

Conway, J. and Hatton, R. (1973). Effects of prostaglandins E$_1$, E$_2$, A$_1$ and A$_2$ on resistance and capacitance vessels in the hindlimb of the dog. *J. Physiol. (Lond.)*, **230**, 56P

Covino, B., Lee, J. B. and McMorrow, J. (1968). Circulatory effects of renal prostaglandins. *Circulation*, **38, Suppl. IV**, 60

Crowshaw, K. and McGiff, J. C. (1973). Prostaglandins in the kidney: a correlative study of their biochemistry and renal function. In *Mechanisms of Hypertension*, Sambhi, M. P. (ed.), pp. 254–273 (Amsterdam: Excerpta Medica)

Crowshaw, K., McGiff, J. C., Strand, J. C., Lonigro, A. J. and Terragno, N. A. (1970). Prostaglandins in dog renal medulla. *J. Pharm. Pharmacol.*, **22**, 302

Crunkhorn, P. and Willis, A. L. (1969). Actions and interactions of prostaglandins administered intradermally in rat and in man. *Br. J. Pharmac.*, **36**, 216P

Csépli, J. and Erdélyi, A. (1973). Circulatory actions of prostaglandin F$_{2\alpha}$ in the rat. *Bibl. Anat.*, **12**, 449

Curnow, R. T. and Nuttall, F. Q. (1971). Effect of prostaglandin E$_1$ (PGE$_1$) on glycogen metabolism in the rat liver and heart *in vivo*. *Fed. Proc.*, **30**, 625

Daniel, P. M., Dawes, J. D. K. and Prichard, M. M. L. (1952–54). Studies of the carotid rete and its associated arteries. *Philosophic Trans.*, **237B**, 173

Daniels, E. G., Hinman, J. W., Leach, B. E. and Muirhead, E. E. (1967). Identification of prostaglandin E$_2$ as the principal vasodepressor lipid of rabbit renal medulla. *Nature (Lond.)*, **215**, 1298

Daugherty, R. M. Jr. (1971). Effects of i.v. and i.a. prostaglandin E$_1$ on dog forelimb skin and muscle blood flow. *Am. J. Physiol.*, **220**, 392

Daugherty, R. M. Jr., Schwinghamer, J. M., Swindall, S. and Haddy, F. J. (1968). The effects of local and systemic infusions of prostaglandin E$_1$ on the skin and muscle vasculature in the dog forelimb. *J. Lab. Clin. Med.*, **72**, 869

Davies, B. N., Horton, E. W. and Withrington, P. G. (1968). The occurrence of prostaglandin E$_2$ in splenic venous blood of the dog following splenic nerve stimulation. *Br. J. Pharmac.*, **32**, 127

Davies, B. N. and Withrington, P. G. (1968). The effects of prostaglandin E$_1$ and E$_2$ on the smooth muscle of the dog spleen and on its responses to catecholamines, angiotensin and nerve stimulation. *Br. J. Pharmac.*, **32**, 136

Davies, B. N. and Withrington, P. G. (1969). Actions of prostaglandins A$_1$, A$_2$, E$_1$, E$_2$, F$_{1\alpha}$ and F$_{2\alpha}$ on splenic vascular and capsular smooth muscle and their interactions with sympathetic nerve stimulation, catecholamines and angiotensin. In *Prostaglandins, peptides and amines*, Mantegazza, P. and Horton, E. W. (eds.), pp. 53–56 (London: Academic Press)

Davies, B. N. and Withrington, P. G. (1971). Actions of prostaglandin F$_{2\alpha}$ on the splenic vascular and capsular smooth muscle in the dog. *Br. J. Pharmac.*, **41**, 1

Davis, H. A. and Horton, E. W. (1972). Output of prostaglandins from the rabbit kidney, its increase on renal nerve stimulation and its inhibition by indomethacin. *Br. J. Pharmac.*, **46**, 658

Denton, I. C. Jr., White, R. P. and Robertson, J. T. (1972). The effects of prostaglandins E$_1$, A$_1$ and F$_{2\alpha}$ on the cerebral circulation of dogs and monkeys. *J. Neurosurg.*, **36**, 34

Dohadwalla, A. M., Freeberg, A. S. and Vaughan Williams, E. M. (1969). The relevance of β-receptor blockade to ouabain induced cardiac arrhythmias. *Br. J. Pharmac.*, **36**, 257

Downing, D. T., Ahern, D. G. and Bachta, M. (1970). Enzyme inhibition by acetylenic compounds. *Biochem. Biophys. Res. Commun.*, **40**, 218

DuCharme, D. W. and Weeks, J. R. (1967). Cardiovascular pharmacology of prostaglandin $F_{2\alpha}$, a unique pressor agent. In *Prostaglandins, Nobel Symposium 2*, Bergström, S. and Samuelsson, B. (eds.), pp. 173–181 (Stockholm: Almqvist and Wiksell)

DuCharme, D. W., Weeks, J. R. and Montgomery, R. G. (1968). Studies on the mechanism of the hypertensive effect of prostaglandin $F_{2\lambda}$. *J. Pharmac. exp. Ther.*, **160**, 1

Dunham, E. W. and Zimmerman, B. G. (1970). Release of prostaglandin-like material from dog kidney during nerve stimulation. *Am. J. Physiol.*, **219**, 1279

Ebashi, S. and Ebashi, F. (1964). A new protein component participating in the super-precipitation of myosin β. *J. Biochem. Tokyo*, **55**, 604

Echlin, F. A. (1968). Current concepts in the etiology and treatment of vasospasm. *Clin. Neurosurg.*, **15**, 133

Einer-Jensen, N. and Scofi, G. (1974). Decreased blood flow through rat testis after intra-testicular injection of $PGF_{2\alpha}$. *Prostaglandins*, **7**, 377

Elliott, R. B. and Starling, M. B. (1972). The effect of prostaglandin $F_{2\alpha}$ in the closure of the ductus arteriosus. *Prostaglandins*, **2**, 399

Ellis, E. and Hutchins, P. (1974). Cardiovascular responses to prostaglandin $F_{2\alpha}$ in spon-taneously hypertensive rats. *Prostaglandins*, **7**, 345

Embrey, M. P. (1970). Induction of abortion by prostaglandin E_1 and E_2. *Br. Med. J.*, **2**, 258

Emerson, T. E. Jr., Jelks, G. W., Daugherty, R. M. Jr. and Hodgmen, R. E. (1971). Effects of prostaglandin E_1 and $F_{2\alpha}$ on venous return and other parameters in the dog. *Am. J. Physiol.*, **220**, 243

Emmons, P. R., Hampton, J. R., Harrison, M. J. G., Honour, A. J. and Mitchell, J. R. A. (1967). Effect of prostaglandin E_1 on platelet behaviour *in vitro* and *in vivo*. *Br. Med. J.*, **2**, 468

Euler, U. S.v. (1934). Zur kenntnis der pharmakologischen Wirkungen von Nativsekreten und Extrackten männlicher accessorischer Geschlechtsdrusen. *Naunyn-Schmiedebergs Arch. Exp. Path. Pharmak.*, **175**, 78

Euler, U. S.v. (1935). Über diě spezifische blutdrucksenkende Substanz des Menschlichen prostata und Samenblasensekretes. *Klin. Wochenschr.*, **14**, 1182

Euler, U. S.v. (1936). On the specific vasodilating and plain muscle stimulating substances from accessory genital glands in man and certain animals (prostaglandin and vesiglandin). *J. Physiol. (Lond.)*, **88**, 213

Euler, U. S.v. (1939). Weitere Untersuchungen über Prostaglandin, die physiologisch aktiv Substanz gewisser Genitaldrüsen. *Skand. Arch. Physiol.*, **81**, 65

Fain, J. N. (1967). Adrenergic blockade of hormone-induced lipolysis in isolated fat cells. *Ann. N.Y. Acad. Sci.*, **139**, 879

Fassina, G., Carpendo, F. and Santi, R. (1969). Effect of prostaglandin E_1 on isolated short-circuited frog skin. *Life Sci.*, **8, Part I**, 181

Fassina, G. and Contessa, A. R. (1967). Digitoxin and prostaglandin E_1 as inhibitors of catecholamine-stimulated lipolysis and their interaction with Ca^{2+} in the process. *Biochem. Pharmacol.*, **16**, 1447

Ferreira, S. H., Moncada, S. and Vane, J. R. (1971). Indomethacin and aspirin abolish prostaglandin release from the spleen. *Nature New Biology*, **231**, 237

Ferreira, S. H., Moncada, S. and Vane, J. R. (1973). Some effects of inhibiting endogenous prostaglandin formation on the responses of the cat spleen. *Br. J. Pharmacol.*, **47**, 48

Ferreira, S. H. and Vane, J. R. (1967). Prostaglandins: their disappearance from and release into the circulation. *Nature (Lond.)*, **216**, 868

Ferris, T. F., Stein, J. H. and Kauffman, J. (1972). Uterine blood flow and uterine renin secretion. *J. Clin. Invest.*, **51**, 2827

Fichman, M. P. (1969). Natriuretic effect of prostaglandin (PGA_1) in man. *Clin. Res.*, **17**, 429

Fichman, M. P. (1970). Natriuretic and vasodepressor effect of prostaglandin (PGA_1) in man. *Clin. Res.*, **18**, 149

Fishburne, J. I., Brenner, W. E., Braaksma, J. T., Staurovsky, L. G., Mueller, R. A., Hoffer, J. L. and Hendricks, C. H. (1972). Cardiovascular and respiratory responses to intravenous infusion of prostaglandin $F_{2\alpha}$ in the pregnant woman. *Am. J. Obstet. Gynecol.*, **114**, 765

Forster, W., Mest, H. J. and Mentz, P. (1973). The influence of $PGF_{2\alpha}$ on experimental arrhythmias. *Prostaglandins*, **3**, 895

Frame, M. H., Hedqvist, P. and Aström, Å. (1974). Effect of prostaglandin E_2 on vascular responses of the rabbit kidney to nerve stimulation and noradrenaline *in vitro* and *in situ*. *Life Sci.*, **15**, 239

Franklin, G. O., Dowd, A. J., Caldwell, B. V. and Speroff, L. (1974). The effect of angiotensin-II intravenous infusion on plasma renin activity and prostaglandin A, E and F levels in the uterine vein of the pregnant monkey. *Prostaglandins*, **6**, 271

Free, M. J. and Jaffe, R. A. (1972). Effect of prostaglandins on blood flow and pressure in the conscious rat. *Prostaglandins*, **1**, 483

Gagnon, D. J., Gauthier, R. and Regoli, D. (1974). Release of prostaglandins from the rabbit perfused kidney: Effects of vasoconstrictors. *Br. J. Pharmac.*, **50**, 553

Gant, N, F., Daley, G. L., Chand, S., Whalley, P. J. and MacDonald, P. C. (1973). A study of angiotensin II pressor response throughout primigravid pregnancy. *J. Clin. Invest.*, **52**, 2682

Geumi, A., Bashour, F. A., Swamy, B. V. and Nafrawi, A. G. (1973). Prostaglandin E_1: Its effects on hepatic circulation in dogs. *Pharmacology*, **9**, 336

Giles, T. D., Quiroz, A. C. and Burch, G. E. (1969). The effects of prostaglandin E_1 on the systemic and pulmonary circulations of intact dogs. The influence of urethane and pentobarbital anesthesia. *Experientia*, **25**, 1056

Gilmore, N., Vane, J. R. and Wyllie, J. H. (1968). Prostaglandins released by the spleen. *Nature (Lond.)*, **218**, 1135

Gilmore, N., Vane, J. R. and Wyllie, J. H. (1969). Prostaglandin release by the spleen in response to infusion of particles. In *Prostaglandins, Peptides and Amines*, Mantegazza, P. and Horton, E. (eds.), pp. 21–29 (London and New York: Academic Press)

Glaviano, V. and Masters, T. (1968). Inhibitory action of prostaglandin E_1 on myocardial lipolysis. *Circulation*, **38, Suppl. VI**, 83

Glaviano, V. and Masters, T. (1971). Inhibitory action of intercoronary prostaglandin E_1 on myocardial lipolysis. *Am. J. Physiol.*, **220**, 1187

Goldblatt, M. W. (1933). A depressor substance in seminal fluid. *J. Soc. Chem. Ind. (Lond.)*, **52**, 1056

Goldblatt, M. W. (1935). Properties of human seminal plasma. *J. Physiol. (Lond.)*, **84**, 208

Goldyne, M. E. and Winkelmann, R. K. (1973). *In vitro* effects of prostaglandin E_2 on cutaneous vascular smooth muscle in the dog and in man. *J. Invest. Dermatol.*, **60**, 258

Greenberg, R. (1974). The effects of indomethacin and eicosa-5,8,11,14-tetraynoic acid on the response of the rabbit portal vein to electrical stimulation. *Br. J. Pharmac.*, **52**, 61

Greenberg, R. A. and Sparks, H. V. (1969). Prostaglandin and consecutive vascular segments of the canine hindlimb. *Am. J. Physiol.*, **216**, 567

Greenberg, S., Engelbrecht, J. A. and Wilson, W. R. (1973). Cardiovascular pharmacology of prostaglandin B_1 and B_2 in the intact dog. *Proc. Soc. Exp. Biol. Med.*, **143**, 1008

Greenberg, S., Engelbrecht, J. A. and Wilson, W. R. (1974a). Prostaglandin B_2-induced cutaneous vasoconstriction of the canine hindpaw. *Circulation Res.*, **34**, 491

Greenberg, S., Engelbrecht, J. A. and Wilson, W. R. (1974b). The role of the autonomic nervous system in the responses of the perfused canine paw to prostaglandins B_1 and B_2. *J. Pharmac. exp. Ther.*, **189**, 130

Greenberg, S., Howard, L., Engelbrecht, J. and Wilson, W. R. (1974). Effects of prostaglandins B_1 and B_2 on vasoconstrictor responses of the canine hindpaw. *J. Pharmac. exp. Ther.*, **190**, 70

Greenberg, S., Howard, L. and Wilson, W. R. (1974). Comparative effects of prostaglandins A_2 and B_2 on vascular and airway resistances and adrenergic neurotransmission. *Can. J. Physiol. Pharmacol.*, **52**, 699

Greenberg, S., Kadowitz, P. J., Diecke, F. P. J. and Long, J. P. (1973). Effect of prostaglandin $F_{2\alpha}$ ($PGF_{2\alpha}$) on arterial and venous contractility and ^{45}Ca uptake. *Archs. int. Pharmacodyn. Ther.*, **205**, 381

Greenberg, S. and Long, J. P. (1973). Enhancement of vascular smooth muscle responses to vasoactive stimuli by prostaglandin E_1 and E_2. *Archs. int. Pharmacodyn. Ther.*, **206**, 94

Greenberg, S., Long, J. P. and Diecke, F. P. J. (1973a). Effect of prostaglandins on arterial and venous tone and calcium transport. *Archs. int. Pharmacodyn. Ther.*, **204**, 373

Greenberg, S., Long, J. P. and Diecke, F. P. J. (1973b). Interaction of prostaglandin A_2 with vascular smooth muscle tone and contractility. *Archs. int. Pharmacodyn. Ther.*, **205**, 399

Hadházy, P., Illés, P. and Knoll, J. (1973). The effects of PGE_1 on responses to cardiac vagus nerve stimulation and acetycholine release. *Eur. J. Pharmacol.*, **23**, 251

Hamberg, M. and Samuelsson, B. (1966). Prostaglandins in human seminal plasma. *J. Biol. Chem.*, **241**, 257

Hansson, E. and Samuelsson, B. (1965). Autoradiographic distribution studies of ^{3}H-labelled prostaglandin E_1 in mice. *Biochem. Biophys. Acta*, **106**, 379

Hauge, A., Lunde, P. K. M. and Waaler, B. A. (1967). Effects of prostaglandin E_1 and adrenaline on the pulmonary vascular resistance (PVR) in isolated rabbit lungs. *Life Sci.*, **6**, 673

Hedqvist, P. (1969). Modulating effect of prostaglandin E_2 on noradrenaline release from the isolated cat spleen. *Acta Physiol. Scand.*, **75**, 511

Hedqvist, P. (1970a). Studies on the effect of prostaglandins E_1 and E_2 on the sympathetic neuromuscular transmission in some animal tissues. *Acta Physiol. Scand.*, **79, Suppl. 345**, 1

Hedqvist, P. (1970b). Control by prostaglandin E_2 of sympathetic neurotransmission in the spleen. *Life Sci. (Part I)*, **9**, 269

Hedqvist, P. (1970c). Antagonism by calcium of the inhibitory action of prostaglandin E_2 on sympathetic neurotransmission in the cat spleen. *Acta Physiol. Scand.*, **80**, 269

Hedqvist, P. (1972). Prostaglandin-induced inhibition of vascular tone and reactivity in the cat's hindleg *in vivo*. *Eur. J. Pharmacol.*, **17**, 157

Hedqvist, P. (1973). Autonomic neurotransmission. In *The Prostaglandins*, Ramwell, P. W. (ed.), pp. 101–131 (New York: Plenum Press)

Hedqvist, P. and Brundin, J. (1969). Inhibition by prostaglandin E_1 of noradrenaline release and of effector responses to nerve stimulation in the cat spleen. *Life Sci. (Part I)*, **8**, 389

Hedqvist, P., Stjärne, L. and Wennmalm, Å. (1970). Inhibition by prostaglandin E_2 of sympathetic neurotransmission in the rabbit heart. *Acta Physiol. Scand.*, **79**, 139

Hedqvist, P., Stjärne, L., and Wennmalm, Å. (1971). Facilitation of sympathetic neurotransmission in the cat spleen after inhibition of prostaglandin synthesis. *Acta Physiol. Scand.*, **83**, 430

Hedqvist, P. and Wennmalm, Å. (1971). Comparison of the effects of prostaglandin E_1, E_2 and $F_{2\alpha}$ on the sympathetically stimulated rabbit heart. *Acta Physiol. Scand.*, **83**, 156

Hedwall, P. R., Abdel-Sayed, W., Schmid, P. G. and Abboud, F. M. (1970). Selective interaction between prostaglandin E_1 (PGE_1) and adrenergic stimuli. *Circulation*, **42, Suppl. III**, 89

Hedwall, P. R., Abdel-Sayed, W. A., Schmid, P. G., Mark, A. L. and Abboud, F. M. (1971). Vascular responses to prostaglandin E_1 in gracilis muscle and hindpaw of the dog. *Am. J. Physiol.*, **221**, 42

Hendricks, C. H., Brenner, W. E., Ekbladh, L., Brotanek, V. and Fishburne, J. I. Jr. (1971). Efficacy and tolerance of intravenous prostaglandins $F_{2\alpha}$ and E_2. *Am. J. Obstet. Gynecol.*, **111**, 564

Higgins, C. B., Vatner, S. F. and Braunwald, E. (1973). Regional hemodynamic effects of prostaglandin A_1 in the conscious dog. *Am. Heart J.*, **85**, 349

Higgins, C., Vatner, S., Franklin, D. and Braunwald, E. (1970). Augmentation of coronary blood flow and cardiac output in conscious dogs by intravenous prostaglandin A_1. *Circulation*, **42, Suppl. III**, 123

Higgins, C. B., Vatner, S. F., Franklin, D. and Braunwald, E. (1972). Effects of prostaglandin A_1 on left ventricular dynamics in the conscious dog. *Am. J. Physiol.*, **222**, 1534

Higgins, C. B., Vatner, S. F., Franklin, D., Patrick, T. and Braunwald, E. (1971). Effects of prostaglandin A_1 on the systemic and coronary circulations in the conscious dog. *Circulation Res.*, **28**, 638

Hillier, K. and Karim, S. M. M. (1968). Effects of prostaglandins E_1, E_2, $F_{1\alpha}$ and $F_{2\alpha}$ on isolated human umbilical and placental blood vessels. *J. Obstet. Gynaecol. Br. Commonwealth*, **75**, 667

Hodgman, R. E., Jelks, G. W., Swindall, S. and Daugherty, R. M. Jr. (1970). Effects of local infusion of $PGF_{2\alpha}$ on the skin and muscle vasculature of the dog forelimb. *Clin. Res.*, **18**, 312

Hollander, W., Kramsch, D. M., Franzblau, C., Paddock, J. and Colombo, M. A. (1974). Suppression of atheromatous fibrous plaque formation by antiproliferative and anti-inflammatory drugs. *Circulation Res.*, **34, Suppl. I**, 131

Hollenberg, M., Walker, R. S. and McCormick, D. P. (1968). Cardiovascular responses to intracoronary infusion of prostaglandin E_1, $F_{1\alpha}$ and $F_{2\alpha}$. *Arch. int. Pharmacodyn. Ther.*, **174**, 66

Holmes, S. W., Horton, E. W. and Main, I. H. M. (1963). The effect of prostaglandin E_1 on responses of smooth muscle to catecholamines, angiotensin and vasopressin. *Br. J. Pharmac.*, **21**, 538

Hornych, A., Safar, M., Papanicolaou, N., Meyer, P. and Milliez, P. (1973). Renal and cardiovascular effects of prostaglandin A_2 in hypertensive patients. *Eur. J. Clin. Invest.*, **3**, 391

Horrobin, D. F., Manku, M. S., Karmali, R. A., Nassar, B. A. and Davies, P. A. (1974). Aspirin, indomethacin, catecholamine and prostaglandin interactions on rat arterioles and rabbit hearts. *Nature (Lond.)*, **250**, 425

Horton, E. W. (1973). Prostaglandins at adrenergic nerve endings. *Br. Med. Bull.*, **29**, 148

Horton, E. W. and Jones, R. L. (1969). Prostaglandins A_1, A_2 and 19-hydroxy A_1; their actions on smooth muscle and their inactivation on passage through the pulmonary and hepatic portal vascular beds. *Br. J. Pharmac.*, **37**, 705

Horton, E. W. and Main, I. H. M. (1963). A comparison of the biological activities of four prostaglandins. *Br. J. Pharmac.*, **21**, 182

Horton, E. W. and Main, I. H. M. (1965a). Differences in the effects of prostaglandin $F_{2\alpha}$, a constituent of cerebral tissue, and prostaglandin E_1 on conscious cats and chicks. *Int. J. Neuropharmacol.*, **4**, 65

Horton, E. W. and Main, I. H. M. (1965b). A comparison of the actions of prostaglandins $F_{2\alpha}$ and E_1 on smooth muscle. *Br. J. Pharmac.*, **24**, 470

Horton, E. W. and Main, I. H. M. (1967). Further observations on the central nervous actions of prostaglandins $F_{2\alpha}$ and E_1. *Br. J. Pharmac.*, **30**, 568

Hubbard, J. I. (1970). Mechanism of transmitter release. *Progr. Biophys. Mol. Biol.*, **21**, 33

Huković, S. and Muscholl, E. (1962). Die Noradrenaline-Abyabe aus dem isolierten Kaninchenherzen bei sympathischer Nerverreizung und ihre pharmakologische Beeinflussung. *Naunyn-Schmiedebergs Arch. Pharmakol. Exp. Pathol.*, **244**, 81

Hyman, A. L. (1969). The active responses of pulmonary veins in intact dogs to prostaglandins F_2 alpha and E_1. *J. Pharmac. exp. Ther.*, **165**, 267

Illés, P., Hadházy, P., Torma, Z., Vizi, E. S. and Knoll, J. (1973). The effect of number of stimuli and rate of stimulation on the inhibition by PGE_1 of adrenergic transmission. *Eur. J. Pharmacol.*, **24**, 29

Jackson, H. R. and Hall, R. C. (1973). The effect of aspirin on the response to the rabbit ear artery. *Eur. J. Pharmacol.*, **21**, 107

Jacobson, E. D. (1970). Comparison of prostaglandin E_1 and norepinephrine on the gastric mucosal circulation. *Proc. Soc. Exp. Biol. Med.*, **133**, 516

Johansson, B., Johnsson, O., Axelsson, J., Phil, D. and Wahlström, B. (1967). Electrical and mechanical characteristics of vascular smooth muscle response to norepinephrine and isoproterenol. *Circulation Res.*, **21**, 619

Jones, R. L. (1972a). Properties of a new prostaglandin. *Br. J. Pharmac.*, **45**, 144P

Jones, R. L. (1972b). 15-hydroxy-9-oxoprosta-11, 13-dienoic acid as the product of a prostaglandin isomerase. *J. Lipid Res.*, **13**, 511

Jones, R. L. and Cammock, S. (1973). Purification, properties and biological significance of prostaglandin A isomerase. *Adv. Biosci.*, **9**, 61

Jones, R. L., Cammock, S. and Horton, E. W. (1972). Partial purification and properties of cat plasma prostaglandin A isomerase. *Biochem. Biophys. Acta*, **280**, 588

Jones, R. L., Kane, K. A. and Ungar, A. (1974). Cardiovascular actions of prostaglandin C in the cat and dog. *Br. J. Pharmac.*, **51**, 157

Jørgensen, H. P. and Søndergaard, J. (1973). Vascular responses to prostaglandin E_1. *Acta Derm. Venerol. (Stockholm)*, **53**, 203

Juhlin, L. and Michaelsson, G. (1969). Cutaneous vascular reactions to prostaglandins in healthy subjects and in patients with urticaria and atopic dermatitis. *Acta Derm. Venerol. (Stockholm)*, **49**, 251

Junstad, M. and Wennmalm, Å. (1973). On the release of prostaglandin E_2 from the rabbit heart following infusion of noradrenaline. *Acta Physiol. Scand.*, **87**, 573

Junstad, M. and Wennmalm, Å. (1974). Release of prostaglandin from the isolated rabbit heart following vagal nerve stimulation or acetylcholine infusion. *Br. J. Pharmac.*, **52**, 375

Kadar, D. and Sunahara, F. A. (1967). The influence of prostaglandins on the effect of autonomic drugs in the superior mesenteric vein. *Proc. Cand. Fed. Biol. Sci.*, **10**, 24

Kadar, D. and Sunahara, F. A. (1969). Inhibition of prostaglandin effects by ouabain in the canine vascular tissue. *Can. J. Physiol. Pharmacol.*, **47**, 871

Kadowitz, P. J. (1972). Effect of prostaglandins E_1, E_2 and A_2 on vascular resistance and responses to noradrenaline, nerve stimulation and angiotensin in the dog hindlimb. *Br. J. Pharmac.*, **46**, 395

Kadowitz, P. J., George, W. J., Joiner, P. D. and Hyman, A. L. (1973). Effect of prostaglandins E_1 and $F_{2\alpha}$ on adrenergic responses in the pulmonary circulation. *Adv. Biosci.*, **9**, 501

Kadowitz, P. J., Sweet, C. S. and Brody, M. J. (1971a). Blockade of adrenergic vasoconstrictor responses in the dog by prostaglandins E_1 and A_1. *J. Pharmac. Exp. Ther.*, **179**, 563

Kadowitz, P. J., Sweet, C. S. and Brody, M. J. (1971b). Potentiation of adrenergic venomotor responses by angiotensin, prostaglandin $F_{2\alpha}$ and cocaine. *J. Pharmac. Exp. Ther.*, **176**, 167

Kadowitz, P. J., Sweet, C. S. and Brody, M. J. (1971c). Differential effects of prostaglandins E_1, E_2, $F_{1\alpha}$ and $F_{2\alpha}$ on adrenergic vasoconstriction in the dog hindpaw. *J. Pharmac. Exp. Ther.*, **177**, 641

Kadowitz, P. J., Sweet, C. S. and Brody, M. J. (1972). Enhancement of sympathetic neurotransmission by prostaglandin $F_{2\alpha}$ in the cutaneous vascular bed of the dog. *Eur. J. Pharmacol.*, **18**, 189

Kaldec, O., Mašek, K. and Šeferna, I. (1974). A modulating role of prostaglandins in contractions of the guinea-pig ileum. *Br. J. Pharmac.*, **51**, 565

Kaley, G. and Weiner, R. (1968). Microcirculatory studies with prostaglandin E_1. In *Prostaglandin Symposium of the Worcester Foundation for Experimental Biology*, Ramwell, P. W. and Shaw, J. E. (eds.), pp. 321–328 (New York: Interscience).

Kalsner, S. (1974) A vasodilator innervation to the central artery of the rabbit ear. *Br. J. Pharmac.*, **52**, 5

Kannegiesser, H. and Lee, J. B. (1971). Difference in haemodynamic response to prostaglandin A and E. *Nature (Lond.)*, **229**, 498

Kaplan, H. R., Grega, G. J., Sherman, G. P. and Buckley, J. P. (1969). Central and reflexogenic cardiovascular actions of prostaglandin E_1. *Int. J. Neuropharmacol.*, **8**, 15

Karim, S. M. M. (1967). The identification of prostaglandins in human umbilical cord. *Br. J. Pharmac.*, **29**, 230

Karim, S. M. M. (1971). Effects of oral administration of prostaglandins E_2 and $F_{2\alpha}$ on the human uterus. *J. Obstet. Gynaec. Br. Commonwealth*, **78**, 289

Karim, S. M. M. and Filshie, G. M. (1970). The use of prostaglandin E_2 for therapeutic abortion. *Br. Med. J.*, **3**, 198

Karim, S. M. M. and Somers, K. (1972) (eds.). The Prostaglandins. (New York: Interscience)

Karim, S. M. M., Hillier, K., Somers, K. and Trussell, R. R. (1971). The effects of prostaglandins E_2 and $F_{2\alpha}$ administered by different routes on uterine activity and the cardiovascular system in pregnant and non-pregnant women. *J. Obstet. Gynaecol. Br. Commonwealth*, **78**, 172

Karim, S. M. M., Hillier, K. and Devlin, J. (1968). Distribution of prostaglandins E_1, E_2, $F_{1\alpha}$ and $F_{2\alpha}$ in some animal tissues. *J. Pharm. Pharmacol.*, **20**, 749

Karim, S. M. M., Sandler, M. and Williams, E. D. (1967). Distribution of prostaglandins in human tissues. *Br. J. Pharmac.*, **31**, 340

Karim, S. M. M. and Sharma, S. D. (1971). Therapeutic abortion and induction of labour by the intravaginal administration of prostaglandins E_2 and $F_{2\alpha}$. *J. Obstet. Gynaecol. Br. Commonwealth*, **78**, 294

Karim, S. M. M., Somers, K. and Hillier, K. (1969). Cardiovascular actions of prostaglandin $F_{2\alpha}$ infusion in man. *Eur. J. Pharmacol.*, **5**, 117

Karim, S. M. M., Somers, K. and Hillier, K. (1971). Cardiovascular and other effects of prostaglandins E_2 and $F_{2\alpha}$ in man. *Cardiovasc. Res.*, **5**, 255

Kataoka, K., Ramwell, P. W. and Jessup, S. (1967). Prostaglandins: localization in subcellular particles of rat cerebral cortex. *Science*, **157**, 1187

Katori, M., Takeda, K. and Imai, S. (1970). Effects of prostaglandins E_1 and $F_{1\alpha}$ on the heart–lung preparation of the dog. *Tohoku. J. Exp. Med.*, **101**, 67

Katsuki, S., Onome, T., Ino, K. and Ito, A. (1969). The effects of prostaglandin E_1 (PGE_1) on brain circulation. (In Japanese). In *The Prostaglandins* (Symp. 20 Sept. 1968, Kyoto), pp. 83–85. (Osaka: Ono Pharmaceutical Co.)

Kaufman, R. G., Freeman, R. K. and Mishell, D. R. Jr. (1971). Abortifacient activity of intravenously administered prostaglandins. *Contraception*, **3**, 121

Kelliher, G. J., and Glenn, T. M. (1973). Effect of prostaglandin E_1 on ouabain-induced arrhythmia. *Eur. J. Pharmacol.*, **24**, 410

Khairallah, P. A., Page, I. H. and Türker, R. K. (1967). Some properties of prostaglandin E_1 action on muscle. *Archs. int. Pharmacodyn. Ther.*, **169**, 328

Kirpekar, S. M. and Misu, Y. (1967). Release of noradrenaline by splenic nerve stimulation and its dependence on calcium. *J. Physiol. (Lond.)*, **188**, 219

Kirtland, S. J. and Baum, H. (1972). Prostaglandin E_1 may act as a 'calcium ionophore'. *Nature (Lond.)*, **236**, 47

Klaus, W. and Piccinini, F. (1967). Über die Wirkung von Prostaglandin E_1 auf den Ca haushalt isolierter Meerschweichenherzen. *Experientia*, **23**, 556

Klein, I. and Levey, G. S. (1971). Effect of prostaglandins on guinea-pig myocardial adenyl cyclase. *Metabolism*, **20**, 890

Koss, M. C., Gray, J. W., Davison, M. and Nakano, J. (1973). Cardiovascular actions of prostaglandins E_1 and $F_{2\alpha}$ in the cat. *Eur. J. Pharmacol.*, **24**, 151

Koss, M. C. and Nakano, J. (1973). Effects of prostaglandins E_1 and $F_{2\alpha}$ on the peripheral circulation in the cat. *Proc. Soc. Exp. Biol. Med.*, **142**, 383

Krakoff, L. R., Guia, D. D., Vlachakis, N., Stricker, J. and Goldstein, M. (1973). Effect of sodium balance on arterial blood pressure and renal responses to prostaglandin A_1 in man. *Circulation Res.*, **33**, 539

Kukovetz, W. R. and Poch, G. (1970). Inhibition of cyclic-3'5'-nucleotide-phosphodiesterase as a possible mode of action of papaverine and similarly acting drugs. *Naunyn-Schmiedebergs Arch. Pharmacol.*, **267**, 189

Kunze, H. and Vogt, W. (1971). Significance of phospholipase A for prostaglandin formation. *Ann. N.Y. Acad. Sci.*, **180**, 123

Laborit, H. and Valette, N. (1974). The action of l-tyrosine and arachidonic acid on the experimental hypertension in rat: Physiopathogenic deductions. *Res. Commun. Chem. Path. Pharmac.*, **8**, 489

Ladner, C., Brinkman III, C. R., Weston, P. and Assali, N. S. (1970). Dynamics of uterine circulation in pregnant and nonpregnant sheep. *Am. J. Physiol.*, **218**, 257

Larsson, C. and Änggård, E. (1973). Arachidonic acid lowers and indomethacin increases the blood pressure of the rabbit. *J. Pharm. Pharmacol.*, **25**, 653

Lavery, H. A., Lowe, R. D. and Scroop, G. C. (1969). Cardiovascular effects of prostaglandins infused into extracranial arteries of the dog. *J. Physiol. (Lond.)*, **204**, 109P

Lavery, H. A., Lowe, R. D. and Scroop, G. C. (1970). Cardiovascular effects of prostaglandins mediated by the central nervous system of the dog. *Br. J. Pharmac.*, **39**, 511

Lavery, H. A., Lowe, R. D. and Scroop, G. C. (1971). Central autonomic effects of prostaglandin $F_{2\alpha}$ on the cardiovascular system of the dog. *Br. J. Pharmac.*, **41**, 454

Leach, B. E., Armstrong, F. B., Germain, G. S. and Muirhead, E. E. (1973). Vasodepressor action of prostaglandins A_2 and E_2 in the spontaneously hypertensive rat (SH rat): Evidence for an action mediated by the vagus. *J. Pharmac. Exp. Ther.*, **185**, 479

Lee, J. B. (1968). Cardiovascular implications of the renal prostaglandins. In *Prostaglandin Symposium of the Worcester Foundation for Exp. Biol.*, Ramwell, P. W. and Shaw, J. E. (eds.), pp. 131–146. (New York: Interscience)

Lee, J. B. (1969). Hypertension, natriuresis and the renal prostaglandins. *Ann. Intern. Med.*, **70**, 1033

Lee, J. B., Covino, B. G., Takman, B. H. and Smith, E. R. (1965). Renomedullary vasodepressor substance, medullin: Isolation chemical characterization and physiological properties. *Circulation Res.*, **17**, 57

Lee, J. B., Crowshaw, K., Takman, B. H., Atrep, K. A. and Gougoutas, J. Z. (1967). The identification of prostaglandins E_2, $F_{2\alpha}$ and A_2 from rabbit kidney medulla. *Biochem. J.*, **105**, 1251

Lee, J. B., Gougoutas, J. Z., Takman, B. H., Daniels, E. G., Grostic, M. F., Pike, J. E., Hinman, J. W. and Muirhead, E. E. (1966). Vasodepressor and antihypertensive prostaglandins of PGE type with emphasis on the identification of medullin as PGE_2-217. *J. Clin. Invest.*, **45**, 1036

Lee, J. B., McGiff, J. C., Kannegiesser, H., Mudd, J. G., Aykent, Y. and Frawley, T. F. (1969). Antihypertensive and natriuretic activity of prostaglandin A_1 in human hypertension. *Clin. Res.*, **17**, 456

Lee, J., Kannegiesser, H., O'Toole, J. and Westura, E. (1971). Hypertension and the renomedullary prostaglandins: Human study of the antihypertensive effects of PGA_1. *Ann. N.Y. Acad. Sci.*, **180**, 218

Lee, S. C. and Levine, L. (1974a). Prostaglandin metabolism: I. Cytoplasmic reduced NADPH-dependent and microsomal reduced NADH-dependent PGE 9-keto reductase activities in monkey and pigeon tissues. *J. Biol. Chem.*, **249**, 1369

Lee, S. C. and Levine, L. (1974b). Purification and properties of chicken heart prostaglandin Δ^{13}-reductase. *Biochem. Biophys. Res. Commun.*, **61**, 14

Lee, S. C., Pong, S. S., Katzen, D., Wu, K. Y. and Levine, L. (1975). Distribution of prostaglandin E 9-ketoreductase and types I and II 15-hydroxyprostaglandin dehydrogenase in swine kidney medulla and cortex. *Biochemistry*, **14**, 142

Leslie, C. A. and Levine, L. (1973). Evidence for the presence of a prostaglandin E_2-9-keto reductase in rat organs. *Biochem. Biophys. Res. Commun.*, **52**, 717

Levey, G. S. and Epstein, S. E. (1969a). Myocardial adenyl cyclase: activation by thyroid hormones and evidence for two adenyl cyclase systems. *J. Clin. Invest.*, **48**, 1663

Levey, G. S. and Epstein, S. E. (1969b). Activation of adenyl cyclase by glucagon in cat and human heart. *Circulation Res.*, **24**, 151

Levy, J. V. (1973a). Chronotropic and inotropic effects of PGE_2 on isolated rat atria from normal and spontaneously hypertensive rats (SHR). *Prostaglandins*, **4**, 731

Levy, J. V. (1973b). Papaverine antagonism of prostaglandin E_2-induced contraction of rabbit aortic strips. *Res. Commun. Chem. Pathol. Pharmacol.*, **5**, 297

Levy, J. V. (1973c). Studies on the contractile effects of prostaglandins on aortic preparations from spontaneously hypertensive rats. *Res. Commun. Chem. Path. Pharmac.*, **6**, 365

Levy, J. V. (1974). Differences in papaverine inhibition of prostaglandin-induced contraction of aortic strips from normal and spontaneously hypertensive rats (SHR). *Eur. J. Pharmac.*, **25**, 117

Levy, J. V. and Killebrew, E. (1971). Inotropic effects of prostaglandin E_2 on isolated cardiac tissue. *Proc. Soc. Exp. Biol. Med.*, **136**, 1227

Levy, B. and Lindner, H. R. (1971). Selective blockade of the vasodepressor response to prostaglandin $F_{2\alpha}$ in the anaesthetized rabbit. *Br. J. Pharmac.*, **43**, 236

Lewis, A. J. and Eyre, P. (1972). Some cardiovascular and respiratory effects of prostaglandin E_1, E_2 and $F_{2\alpha}$ in the calf. *Prostaglandins*, **2**, 55

Limas, C. J. and Cohn, J. N. (1973). Isolation and properties of myocardial and prostaglandin synthetase. *Cardiovasc. Res.*, **7**, 623

Lonigro, A. J., Terragno, N. A., Malik, K. U. and McGiff, J. C. (1973). Differential inhibition by prostaglandins of the renal actions of pressor stimuli. *Prostaglandins*, **3**, 595

Main, I. H. M. and Whittle, B. J. R. (1973a). The effects of E and A prostaglandins on gastric mucosal blood flow and acid secretion in the rat. *Br. J. Pharmac.*, **49**, 428

Main, I. H. M. and Whittle, B. J. R. (1973b). Effects of indomethacin on rat gastric acid secretion and mucosal blood flow. *Br. J. Pharmac.*, **47**, 666P

Malik, K. U. and McGiff, J. C. (1972). Effects of ganglionic blocking agents on adrenergic transmission in rat mesenteric arteries. *Am. J. Physiol.*, **223**, 1210

Malik, K. U. and McGiff, J. C. (1974). Relationship of glucose metabolism to adrenergic transmission in rat mesenteric arteries. Effect of glucose deprivation, glucose metabolites and changes in ionic composition on adrenergic mechanisms. *Circulation Res.*, **35**, 553

Malik, K. U. and McGiff, J. C. (1975). Modulation by prostaglandins of adrenergic transmission in isolated perfused rabbit and rat kidneys. *Circulation Res.* (accepted for publication)

Mandel, L. R. and Kuehl, F. A. Jr. (1967). Lipolytic action of 3, 3′5-tri-iodo *l*-thyronine, a cyclic AMP phosphodiesterase inhibitor. *Biochem. Biophys. Res. Commun.*, **28**, 13

Mantegazza, P. (1965). La prostaglandin E_1 come sostanza sensibilizzatrice per il calcio a livello del cuore isolato di cavia. *Atti. Accad. Med. Lomb.*, **20**, 66

Mantegazza, P. and Naimzada, M. K. (1965). Attivita della prostaglandin E_1 sul preparato nervo ipogastrico-deferente di varie specie animali. *Atti. Accad. Med. Lomb.*, **20**, 58

Mark, A. L., Schmid, P. G., Eckstein, J. W. and Wendling, M. G. (1971). Venous responses to prostaglandin $F_{2\alpha}$. *Am. J. Physiol.*, **220**, 222

Mathé, A. A., Strandberg, K. and Fredholm, B. (1972). Antagonism of prostaglandin $F_{2\alpha}$-induced bronchoconstriction and blood pressure changes by polyphloretin phosphate in the guinea-pig and cat. *J. Pharm. Pharmacol.*, **24**, 378

Maxwell, G. M. (1967). The effect of prostaglandin E_1 upon the general and coronary haemodynamics and metabolism of the intact dog. *Br. J. Pharmac.*, **31**, 162

Maxwell, G. M. (1969). The effect of prostaglandin $F_{2\alpha}$ upon coronary venous flow and myocardial metabolism. *Austr. J. Exp. Biol. Med. Sci.*, **47**, 713

Mayer, H. E., Abboud, F. M., Schmid, P. G. and Mark, A. L. (1970). Release of norepinephrine by prostaglandin E_1. *Clin. Res.*, **18**, 594

McGiff, J. C., Crowshaw, K. and Itskovitz, H. D. (1974). Prostaglandins and renal function. *Fed. Proc.*, **33**, 39

McGiff, J. C., Crowshaw, K., Terragno, N. A. and Lonigro, A. J. (1970). Release of a prostaglandin-like substance into renal venous blood in response to angiotensin II. *Circulation Res.*, **27, Suppl. I**, 121

McGiff, J. C., Crowshaw, K., Terragno, N. A., Lonigro, A. J., Strand, J. C., Williamson, M. A., Lee, J. B. and Ng, K. K. F. (1970). Prostaglandin-like substances appearing in canine renal venous blood during renal ischemia. Their partial characterization by pharmacologic and chromatographic procedures. *Circulation Res.*, **27**, 765

McGiff, J. C., Crowshaw, K., Terragno, N. A., Malik, K. U. and Lonigro, A. J. (1972). Differential effect of noradrenaline and renal nerve stimulation on vascular resistance in the dog kidney and the release of a prostaglandin E-like substance. *Clin. Sci.*, **42**, 223

McGiff, J. C. and Itskovitz, H. D. (1973). Prostaglandins and the kidney. *Circulation Res.*, **33**, 479

McGiff, J. C., Terragno, N. A., Malik, K. U. and Lonigro, A. J. (1972). Release of a prostaglandin E-like substance from canine kidney by bradykinin. *Circulation Res.*, **31**, 36

McGiff, J. C., Terragno, N. A., Strand, J. C., Lee, J. B., Lonigro, A. J. and Ng, K. K. F. (1969). Selective passage of prostaglandins across the lung. *Nature (Lond.)*, **223**, 742

McQueen, D. S. (1973). The effects of prostaglandin E_2, prostaglandin $F_{2\alpha}$ and polyphloretin phosphate on respiration and blood pressure in anaesthetized guinea-pigs. *Life Sci. (Part I)*, **12**, 163

Messina, E. J., Weiner, R. and Kaley, G. (1974). Microcirculatory effects of prostaglandins E_1, E_2 and A_1 in the rat mesentery and cremaster muscle. *Microvasc. Res.*, **8**, 77

Mest, H. J., Schrör, K. and Förster, W. (1973). Anti-arrhythmic properties of PGE_2: preliminary results. *Adv. Biosci.*, **9**, 385

Metcalfe, J., Romney, S. L., Swartout, J. R., Pitcairn, D. M., Lethin, A. N. Jr. and Barron, D. H. (1959). Uterine blood flow and oxygen consumption in pregnant sheep and goats. *Am. J. Physiol.*, **197**, 929

Murad, F., Chi, Y. M., Rall, T. W. and Sutherland, E. W. (1962). Adenyl cyclase. III. Effect of catecholamines and choline esters on the formation of adenosine 3'5'-phosphate by preparations from cardiac muscle and liver. *J. Biol. Chem.*, **237**, 1233

Murphy, G. P., Hesse, V. E., Evers, J. L., Hobika, G., Mostert, J. W., Szolnoky, A., Schoonees, R., Abramczyk, J. and Grace, J. T. Jr. (1970). The renal and cardiodynamic effects of prostaglandins (PGE_1, PGA_1) in renal ischemia. *J. Surg. Res.*, **10**, 533

Nagasawa, M., Chan, J. A. and Sih, C. J. (1974). Prostaglandin-sepharose: Application to the purification of bovine lung 15 (S) hydroxyprostaglandin dehydrogenase. *Prostaglandins*, **8**, 221

Nakano, J. (1964). Studies on the cardiovascular effects of synthetic eledoişin. *J. Pharmac. exp. Ther.*, **145**, 71

Nakano, J. (1965a). Effects of eledoisin on the systemic venous return. *Proc. Soc. Exp. Biol. Med.*, **118**, 108

Nakano, J. (1965b). Effect of synthetic bradykinin on the cardiovascular system. *Archs. int. Pharmacodyn. Ther.*, **157**, 1

Nakano, J. (1968a). Effects of prostaglandin E_1, A_1 and $F_{2\alpha}$ on the coronary and peripheral circulations. *Proc. Soc. Exp. Biol. Med.*, **127**, 1160

Nakano, J. (1968b). Effect of prostaglandins E_1, A_1 and $F_{2\alpha}$ on cardiovascular dynamics in dogs. In *Prostaglandin Symposium of the Worcester Foundation for Exp. Biol.*, Ramwell, P. W. and Shaw, J. E. (eds.), pp. 201–214 (New York: Interscience)

Nakano, J. (1969). Cardiovascular effect of a prostaglandin isolated from a gorgonian *Plexaura homomalla*. *J. Pharm. Pharmacol.*, **21**, 782

Nakano, J. (1971). Effects of the metabolites of prostaglandin E_1 on the systemic and peripheral circulation in dogs. *Proc. Soc. Exp. Biol. Med.*, **136**, 1265

Nakano, J. (1973). Cardiovascular actions. In *The Prostaglandins*, Ramwell, **P. W.** (ed.), pp. 238–316 (New York: Plenum Press)

Nakano, J., Änggård, E. and Samuelsson, B. (1969). 15-Hydroxy-prostanoate dehydrogenase. Prostaglandins as substrates and inhibitors. *Eur. J. Biochem.*, **II**, 386

Nakano, J., Chang, A. C. K. and Fisher, R. G. (1973). Effects of prostaglandins E_1, E_2, A_1, A_2 and $F_{2\alpha}$ on canine carotid arterial blood flow, cerebrospinal fluid pressure, and intraocular pressure. *J. Neurosurg.*, **38**, 32

Nakano, J. and Cole, B. (1969). Effects of prostaglandins E_1 and $F_{2\alpha}$ on systemic, pulmonary and splanchnic circulation in dogs. *Am. J. Physiol.*, **217**, 222

Nakano, J. and Kessinger, J. M. (1970). Effects of 8-isoprostaglandin E_1 on the systemic and pulmonary circulation in dogs. *Proc. Soc. Exp. Biol. Med*, **133**, 1314

Nakano, J , McCloy, R B. and Prancan, A. V. (1973). Circulatory and pulmonary airway responses to different mixtures of prostaglandins E_2 and $F_{2\alpha}$ in dogs. *Eur. J. Pharmacol.*, **24**, 61

Nakano, J. and McCurdy, J. R. (1967). Cardiovascular effects of prostaglandin E_1. *J. Pharmac. exp. Ther.*, **156**, 538

Nakano, J. and McCurdy, J. R. (1968). Hemodynamic effects of prostaglandin E_1, A_1 and $F_{2\alpha}$ in dog. *Proc. Soc. Exp. Biol. Med.*, **128**, 39

Nakano, J. and Prancan, A. V. (1971). Metabolic degradation of prostaglandin E_1 in the rat plasma and rat brain, heart, lung, kidney and testicle homogenates. *J. Pharm. Pharmac.*, **23**, 231

Nakano, J., Prancan, A. V. and Kessinger, J. M. (1971). Effect of prostaglandin E_1 and A_1 on the gastric circulation in dogs. *Clin. Res.*, **19**, 399

Needleman, P., Douglas, J. R. Jr., Jakschik, B., Stoexklein, P. B. and Johnson, E. M. Jr. (1974). Release of renal prostaglandin by catecholamines: relationship to renal endocrine function. *J. Pharmac. exp. Ther.*, **188**, 453

Needleman, P., Kauffman, A. H., Douglas, J. R. Jr., Johnson, E. M., Jr. and Marshall, G. R. (1973). Specific stimulation and inhibition of renal prostaglandin release by angiotensin analogs. *Am. J. Physiol.*, **224**, 1415

Needleman, P., Minkes, M. S. and Douglas, J. R. Jr. (1974). Stimulation of prostaglandin biosynthesis by adenine nucleotides. *Circulation Res.*, **34**, 455

Nutter, D. O. and Crumly, H. (1970). Coronary-myocardial responses to prostaglandins E_1 and A_1. *Circulation, Suppl. III*, **42**, 124

Nutter, D. O. and Crumly, H. R. Jr. (1972). Canine coronary vascular and cardiac responses to the prostaglandins. *Cardiovasc. Res.*, **6**, 217

Okada, F., Nukada, T., Yamauchi, Y. and Abe, H. (1974). The hypotensive effect of prostaglandin E_1 on hypertensive cases of various types. *Prostaglandins*, **7**, 99

Okpako, D. T. (1972). The actions of histamine and prostaglandins $F_{2\alpha}$ and E_2 on pulmonary vascular resistance of the lung of the guinea-pig. *J. Pharm. Pharmac.*, **24**, 40

Page, E. W. (1947). Relation of the fetus and placenta to the decline of hypertension. *Am. J. Obstet. Gynec.*, **53**, 275

Papanicolaou, N., Makrakis, S., Bariety, J. and Milliez, P. (1974). Prostaglandins in rat tissues. *J. Pharm. Pharmac.*, **26**, 270

Park, M. K., Dyer, D. C. and Vincenzi, F. F. (1973). Prostaglandin E_2 and its antagonists: Effects on autonomic transmission in the isolated sino-atrial node. *Prostaglandins*, **4**, 717

Park, M. K., Rishor, C. and Dyer, D. C. (1972). Vasoactive actions of prostaglandins and serotonin on isolated human umbilical arteries and veins. *Can. J. Physiol. Pharmacol.*, **50**, 393

Pelofsky, S., Jacobson, E. D., and Fisher, R. G. (1972). Effects of prostaglandin E_1 on experimental cerebral vasospasm. *J. Neurosurg.*, **36**, 634

Pennink, M., White, R. P., Crockarell, J R and Robertson, J. T. (1972). Role of prostaglandin $F_{2\alpha}$ in the genesis of experimental cerebral vasospasm. Angiographic study in dogs. *J. Neurosurg.*, **37**, 398

Peskar, B. and Hertting, G. (1973). Release of prostaglandins from isolated cat spleen by angiotensin and vasopressin. *Naunyn-Schmiedeberg's Arch. Pharmacol.*, **279**, 227

Pharriss, B. B., Cornette, J. C. and Gutknecht, G. D. (1970). Vascular control of luteal steroidogenesis. *J. Reprod. Fert. (Suppl 10)*, 97

Piccinini, F., Pomarelli, P. and Chiarra, A. (1969). Further investigations on the mechanism of the inotropic action of prostaglandin E_1 in relation to the ion balance in the frog heart. *Pharmacol. Res. Commun.*, **1**, 381

Pickard, J. D. (1973). The mechanism of action of prostaglandin $F_{2\alpha}$ on cerebral blood flow in the baboon. *J. Physiol. (Lond.)*, **234**, 46P

Pike, J. E., Kupiecki, F. P. and Weeks, J. R. (1967). Biological activity of the prostaglandins and related analogs. In *Prostaglandins, Nobel Symposium 2*, Bergström, S., and Samuelsson, B. (eds.), pp. 161–171 (Stockholm: Almqvist and Wiksell)

Pöch, G. and Kukovetz, W. (1972). Studies on the possible role of cyclic AMP in drug induced coronary vasodilation. In *Advances in Cyclic Nucleotide Research, Vol. 1*, Greenyard, R., Paoletti, R. and Robison, G. (eds.), pp. 195–211 (New York: Raven Press)

Powell, J. R. and Brody, M. J. (1973). Peripheral facilitation of reflex vasoconstriction by prostaglandin $F_{2\alpha}$. *J. Pharmac. exp. Ther.*, **187**, 495

Ramwell, P. W. and Shaw, J. E. (1966). Spontaneous and evoked release of prostaglandins from the cortex of anesthetized cats. *Am. J. Physiol.*, **211**, 125

Ramwell, P. W. and Shaw, J. E. (1970). Biological significance of the prostaglandins. *Recent Prog. Horm. Res.*, **26**, 139

Roberts, J., Ito, R., Reilly, J. and Cairoli, V. (1963). Influence of reserpine and βTM 10 on digitalis-induced ventricular arrhythmia. *Circulation Res.*, **13**, 149

Robinson, B. F., Collier, J. G., Karim, S. M. M. and Somers, K. (1973). Effect of prostaglandins A_1, A_2, B_1, E_2 and $F_{2\alpha}$ on forearm arterial bed and superficial hand veins in man. *Clin. Sci.*, **44**, 367

Robison, G. A., Butcher, R. and Sutherland, E. W. (1971). Cyclic AMP and the function of eukaryotic cells: an introduction. *Ann. N.Y. Acad. Sci.*, **185**, 5

Roth-Brandel, U., Bygdeman, M., Wiqvist, N. and Bergström, S. (1970). Prostaglandins for induction of therapeutic abortion. *Lancet*, **i**, 190

Rowe, G. G. and Afonso, S. (1974). Systemic and coronary hemodynamic effects of intracoronary administration of prostaglandin E_1 and E_2. *Am. Heart. J.*, **88**, 51

Rubin, R. P. (1970). The role of calcium in the release of neurotransmitter substances and hormones. *Pharmac. Rev.*, **22**, 389

Ryan, M. J. and Zimmerman, B. G. (1974). Effect of prostaglandin precursors, dihomo-gamma-linolenic acid and arachidonic acid on the vasoconstrictor response to nore-pinephrine in the dog paw. *Prostaglandins*, **6**, 179

Sabatini-Smith, S. (1970). Action of prostaglandins E_1 and $F_{2\alpha}$ on calcium (Ca) flux in the isolated guinea-pig atria and fragmented cardiac sarcoplasmic reticulum. *Pharmacologist*, **12**, 239

Said, S. I. (1968). Some respiratory effects of prostaglandins E_2 and $F_{2\alpha}$. In *Prostaglandin Symposium of Worcester Foundation for Experimental Biology*, Ramwell, P. W. and Shaw, J. E. (eds.), pp. 267–277 (New York: Interscience)

Samuelsson, B. (1970). Biosynthesis and metabolism of prostaglandins. *Proc. 4th Internat. Congr. Pharmacol.*, **4**, 12

Samuelsson, B. (1972). Biosynthesis of prostaglandins. *Fed. Proc. Fedn. Am. Soc. Exp. Biol.*, **31**, 1442

Samuelsson, B., Granström, E., Gréen, K. and Hamberg, M. (1971). Metabolism of prostaglandins. *Ann. N.Y. Acad. Sci.*, **180**, 138

Samuelsson, B., Granström, E. and Hamberg, M. (1967). On the mechanism of the bio-synthesis of prostaglandins. In *Prostaglandins, Proceedings of the Second Nobel Sympo-sium, Stockholm, 1966*. Bergström, S. and Samuelsson, B. (eds.), pp. 31–44 (Stockholm: Almqvist and Wiksell)

Samuelsson, B. and Wennmalm, Å. (1971). Increased nerve stimulation induced release of noradrenaline from the rabbit heart after inhibition of prostaglandin synthesis. *Acta Physiol. Scand.*, **83**, 163

Saunders, R. N. and Moser, C. A. (1972a). Changes in vascular resistance induced by prostaglandins E_2 and $F_{2\alpha}$ in the isolated rat pancreas. *Archs. int. Pharmacodyn. Ther.*, **197**, 86

Saunders, R. N. and Moser, C. A. (1972b). Increased vascular resistance by prostaglandins B_1 and B_2 in the isolated rat pancreas. *Nature New Biology*, **237**, 285

Schlegel, W., Demers, L. M., Hildebrandt-Stark, H. E., Behrman, H. R. and Greep, R. O. (1974). Partial purification of human placental 15-hydroxy-prostaglandin dehydrogenase kinetic properties. *Prostaglandins*, **5**, 417

Sen, A. K., Sunahara, F. A. and Talesnik, J. (1972). Cyclic AMP and metabolically-induced coronary vasodilation in the isolated perfused rat heart. *Abstr. Fifth Int. Congr. Pharmacol.*, No. 208 (San Francisco)

Shalit, M. N., Shimojyo, S., Reinmuth, O. M., Lockhart, N. S. Jr. and Scheinberg, P.

(1968). The mechanism of action of carbon dioxide in the regulation of cerebral blood flow. In *Progress in Brain Research, Vol. 30*, Luyendyk, W. (ed.), pp. 103–106 (New York: Elsevier Publ. Co.)

Shehadeh, Z., Price, W. E. and Jacobson, E. D. (1969). Effects of vasoactive agents on intestinal blood flow and motility in the dog. *Am. J. Physiol.*, **216**, 386

Simpson, L. L. (1974). The effect of prostaglandin E_2 on the rterial blood pressure of normotensive and spontaneously hypertensive rats. *Br. J. Pharmac.*, **51**, 559

Skovsted, P., Price, M. L. and Price, H. L. (1969). The effects of halothane on arterial pressure, preganglionic sympathetic activity and barostatic reflexes. *Anesthesiology*, **31**, 507

Slotkoff, L. M. (1974). Prostaglandin A_1 in hypertensive crisis. *Ann. N. Y. Acad. Sci.*, **81**, 345

Smith, E. R., McMorrow, J. V. Jr., Covino, B. G. and Lee, J. B. (1968). Studies on the vasodilator actions of prostaglandin E_1. In *Prostaglandins, Symposium of Worcester Foundation for Exp. Biol.*, Ramwell, P. W. and Shaw, J. E. (eds.), pp. 259–266 (New York: Interscience)

Sobel, B. E. and Robison, A. K. (1969). Activation of guinea-pig myocardial adenyl cyclase by prostaglandins. *Circulation*, **40, Suppl. III**, 189

Solomon, L. M., Juhlin, L. and Kirschenbaum, M. B. (1968). Prostaglandin on cutaneous vasculature. *J. Invest. Dermat.*, **51**, 280

Somlyo, A. V. and Somlyo, A. P. (1968a), Electromechanical and pharmacomechanical coupling in vascular smooth muscle. *J. Pharmac. exp. Ther.*, **159**, 129

Somlyo, A. P. and Somlyo, A. V. (1968b). Vascular smooth muscle. I. Normal structure, pathology, biochemistry, and biophysics. *Pharmac. Rev.*, **20**, 197

Somova, L. (1972). Effect of prostaglandin E_1 and E_2 on the vascular responsiveness to adrenaline, noradrenaline, angiotensin and vasopressin. *Cor. Vasa.*, **14**, 213

Somova, L. I. and Dochev, D. (1971). The effect of prostaglandins (PGE_1, PGE_2, PGA_1 and PGA_2) on the electrolyte balance in animals with experimental hypertension. *C. R. Acad. Bulg. Sci.*, **24**, 1275

Sperelakis, N. and Lehmkuhl, D. (1965). Insensitivity of cultured chick heart cells to autonomic agents and tetrodotoxin. *Am. J. Physiol.*, **209**, 693

Steinberg, D. and Pittman, R. (1966). Depression of plasma FFA levels in unanesthetized dogs by single intravenous doses of prostaglandin E_1. *Proc. Soc. Exp. Biol. Med.*, **123**, 192

Steinberg, D., Vaughan, M., Nestel, P. J. and Bergström, S. (1963). Effects of prostaglandin E opposing those of catecholamines on blood pressure and on triglyceride breakdown in adipose tissue. *Biochem. Pharm. Pharmacol.*, **12**, 764

Steinberg, D., Vaughan, M., Nestel, P. J., Strand, O. and Bergström, S. (1964). Effects of prostaglandin on hormone-induced mobilization of free fatty acids. *J. Clin. Invest.*, **43**, 1533

Steiner, L., Forster, D. M. C., Bergvall, U. and Carlson, L. A. (1972). Effect of prostaglandin E_1 on cerebral circulatory disturbances. *Eur. Neurol. (Part II)*, **8**, 23

Stjärne, L. (1973). Prostaglandin versus alpha-adrenoceptor-mediated control of sympathetic neurotransmitter secretion in guinea-pig isolated vas deferens. *Eur. J. Pharmacol.*, **22**, 233

Stjärne, L. and Gripe, K. (1973). Prostaglandin-dependent and independent feedback control of noradrenaline secretion in vasoconstrictor nerves of normotensive human subjects. *Naunyn-Schmiedeberg's Arch. Pharmacol.*, **280**, 441

Strand, J. C., Miller, M. P. and McGiff, J. C. (1974), Biological activity of the methyl esters of prostaglandin E_2 and its (15S)-15-methyl analogue. *Eur. J. Pharmacol.*, **26**, 151

Strong, C. G. and Bohr, D. F. (1967). Effects of prostaglandins E_1, E_2, A_1 and $F_{1\alpha}$ on isolated vascular smooth muscle. *Am. J. Physiol.*, **213**, 725

Strong, C. G. and Chandler, J. T. (1972). Interactions of prostaglandin E_1 and catecholamines in isolated vascular smooth muscle. In *Prostaglandins in Cellular Biology*, Ramwell, P. W., and Pharriss, B. B. (eds.), pp. 369–383 (New York and London: Plenum Press)

Su, J. Y., Higgins, C. B. and Friedman, W. F. (1973). Chronotropic and inotropic effects of prostaglandins E_1, A_1 and $F_{2\alpha}$ on isolated mammalian cardiac tissue. *Proc. Soc. Exp. Biol. Med.*, **143**, 1227

Sunahara, F. A. and Kadar, D. (1968). Effects of ouabain on the interaction of autonomic drugs and prostaglandins on isolated vascular tissue. In *Prostaglandin Symposium of the Worcester Foundation for Experimental Biology*, Ramwell, P. W. and Shaw, J E. (eds.), pp. 247–257 (New York: Interscience)

Sunahara, F. A. and Talesnik, J. (1974). Prostaglandin inhibition of metabolically induced coronary vasodilation. *J. Pharmac. exp. Ther.*, **188**, 135

Sunahara, F. A., Talesnik, J. and Sen, A. K. (1972). Effects of prostaglandin and diazoxide on coronary circulation of norepinephrine and calcium stimulated heart. *Proc. Fifth Int. Congr. Pharmacol.*, Abs. No. 1350, p. 225 (San Francisco)

Suzuki, T., Abiko, Y. and Funaki, T. (1969). Effects of prostaglandin E_1 on the cardiovascular system in dogs. *Folia. Pharmacol.*, *Jap.*, **65**, 1

Sweet, C. S., Kadowitz, P. J. and Brody, M. J. (1971). A hypertensive response to infusion of prostaglandin $F_{2\alpha}$ into the vertebral artery of the conscious dog. *Eur. J. Pharmacol.*, **16**, 229

Sweet, C. S., Kadowitz, P. J., Forker, E. L. and Brody, M. J. (1972). Depression of adrenergic transmission by a factor in renal venous blood: New evidence for an antihypertensive function of the kidney. *Archs. int. Pharmacodyn. Ther.*, **198**, 229

Talesnik, J. and Sunahara, F. A. (1973). Enhancement of metabolic coronary dilatation by aspirin-like substances by suppression of prostaglandin feedback control. *Nature (Lond.)*, **244**, 351

Talledo, O. E., Chesley, L. C. and Zuspan, F. P. (1968). Renin–angiotensin system in normal and toxemic pregnancies. Differential sensitivity to angiotensin II and toxemia of pregnancy. *Am. J. Obstet. Gynecol.*, **100**, 218

Tanz, R. D. (1974). Mechanism of aconitine-induced tachycardia and the antiarrhythmic activity of certain prostaglandins. *Proc. West. Pharmacol. Soc.*, **17**, 22

Terragno, D. A., Crowshaw, K., Terragno, N. A. and McGiff, J. C. (1975). Prostaglandin synthesis by bovine mesenteric arteries and veins. *Circulation Res. Suppl.* (accepted for publication)

Terragno, N. A., Terragno D. A. and McGiff, J. C. (1974). Prostaglandin E–angiotensin II interactions in the gravid uterus. *Acta Physiol. Latinoamer.* (accepted for publication)

Terragno, N. A., Terragno, D. A., Pacholczyk, D. and McGiff, J. C. (1974). Prostaglandins and the regulation of uterine blood flow in pregnancy. *Nature (Lond.)*, **249**, 57

Thompson, J. H. and Angulo, M. (1968). The effect of prostaglandins on gastrointestinal serotonin in the rat. *Eur. J. Pharmacol.*, **4**, 224

Thompson, J. H. and Angulo, M. (1969). Prostaglandin-induced serotonin release. *Experientia*, **25**, 721

Tobian, L. and Viets, J. (1970). Potentiation of *in vitro* norepinephrine vasoconstriction with prostaglandin E_1. *Fed. Proc.*, **29**, 387

Torre, E. L., Patrono, C., Fortuna, A. and Grossi-Belloni, D. (1974). Role of prostaglandin F_2 in human cerebral vasospasm. *J. Neurosurg.*, **41**, 293

Türker, R. K., Kaymakcalan, S. and Ayhan, I. H. (1968). Effect of prostaglandin E_1 (PGE_1) on the vascular responsiveness to norepinephrine and angiotensin in the anesthetized rat. *Arzneim. Forsch.*, **18**, 1310

Türker, R. K., Kiran, B. K. and Vural, H. (1971). Dual effects of prostaglandin E_1 on the cat isolated papillary muscle. *Arzneim. Forsch.*, **21**, 989

Tuttle, R. S. and Skelly, M. M. (1968). Interaction of prostaglandin E_1 and ouabain on contractility of isolated rabbit atria and intracellular cation concentration. In *Prostaglandin Symposium of the Worcester Foundation for Experimental Biology*, Ramwell, P. W. and Shaw, J. E. (eds.), pp. 309–320 (New York: Interscience)

Ulano, H. B., Treat, E., Shanbour, L. L. and Jacobson, E. D. (1972). Selective dilation of the constricted superior mesenteric artery. *Gastroenterology*, **62**, 39

Vane, J. R. (1971). Inhibition of prostaglandin synthesis as a mechanism of action of aspirin-like drugs. *Nature New Biology*, **231**, 232

Vatner, S. F., Franklin, D. and Braunwald, E. (1971). Effects of anesthesia and sleep on circulatory response to carotid sinus nerve stimulation. *Am. J. Physiol.*, **220**, 1249

Venuto, R., O'Dorisio, T., Stein, J. H. and Ferris, T. F. (1975). Uterine prostaglandin E (PGE) secretion and uterine blood flow in the pregnant rabbit. *J. Clin. Invest.*, **55**, 193

Vergroesen, A. J. and de Boer, J. (1968). Effects of prostaglandins E_1 and $F_{1\alpha}$ on isolated frog and rat hearts in relation to the potassium–calcium ratio of the perfusion fluid. *Eur. J. Pharmacol.*, **3**, 171

Vergroesen, A. J., de Boer, J. and Gottenbos, J. J. (1967). Effects of prostaglandins on perfused isolated rat hearts. In *Prostaglandins, Nobel Symposium 2*, Bergström, S. and Samuelsson, B. (eds.), pp. 211–218 (Stockholm: Almqvist and Wiksell)

Viguera, M. G. and Sunahara, F. A. (1969). Microcirculatory effects of prostaglandins. *Can. J. Physiol. Pharmac.*, **47**, 627

Villanueva, R., Hinds, L., Katz, R. L. and Eakins, K. E. (1972). The effect of polyphloretin phosphate on some smooth muscle actions of prostaglandins in the cat. *J. Pharmac. exp. Ther.*, **180**, 78

Wagner, S. L., Terragno, N. A., Terragno, D. A. and McGiff, J. C. (1974). Modulation of prostaglandin synthesis by an NADPH dependent enzyme in rabbit kidney. *Clin. Res.*, **22**, 627a

Weeks, J. R. (1969). The prostaglandins: Biologically active lipids with implications in circulatory physiology. *Circulation Res.*, **24**, Suppl. *I*, 123

Weeks, J. R. (1972). Prostaglandins. *Ann. Rev. Pharmacol.*, **12**, 317

Weeks, J. R., DuCharme, D. W., Magee, W. E. and Miller, W. L. (1973). The biological activity of the (15S)-15-methyl analogs of prostaglandins E_2 and $F_{2\alpha}$. *J. Pharmac. exp. Ther.*, **186**, 67

Weeks, J. R., Sekhar, N. C. and DuCharme, D. W. (1969). Relative activity of prostaglandins E_1, A_1, E_2 and A_2 on lipolysis, platelet aggregation, smooth muscle and the cardiovascular system. *J. Pharm. Pharmac.*, **21**, 103

Weeks, J. R. and Wingerson, F. (1964). Cardiovascular action of prostaglandin E_1 evaluated using unanesthetized relatively unrestrained rats. *Proc. Fed. Am. Soc. Exptl. Biol.*, **23**, 327

Weiner, R. and Kaley, G. (1969). Influence of prostaglandin E_1 on the terminal vascular bed. *Am. J. Physiol.*, **217**, 563

Welch, K. M. A., Knowles, L. and Spira, P. (1974). Local effect of prostaglandins on cat pial arteries *Eur. J. Pharmacol.*, **25**, 155

Welch, K. M. A., Spira, P. J., Knowles, L. and Lance, J. W. (1974). Effects of prostaglandins on the internal and external carotid blood flow in the monkey. *Neurolog.*, **24**, 705

Wendling, M. G. and DuCharme, D. W. (1974). Effects of chronic administration of prostaglandin E_1 (PGE_1) on arterial blood pressure of unanesthetized hypertensive rats. *Prostaglandins*, **7**, 71

Wendt, R. L. and Baum, T. (1972). Aerosol administration of prostaglandins E_1 and E_2 and isoproterenol: Studies on the cardiovascular system. *Eur. J. Pharmacol.*, **17**, 141

Wennmalm, Å. (1971). Studies on mechanisms controlling the secretion of neurotransmitters in the rabbit heart. *Acta Physiol. Scand.*, **83**, Suppl. 365, 1

Wennmalm, Å. and Hedqvist, P. (1970). Prostaglandin E_1 as inhibitor of the sympathetic neuroeffector system in the rabbit heart. *Life Sci. (Part I)*, **9**, 931

Wennmalm, Å. and Hedqvist, P. (1971). Inhibition by prostaglandin E_1 of parasympathetic neurotransmission in the rabbit heart. *Life Sci. (Part I)*, **10**, 465

Wennmalm, Å. and Stjärne, L. (1971). Inhibition of the release of adrenergic transmitter by a fatty acid in the perfusate from sympathetically stimulated rabbit heart. *Life Sci. (Part I)*, **10**, 471

Westura, E. E., Kannegiesser, H., O'Toole, J. D. and Lee, J. B. (1970). Antihypertensive effects of prostaglandin A_1 in essential hypertension. *Circulation Res. (Suppl. I)*, **27**, 131

White, R. P., Heaton, J. A. and Denton, I. C. (1971). Pharmacological comparison of prostaglandin $F_{2\alpha}$, serotonin and norepinephrine on cerebrovascular tone of monkey. *Eur. J. Pharmacol.*, **15**, 300

White, R. P. and Pennink, M. (1972). Reversal of the pressor response of prostaglandin $F_{2\alpha}$ by polyphloretin phosphate in dogs. *Archs. int. Pharmacodyn. Ther.*, **197**, 274

Willebrands, A. F. and Tasseron, S. J. A. (1968). Effect of hormones on substrate preference in isolated rat heart. *Am. J. Physiol.*, **215**, 1089

Willoughby, D. A. (1968). Effects of prostaglandins $PGF_{2\alpha}$ and PGE_1 on vascular permeability. *J. Pathol. Bacteriol.*, **96**, 381

Wilson, D. E. and Levine, R. A. (1969). Decreased canine gastric mucosal blood flow induced by prostaglandin E_1. A mechanism for its inhibitory effect on gastric secretion. *Gastroenterology*, **56**, 1268

Wilson, D. E. and Levine, R. A. (1972). The effect of prostaglandin E_1 on canine gastric acid secretion and gastric mucosal blood flow. *Am. J. Dig. Dis.*, **17**, 527

Wong, P. Y. K., Terragno, D. A., Terragno, N. A. and McGiff, J. C. (1975). Prostaglandin 9-ketoreductase in bovine mesenteric blood vessels. The role of bradykinin and angiotensin. (In press)

Yamamoto, Y. L., Feindel, W., Wolfe, L. S., Katoh, H. and Hodge, C. P. (1971–72). Effects of prostaglandins on cerebral blood flow. *Eur. Neurology*, **6**, 144

Yamamoto, Y. L., Feindel, W., Wolfe, L. S., Katoh, H. and Hodge, C. P. (1972). Experimental vasoconstriction of cerebral arteries by prostaglandins. *J. Neurosurg.*, **37** 385

Zijlstra, W. G., Brunsting, J. R., Ten Hoor, F. and Vergroesen, A. J. (1972). Prostaglandin E_1 and cardiac arrhythmia. *Eur. J. Pharmacol.*, **18**, 392

Zimmerman, B. G., Ryan, M. J., Gomer, S. and Kraft, E. (1973). Effect of the prostaglandin synthesis inhibitors indomethacin and eicosa-5,8,11,14-tetraynoic acid on adrenergic esponses in dog cutaneous vasculature. *J. Pharmac. exp. Ther.*, **187**, 315

6

Renal Prostaglandins

JOHN C. McGIFF and KAFAIT U. MALIK

6.1 IDENTIFICATION, SYNTHESIS AND DEGRADATION   202
     6.1.1 IDENTIFICATION   202
     6.1.2 SYNTHESIS AND DEGRADATION   203

6.2 PROSTAGLANDINS AS TISSUE HORMONES   207

6.3 ASSAY OF PROSTAGLANDINS: THE BLOOD-BATHED ORGAN
     TECHNIQUE   211

6.4 RENAL PROSTAGLANDINS: RANGE OF ACTIVITIES   214
     6.4.1 *Modulators*   215
         6.4.1.1 Attenuation of pressor hormones   215
         6.4.1.2 Amplification   221
         6.4.1.3 Paradoxical effect of PGE_2 in the rat   223
     6.4.2 *Mediators*   225
         6.4.2.1 Kinin-induced water excretion   225
         6.4.2.2 Prostaglandins as possible mediators of renal
                 autoregulation   228
     6.4.3 *Stimulation of prostaglandin synthesis*   229

6.5 PROSTAGLANDINS AND THE RENAL CIRCULATION   231
     6.5.1 *Resting renal blood flow*   231
     6.5.2 *Distribution of renal blood flow*   233

6.6 MECHANISM OF THE BASAL OUTPUT OF RENAL PROSTAGLANDINS   237

6.7 $PGF_{2\alpha}$: A VENOUS HORMONE?   238

6.8 CLINICAL STUDIES   238
     REFERENCES   239

6.1 IDENTIFICATION, SYNTHESIS AND DEGRADATION

6.1.1 Identification

Muirhead *et al.* (1960) isolated a low-molecular weight lipid with anti-hypertensive properties from the renal medulla which inaugurated an intense search for the isolation and identification of renal vasodepressor lipids. In this study as well as in those of Lee and his associates (Lee *et al.*, 1963, 1965) the search for the mediator(s) of the antihypertensive function of the kidney provided the motivating force. Lee *et al.* (1965) isolated three prostaglandin-like compounds from rabbit renal medulla. The first lipid was not vaso-depressor and demonstrated chromatographic and biologic properties indistinguishable from prostaglandin F (PGF) compounds; the second was vasodepressor and was prostaglandin E (PGE)-like, while the third was vaso-depressor with negligible smooth muscle stimulating properties and was termed 'medullin'. The material referred to as 'medullin' by Lee was con-sidered by Strong *et al.* (1966) to be PGA_1 on the basis of its relative inac-tivity on smooth muscle when compared to its vasodepressor properties. Final clarification of 'medullin' as PGA_2 resulted from the isolation of three prostaglandins, PGE_2, $PGF_{2\alpha}$ and PGA_2 (Figure 6.1) from rabbit renal medulla in a chromatographically pure state (Lee *et al.*, 1967). Their identi-ties were established by mass spectroscopy of the free acids and their methyl esters, comparison of their biologic and chromatographic properties with standard prostaglandins and by infrared and ultraviolet spectroscopy. This work also strongly suggested that the bulk of PGA_2 isolated from renal medulla was an artifact but did not exclude the natural occurrence of PGA_2 within the renal medulla. Daniels *et al.* (1967) identified PGE_2 as the principal vasodepressor lipid in rabbit renal medulla. These workers also considered that the small amount of PGA_2 isolated was probably an artifact.

STRUCTURE	ACTIVITY ON SMOOTH MUSCLE (NONVASCULAR)	BLOOD PRESSURE	RENAL BLOOD FLOW	SODIUM EXCRETION	REMOVAL BY LUNG
PGE_2 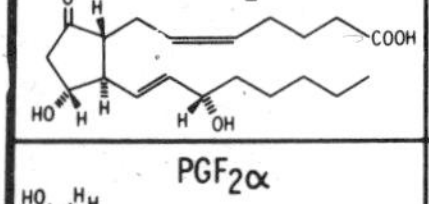	CONTRACT	↓	↑	↑	YES
$PGF_{2\alpha}$ 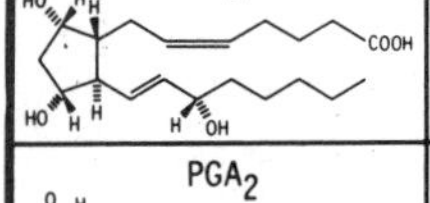	CONTRACT	↑	?	?	YES
PGA_2 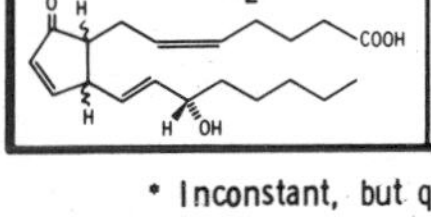	NO EFFECT*	↓	↑	↑	NO

* Inconstant, but qualitatively similar, effects to E_2 and $F_{2\alpha}$ at high doses

(>50 fold threshold dose of E_2)

Figure 6.1   Comparative biological activity of renal prostaglandins

6.1.2 Synthesis and degradation

The presence within the renal medulla of the prostaglandin-synthesizing enzyme system (prostaglandin synthetase) was demonstrated by Hamberg (1969) who added to medullary homogenates tritiated arachidonic acid, the natural precursor of PGE_2 and $PGF_{2\alpha}$. After incubation of homogenates with tritiated arachidonic acid, the bulk of the radioactivity recovered (22–47%) was identified as PGE_2, while a lower yield (5–7%) of $PGF_{2\alpha}$ was obtained. Only traces of a labelled compound, tentatively identified as PGA_2, were isolated from these homogenates.

Blackwell *et al.* (1975) have recently identified PGD_2 as a major product of the synthesizing system of a microsomal preparation obtained from rabbit renal medulla. They have shown that stimulation of prostaglandin synthesis by endogenous cofactors resulted in the production of more PGD_2 than either PGE_2 or $PGF_{2\alpha}$, suggesting that *in vivo* PGD_2 is the principal renal prostaglandin. In this study important and distinguishing characteristics of the renomedullary prostaglandin synthetase emerged when compared to those of bovine seminal vesicular synthetase. Perhaps the most important difference was the pH sensitivity of the medullary synthetase which demonstrated a very narrow optimal pH range, 7.5–7.6. Thus, a pH of less than 7.3 or more than 7.7 resulted in a reduction of its reaction velocity by about 50%, whereas the vesicular synthetase showed a wider optimal pH range, 7.8–8.2, and a relative insensitivity to changes in pH between 7.3 and 8.2. The two synthetase systems also differ in the shapes and optima of the substrate/velocity curves; arachidonic acid inhibited prostaglandin formation by vesicular but not by renal synthetases. A considerable difference in the synthetic capacity of various synthetases was also evident from this and other studies: the prostaglandin synthetase of dog spleen (Flower *et al.*, 1972) has a capacity one-tenth that of the rabbit renomedullary enzyme, which in turn has one-tenth the prostaglandin biosynthetic capacity of bovine seminal vesicles (Flower *et al.*, 1973). This study also strongly supports the proposal of Flower and Vane (1972) that prostaglandin synthetases demonstrate species- and tissue-dependent differences in their biochemical and pharmacological profiles.

Differences between prostaglandin synthetase of renal medulla and cortex may be expected and should explain the variability of results in the renal haemodynamic studies which have appeared since 1971, the year of the important discovery by Vane that aspirin inhibits prostaglandin synthetase. This finding set the haemodynamic studies in motion by providing physiologists with a tool to explore the relationship between prostaglandin synthesis and function. Thus, a differential susceptibility of medullary and cortical enzymes to stimulation by experimental procedures and to inhibition by anti-inflammatory acids appears mandatory to explain seeming discrepancies of several groups who have studied the contribution of prostaglandins to renal circulatory autoregulation.

In the study of Blackwell *et al.* (1975), it was also observed that phenylbutazone did not inhibit PGD_2 formation and that another anti-inflammatory agent, benzydamine, facilitated PGE_2 production; findings which may prove useful to those attempting to influence the end-product, after stimulation of prostaglandin synthetase by vasoactive agents. In this study, as in previous biochemical studies, the small amount of PGA_2 which was detected was considered to arise non-enzymatically. Indeed, even in the presence of NAD^+ or pyridoxal phosphate which stimulates other dehydratase enzymes, the only PGA_2 which was formed arose non-enzymatically from PGE_2.

Either absence of prostaglandin synthetase in the renal cortex or degradation of prostaglandins to inactive metabolites after synthesis in the cortex could have accounted for the failure of Crowshaw and Szylk (1970) to recover appreciable quantities of prostaglandins from the renal cortex. However, their inability to detect the major metabolites of PGE_2 and $PGF_{2\alpha}$ in extracts of pooled rabbit renal cortices, probably resulted from the absence of one or more cofactors, such as NAD^+, in the incubation medium. Larsson and Änggård (1973a) using a microsomal fraction obtained from rabbit renal medulla, reported that the capacity of the cortex to biosynthesize a tritium-labelled PGE-like material from added arachidonic acid was 10% that of the renal medulla and papilla. However, the formation of biologically active PGE_2 from endogenous precursors and added unlabelled arachidonic acid was much smaller, perhaps only 1-2% of that formed by either the medullary or the papillary enzyme preparations. None the less, this level of cortical biosynthetic activity cannot be considered trivial in view of the considerable prostaglandin biosynthetic activity of the renal medulla, surpassed only by that of seminal vesicles (Samuelsson, 1963). Further, the presence of prostaglandin synthetase in the cortex, however meagre, may have important functional implications in terms of regulation of the renal circulation, particularly autoregulation of blood flow to the kidney (Herbaczynska-Cedro and Vane, 1973). Although primary localization of prostaglandin synthetase in the renal medulla is established, zonal localization of the synthetase within the medulla is uncertain. Thus, the work of Larsson and Änggård indicated the highest concentration of PGE_2 to be in the *papilla* of the rabbit kidney, whereas, Van Dorp (1971) found that the mid- and inner *medulla* have the highest concentration.

Änggård *et al.* (1972), studied in detail the subcellular localization of the prostaglandin synthetase and 15-hydroxyprostaglandin dehydrogenase in the papilla of rabbit renal medulla. Prostaglandin synthetase was associated mainly with microsomes, in agreement with the observations of Samuelsson *et al.* (1967) on sheep vesicular glands. The precise subcellular site of prostaglandin synthetase has awaited the study of Bohman and Larsson (1975) who found the greatest concentration of synthetase activity in the cytomembrane fraction of cells obtained from the rabbit renal medulla. Although plasma membranes and mitochondria showed lower concentrations, this was considered to result from cross-contamination. In contrast to the localization of synthetase, prostaglandins themselves were located mainly in the supernatant fraction (Änggård *et al.*, 1972). These observations suggest that prostaglandins are synthesized by enzymes located in the endoplasmic reticulum and possibly the Golgi apparatus and then are released either into the cytoplasm or into the extracellular fluid. The small portion of prostaglandins associated with microsomes, mitochondria and lipid droplets suggests that there are no sites of storage within the renal medulla. These conclusions have been confirmed by Crowshaw (1973) who demonstrated that prostaglandins synthesized from [1-^{14}C]arachidonic acid by rabbit renomedullary slices were all located in the incubation medium. None was present in the tissue slice even though the slice had incorporated large quantities of arachidonic acid into tissue phospholipids and neutral lipids. Thus, appreciable storage of renal prostaglandins in a cellular element is unlikely. This interpretation is confirmed by tissue levels of prostaglandins, which vary according to experimental conditions. In the rabbit renal medulla, the concentration of PGE_2 may be as high as 24 μg/g (Crowshaw, 1971), a value approaching that of human seminal fluid where the highest concentrations occur (Samuelsson, 1963). In contrast, if the kidney was quick-frozen, the concentration decreased to 0.005 μg/g (Änggård et al., 1972). Thus, reported concentrations of prostaglandins in a tissue are more an index of the biosynthetic activity of the tissue rather than endogenous content of prostaglandins. The demonstration by Muirhead et al. (1972) that tissue cultures of renomedullary interstitial cells synthesize prostaglandins should not be interpreted to mean that interstitial cells are the sole sites of prostaglandin synthesis intrarenally, since interstitial cells have less biosynthetic capacity than renomedullary homogenates and slices (Hamberg, 1969). Janszen and Nugteren (1971) using a histochemical method have identified several cellular elements, primarily the collecting ducts, as possible sites of prostaglandin synthesis.

The relative exclusion from the rabbit renal papilla of the primary metabolizing enzyme, 15-hydroxyprostaglandin dehydrogenase (Larsson and Änggård, 1973a) indicates a dissociation between sites of synthesis and degradation. This separation has major functional implications. Thus, the major prostaglandin-metabolizing enzyme, the dehydrogenase, achieves its highest activity in the cortex, more than ten-fold that of the medulla. Further, histochemical methods have localized prostaglandin dehydrogenase in a cortical structure, the distal convolution of the nephron (Nissen and Andersen, 1968). Although most of these biochemical studies were conducted in the rabbit, it has been shown that for the dog kidney, the same prostaglandins are also present in the renal medulla (Crowshaw et al., 1970). It has also been shown that renomedullary homogenates do not synthesize PGA_2 from endogenous arachidonic acid, and the optimum conditions for synthesis are the same as those for rabbit; also that synthesis and degradation of prostaglandins are relatively segregated (synthesis to the medulla and degradation to the cortex) (Crowshaw and McGiff, 1973).

The initial step in the synthesis of prostaglandins is presumably activation of an acylhydrolase, such as phospholipase A_2 which releases arachidonic acid, the precursor of PGE_2 and $PGF_{2\alpha}$, from phospholipids. Although widely accepted, there was no direct evidence for the involvement of one or more acylhydrolases in the synthesis of prostaglandins until Flower and Blackwell (1975) showed that phospholipase A_2 was the key enzyme which mobilizes free fatty acids for prostaglandin synthesis in response to cell injury in slices of guinea pig spleen. They also showed that substrate availability was not the only requirement for stimulation of prostaglandin synthesis; activation of the synthetase complex seems necessary (alternatively inhibition of a synthetase repressor). Arachidonic acid is rapidly converted to

PGE_2 and $PGF_{2\alpha}$ after undergoing oxidative cyclization. Two of the inter-mediates in the synthesis of prostaglandins, the cyclic endoperoxides, may possess independent biological activity within the kidney. Gryglewski and Vane (1972) had suggested that a series of vasoactive substances results from activation of acylhydrolases of which prostaglandins are the end-products. Their proposal has been confirmed by the studies of Hamberg and Samuelsson (1974) and Hamberg, Svensson and Samuelsson (1974) who reported that the cyclic endoperoxides differ in their potencies, metabolic degradation, and range of biological activities from PGE and PGF compounds. Indeed cyclic endoperoxides are the major products of prostaglandin synthetase in some tissues. Thus, it is possible that one or more of the aforementioned products of prostaglandin synthetase will prove to be of greater importance than PGE_2 in mediating some of the functional changes associated with increased activity of prostaglandin synthetase within the kidney.

In addition, a by-product, the lysophospholipid, resulting from phospholi-pase-induced release of prostaglandin precursors from phospholipids possesses potent biological actions. A lysophospholipid has been proposed to be a naturally occurring inhibitor of renin (Smeby et al., 1967). These factors operating in vivo which determine the major product(s) of prostaglandin synthetase have recently been studied by Lee and Levine (1974) in terms of enzymic reduction of the 9-keto group of PGE to form PGF. They suggested that this enzyme, PGE 9-ketoreductase, constitutes the major determinant of the effects of changes in prostaglandin synthetase activity since it will affect the ratio of PGE to PGF. PGE_2 and $PGF_{2\alpha}$ differ considerably in their biological properties and their effects on renal function. Some vasoactive hormones are capable of activating the PGE 9-ketoreductase as well as the synthetase thereby affecting not only prostaglandin production but also the functional consequences of increased synthesis.

Those aspects of the biochemistry of prostaglandins having major func-tional implications will be recapitulated. Since prostaglandins are not stored intrarenally, release of prostaglandins from the kidney in response to a stimulus such as angiotensin II denotes increased prostaglandin synthesis which results in the immediate entry of newly synthesized prostaglandins into the extracellular compartment. After their release within the renal medulla, prostaglandins will not be degraded appreciably locally because of the relative exclusion of the degrading enzymes from this zone. The absence of the major metabolizing enzyme, 15-hydroxyprostaglandin dehydrogenase from the inner medulla, where synthesizing enzymes have been shown to be most active, has intriguing implications concerning duration and sites of activity of prostaglandins after their release intrarenally, and is directly related to the proposal that PGE_2 is a major, but not exclusive, determinant of medullary and juxtamedullary blood flow, thereby participating in the distribution of blood flow within the kidney. An additional finding which may be related to the maintenance and distribution of resting renal blood flow is the uninterrupted synthesis of PGE_2 as reflected by sustained efflux of prostaglandins from the kidney under 'basal' conditions which is greatest in those experimental preparations subjected to the most extensive surgery and least in the resting unanaesthetized animal.

6.2 PROSTAGLANDINS AS TISSUE HORMONES

Qualitative differences between prostaglandins of the F series and those of the E and the A series are the rule. The latter two groups of prostaglandins resemble each other in their biological actions. However, PGE compounds are more potent than PGA compounds and, unlike the PGA compounds, they, as well as the PGF compounds, are almost entirely removed from the blood on passage across the lung (Ferreira and Vane, 1967a). PGE_2 and PGA_2 have equivalent renal vasodilator potencies in dogs when infused into the renal artery at rates of 100 ng/min or less, whereas at higher infusion rates PGE_2 is several times more potent (Lonigro et al., 1973; Fülgraff et al., 1974). In contrast, $PGF_{2\alpha}$ does not affect renal blood flow under the same conditions. The renal vasodilator actions of prostaglandins of the E and the A series have not been dissociated from the concurrent natriuresis. The demonstration that PGE compounds oppose vasoconstrictor stimuli is vital to the proposal that endogenous prostaglandins modulate autonomic nervous activity generally (Hedqvist, 1970a) and renal pressor systems specifically (McGiff et al., 1970b). In contrast, $PGF_{2\alpha}$ augments vasoconstriction produced by pressor stimuli in some vascular beds, although the renal vascular bed is exempted from this action. Since PGE_2 and $PGF_{2\alpha}$ are inactivated in the lung, these are like tissue hormones synthesized or activated elsewhere in the body; their activity would be limited largely to sites of formation and degradation, in this case the kidney, and those cardiovascular structures—great veins and right heart—proximal to the lung. PGA_2 could function as a circulating hormone since it escapes destruction in the lung (McGiff et al., 1969). The issue of biologically significant blood levels of a prostaglandin of the A series is an important one, since if established, it would indicate a role for prostaglandins beyond that of local hormones. PGA_2 must originate from enzymic conversion of PGE_2, since the breakdown of the biosynthetic intermediate, the cyclic endoperoxide, results in PGD_2, PGE_2 and $PGF_{2\alpha}$, not PGA_2. The proposal that PGA_2 of renal origin is a circulating hormone should, in the very least, be examined in terms of the ability of the kidney to synthesize PGA_2. The evidence against this likelihood is:

(1) Crowshaw and McGiff (1973) using rabbit and dog renomedullary slices and homogenates, have consistently failed to demonstrate biosynthesis of PGA_2 after addition of either labelled arachidonic acid, the natural substrate for prostaglandin synthetase, or labelled PGE_2, the immediate precursor of PGA_2. These observations support the studies of Hamberg (1969) and Blackwell et al. (1975) which were referred to previously.

(2) Davis and Horton (1972) have found relatively high concentrations of PGE_2 and $PGF_{2\alpha}$ in rabbit renal venous blood. Another prostaglandin which could have been either a PGA or PGC or a PGB was not recovered by these investigators from renal venous blood in sufficient quantity to permit its definitive identification. If one assumed that the PGA-like material was PGA_2, then its concentration was

considerably less than one-tenth that of PGE_2. Since the renal vasodilator–diuretic activity of PGA_2 is less than that of PGE_2, differences in concentrations in renal venous blood between PGE_2 and a PGA-like substance, expressed in terms of equivalency of their vasodilator–diuretic actions, approaches fifty-fold.

(3) Larsson and Änggård (1975) used quantitative mass fragmentography to determine regional distribution of prostaglandins in rabbit kidney. Recoveries were checked by the addition of $^{14}C\text{-}PGE_2$, $^{3}H\text{-}PGF_{2\alpha}$ and $^{3}H\text{-}PGA_2$. The amount of PGE_2 converted to PGA_2 during isolation was calculated by determining the amount of $^{14}C\text{-}PGA_2$ and $^{3}H\text{-}PGA_2$ recovered. Levels of PGE_2 and $PGF_{2\alpha}$ were respectively, 2.8 and 1.8 $\mu g/g$ in the medulla and 0.16 and 0.14 $\mu g/g$ in the cortex. PGA_2 was not detected in the medulla and only a trace was found in the cortex, 0.005 $\mu g/g$.

Further evidence occurs from the isolated blood-perfused canine kidney in which concentrations of PGE and PGF compounds increased progressively in the blood perfusate, such that after 3 h of perfusion, their concentrations exceeded by ten-fold those values observed in venous effluent of the *in situ* canine kidney (McGiff *et al.*, 1974). In part, the increased levels of prostaglandins of the E and F series in the blood perfusing the isolated kidney are determined by exclusion of the lungs from the circuit. Under these conditions, prostaglandins of the E, F and A series were measured simultaneously using radioimmunoassay and bioassay (Figure 6.2). Although PGE and PGF compounds increased to high levels as expected, PGA, as measured by radioimmunoassay, remained depressed throughout the 6 h period of observation. Further, the levels of a PGA compound are at the threshold of sensitivity of the method and may represent material other than a prostaglandin of the A series. Indeed its being unaffected by indomethacin administration in view of the precipitous decline in PGE and PGF compounds produced by the anti-inflammatory agent suggests this is the case. Thus, PGA_2, if present in the kidney, is present in amounts which are not detected readily and this problematic renal production of PGA_2 (much less than 10% that of PGE_2) could not account for the high peripheral blood levels (> 1.0 ng/ml) reported for PGA compounds in man (Zusman *et al.*, 1972), although the possibility of species difference should be considered. None the less, the proposal of Lee (1967) that a prostaglandin of the A series is a circulating hormone should be considered an open issue, since demonstration of enzymic conversion of PGE_2 to PGA_2 intrarenally may be determined by the state of sodium balance or experimental conditions different from those which have obtained in the biochemical studies. Alternatively, the release of PGE_2 either from the cortex or outer medulla into the descending limb of the vasa recta or loop of Henle would result in PGE_2 making contact with the more acidic environment of the inner medulla which could result in the non-enzymic conversion of PGE_2 to $PGF_{2\alpha}$. In addition, a PGA isomerase which has been described in plasma converts PGA to PGC compounds (Jones and Cammock, 1972). PGC compounds are more potent than their PGA precursors and like them, escape degradation on passage across the lungs. However, the activity of the isomerase in many species, including man, is undetectable. Furthermore, two

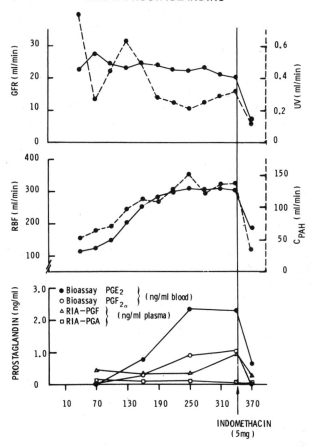

Figure 6.2 Effect of indomethacin in the isolated dog kidney. From the top: GFR (glomerular filtration rate, solid line); UV (urine flow rate, broken line); RBF (renal blood flow, solid line); C_{PAH} (renal plasma flow, broken line); RIA (radioimmunoassay) and bioassay prostaglandin concentrations in blood perfusate. Indomethacin, 5 mg, was administered at time indicated by the arrow, 340 min after perfusion began

laboratories have reported a substance, immunoreactive with PGA antibodies in concentrations of *ca.* 1.5 ng/ml plasma, several-fold greater than the concentrations of PGE compounds (Jaffe *et al.*, 1973). In one of these studies (Zusman *et al.*, 1973), this substance unexpectedly increased in response to sodium deprivation and decreased on sodium repletion, changes which should occur if it played a role in conservation of salt and water. Since prostaglandins of the A series possess vasodilator and diuretic properties, there are obvious difficulties in assigning a role in salt and water conservation to a PGA compound of renal origin, despite the report that PGA has been shown to increase aldosterone secretion (Fichman *et al.*, 1972). In the absence of complete information on prostaglandin metabolism, claims of specificity for radioimmunoassay of prostaglandins should be cautiously received, since the issue of one or more metabolites, or closely related substances, cross-reacting with antibody to the substance being measured is unsettled. Thus, the plasma concentration of the metabolites of the major prostaglandins has been estimated to be ten- to seventy-fold that of the parent compound (Samuelsson, 1973).

Although arterial concentrations of prostaglandins of the E and F series are probably less than 0.02 ng/ml under resting conditions (Lonigro et al., 1973) precipitous increases in the arterial levels of prostaglandins may occur, such as in response to pulmonary embolism (Lindsey and Wyllie, 1970). Chronic increases would be expected in advanced lung disease in the presence of extensive shunting of blood between the pulmonary and systemic circulations. There are species, such as the rabbit (Venuto et al., 1975), in which mixed venous levels of prostaglandins, and perhaps arterial levels as well, may be higher than in dog or man, probably reflecting the greater biosynthetic capacity of the rabbit. In addition, decreased degradation of prostaglandins will elevate their levels. The study of Blackwell et al. (1975) indicates that the rate of turnover of the major metabolizing enzyme, prostaglandin 15-hydroxydehydrogenase is rapid and is susceptible to repression by cycloheximide and puromycin, inhibitors of protein synthesis, which prevent synthesis of the enzyme. Changes in enzyme activity with pregnancy have also been reported (Bedwani and Marley, 1975). Thus, the hormonal background and intake of drugs could affect the tissue and circulating levels of prostaglandins by interfering with their degradation as well as their synthesis. The localization of the major prostaglandin-metabolizing enzymes in the renal cortex (Larsson and Änggård, 1973a) reduces the threat to body fluid homeostasis presented by sudden increase in the arterial levels of prostaglandins. Of fifteen different swine tissues studied, the renal cortex contained the highest activity of prostaglandin dehydrogenase (Änggård, Larsson and Samuelsson, 1971) which is in agreement with the histochemical studies of Nissen and Andersen (1968) who found the highest activity in the distal nephron and media of cortical arterioles, sites which would affect the levels of prostaglandins in both blood and urine. The heavy concentration of dehydrogenase in the cortex prevents systemic prostaglandins from reaching the medulla, since medullary blood vessels arise from those of the inner cortex, and circumscribes the activity of prostaglandins synthesized in the cortex to those structures at or near their sites of synthesis. Thus, a picket line of prostaglandin dehydrogenase stands ready to intercept systemic and renal cortical prostaglandins from gaining access to the renal medulla. Viewed in another way this line also defends the cortex from prostaglandins of medullary origin that might reach the cortex via the ascending vasa recta or the loop of Henle.

In view of the high level of activity of the renal kallikrein–kinin system (Margolius et al., 1974) and the interactions between it and prostaglandins within the kidney, i.e. prostaglandins mediate and amplify its effects (McGiff et al., 1975), the prostaglandin degradative enzymes would also serve the additional purpose of containing or modulating the effects of the kallikrein–kinin system.

Since prostaglandins possess diverse actions and affect most biological systems, construction of their intrarenal actions based on their intravascular administration demands recognition that blood levels rarely, if ever, exceed 10^{-10} moles/ml (< 35 ng/ml). Concentrations of this magnitude would be expected only in the venous effluent from organs having large biosynthetic capacity, representing peak levels which are not maintained, although a study based on radioimmunoassay claims prostaglandin levels in the venous effluent of the gravid uterus of the rabbit to be in excess of 100 ng/ml (Venuto *et al.*, 1975). Arterial levels, which are less than one-fiftieth those occurring in renal venous blood, probably rarely exceed 20 pg/ml blood (with the possible exceptions noted above). When blood levels of administered prostaglandins are excessive, a sought-for direct renal action may be superseded or obscured by their systemic effects. Questionable purposes are served by studies of the effects of administration of prostaglandins by bolus injection or in amounts which establish blood levels in excess of 100 ng/ml. Furthermore, no route of administration of prostaglandins reproduces the effects evoked by release of endogenous prostaglandins from an organ in terms of either concentrations achieved at their sites of action, structures initially affected or the sequence of tubular and vascular elements affected. These considerations are frequently overlooked when physiological roles are inferred on the basis of the reported effects of exogenous prostaglandins on renal function. For example, since administration of a PGA compound reduced renal medullary blood flow and increased cortical blood flow, it has been reasoned that a deficiency of prostaglandins intrarenally will result in cortical ischaemia (Lee, 1967). On the contrary, release of prostaglandins within the renal medulla where metabolizing enzymes are deficient or absent should primarily increase medullary blood flow. Furthermore, the presence of the major prostaglandin-metabolizing enzymes in the cortex should assure a primary local action for prostaglandins of medullary origin, the site of the most active renal synthetase. Thus, deficiency of renal prostaglandins induced by inhibition of prostaglandin synthetase should result primarily in ischaemia of the renal medulla, not the renal cortex. Studies directed towards examination of the physiological roles of renal prostaglandins are scarce because of the considerable difficulties involved in measuring levels of prostaglandins in biological fluids and also the absence of agents which block effector responses efficiently and predictably. However, the important discovery that non-steroidal anti-inflammatory drugs such as salicylates and indomethacin inhibit synthesis of prostaglandins (Vane, 1971) has resulted in important findings on the role of renal prostaglandins as modulators and mediators of the effects of vasoactive hormones.

6.3 ASSAY OF PROSTAGLANDINS: THE BLOOD-BATHED ORGAN TECHNIQUE

In various experimental manoeuvres aimed at studying prostaglandin release by the kidney, McGiff *et al.* (1970) employed the sensitive bioassay developed by Vane (1969) for identifying hormones released from an organ into its venous effluent. The method, which is capable of detecting prostaglandin in subnanogram quantities, utilizes the principle of parallel pharmacologic assay. Specificity is achieved by including in the assay system several kinds of tissues obtained from organs of known sensitivity to the hormone. The tissues are superfused in series by blood or other body fluid to be analysed for

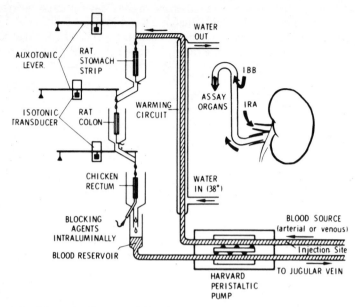

Figure 6.3 Schematic diagram of blood-bathed organ system (one bank). Blood was withdrawn at the rate of 10–15 ml/min by a pump. After traversing a constant-temperature circuit, the blood cascaded over three assay organs arranged in series. Changes in the length of the assay organs were transduced and recorded on a multichannel recorder. The blood was collected in a reservoir and returned to the animal at the same rate as it was withdrawn. Selective blockade of assay organs is possible by direct intraluminal application of a blocking agent. A major use of this method is shown by the schematized kidney on the right. Thus, a substance may be given into the renal artery (IRA) and its effects on assay organs compared with its direct effects by administration into the extra-corporeal circuit (IBB = into the bathing blood), indicated by 'injection site' in the diagram of the assay system. Indirect effects of hormones may thereby be determined, e.g. release of intrarenal substances by angiotensin II

hormone content (Figure 6.3). In the case of prostaglandins, the 'bank' of assay tissues comprises rat stomach strip, rat colon and chick rectum. Three banks of assay tissues were used to monitor venous effluents of the kidneys and aortic blood simultaneously for changes in concentrations of prostaglandins, thereby determining the time course of release and fate of prostaglandins in response to a stimulus.

Consider the results in dogs subjected to unilateral renal ischaemia (Figure 6.4). Prostaglandin release into renal venous blood was evident within 2 to 4 min; the absence of prostaglandins at this time in aortic blood suggested its prompt inactivation on passage across the lung. Within 7 minutes prostaglandins were also released into venous blood of the contralateral kidney. Unexpectedly, this seemed to have occurred via a mediating effect of angiotensin II on prostaglandin release. Several findings suggested this to be so; for example, an increase in arterial angiotensin concentration always occurred shortly before prostaglandin release, and plasma renin activity increased ten-fold at the time of the elevated prostaglandin levels in the venous blood of the contralateral kidney. These results were explained as follows: the

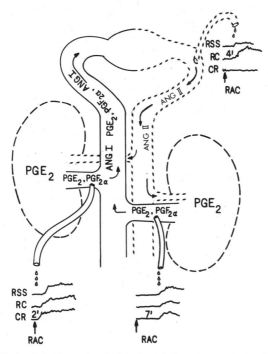

Figure 6.4 Effect of right renal arterial constriction on prostaglandin release by the ischaemic and contralateral kidneys. Three banks of organs continuously sampled venous blood of each kidney and aortic blood for changes in concentrations of prostaglandins. Within 2 min (2′) after constriction of the renal artery, prostaglandins (PGE_2 and $PGF_{2\alpha}$ appeared in venous blood of the ischaemic kidney as indicated by contraction of the three assay organs (lower left; RSS = rat stomach strip, RC = rat colon, CR = chick rectum). Within 7 min (7′) after induction of renal ischaemia, the contralateral kidney released prostaglandin-like substances probably mediated by angiotensin II (lower right). The assay organs monitoring aortic blood (upper right) contracted in a manner consistent with increased generation of angiotensin(s) (contraction of RC primarily). Thoracic caval and renal venous blood, obtained at the time of peak activity of the assay organs, was extracted and purified: PGE_2 and $PGF_{2\alpha}$ were recovered from samples of renal venous blood, and caval plasma showed greater than 10-fold increase in renin activity

initial response to unilateral renal ischaemia included release of both renin and prostaglandin into the venous blood of the ischaemic kidney. Most of the released prostaglandin is removed on passage across the lung. However, continued release of renin from the ischaemic kidney accelerates formation of angiotensin I; the latter, on passage across the lung and perhaps within the ischaemic kidney, being converted to angiotensin II, which in turn stimulates prostaglandin release from the contralateral kidney.

Thus, the blood-bathed organ technique allows an integrated description of the cardiorenal response to a stimulus which no other method nor combination of methods permits; providing as it does an 'on line' assay of blood levels of prostaglandins simultaneously for several sampling sites. It also indicates the optimal time for collection of blood during application of a stimulus. Blood obtained during peak contractions of the assay tissues can be

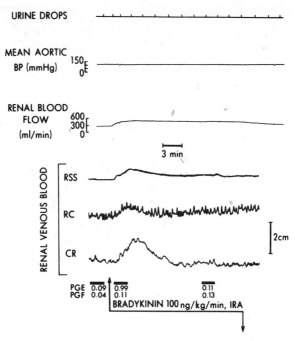

Figure 6.5 Effects of bradykinin infused for 20 min into the renal artery (IRA), on urine flow, mean aortic blood pressure (BP), renal blood flow, and assay organs (rat stomach strip (RSS), rat colon (RC), and chick rectum (CR)) superfused by venous blood of the same kidney in a chloralose-anaesthetized dog. Each mark on the urine drop scale represents every tenth drop. The time of collection of a sample of renal venous blood for assay is indicated by the back bar, and the concentrations of prostaglandins (ng/ml blood) in that sample are indicated below the bar

extracted for acidic lipids and subjected to purification to verify the identification of prostaglandins provided by the *in vivo* assay system which must be regarded as tentative. For example in Figure 6.5, the first collection of blood obtained during bradykinin infusion was timed to coincide with peak contractions of the assay organs. The unsustained contraction of the assay organs suggested a waning of the concentration of prostaglandins in renal venous effluent during infusion of bradykinin. This analysis was confirmed by the results of the *in vivo* assay: an initial eleven-fold increase in the concentration of PGE_2 was unsustained, declining to lower levels within 6 min despite continued infusion of bradykinin (McGiff *et al.*, 1972).

6.4 RENAL PROSTAGLANDINS: RANGE OF ACTIVITIES

Renal prostaglandins may be considered in terms of three types of actions:

First, as MODULATORS, whereby PGE_2 and perhaps PGD_2 blunt the renal vasoconstrictor–antidiuretic activity of pressor hormones and augment the renal vasodilator activity of kinins. That is, prostaglandins as modulators AMPLIFY the renal kallikrein–kinin system and ATTENUATE the renin–

angiotensin and adrenergic nervous systems. Modulation requires that the rate of synthesis of PGE_2 is capable of increasing rapidly above the basal rate when stimulated by a vasoactive hormone.

Second, as MEDIATORS, renal prostaglandins may affect some of the actions of other hormones. For example PGE_2 mediates the effects of bradykinin on excretion of solute free water, and thereby on the concentration of the urine, and may subserve one or more components of autoregulation of renal blood flow.

Third, prostaglandins (since they are synthesized continuously by the kidney) may contribute to the MAINTENANCE of resting renal blood flow and basal excretion of salt and water.

In order to examine possible actions of renal prostaglandins, it is useful to alter their level of activity by inhibiting their synthesis with anti-inflammatory acids or by enhancing their synthesis by providing substrate, arachidonic acid, to renal prostaglandin synthetase. The discovery by Vane (1971) that aspirin-like drugs inhibit prostaglandin synthesis has resulted in the identification of those components of the renal actions of vasoactive hormones which are contributed to, mediated and attenuated by the released prostaglandin. There is evidence for all of these interactions within the kidney.

6.4.1 Modulators

6.4.1.1 Attenuation of pressor hormones

The study cited above (McGiff et al., 1970) suggested that angiotensin II released prostaglandins from the contralateral kidney. This hypothesis was tested by infusing angiotensin II into the renal artery (McGiff et al., 1970a) at a rate which established blood levels of angiotensin II similar to those reported in renovascular hypertension, 0.1–0.5 ng/ml (Gocke et al., 1969). Renal venous blood was assayed continuously for changes in prostaglandin concentration with the blood-bathed organ method of Vane (1969). Renal blood flow and urine flow were decreased by angiotensin, but within 2–5 min both blood flow and urine flow returned towards control levels despite continued infusion of angiotensin (Figure 6.6). This recovery phase coincided with prostaglandin release. In several experiments infusion of angiotensin did not release prostaglandins from the kidney, and vasoconstriction and decreased urine flow were maintained throughout the period of infusion (Figure 6.6). Aiken and Vane (1973) confirmed release of prostaglandins in response to infusion of angiotensin into the renal artery and further showed that when release was prevented by a prostaglandin synthetase inhibitor, indomethacin, the vasoconstrictor effect of angiotensin II in the kidney, but not that in the hindleg, was substantially potentiated. In the resting state, synthesis of prostaglandins by the limb is negligible (Lonigro et al., 1973). Thus, the inability of indomethacin to potentiate the vasoconstrictor action of angiotensin in the hindlimb is a reflection of the low prostaglandin biosynthetic capacity of the resting limb. On the other hand, in those organs that exhibit a high prostaglandin biosynthetic capacity, such as the gravid uterus (Terragno et al., 1974) and kidney (Itskovitz et al., 1974), there is a

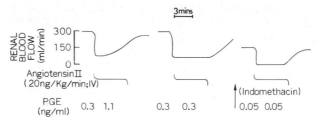

Figure 6.6 In an anaesthetized dog, the renal vasoconstrictor action of angiotensin II, infused for 10 min, may be related to changes in the renal venous concentration of PGE_2. From left to right: 1. infusion of angiotensin II decreased renal blood flow which recovered partially despite continued infusion of the pressor agent. Coincident with recovery of renal blood flow, the concentration of PGE_2 in renal venous blood increased almost fourfold. 2. In contrast, angiotensin II produced a sustained decrease in renal blood flow whenever the renal venous concentration of PGE_2 did not increase. 3. After inhibition of prostaglandin synthesis with indomethacin, renal blood flow fell below the pre-indomethacin level as the renal venous concentration of PGE_2 decreased from 0.3 to 0.05 ng/ml. Post-indomethacin infusion of angiotensin II resulted in a sustained decrease in renal blood flow

corresponding reduction or even loss of the vasoconstrictor potency of pressor hormones which can be restored by inhibiting prostaglandin synthesis. Indeed, in canine isolated blood-perfused kidneys, doses of angiotensin II, which were previously without effect, decreased renal blood flow after inhibition of prostaglandin synthetase. The relationship between the vaso-constrictor activity of pressor hormones in an organ and the prostaglandin biosynthetic capacity of that organ has been investigated by Terragno *et al.* (1974) in the uterine vascular bed. In late pregnancy in the chloralose-anaesthetized dog, infusion of angiotensin II increased uterine blood flow and concomitantly resulted in a two- to three-fold increased uterine efflux of a PGE compound in the venous effluent. In the non-gravid state and in early pregnancy, when prostaglandins could not be detected in uterine venous blood, either before or during administration of angiotensin, constriction of the uterine vascular bed in response to angiotensin was rapidly demonstrated. Thus, the capacity of the kidney and of the gravid uterus to synthesize prostaglandin E_2 seems to protect these organs against the vasoconstrictor action of angiotensin II.

These studies also strongly suggested that prostaglandins might function as regulators of blood flow to the kidney and gravid uterus since a basal efflux of a PGE persisted in the absence of pressor hormonal stimulation. Further, the findings could account for the development of tachyphylaxis to angio-tensin which is usually observed at high doses. The conventional explanation invokes receptor theory; tachyphylaxis to the vasoconstrictor action of angiotensin occurs when all receptor sites are occupied so that none remains accessible to the hormone (Thurston and Laragh, 1975). For those tissues having a large capacity to synthesize prostaglandins, tachyphylaxis results at least in part from stimulation of PGE_2 synthesis by angiotensin II; the newly generated PGE_2 opposes the pressor hormone's vasoconstrictor action. This hypothesis received support from Aiken (1974) who studied the contractile effects of angiotensin II on spirally cut strips of femoral and celiac arteries and distinguished two components of tachyphylaxis to angiotensin. The first component was dependent on angiotensin-induced generation of prosta-glandins within the vascular wall. Doses of angiotensin II repeated every half-hour induced reproducible contractions of femoral arterial strips, but with strips of celiac artery, successive doses of angiotensin II gave smaller and smaller responses. Tachyphylaxis of the celiac artery was prevented by prostaglandin synthetase inhibitors and correlated with a high sensitivity of the artery to relaxation evoked by PGE compounds. Thus, addition of minute concentrations of PGE_2, less than 1 ng/ml, together with angiotensin II did not affect angiotensin-induced contractions of the femoral arterial strips, but substantially reduced those of the celiac artery. The second component of tachyphylaxis was independent of prostaglandin synthesis by the blood vessels and therefore could be shown in either femoral or celiac arterial strips. It is this component that is explainable on the basis of receptor occupancy by the pressor hormone and for its demonstration requires administration of angiotensin at more frequent intervals. Thus, administra-tion of angiotensin II at 5 or 10 min intervals to the tissue bath resulted in diminishing contractile responses of celiac arterial strips despite prior treat-ment with indomethacin. Aiken concluded that angiotensin II induced synthesis of prostaglandins intra-murally in celiac arterial strips which also relaxed in response to small doses of PGE compounds and that tachyphylaxis was most readily produced in arteries exhibiting these characteristics. Prostaglandins synthesized in the walls of the major resistance blood vessels where they can influence hormonal and neural induced vasoconstriction directly may, thereby, affect the state of constriction of blood vessels. This capacity of blood vessels to generate prostaglandins within their wall is directly related to regulation of vascular tone and reactivity. It has not been defined for the renal vasculature, although there is indirect evidence that the main renal artery has a low or negligible capacity for prostaglandin synthesis (Aiken, 1974) which is not likely to be the case for the smaller renal blood vessels.

On exploring the relationship of prostaglandins to other pressor hormones, it was found that norepinephrine shares with angiotensin II the ability to release PGE_2 from the kidney and that when this occurs the vasoconstrictor–antidiuretic effect of the amine is blunted (McGiff et al., 1972). As with angiotensin, the amount of prostaglandin released by norepinephrine was unrelated to the dose of the pressor agent. A few details of these experiments are worth citing: mean concentration of PGE_2 in renal venous blood increased to 6.5 ng/ml from a control of 0.2 (the range of peak concentration was 0.5–24.2 ng/ml, and while the prostaglandin response appeared un-related to the norepinephrine dose, it was related in each animal to plasma renin activity (McGiff and Itskovitz, 1973). Norepinephrine released the largest amount of PGE_2 when plasma renin activity was low and the least when plasma renin activity was high (Figure 6.7). Plasma renin activity may be used as an index of the states of sodium balance, since the two correlate inversely. According to these findings, then, renal vascular reactivity to norepinephrine was potentiated by negative sodium balance, attenuated when the balance was positive. This was unexpected inasmuch as the degree of vasoconstriction in response to a pressor stimulus is thought to be greater during sodium excess. At least this is the accepted view, although it is of

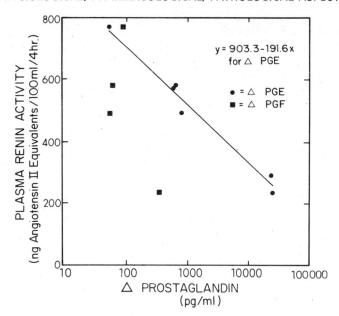

Figure 6.7 Relationship between the increase in concentration of PGE_2 and $PGF_{2\alpha}$ in renal venous blood produced by norepinephrine and the control plasma renin activity in six experiments in chloralose-anaesthetized dogs. Ordinate = control plasma renin activity (expressed as ng angiotensin II equivalents per 100 ml plasma per 4 h incubation): abscissa = log scale of the increase in renal venous concentrations of PGE_2 and $PGF_{2\alpha}$

interest that Kilcoyne and Cannon (1971) showed similar enhancement of renal vascular reactivity to norepinephrine during negative sodium balance and diminished responsiveness when sodium balance was positive.

It appears that the state of sodium balance affects the responses to norepinephrine by influencing both the amount of prostaglandin released by the pressor hormone and the threshold dose of the amine. Evidently, more prostaglandin is released in the face of sodium excess, which curbs the vasoconstriction induced by norepinephrine. Might this relationship apply to other pressor hormones? In studying renal vascular response to angiotensin II, Hollenberg *et al.* (1972) found that vascular reactivity was potentiated, not diminished, by positive sodium balance. Thus, angiotensin II may differ from norepinephrine in its relationship to those factors, such as sodium, which determines its capacity to release prostaglandins and thereby, vascular reactivity to the pressor hormone. However, in related work in anaesthetized dogs, a linear relationship was observed between sodium balance (plasma renin activity) and the dose of angiotensin that released renal prostaglandins (McGiff *et al.*, 1971); threshold angiotensin II doses were smallest during positive sodium balance, suggesting similarities between angiotensin II and norepinephrine.

With norepinephrine, and perhaps angiotensin II as well, the capacity to release prostaglandins from the renal vascular bed—as affected by sodium balance—may determine the degree of residual vasoconstriction. Release of prostaglandins from the ischaemic kidney on removal of arterial occlusion may be affected similarly. Herbaczynska-Cedro and Vane (1974) measured renal blood flow in anaesthetized dogs before and after occlusion of the renal artery for 3 min. The reactive hyperaemia which ensued and the amount of prostaglandin released were increased by 0.9% sodium chloride, infused before the period of ischaemia. After indomethacin, all but the initial brief overshoot of the reactive hyperaemia was abolished.

Sympathetic nerve stimulation also leads to prostaglandin release in many tissues (Hedqvist, 1970a). The released prostaglandin moderates the effects of sympathetic nerve stimulation not only by counteracting vasoconstriction, but also by inhibiting the release of norepinephrine from the nerve endings. This negative feedback mechanism, by which the innervated tissue cells call on prostaglandin to brake the release of the sympathetic transmitter has been demonstrated in the kidney by Frame et al. (1974) and Malik and McGiff (1975). Thus, local prostaglandin release may be a major determinant of vascular reactivity not only to circulating pressor hormones, but also to locally released neurotransmitters.

In all these studies release of a PGE compound during application of a pressor stimulus was associated with attenuation of the vasoconstrictor action of the stimulus, be it angiotensin II, norepinephrine or adrenergic nerve excitation. If release of renal PGE_2, as reflected by increasing concentrations of PGE_2 in renal venous blood, blunts the effect of pressor stimuli, then it should be possible to antagonize their actions with exogenous PGE_2. Lonigro et al. (1973) infused PGE_2 into the renal artery at a rate which established a concentration of 0.5 ng/ml blood, comparable to the lower range of levels found to be present during attenuation of the renal vasoconstrictor action of pressor hormones. Infusion of PGE_2 into the renal artery reversibly inhibited the renal effects of pressor stimuli. Contribution of endogenous prostaglandins to this inhibition was at most slight, since the intensity of pressor stimuli was moderated to reduce renal blood flow by no more than 30%, a decrease usually not associated with release of renal prostaglandins. The vascular response of the contralateral kidney, which was exposed to the pressor stimulus but not to exogenous prostaglandins, confirmed the absence of significant release of endogenous prostaglandins under these experimental conditions.

At this point, examination of the wide range of inhibitory actions of PGE_2 in terms of its interaction with ionic calcium is useful for the insights it affords into an understanding of vascular reactivity. Inhibition by PGE compounds of nerve mediated norepinephrine release may be overridden by increasing the calcium concentration (Hedqvist, 1970b) whearease release of norepinephrine from nerve endings by tyramine, which is independent of calcium, is unaffected by PGE_2 (Hedqvist, 1970a). Involvement of prostaglandins at this level of neuroeffector activity, translocation of ionic calcium or affecting its passage across cellular membranes, provides an explanation for another aspect of prostaglandin interactions with vasoactive substances; viz. the relative non-specificity of modulation by prostaglandins with respect to stimuli and systems. Thus, prostaglandins of the E series not only inhibit adrenergic-induced vasoconstriction, but also that effected by angiotensin II and norepinephrine as well as annulling the cardiodecelerator response to stimulation of cholinergic nerves (Wennmalm and Hedqvist, 1971). Since the vasoconstrictor action of angiotensin II is apparently mediated by displacement of calcium from cellular binding sites (Baudouin et al., 1972) and the release of acetylcholine from nerves is calcium-dependent (Rasmussen, 1970), the demonstration that an E prostaglandin affects the access of calcium ions to cellular binding sites (Kirtland and Baum, 1972) seems to be related to the varied actions of prostaglandins. Because ionic calcium is required for expression of activity of hormones and is involved in the initial hormone-receptor interaction (Rasmussen, 1970) the importance of a substance which affects disposition of calcium ions cannot be overemphasized. Changes in cellular binding of ionic calcium produced by prostaglandins, may be the vital link in prostaglandin–adenyl or guanyl cyclase interactions (Marumo and Edelman, 1971). However, failure of E prostaglandins to modify release of catecholamines from the adrenal medulla (Hedqvist, 1970a) in view of the dependence of this event on calcium (Douglas and Rubin, 1963) should serve as a warning that the mechanism of the modulatory action of prostaglandins is not settled.

Since increased vascular reactivity precedes the onset of hypertension (Doyle and Fraser, 1961), the contribution of prostaglandins to changes in vascular reactivity should be of importance to the pathogenesis of hypertension. Specifically, if a deficiency in prostaglandin production initiates or exaggerates hypertension, chronic administration of prostaglandin synthetase inhibitors should result in hypertension. An elevated blood pressure has not been reported in heavy users of non-steroidal anti-inflammatory agents, but in at least two species, the dog (Lonigro et al., 1973) and rabbit (Larsson and Änggård, 1973b), acute administration of indomethacin leads to hypertension. In the chloralose-anaesthetized dog the immediate haemodynamic effects of indomethacin resemble those of uncomplicated essential hypertension: elevated blood pressure, unchanged cardiac output, marked increase in renovascular resistance and a smaller increase in vascular resistance of the limbs. Most attempts to reproduce chronic hypertension with anti-inflammatory agents have failed. However, Colina et al. (1975) have recently succeeded in producing 25 mmHg or more increases in mean aortic blood pressure in the unanaesthetized rabbit treated daily for several weeks with indomethacin, 10–20 mg/kg per day. This study resulted in several important observations: the dose of indomethacin required to elevate blood pressure is greater, and takes a much longer period (often several days) than the dose required to produce these effects in anaesthetized animals. A reliable index of the efficacy of indomethacin was found to be the change in urinary excretion of PGE. Only after a reduction of 80% or more in PGE excretion were elevations in blood pressure noted. Since urinary prostaglandins probably arise primarily, if not exclusively, within the kidney (Frolich et al., 1973) decreased urinary excretion reflects reduced prostaglandin synthesis intrarenally. This interpretation was supported by the study of Colina et al. (1975). Thus, the conversion of radiolabelled arachidonic acid to PGE_2 and $PGF_{2\alpha}$ by medullary homogenates was reduced by about 80% in those kidneys obtained from rabbits after 17 days of indomethacin treatment, at a time when urinary excretion of prostaglandins showed a similar reduction. This study is the most convincing to date which links deficient PGE production to the pathogenesis of hypertension.

6.4.1.2 Amplification

PGE$_2$ modulates the effects of vasoactive hormones, not only attenuating the vasoconstrictor actions of pressor hormones, but also amplifying the vasodilator action of kinins.

The finding that bradykinin released prostaglandins from the kidney (Terragno et al., 1972) challenged the concept that prostaglandins function primarily as agents of bodily defence, as their release by angiotensin II and norepinephrine suggested (McGiff et al., 1970b). This hypothesis, if applicable to the kidney, required the demonstration of selective release of prostaglandins only when renal function was depressed. In this study canine isolated blood-perfused kidneys were used in order to restrict the study to those factors of renal origin which affect the interactions of kinins and prostaglandins (McGiff et al., 1975). Circulating vasoactive substances of extrarenal origin were thus excluded and variations in perfusion pressure and cardiopulmonary performance which might obscure definition of these hormonal relationships were prevented. The effects of bradykinin on renal function were studied before and after inhibition of prostaglandin synthesis by indomethacin (Vane, 1971) and the changes compared with those produced by another vasodilator polypeptide, eledoisin which does not release prostaglandins from the kidney (McGiff et al., 1972). Both polypeptides were infused at rates which produced a similar degree of renal vasodilatation. Comparison of the renal response to bradykinin before and after administration of indomethacin, should relate to the inability of the kinin to release prostaglandins after inhibition of their synthesis. In contrast, the action of eledoisin should be unaffected by indomethacin. After administration of indomethacin, the renal vasodilator action of bradykinin was reduced, whereas the vasodilator action of eledoisin was unaffected (Figure 6.8). That component of the renal vasodilator action of the kinin related to release of PGE$_2$ from the kidney and revealed after inhibition of prostaglandin synthesis was found to be about 30% in the canine isolated kidney. A corollary of this conclusion is that attenuation of the renal vasodilator action of kinins should be possible by diminishing their capacity to generate PGE$_2$. This effect could be achieved in several ways which can be reduced to two primary objectives.

The first is inhibition of prostaglandin production by the use of anti-inflammatory agents (Vane, 1971). The same effect also can be realized by inhibiting the acylhydrolase, the presumed first step in activation of the prostaglandin synthesizing system by kinins. Mepacrine has been suggested to act at this site through inhibition of phospholipase (Vargaftig and Dao Hai, 1972). It is possible that those ions associated with altered vascular reactivity operate at this level, thereby affecting the sensitivity of the acylhydrolase or one of the components of the synthetase complex.

The second means of modifying those renal actions of kinins to which released PGE$_2$ contributes, is to accelerate degradation of PGE$_2$ or to convert it to a compound which is either inactive intrarenally or which possesses properties antagonistic to kinins. Since there is dissociation between major sites of synthesis and degradation of prostaglandins within the kidney

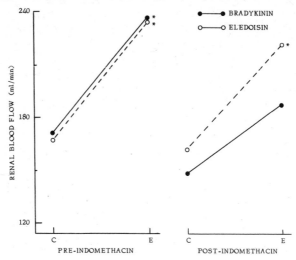

Figure 6.8   Canine isolated blood perfused kidney. Means for periods of 30 min duration each. After control observations (C) either bradykinin or eledoisin was infused during the experimental (E) period. Between the first and second set of observations, indomethacin was administered, then control observations were repeated and the same dose of the polypeptide was infused as before indomethacin. Significant differences between control and experimental periods are indicated by the asterisk

(Larsson and Änggård, 1973a), synthesis occurring predominantly in the medulla and degradation in the cortex, there is less opportunity within the kidney to influence the effects of released PGE_2 by accelerating its metabolism. However, conversion of PGE_2 to $PGF_{2\alpha}$ would result in effective termination of the activity of PGE_2 since $PGF_{2\alpha}$ affects neither renal blood vessels nor salt and water excretion (Lonigro *et al.*, 1973; Tannenbaum *et al.*, 1975), although an extrarenal action on major capacitance vessels (DuCharme, Weeks and Montgomery, 1968), the great veins, seems probable. In addition, the opportunities for PGE–PGF interconversion within the kidney are considerable since the responsible enzyme, 9-ketoreductase, is not segregated in the cortex (Lee and Levine, 1974), as is the prostaglandin dehydrogenase, but rather is equally distributed between the medulla and cortex. Thus, the final determinant of kinin–prostaglandin interactions may be the level of activity of the PGE 9-ketoreductase which determines whether a PGE or PGF compound results from increased prostaglandin synthesis evoked by kinins (Figure 6.9). For example, if PGE 9-ketoreductase activity was low, as may be the case during excess salt intake, kinins generated intrarenally (in the absence of any change in the amount of kallikrein released) would favour synthesis of PGE_2 (none is converted to $PGF_{2\alpha}$) which results in increased renal blood flow, particularly to the inner cortex and medulla (Itskovitz *et al.*, 1974). The latter change has been associated with increased salt and water excretion (Stein *et al.*, 1973). Thus, increased generation of kinins intrarenally need not occur, as reflected by increased excretion of kallikrein (an index of changes in renal kinin activity), to enhance the level of kallikrein–kinin activity within the kidney. All that is required is inhibition of 9-ketoreductase (or failure to activate it) which thereby favours production

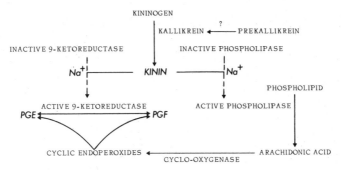

Figure 6.9   Kinin increases prostaglandin synthesis by making more substrate available to the synthetase complex. Kinin also may regulate production of the major end-product, a PGE or PGF, by activating a PGE 9-ketoreductase. These two steps, activation of the phospholipase and the 9-ketoreductase, are possibly sensitive to sodium ions which promote the former and inhibit the latter

of PGE_2. Conversely, in the face of loss of extracellular fluid volume increased activity of 9-ketoreductase should result in greater formation of $PGF_{2\alpha}$ and consequently less PGE_2. The latter by itself would reduce the haemodynamic effects and accompanying diuresis, resulting from generation of kinins intrarenally in the absence of any decrease in their formation.

There are other factors affecting the activity of the renal kallikrein–kinin system. Thus, release of kallikrein or activation of pre-kallikrein may have one or more neural or hormonal determinants. Substance P, a polypeptide hormone originally isolated from the intestines was found to be a potent stimulus to kallikrein excretion (Mills *et al.*, 1974). A parallel system, renin–angiotensin, is subject to regulation by neural and hormonal as well as by local factors. A similar regulatory network seems probable for the kallikrein–kinin system which may be considered, when linked to renal prostaglandins, the vasodilator–diuretic protagonist much as the renin–angiotensin–aldosterone–ADH system is the vasoconstrictor, salt and water conserving protagonist. Kinin generation may also be effectively regulated by altering its degradation. However, renal kininases may, under most conditions, be operating at close to maximal activity. Thus, the renal degradation of infused bradykinin is in excess of 80% in the cat (Ferreira and Vane, 1967b) and approaches 95% in the dog (Nasjletti *et al.*, 1975). There remain other alternatives of which the most important appears to be the undefined role of products of renal prostaglandin synthetase, other than PGE_2 and $PGF_{2\alpha}$, which may modify the actions of kinins. Thus, the cyclic endoperoxide intermediates, PGG_2 and PGH_2 as well as another renal prostaglandin PGD_2, which differ in their potencies and range of biological activities from PGE and PGF compounds, could contribute to or even determine the end-result of increased kallikrein–kinin activity within the kidney.

6.4.1.3 Paradoxical effect of PGE_2 in the rat

In the rat production of PGE and PGA compounds was reported to increase in response to sodium deprivation (Tobian *et al.*, 1974). If these hormones

dilate the renal vasculature of the rat as they do in other species, then enhanced synthesis of prostaglandins of the E and A series should result in
increasing negative sodium balance, whereas body economy calls for salt and
water conservation under these conditions. However, prostaglandins of the
E and A series were shown to augment the vasoconstrictor response of the
isolated perfused kidney of the rat to nerve stimulation in concentrations
which did not affect vascular tone (100 pg/ml) and to constrict the renal
vasculature in higher concentrations (Malik and McGiff, 1975). Under
identical conditions in the isolated perfused kidney of the rabbit, PGE and
PGA compounds inhibited adrenergic vasoconstriction and dilated blood
vessels (Figure 6.10). Further, endogenous prostaglandins of the rat presumably have the same effect as exogenous prostaglandins since enhanced
synthesis of renal prostaglandins, induced by arachidonic acid, resulted in
vasoconstriction, whereas inhibition of their synthesis promoted vasodilatation. This study suggests that, in the rat, PGE and PGA compounds participate in sodium conservation and that their increased synthesis in response to

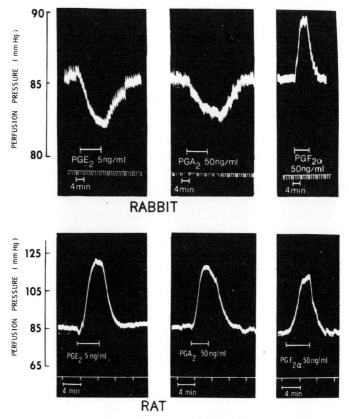

Figure 6.10 In the isolated Krebs-perfused kidneys of rabbits and rats infusion of PGE₂
and PGA₂ in the indicated concentrations results in vasoconstriction (elevated perfusion
pressure in the rat) and vasodilatation (decreased perfusion pressure in the rabbit). (after
Malik, K.U.)

sodium deprivation is appropriate. In this connection the experiments of Leary *et al.* (1974) are of interest. Kidneys of rats were perfused with Krebs' solution and prostaglandin release into the venous effluent was measured. There was no basal output of PGE-like activity but norepinephrine injection stimulated release, which reached a mean concentration of 9 ng/g per ml perfusate in the kidneys of rats drinking water. In kidneys of rats drinking 1.5% sodium chloride, injection of norepinephrine produced prostaglandin concentrations of only 2.9 ng/g per ml. Prostaglandin release by norepinephrine was also much lower in kidneys of rats which had developed hypertension due to constriction of renal artery, coupled with uninephrectomy. This study, when interpreted in terms of the findings of Malik and McGiff (1975), questions the suitability of the rat as a model for investigating the anti-hypertensive role of endogenous prostaglandins.

It should be recalled that $PGF_{2\alpha}$ has pressor properties in most species examined thus far, including the rat. $PGF_{2\alpha}$ facilitates the release of the adrenergic transmitter (Kadowitz *et al.*, 1971), affects the rate of discharge of the vasomotor centre (Sweet *et al.*, 1971) and increase venomotor tone and thereby cardiac output (DuCharme *et al.*, 1968). In some tissues the presence of a PGE 9-ketoreductase which transforms PGE to PGF (Lee and Levine, 1974), if activated, would result primarily in pressor effects on stimulation of prostaglandin synthesis. These considerations demonstrate the inadvisability of reducing changes in prostaglandin production to a simple equation. Thus, increased prostaglandin production need not result in decreased renal vascular resistance nor decreased production in increased vascular resistance.

6.4.2 Mediators

6.4.2.1 Kinin-induced water excretion

Possible mediation by prostaglandins of the effects of vasoactive hormones on renal function was studied in terms of the actions of a known releaser of renal prostaglandins, bradykinin, on salt and water excretion. In this study conducted in the canine isolated blood-perfused kidney by McGiff *et al.* (1975), the effects of bradykinin were compared, for the reasons cited previously, to those of eledoisin. Each polypeptide was infused at a rate which increased blood flow to the isolated kidney by about one-third, from control values of 170 ml/min to 230 ml/min; simultaneously, fractional blood flow to the inner cortex increased by 12%. Despite similar haemodynamic responses to these agents, only the kinin increased solute free water excretion (Figure 6.11). A time-dependent decrease in urinary osmolality and increase in free water clearance (C_{H_2O}) occur in the isolated kidney (Berkowitz *et al.*, 1967). These changes were enhanced by the infusion of bradykinin. In contrast, infusion of eledoisin was associated with changes in urinary osmolality and solute free water excretion indistinguishable from the time-dependent alterations in the concentration of the urine. When changes in C_{H_2O} were expressed per 100 ml of glomerular filtration rate (GFR), differences between the effects of bradykinin and eledoisin before indomethacin administration became more pronounced; $C_{H_2O}/100$ ml GFR increased by a

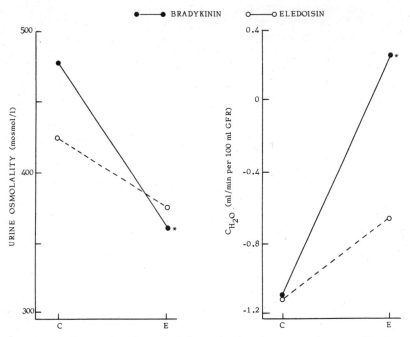

Figure 6.11 Changes in urine osmolality and solute free water clearance (C_{H_2O}) produced by either bradykinin or eledoisin. Refer to Figure 6.8 for explanation

mean of 1.31 ml/min ($p < 0.01$) during infusion of bradykinin, whereas an increase of 0.45 ml/min ($p > 0.05$) occurred during infusion of eledoisin (Figure 6.11). Mean plasma osmolality was unaffected by either agent. After administration of indomethacin, eledoisin and bradykinin either did not affect urinary osmolality or produced slight increases, although the low level of urinary osmolality at this time contributed to the failure of bradykinin to affect excretion of solute free water.

The effect of bradykinin on excretion of water was first described by Webster and Gilmore (1964). If these changes are related to the release of PGE-like substances within the kidney by the kinin, then inhibition of anti-diuretic hormone (ADH) by PGE_2 may contribute to the effects of bradykinin on water excretion. The ability of PGE to antagonize the effects of ADH on isolated collecting ducts was among the first demonstrations of modulation by a prostaglandin of the biological activity of a polypeptide (Grantham and Orloff, 1968). In the study of McGiff et al. (1975) ADH was added continuously in excess to the perfusate. This study also supports the proposal of Adetuyibi and Mills (1972) that there are two mechanisms affecting kallikrein release and hence kinin generation within the kidney. The first mechanism for which this study provides support is related to ex-cretion of water and is independent of changes in sodium excretion. Thus, before administration of indomethacin, bradykinin increased water excretion independently of sodium excretion; indeed in the face of a large reduction in sodium excretion urine flow increased,

The study also provides information on the contribution of renal prostaglandins to the natriuretic action of kinins. Although increased excretion of
sodium has been reported by many workers to occur in response to exogenous
prostaglandins of the E and A series (Johnston *et al.*, 1967; Vander, 1968;
Sinclair *et al.*, 1974; Fülgraff *et al.*, 1974), it need not follow that after the
release intrarenally of endogenous PGE_2 natriuresis will result. Indeed, there
is evidence to the contrary which suggests that in the distal nephron, and
particularly the collecting ducts, PGE_2 may promote sodium absorption.
Thus, stimulation of sodium transport by PGE_2 has been shown in the
isolated toad bladder (Lipson and Sharp, 1971) and mammalian collecting
ducts (Grantham and Orloff, 1968). As to the difficulties of reconstructing
the actions of an endogenous prostaglandin from the effects of the administered prostaglandin, it should be recalled that no route of administration
can reproduce the effects evoked by release of endogenous prostaglandins in
terms of concentrations achieved at their sites of action, vascular and tubular
elements initially affected, and the sequence of vascular and tubular elements
affected. For example, it is likely that release of prostaglandins from the
major sites of synthesis in the renal medulla effectively circumscribes their
activities to the distal nephron and medullary circulation under most conditions. In contrast, infused PGE_2 'sees' the proximal tubule first, a site which
may possibly be 'off-bounds' to most renal prostaglandins, although possibly not all, in view of the study of Larsson and Änggård (1973a) showing

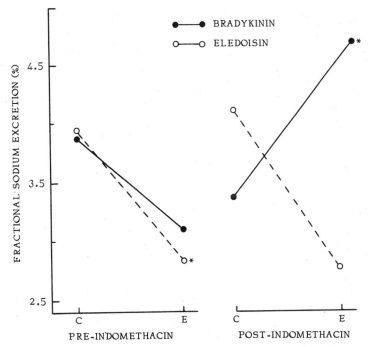

Figure 6.12 Changes in fractional sodium excretion expressed as percentage produced
by either bradykinin or eledoisin pre- and post-indomethacin. Refer to Figure 6.8 for
explanation

synthesis of prostaglandins by the renal cortex. The studies in the canine isolated kidney provide important clues to the possible contribution of prostaglandins to the changes in sodium excretion evoked by kinins. Before inhibition of prostaglandin synthesis, bradykinin usually did not affect sodium excretion, although decreases occurred due to decreased GFR. Thus, fractional excretion of sodium was not increased by bradykinin before indomethacin (Figure 6.12). Expression of sodium excretion in these terms i.e., as the fraction of the filtered load (Sodium excretion/GFR × plasma sodium concentration), takes into account variability of GFR. However, after inhibition of prostaglandin synthesis with indomethacin, bradykinin significantly increased both fractional, (3.3–4.7%) and total sodium excretion, the latter by two-fold. On the basis of this study it appears that under some conditions the prostaglandin released during administration of bradykinin, and presumably in response to increased intrarenal generation of kinins, will oppose the natriuretic effect of the kinin. The latter, in part at least, derives from the renal haemodynamic action of the kinin to which the released prostaglandin contributes, although the direct effect of the prostaglandin, perhaps at the level of the collecting ducts, is to promote sodium reabsorption. Despite the complexities of postulating a substance, PGE_2, released by renal kinins, having a haemodynamic action which amplifies, and a direct tubular action which could reduce the natriuretic–diuretic effects of kinins, the possibility exists that PGE_2 may contribute to modulation of the diuretic actions of kinins.

6.4.2.2 Prostaglandins as possible mediators of renal autoregulation

In the anaesthetized dog there is a continuous output of PGE_2 into the renal vein. The output is increased by various manoeuvres, including ischaemia (McGiff et al., 1970a), reduction in perfusion pressure (McGiff et al., 1970) and during reactive hyperaemia following release of renal arterial occlusion (Herbaczynska-Cedro and Vane, 1974). Reactive hyperaemia is increased by prior infusion of 0.9% sodium chloride and all but the initial brief overshoot is abolished by treatment with indomethacin. The contribution of intrarenal generation of prostaglandins to autoregulation of renal blood flow was studied by Herbaczynska-Cedro and Vane (1973). They found that the output of PGE material into venous blood increased as perfusion pressure decreased. Furthermore, the increase coincided with the vasodilatation which was associated with autoregulation. After indomethacin, the prostaglandin output and the autoregulatory vasodilatation were abolished.

If rapid biosynthesis and release of a prostaglandin contributes to renal autoregulation, what are the mechanisms involved? Blood flow to the cortex accounts for 85 to 95% of the total renal blood flow and autoregulation takes place primarily in the preglomerular resistance vessels (Thurau, 1964). However, most of the prostaglandin synthesizing enzyme is located in the renal medulla (Larsson and Änggård, 1973a). In discussing this point, Herbaczynska-Cedro and Vane (1974) suggest that a system may exist for transport of prostaglandins generated in the medulla to the cortex and put forward the possibility that the urine travelling up the ascending limb of the loop of Henle may be the transport system. There is evidence supporting this suggestion. Thus, prostaglandins, as well as their metabolites, have been definitively identified in the urine (Frölich *et al.*, 1973) and stimulation of prostaglandin synthesis in the isolated kidney by kinins results in an equivalent efflux of prostaglandins into urinary and venous effluents (Colina *et al.*, 1974). An alternative explanation is provided by the finding of Larsson and Änggård (1973a), viz. the renal cortex can synthesize prostaglandins, although at much lower rates than the renal medulla. In view of the potency of PGE_2, a small rate of production is all that is required, particularly if the site of synthesis is located near or within the vascular element, the afferent arteriole, which mediates autoregulation.

One criticism of the experiments of Herbaczynska-Cedro and Vane is that the majority of them were performed using kidney perfused with blood by an artificial pumping system. Under these experimental conditions the perfusion system may in some way exaggerate the contribution that prostaglandins make to renal autoregulation. Certainly, Ferreira *et al.* (1973) noted that in saline-perfused spleens, basal prostaglandin generation gradually increased as the experiment progressed. Similarly, Itskovitz and McGiff (1974) using blood-perfused kidneys, have shown that blood levels of prostaglandins increased considerably over a period of several hours; indeed, it is this increase in prostaglandin generation that enables renal perfusion to continue at high blood flows. Thus, the higher the background levels of vasodilator prostaglandins, the more likely the demonstration of a haemodynamic effect related to inhibition of their production. This explanation received support from a recent study of Terragno *et al.* (1975) who showed a PGE substance in renal venous blood of unanaesthetized resting dogs to be considerably less than in anaesthetized animals after surgery. The failure of McNay and Miyazaki (1973) to substantially influence renal autoregulation with indomethacin presumably is partially dependent on differences in renal levels of prostaglandins between their study and that of Herbaczynska-Cedro and Vane (1973). Thus, the study of McNay and Miyazaki (1973) did distinguish one component of the autoregulatory response of the kidney which was affected by indomethacin; namely, blood flow to the inner or juxtamedullary cortex which has important implications relative to a prostaglandin mechanism regulating, in concert with other factors, the intrarenal distribution of blood flow. This and other aspects of the renal haemodynamic actions of prostaglandins will be discussed again after a reconsideration of those mechanisms leading to activation of renal prostaglandins.

6.4.3 Stimulation of prostaglandin synthesis

That mechanical and hormonal stimuli which depress renal function are capable of stimulating prostaglandin synthesis was evident from most of the studies on the determinants of release of renal prostaglandins. The notable exceptions were the study by Terragno *et al.* (1972) on prostaglandin release by a potent renal vasodilator, bradykinin, and that by Needleman, Minkes and Douglas (1974) on stimulation of renal prostaglandin synthesis by adenosine nucleotides. Gagnon *et al.* (1974) showed in the rabbit isolated perfused kidney that the amount of prostaglandins released by angiotensin II was highly correlated with the elevation in perfusion pressure, although McGiff *et al.* (1970a, 1972) failed to show a high degree of correlation in the dog between the renal vasoconstrictor activity of either angiotensin II or norepinephrine and their capacity to release prostaglandins. Indeed the closest correlation, a negative one, exists between the amount of PGE_2 released and plasma renin activity suggesting that this step, activation of an acylhydrolase by the vasoactive hormone, is sodium-sensitive. Moreover, prostaglandins may be released by pressor hormones into the incubating medium from renomedullary tissue slices (Kalisker and Dyer, 1972) indicating that vaso-constriction is not indispensable to this action. Nonetheless, the importance of elevations in renal perfusion pressure as a stimulus to increased prosta-glandin production is seen on close inspection of three studies. In the first dopamine was shown to release prostaglandins from the rabbit isolated per-fused kidney only when substantial increases in renal perfusion pressure occurred, i.e. in concentrations one thousand times that of epinephrine (Needleman *et al.*, 1974). Comparison of two other studies revealed that nerve stimulation released renal prostaglandins only when renal perfusion pressure increased considerably. Thus, when renal blood flow was allowed to vary during renal nerve stimulation, the resulting moderate decreases in blood flow were not associated with prostaglandin release (McGiff *et al.*, 1972) although increasing the intensity of nerve stimulation under these experi-mental conditions will release prostaglandins (McGiff *et al.*, 1971). In the third study (Dunham and Zimmerman, 1970), renal blood flow was kept constant and perfusion pressure varied. Under these conditions, nerve stimulation greatly increased renal perfusion pressure which was associated with increased efflux of prostaglandins from the kidney. Inasmuch as renal nerve stimulation activates the renin–angiotensin system and releases nor-epinephrine from renal nerve endings, the possibility that one or more vaso-active hormones contributes to its effects on prostaglandin output seems likely.

The demonstration that vasoactive hormones induced release of prosta-glandins from an organ, i.e. result in *de novo* synthesis of prostaglandins, does not permit the conclusion that they directly affect prostaglandin synthesizing enzymes. Thus, a direct action of bradykinin on prostaglandin synthesis in the seminal vesicles could not be demonstrated (Damas *et al.*, 1973). Further, mepacrine, an anti-malarial agent which inhibits phospholipase A, prevented release of the products of prostaglandin synthetase from guinea pig lung, evoked by bradykinin, although the release evoked by arachidonic acid was not affected (Vargraftig and Dao Hai, 1972). These studies and that of Kunze and Vogt (1971), suggest that vasoactive hormones activate one or more acylhydrolases, such as phospholipase A, which results in substrate being made available to synthetase, thereby increasing synthesis of prostaglandins (Figure 6.9). Kalisker and Dyer (1972) have shown that phospholipase A stimulated the rate of release of prostaglandins from slices of rabbit renal inner medulla. An additional step has been suggested by Oates according to Zins (1975), whereby vasoactive hormones first increase adenylate cyclase activity which in turn results in phosphorylation and thereby activation of the lipase consequent to generation of cyclic AMP. Since most of the arachi-donic acid in the kidney is incorporated in phospholipids, there is good reason to consider induction of prostaglandin synthesis in terms of activation of phospholipase. However, the possibility of a triglyceride lipase having an important role in affecting the rate of renal prostaglandin synthesis cannot be dismissed since renal lipases may differ in their zonal or cellular distribution within the kidney as well as in their capacity to respond to different vasoactive hormones; e.g. bradykinin may activate a lipase which is unresponsive to norepinephrine.

The renal interstitial cells are extremely rich in lipid droplets containing arachidonic acid esterified to triglyceride (Nissen and Bojessen, 1969) and have been shown by Muirhead et al. (1972) to synthesize prostaglandins when they are grown in tissue culture. However, Larsson (1975) did not find either prostaglandins or synthetase activity in the lipid droplets, thus calling into question the significance of changes in granularity of the cells as an index of alterations in prostaglandin biosynthetic rate. Further, as indicated previously, there are other renal structures which are capable of synthesizing prostaglandins. Janszen and Nugteren (1971), using a histochemical method, identified the collecting ducts as the most active site of prostaglandin synthesis within the kidney. In addition, renal blood vessels are a potential site of prostaglandin synthesis in view of the high synthetic activity of bovine mesenteric blood vessels found by Terragno et al. (1975).

Vasoactive hormones may not only affect synthesis but also the functional consequences of enhanced prostaglandin production by activating an enzyme, PGE 9-ketoreductase, which determines the ratio of PGE_2 to $PGF_{2\alpha}$ (Figure 6.9). This additional action of kinins became apparent when bradykinin was shown by Terragno et al. (1975) to result in a selective increase of PGE in mesenteric arteries and of PGF in mesenteric veins. Simultaneous activation of an acylhydrolase and PGE 9-ketoreductase (converting PGE to PGF) provides the best explanation for increased production of PGF in veins, whereas in arteries activation of the acylhydrolase results in increased PGE which is not reduced since the 9-ketoreductase is not activated.

The capacity to stimulate renal prostaglandin synthesis has also been related to the renal vasodilator action of ethacrynic acid (Williamson et al., 1974) and has been suggested to contribute to the circulatory changes induced by endotoxin (Herman and Vane, 1974). Prostaglandins do not contribute to the renal vasodilator action of dopamine (Dressler et al., 1974).

6.5 PROSTAGLANDINS AND THE RENAL CIRCULATION

6.5.1 Resting renal blood flow

Renal prostaglandins are clearly capable of a defensive role, one that can protect renal function against excessive activity of pressor hormones. From this it has been assumed that the renal prostaglandin system remains dormant until challenged; in any event it could not be assigned a physiological role. On the other hand, a phenomenon that may be physiologically significant is that basal efflux of prostaglandins from the kidney of the chloralose-anaesthetized dog occurs in the absence of depressed renal function (McGiff et al., 1972). Concentrations of PGE_2 in renal venous blood were approximately 0.5 to 1.0 ng/ml in control periods after correction for losses incurred on solvent extraction and chromatographic separation. Since prostaglandins were assayed by their biological properties and in later studies by their immunoreactive properties, their identification cannot be considered certain; therefore the values are expressed as PGE_2 or $PGF_{2\alpha}$ equivalents. Renal venous concentrations of PGF were about one-half those of PGE in control periods and were not significantly affected by vasoactive hormones, unlike PGE which increased by as much as fifty-fold (McGiff et al., 1972). The presence of prostaglandins in renal venous blood in the 'resting' state in chloralose-anaesthetized dogs suggested that one or more prostaglandins may contribute to the regulation of the renal circulation.

Blood flow to any organ depends on the level of vascular tone, and generally speaking tone reflects the net effect of neurogenic vasoconstrictor discharge and metabolic activity. However, neither of these factors plays a major role in the kidney: neurogenic vasoconstrictor activity is negligible and blood flow is far in excess of metabolic needs (Smith et al., 1939). But might resting vasocular tone be dependent, at least partially, on continued production of renal PGE_2? Inhibition of prostaglandin synthesis with either indomethacin or meclofenamate was used to define a possible dependency of the resting renal circulation on the capacity of the kidney to synthesize prostaglandins in chloralose-anaesthetized dogs. Changes in renal blood flow measured with an electromagnetic flowmeter, were then correlated with renal prostaglandin efflux (efflux = blood flow × venous prostaglandin concentration). Within 15 min of administration of either synthetase inhibitor, mean concentrations of prostaglandin E and F had markedly declined; during the same period renal blood flow decreased by a mean of 45%, despite increased aortic blood pressure. Changes in renal blood flow and efflux of PGE (but not PGF) were correlated closely. The experiments were repeated by Itskovitz using the isolated kidney in which pulse rate, pulsatile perfusion pressure, blood gases, and chemical composition of the blood can be regulated to simulate physiologic conditions. Since extrarenal factors, i.e. humoral, venous or cardiac, that could contribute to changes in renal blood flow are eliminated, any change is attributable to factors of renal origin. The observed reduction in blood flow in the isolated preparation supported the suggestion that PGE_2 of renal origin contributes to resting blood flow to the kidneys through its effects on renal vascular tone (Lonigro et al., 1973).

This study has been confirmed by Kirschenbaum et al. (1974) in pentobarbital-anaesthetized dogs. However, in unanaesthetized resting dogs, indomethacin in similar doses to those used in the aforementioned studies did not reduce renal blood flow (Zins, 1975; Terragno et al., 1975). The study of Zins (1975) failed to give evidence of having achieved the desired effect with indomethacin: reduction in blood or tissue levels of prostaglandins. Thus, in the absence of these measurements, there is no reason to conclude that the unanaesthetized animal should respond to synthetase inhibitors as the anaesthetized surgically-prepared animal. Indeed, Terragno et al. (1975) have provided evidence that they do not, although in this study they show that the unanaesthetized dog has renal venous levels of PGE about one-sixth those of the anaesthetized dog, viz. 100–150 pg/ml versus 600–1000 pg/ml, respectively (values corrected for losses incurred on extraction and purification). However, this study does not answer the important question as to why prostaglandin synthetase inhibitors are unable to affect renal prostaglandin production in unanaesthetized dogs in doses which do so in the anaesthetized state after surgical manipulation.

It should be recalled that the prostaglandin synthetase complex varies in its biochemical and pharmacological profile (Flower and Vane, 1972). This may be decisive in determining its susceptibility to pharmacological interventions in those organs having several possible types of synthetases, i.e. renal cortical and medullary, or viewed differently: tubular, mesenchymal and vascular. Thus, prostaglandins may originate from one synthetase complex in the resting state, whereas under surgical stress another may be activated and make the largest contribution to an organ's output. This seems to be the case in the anaesthetized surgically-prepared dog in which blood flow to the inner cortex and thereby the renal medulla appears to be greatly increased (Itskovitz and McGiff, 1974) over that of the unanaesthetized dog at rest (Zins, 1975), presumably as a result of increased activity of renomedullary prostaglandin synthetase.

6.5.2 Distribution of renal blood flow

In view of the major localization of prostaglandin synthetase in the renal medulla and the relative absence of metabolizing enzymes in this zone (Larsson and Änggård, 1973a), it was hypothesized (McGiff and Nasjletti, 1973) that changes in prostaglandin synthetase affect blood flow primarily to the medulla and inner cortex. To define the zonal localization within the kidney of the vascular effects of altered synthesis of renal prostaglandins and thereby, to identify a possible determinant of the distribution of renal blood flow, use of inhibitors of prostaglandin synthesis allowed the intrarenal role of prostaglandins to be studied by subtraction methods: measurements of renal blood flow and its distribution before and after the addition of an inhibitor permitted the assessment of renal haemodynamics in the presence and in the absence of endogenous prostaglandins (Itskovitz et al., 1973). Furthermore, measurements of renal haemodynamics during infusions of PGE_2 after inhibition of prostaglandin synthesis provided insight into the separate activities of PGE_2 as a local hormone and a circulating hormone (Itskovitz et al., 1974). The infused prostaglandin would substitute for the loss of a circulating prostaglandin but not for the loss of a prostaglandin functioning as a local hormone, since, presumably, an exogenous prostaglandin cannot mimic the intrarenal actions of the corresponding endogenous prostaglandin in terms of specific localization of activity, sequence of vascular elements affected, or concentrations that can be achieved at sites of synthesis and release.

Concentrations of the PGE-like substance in the blood perfusing the isolated kidney increased during the first 3–4 h of perfusion and were associated with a progressive increase in renal blood flow, particularly the fraction to the inner cortex. The greatest rate of increase in renal blood flow and its inner cortical component occurred when the rate of increase in the perfusate concentration of the PGE-like substance was most rapid. Administration of either indomethacin or meclofenamate decreased the concentrations of

PGE in the perfusing blood by over 70%, associated with a decline in renal blood flow particularly its inner cortical component, the latter declining from 34% to 19%. Exogenous PGE_2 did not prevent the major haemodynamic effects of indomethacin, i.e. decreased blood flow to the inner cortex, indicating that loss of the local action of endogenous PGE_2 is the predominant factor in determining the effect of inhibition of prostaglandin synthesis on the distribution of renal blood flow.

A possible explanation for the decreased blood flow to the inner cortex produced by indomethacin becomes apparent on considering the anatomy of the renal circulation and loci of synthesis (medulla) and degradation (cortex) of prostaglandins in the kidney (Figure 6.13). This anatomic arrangement ensures high renomedullary concentrations of prostaglandins and favours the action of prostaglandins at these sites as local renal hormones. The efferent arterioles of the inner cortex, but not those of the outer cortex, extend into the medulla and give rise to the vasa recta (Fourman and Moffat, 1971). Thus, the inner cortical and the medullary circulations are interrelated and might be subject to the same vasodilator action of PGE_2 acting as a local hormone. In this regard, those influences which affect medullary synthesis of PGE_2, as indomethacin does in the present study, should preferentially alter inner cortical blood flow as well as medullary blood flow.

Further support for the finding that prostaglandins formed intrarenally affect primarily the vascular resistance of the inner cortical nephrons

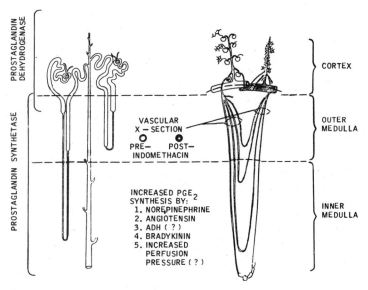

Figure 6.13 Nephrons having long and short loops of Henle are shown on the left. The origin of the renomedullary blood vessels (vasa recta) from the efferent arterioles of the juxtamedullary glomeruli is schematized on the right (after Fourman, J. and Moffat, D. B. (1971). Blood Vessels of the Kidney. Courtesy of Blackwell Scientific Publications, Oxford). The primary effect of inhibition of prostaglandin synthesis is indicated by a decrease in the diameter of the vasa recta as schematized in the vascular cross-sections. The prostaglandin-metabolizing and the prostaglandin-synthesizing enzymes are segregated, the former to the cortex and the latter to the medulla

(Itskovitz et al., 1973) was obtained by Larsson and Änggård (1974) in the rabbit, and by Chang et al. (1975) in the dog. In these studies arachidonic acid increased inner cortical blood flow selectively and this effect was abolished by indomethacin (Larsson and Änggård, 1974). In contrast infusions of PGE_2 increased blood flow to the outer as well as the inner cortex (Chang et al., 1975) associated with (in contrast to arachidonic acid) large increases in renal blood flow. These studies demonstrate once again the limitations of attempting to reconstruct the physiological roles of renal prostaglandins by administration of prostaglandins. The renin–angiotensin system was shown by Itskovitz and McGiff (1974) to participate in the regulation of blood flow to the same zone, the inner cortex, as affected by PGE_2. However, angiotensin I, rather than angiotensin II, is the renal hormone resulting from release of renin which affects the distribution of renal blood flow by decreasing blood flow to the inner cortex and medulla, the zones to which PGE_2 increases blood flow. In addition to antagonizing the haemodynamic effects of the renin–angiotensin system, one or more products of prostaglandin synthetase may affect the rate of angiotensin generation. Prostaglandins of the A series were reported to inhibit the rate of angiotensin production (Kotchen and Miller, 1974), whereas arachidonic acid was reported to increase its generation as indicated by increased plasma renin activity (Larsson et al., 1974). In contrast, indomethacin was found to decrease plasma renin activity. Thus, the findings of Larsson et al. (1974) that enhanced prostaglandin synthetase activity has an effect different from that of prostaglandins urges consideration that this action may be related to a cyclic endoperoxide (Änggård, personal communication) inasmuch as endoperoxides may differ from prostaglandins in their biological activities (Hamberg et al., 1974).

The capacity of angiotensin II in high doses to increase medullary blood flow coincidentally with reduction in total renal blood flow (Cross et al., 1974) may be related to increased release of medullary prostaglandins. A similar mechanism has been invoked by Itskovitz and McGiff (1974) to explain the effects of indomethacin on the renal haemodynamic response to angiotensin II. Before indomethacin, although angiotensin II decreased total renal blood flow, that component to the inner cortex sometimes increased. It is this component which connects with the medullary circulation. After indomethacin angiotensin II decreased blood flow to both the inner and outer cortex uniformly. Thus, the vasoconstrictor effects of angiotensin II on the inner cortical and medullary circulation are modified by the local prostaglandin level which is in part set by the amount of prostaglandin released by the pressor hormone. However, the usual response to angiotensin II is a decreased blood flow to both zones. On the other hand, the fact that angiotensin I selectively diminishes the fraction of blood flow to the inner cortex, as does renin substrate, suggests that it participates along with locally synthesized PGE_2 in regulating the renal circulation. In support of this proposal angiotensin I has been shown by Needleman et al. (1973) to have weak prostaglandin releasing activity as compared to angiotensin II. One arrives at a balanced mechanism to regulate the intrarenal circulation, with local PGE_2 increasing flow to the inner cortex and medulla, angiotensin I decreasing it. The two may thus be complementary intrarenal hormones—

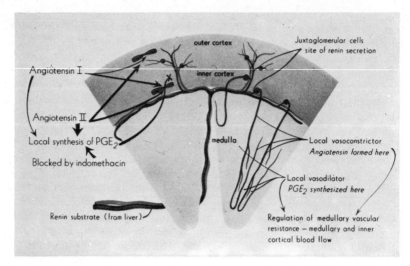

Figure 6.14   Schematic representation denoting potential roles of PGE_2 and the renin–angiotensin system as complementary regulators of the renal circulation

angiotensin I functioning as a local vasoconstrictor hormone, PGE_2 as a vasodilator (Figure 6.14).

The operation of a similar intrarenal mechanism during haemorrhage, as well as in response to other hypovolemic stimuli, seems likely whereby redistribution of renal blood flow follows stimulation of medullary prostaglandin synthesis mediated by one or more vasoactive substances arising within the kidney. Thus, in the dog haemorrhagic hypotension results in redistribution of renal blood flow from the outer to inner cortex effected by a mechanism intrinsic to the kidney (Stein *et al.*, 1973), conditions satisfied by activation of renal prostaglandin synthetase. The activity of renal prostaglandin synthetase under resting conditions is probably low which explains the considerable differences between inner cortical (and presumably medullary) blood flow in the unanaesthetized dog (Zins, 1975) and in the dog subject to anaesthesia and surgery (Kirschenbaum *et al.*, 1974; Itskovitz and McGiff, 1974). In this regard, those drugs which affect medullary synthesis of PGE_2, such as aspirin, indomethacin and other anti-inflammatory acids, preferentially decrease inner cortical and medullary blood flow. Indeed, the pathogenesis of the nephropathy and papillary necrosis associated with excessive use of analgesics has been related to medullary ischaemia resulting from inhibition of prostaglandin synthesis by the non-steroid anti-inflammatory analgesics (Nanra *et al.*, 1973).

Increased renal medullary blood flow may be a sufficient condition for the natriuresis which accompanies renal prostaglandin release (Tennenbaum *et al.*, 1975). Thus, an effect of PGE_2 could not be demonstrated on sodium reabsorption in the proximal tubules (Strandhoy *et al.*, 1974), although this demonstration may require selective application of the prostaglandin to one or the other surfaces of the tubular cells, mucosal or serosal, such as could only follow endogenous release (Leyssac *et al.*, 1974). The relevance of the demonstration that exogenous PGE_2 inhibits distal tubular sodium re-absorption (Fülgraff and Meiforth, 1971) in the rat to a possible direct action of endogenous PGE_2 on tubular transport is uncertain. Thus, large doses of PGE_2 were required: if smaller doses were effective, it took 30 min for this effect to be produced. Dunn (personal communication) could not show a direct effect of prostaglandins E_1, E_2 or A_1 on net fluxes of sodium, chloride and potassium in rabbit isolated renal cortical tubules. In addition the possibility of an action of prostaglandins which promotes sodium re-absorption in the collecting ducts must be considered, as indicated previously. At this time the most likely explanation for the natriuresis associated with endogenous prostaglandin release is based on the changes effected by PGE_2 in renal medullary blood flow. However, a direct renal tubular effect cannot be ruled out, although this action may even serve to mitigate the natriuresis associated with increased medullary blood flow.

6.6 MECHANISM OF THE BASAL OUTPUT OF RENAL PROSTAGLANDINS

The antecedents, hormonal or functional, which determine the basal efflux of renal prostaglandins remain to be identified. Synthesis of renal prosta-glandins under basal conditions is continuous and may contribute to the level of resting renal blood flow, particularly that component to the juxtamedullary cortex (Itskovitz et al., 1973). Two major vasoactive systems located intra-renally, the renin–angiotensin and kallikrein–kinin systems have been shown to affect the efflux of renal prostaglandins (McGiff et al., 1970b; McGiff et al., 1972). Of the two, the kallikrein–kinin system probably determines the level of activity of prostaglandin synthetase within the kidney under physiological conditions for several reasons:

(1) In the isolated kidney, at a time when renin substrate was deficient, and generation of angiotensin impaired, the concentration of PGE_2 in the perfusate continued to increase (Itskovitz and McGiff, 1974).

(2) Some of the renal actions of bradykinin, e.g. its effects on free water clearance are dependent on release of PGE_2. Since this action of bradykinin is 'physiological', functional coupling of prostaglandins and kinins intrarenally is suggested.

(3) The urinary excretion of PGE-like material in unanaesthetized rats, is reduced following administration of Trasylol, an inhibitor of kallikrein (Nasjletti, personal communication).

(4) A priori, a vasodilator–diuretic hormone, such as PGE_2, should be under the primary control of a system, the actions of which it may either support or amplify.

The coupling of these systems within the kidney may be unique: prosta-glandins mediate some of the actions of kinins and modulate others, while depending on the intrarenal generation of kinin to set their level and type of activity (Figure 6.9). Thus, not only production of prostaglandins but, the functional consequences within the kidney of their enhanced production as determined by the ratio of PGE_2 to $PGF_{2\alpha}$ may be subject to regulation by kinin originating intrarenally. It is here that a sodium-sensitive step is postulated, i.e. the capacity of kinin to activate PGE 9-ketoreductase is determined by the state of sodium balance. Whether or not a PGE or PGF compound primarily results from kinin generation intrarenally will be a major determinant of the effects of any given level of activity of the renal kallikrein–kinin system on salt and water excretion.

6.7 PGF$_{2\alpha}$: A VENOUS HORMONE?

Any comprehensive scheme of the role of renal prostaglandins should consider the relative inactivity of PGF$_{2\alpha}$ within the kidney (Tannenbaum *et al.*, 1975) as well as its capacity to constrict systemic veins (DuCharme *et al.* 1968), whereby, it may fulfil a coupling role between renal function and cardiac performance (Hinman, 1967). That is, PGF$_{2\alpha}$ may be released in response, to altered renal function in order to increase cardiac output. The determinants of PGF$_{2\alpha}$ synthesis intrarenally also remain undefined, since both pressor and depressor hormones result in selective release of PGE$_2$. The recent demonstration of a PGE 9-ketoreductase in the kidney (Lee *et al.*, 1975) suggests that conversion of PGE$_2$ to PGF$_{2\alpha}$ may effectively terminate the action of the former and provide an additional means of increasing the level of a prostaglandin, PGF$_{2\alpha}$, which elevates blood pressure. The systemic pressor action of PGF$_{2\alpha}$ is most probably due to increased cardiac output consequent to enhanced venous return resulting from an increase in venomotor tone although direct and reflex cardiovascular effects of PGF$_{2\alpha}$ may contribute to its pressor action. For example, PGF$_{2\alpha}$ facilitates release of the adrenergic neurotransmitter (Kadowitz *et al.*, 1971). In this regard, a substance affecting venous return and synthesized intrarenally may account for the earliest haemodynamic changes produced by ischaemia, i.e. increased cardiac output precedes heightened arteriolar tone (Ferrario *et al.*, 1970). In addition, local synthesis of PGF$_{2\alpha}$ by veins under the control of vasoactive hormones such as an angiotensin may supplement the effects on venomotor tone of PGF$_{2\alpha}$ released from the kidney, or provide an alternative means to regulate venomotor tone (Terragno *et al.*, 1975).

There are intriguing potential relationships which are only beginning to be explored between prostaglandins and other endocrine aspects of renal function. In view of the importance of prostaglandins as mediators and modulators of other hormones, one can predict a surge of interest in areas such as calcium metabolism and parathyroid hormones which are more elusive than those served by vasoactive hormones. Indeed important observations on the role of renal prostaglandins in the generation of erythropoietin have been made recently by Mujovic and Fisher (1974).

6.8 CLINICAL STUDIES

Most of these studies have been performed in hypertensive subjects in whom PGA$_1$ was infused intravenously (Carr, 1970; Lee *et al.*, 1971; Fichman *et al.*, 1972). Increased renal plasma flow without significant changes in GFR, accompanied by diuresis, natriuresis and kaliuresis, occurred during infusion of PGA$_1$. If large reductions in blood pressure occurred, the diuresis was attenuated or abolished (Lee *et al.*, 1971). The effects of PGA$_1$ have also been studied by Krakoff *et al.* (1973) in hypertensive man during salt depletion. Volume depletion diminished the systemic and renal haemodynamic responses to PGA$_1$ while enhancing its effects on plasma renin activity.

Thus, large increases in plasma renin activity probably contributed to blunting of the renal haemodynamic and excretory responses to PGA$_1$ which occurred during sodium depletion.

References

Adetuyibi, A. and Mills, I. H. (1972). Relation between urinary kallikrein and renal function, hypertension, and excretion of sodium and water in man. *Lancet*, 15, 203

Aiken, J. W. and Vane, J. R. (1973). Intrarenal prostaglandin release attenuates the renal vasoconstrictor activity of angiotensin. *J. Pharmac. Exp. Ther.*, 184, 678

Aiken, J. W. (1974). Effects of prostaglandin synthesis inhibitors on angiotensin tachyphylaxis in the isolated coeliac and mesenteric arteries of the rabbit. *Pol. J. Pharmacol. Pharm.*, 26, 217

Änggård, E., Bohman, S. O., Griffin III, J. E., Larsson, C. and Maunsbach, A. B. (1972). Subcellular localization of the prostaglandin system in the rabbit renal papilla. *Acta Physiol. Scand.*, 84, 231

Änggård, E., Larsson, C. and Samuelsson, B. (1971). The distribution of 15-hydroxy prostaglandin dehydrogenase and prostaglandin Δ^{13}-reductase in tissues of the swine. *Acta Physiol. Scand.*, 81, 396

Baudouin, M., Meyer, P., Fermandjian, S. and Morgat, J. L. (1972). Calcium release. induced by interaction of angiotensin with its receptors in smooth muscle cell microsomes. *Nature (Lond.)*, 235, 336

Bedwani, J. R. and Marley, P. B. (1975). Enhanced inactivation of prostaglandin E$_2$ by the rabbit lung during pregnancy or progesterone treatment. *Br. J. Pharmacol.*, 53, 547

Berkowitz, H. D., Miller, L. D. and Itskovitz, H. D. (1967). Renal function and the renin angiotensin system in the perfused kidney. *Am. J. Physiol.*, 213, 928

Blackwell, G. J., Flower, R. J. and Vane, J. R. (1975). Studies on the prostaglandin synthesizing system in rabbit kidney microsomes. *Biochem. Biophys. Acta.* (In press)

Bohman, S. O. and Larsson, C. (1975). Prostaglandin synthesis in membrane fractions from the rabbit medulla. *Acta Physiol. Scand.* (In press)

Carr, A. A. (1970). Hemodynamic and renal effects of prostaglandin, PGA$_1$, in subjects with essential hypertension. *Am. J. Med. Sci.*, 259, 21

Chang, L. C. T., Splawinski, J. A., Oates, J. A. and Nies, A. S. (1975). Enhanced renal prostaglandin production in the dog. *Circulation Res.*, 36, 204

Colina-Chourio, J., McGiff, J. C. and Nasjletti, A. (1975). Development of high blood pressure following inhibition of prostaglandin synthesis. *Fed. Proc.* (In press)

Colina, J., Miller, M. P., McGiff, J. C. and Nasjletti, A. (1974). Dependency of prostaglandin (PG) release on intrarenal generation of kinins. *Fed. Proc.*, 33, 339

Cross, R. B., Trace, J. W. and Vattuone, J. R. (1974). The effect of angiotensin upon the vasculature of the isolated perfused rat kidney. *Cl. Sci. Mol. Med.*, 46, 647

Crowshaw, K. (1971). Prostaglandin biosynthesis from endogenous precursors in rabbit kidney. *Nature New Biology*, 231, 240

Crowshaw, K. (1973). The incorporation of (1-^{14}C) arachidonic acid into the lipids of rabbit renal slices and conversion to prostaglandins E$_2$ and F$_{2\alpha}$. *Prostaglandins*, 3, 607

Crowshaw, K. and McGiff, J. C. (1973). Renal prostaglandins. Proc. Int. Conf. Mechan. Hypertension. In *Excerpta Medica*, M. P. Sambhi (ed.) (Excerpta Medica Foundation)

Crowshaw, K., McGiff, J. C., Strand, J. C., Lonigro, A. J. and Terragno, N. A. (1970). Prostaglandins in dog renal medulla. *J. Pharm. Pharmacol.*, 22, 302

Crowshaw, K. and Szlyk, J. Z. (1970). Distribution of prostaglandins in rabbit kidney. *Biochem. J.*, 116, 421

Damas, J., Bouridon, V., Neuray, J. et Deby, C. (1973). Bradykinine et biosynthese des prostaglandines *in vitro*. *Compte Rendus Soc. Biol.*, **167**, 787

Daniels, E. G., Hinman, J. W., Leach, B. E. and Muirhead, E. E. (1967). Identification of prostaglandin E_2 as the principal vasodepressor lipid of rabbit renal medulla. *Nature (Lond.)*, **215**, 1298

Davis, H. A. and Horton, E. W. (1972). Output of prostaglandins from the rabbit kidney: Its increase on renal nerve stimulation and its inhibition by indomethacin. *Br. J. Pharmacol.*, **46**, 658

Douglas, W. W. and Rubin, R. P. (1963). The mechanism of catecholamine release from the adrenal medulla and the role of calcium in stimulus–secretion coupling. *J. Physiol. (Lond.)*, **167**, 288

Doyle, A. E. and Fraser, J. R. E. (1961). Vascular reactivity in hypertension. *Circulation Res.*, **9**, 755

Dressler, W. E., Rossi, G. V. and Orzechowski, R. F. (1974). Evidence that renal vasodilation by dopamine in dogs does not involve release of prostaglandin. *J. Pharm. Pharmacol.*, **27**, 203

DuCharme, D. W., Weeks, J. R. and Montgomery, R. G. (1968). Studies on the mechanism of the hypertensive effect of prostaglandin $F_{2\alpha}$. *J. Pharmacol. Exp. Ther.*, **160**, 1

Dunham, E. W. and Zimmerman, B. G. (1970). Release of prostaglandin-like material from dog kidney during nerve stimulation. *Am. J. Physiol.*, **219**, 1279

Ferrario, C. M., Page, I. H. and McCubbin, J. W. (1970). Increased cardiac output as a contributory factor in experimental renal hypertension in dogs. *Circulation Res.*, **27**, 799

Ferreira, S. H., Moncada, S. and Vane, J. R. (1973). Some effects of inhibiting endogenous prostaglandin formation on the responses of the cat spleen. *Br. J. Pharmacol.*, **47**, 48

Ferreira, S. H. and Vane, J. R. (1967a). Prostaglandins: their disappearance from and release into the circulation. *Nature (Lond.)*, **216**, 868

Ferreira, S. H. and Vane, J. R. (1967b). The detection and estimation of bradykinin in the circulating blood. *Br. J. Pharmacol.*, **29**, 367

Fichman, M. P., Littenburg, B. A., Brooker, G. and Horton, R. (1972). Effect of prostaglandin A_1 on renal and adrenal function in man. *Circulation Res.*, **31 (Suppl. II)**, 19

Flower, R. J. and Blackwell, G. J. (1975). The importance of phospholipase-A_2 in prostaglandin biosynthesis. *Biochem. Pharmac.* (In press)

Flower, R. J., Cheung, H. S. and Cushman, D. W. (1973). Quantitative determination of prostaglandins and malondialdehyde formed by the arachidonate oxygenase (prostaglandin synthetase) system of bovine seminal vesicle. *Prostaglandins*, **4**, 325

Flower, R. J., Gryglewski, R., Herbaczynska-Cedro, K. and Vane, J. R. (1972). Effects of anti-inflammatory drugs on prostaglandin synthesis. *Nature New Biology*, **238**, 104

Flower, R. J., and Vane, J. R. (1972). Inhibition of prostaglandin synthetase in brain explains the anti-pyretic activity of paracetamol (4-acetamidophenol). *Nature (Lond.)*, **40**, 410

Fourman, J. and Moffat, D. B. (1971). Blood Vessels of the Kidney. p. 58 (Oxford: Blackwell Scientific Publications)

Frame, M. H., Hedqvist, P. and Åström, A. (1974). Effect of prostaglandin E_2 on vascular responses of the rabbit kidney to nerve stimulation and noradrenaline, *in vitro* and *in situ*. *Life Sci.*, **15**, 239

Frölich, J. C., Sweetman, B. J., Carr, K., Splawinski, J., Watson, J. T., Änggård, E. and Oates, J. A. (1973). Occurrence of prostaglandins in human urine. *Adv. Biosci.*, **9**, 321

Fülgraff, G., Brandenbusch, G. and Heintze, K. (1974). Dose response relation of the renal effects of PGA_1, PGE_2, and $PGF_{2\alpha}$ in dogs. *Prostaglandins*, **8**, 21

Fülgraff, G. and Meiforth, A. (1971). Effects of prostaglandin E_2 on excretion and reabsorption of sodium and fluid in rat kidneys (micropuncture studies). *Pflügers Arch.*, **330**, 243

Gagnon, D. J., Gauthier, R. and Regoli, D. (1974). Release of prostaglandins from the rabbit perfused kidney; effects of vasoconstrictors. *Br. J. Pharmacol.*, **50**, 553

Gocke, D. J., Gerten, J. Sherwood, L. M. and Laragh, J. H. (1969). Physiological and pathological variations of plasma angiotensin II in man. *Circulation Res.*, **24, (Suppl. 1)**, 131

Grantham, J. J. and Orloff, J. (1968). Effect of prostaglandin E_1 on the permeability response of the isolated collecting tubule to vasopressin, adenosine $3', 5'$-monophosphate, and theophylline. *J. Clin. Invest.*, **47**, 1154

Gryglewski, R. and Vane, J. R. (1972). The release of prostaglandins and rabbit aorta contracting substance (RCS) from rabbit spleen and its antagonism by anti-inflammatory drugs. *Br. J. Pharmacol.*, **45**, 37

Hamberg, M. (1969). Biosynthesis of prostaglandins in the renal medulla of rabbit. *FEBS Letters*, **5**, 127

Hamberg, M. and Samuelsson, B. (1974). Prostaglandin endoperoxides. Novel transformations of arachidonic acid in human platelets. *Proc. Nat. Acad. Sci. (USA)*, **71**, 3400

Hamberg, M. Svensson, J. and Samuelsson, B. (1974). Prostaglandin endoperoxides. A new concept concerning the mode of action and release of prostaglandins. *Proc. Nat. Acad. Sci. (USA)*, **71**, 3824

Hedqvist, P. (1970a). Studies on the effect of prostaglandins E_1 and E_2 on the sympathetic neuromuscular transmission in some animal tissues. *Acta Physiol. Scand. (Suppl.)*, **345** 1

Hedqvist, P. (1970b). Antagonism by calcium of the inhibitory action of prostaglandin E_2 on sympathetic neurotransmission in the cat spleen. *Acta Physiol. Scand.*, **80**, 269

Herbaczynska-Cedro, K. and Vane, J. R. (1973). Contribution of intrarenal generation of prostaglandin to autoregulation of renal blood flow in the dog. *Circulation Res.*, **33**, 428

Herbaczynska-Cedro, K. and Vane, J. R. (1974). Prostaglandins as mediators of reactive hyperaemia in the kidney. *Nature (Lond.)*, **247**, 402

Herman, A. G. and Vane, J. R. (1974). On the mechanism of the release of prostaglandins E_2 and $F_{2\alpha}$ in renal venous blood during endotoxin-hypotension. *Archs. int. Pharmacodyn. Ther.*, **208**, 365

Hinman, J. W. (1967). The prostaglandins. *Bioscience*, **17**, 779

Hollenberg, N. K., Solomon, H. S., Adams, D. F., Abrams, H. L. and Merrill, J. P. (1972). Renal vascular responses to angiotensin and norepinephrine in normal man. *Circulation Res.*, **31**, 750

Itskovitz, H. D. and McGiff, J. C. (1974). Hormonal regulation of the renal circulation. *Circulation Res. (Suppl. 1)*, **34 and 35**, 65

Itskovitz, H. D., Stemper, J., Pacholczyk, D. and McGiff, J. C. (1973). Renal prostaglandins: determinants of intrarenal distribution of blood flow. *Clin. Sci. Mol. Med.*, **45, (Suppl. 1)**, 321

Itskovitz, H. D., Terragno, N. A. and McGiff, J. C. (1974). Effect of a renal prostaglandin on distribution of blood flow in the isolated canine kidney. *Circulation Res.*, **34**, 770

Jaffe, B. M., Behrman, H. R. and Parker, C. W. (1973). Radioimmunoassay measurement of prostaglandins E, A, and F in human plasma. *J. Clin. Invest.*, **52**, 398

Janszen, F. H. A. and Nugteren, D. H. (1971). Histochemical localisation of prostaglandin synthetase. *Histochemie*, **27**, 159

Johnston, H. H., Herzog, J. P. and Lauler, D. P. (1967). Effect of prostaglandin E_1 on renal hemodynamics, sodium and water excretion. *Am. J. Physiol.*, **213**, 939

Jones, R. L. and Cammock, S. (1972). Purification, properties and biological significance of prostaglandin A isomerase. *Adv. Biosci.*, **9**, 61

Kadowitz, P. J., Sweet, C. S. and Brody, M. J. (1971). Potentiation of adrenergic venomotor responses by angiotensin, prostaglandin $F_{2\alpha}$ and cocaine. *J. Pharmacol. Exp. Ther.*, **176**, 176

Kalisker, A. and Dyer, D. C. (1972). *In vitro* release of prostaglandin from the renal medulla. *Eur. J. Pharmacol.*, **19**, 305

Kilcoyne, M. M. and Cannon, P. J. (1971). Neural and humoral influences on intrarenal blood flow distribution during thoracic caval occlusion. *Am. J. Physiol.*, **220**, 1231

Kirschenbaum, M. A., White, N., Stein, J. H. and Ferris, T. F. (1974). Redistribution of renal cortical blood flow during inhibition of prostaglandin synthesis. *Am. J. Physiol.*, **227**, 801

Kirtland, S. J. and Baum, H. (1972). Prostaglandin E_1 may act as a 'calcium ionophore'. *Nature New Biology*, **236**, 47

Kotchen, T. A. and Miller, M. C. (1974). Effect of prostaglandins on renin reactivity. *Am. J. Physiol.*, **226**, 314

Krakoff, L. R., De Guia, D., Vlachakis, N., Stricker, J. and Goldstein, M. (1973). Effect of sodium balance on arterial blood pressure and renal responses to prostaglandin A_1 in man. *Circulation Res.*, **33**, 539

Kunze, H. and Vogt, W. (1971). Significance of phospholipase A for prostaglandin formation. *Ann. N.Y. Acad. Sci.*, **180**, 123

Larsson, C. (1975). The renal prostaglandins. An experimental study in the rabbit. *Dept. Pharm., Karolinska Inst., Stockholm, Sweden*

Larsson, C. and Änggård, E. (1973a). Regional differences in the formation and metabolism of prostaglandins in the rabbit kidney. *Eur. J. Pharmacol.*, **21**, 30

Larsson, C. and Änggård, E. (1973b). Arachidonic acid lowers and indomethacin increases the blood pressure of the rabbit. *J. Pharm. Pharmacol.*, **25**, 653

Larsson, C. and Änggård, E. (1974). Increased juxtamedullary blood flow on stimulation of intrarenal prostaglandin biosynthesis. *Eur. J. Pharmacol.*, **25**, 326

Larsson, C. and Änggård, E. (1975). The renal prostaglandins. An experimental study in the rabbit. *Dept. Pharm., Karolinska Inst. Stockholm, Sweden*

Larsson, C., Weber, P. and Änggård, E. (1974). Arachidonic acid increases and indomethacin decreases plasma renin activity in the rabbit. *Eur. J. Pharmacol.*, **28**, 391

Leary, W. P., Ledingham, J. E. and Vane, J. R. (1974). Impaired prostaglandin release from the kidneys of salt-loaded hypertensive rats. *Prostaglandins*, **7**, 425

Lee, J. B. (1967). Antihypertensive activity of the kidney: The renomedullary prostaglandins. *New Engl. J. Med.*, **277**, 1073

Lee, J. B., Covino, B. G., Takman, B. H. and Smith, E. R. (1965). Renomedullary vaso-depressor substance, medullin: isolation, chemical characterization and physiological properties. *Circulation Res.*, **17**, 57

Lee, J. B., Crowshaw, K., Takman, B. H., Attrep, K. A. and Gougoutas, J. Z. (1967). Identification of prostaglandins E_2, $F_{2\alpha}$ and A_2 from rabbit kidney medulla. *Biochem. J.*, **105**, 1251

Lee, J. B., Hickler, R. B., Saravis, C. A. and Thorn, G. W. (1963). Sustained depressor effect of renal medullary extract in the normotensive rat. *Circulation Res.*, **13**, 359

Lee, J. B., McGiff, J. C., Kannegiesser, H., Aykent, Y. Y., Mudd, J. G. and Frawley, T. F. (1971). Prostaglandin A_1: antihypertensive and renal effects. *Ann. Intern. Med.*, **74**, 703

Lee, S. C. and Levine, L. (1974). Prostaglandin metabolism: I. Cytoplasmic reduced nicotinamide adenine dinucleotide phosphate-dependent and microsomal reduced nicotin-amide adenine dinucleotide-dependent prostaglandin E 9-ketoreductase activities in monkey and pigeon tissues. *J. Biol. Chem.*, **249**, 1369

Lee, S. C., Pong, S. S., Katzen, D., Wu, K. Y. and Levine, L. (1975). Distribution of prostaglandin E 9-ketoreductase and types I and II 15-hydroxyprostaglandin dehydro-genase in swine kidney medulla and cortex. *Biochemistry*, **14**, 142

Leyssac, P. P., Bukhave, K. and Frederiksen, O. (1974). Inhibitory effect of prostaglandins on isosmotic fluid transport by rabbit gall-bladder *in vitro* and its modification by blockade of endogenous PGE-biosynthesis with indomethacin. *Acta Physiol. Scand.*, **92**, 496

Lindsey, H. E. and Wyllie, J. H. (1970). Release of prostaglandins from embolized lungs. *Br. J. Surg.*, **57**, 738

Lipson, L. C. and Sharp, G. W. G. (1971). The effect of prostaglandin E_1 on sodium transport and osmotic water flow in the toad bladder. *Am. J. Physiol.*, **220**, 1046

Lonigro, A. J., Itskovitz, H. D., Crowshaw, K. and McGiff, J. C. (1973). Dependency of renal blood flow on prostaglandin synthesis in the dog. *Circulation Res.*, **32**, 712

Lonigro, A. J., Terragno, N. A., Malik, K. U. and McGiff, J. C. (1973). Differential inhibi-tion by prostaglandins of the renal actions of pressor stimuli. *Prostaglandins*, **3**, 595

Malik, K. U. and McGiff, J. C. (1975). Modulation by prostaglandins of adrenergic trans-mission in the isolated perfused rabbit and rat kidney. *Circulation Res.*, **36**, 599

Margolius, H. S., Horwitz, D., Geller, R. G., Alexander, J. R., Gill, J. R., Pisano, J. J. and Keiser, H. R. (1974). Urinary kallikrein excretion in normal man: relationships to sodium intake and sodium-retaining steroids. *Circulation Res.*, **35**, 812

Marumo, F. and Edelman, I. S. (1971). Effects of Ca^{++} and prostaglandin E_1 on vasopressin activation of renal adenyl cyclase. *J. Clin. Invest.*, **50**, 1613

McGiff, J. C., Crowshaw, K. and Itskovitz, H. D. (1974). Prostaglandins and renal function. *Fed. Proc.*, **33**, 39

McGiff, J. C., Crowshaw, K., Terragno, N. A. and Lonigro, A. J. (1970a). Release of a prostaglandin-like substance into renal venous blood in response to angiotensin II. *Circulation Res.*, **27 (Suppl. 1)**, 1073

McGiff, J. C., Crowshaw, K., Terragno, N. A. and Lonigro, A. J. (1970b). Renal prosta-glandins: possible regulators of the renal actions of pressor hormones. *Nature (Lond.)*, **227**, 1255

McGiff, J. C., Crowshaw, K. Terragno, N. A. and Lonigro, A. J. (1971). Renal prostaglandins: their biosynthesis, release, effects and fate. In *Renal Pharmacology*, Fisher, J. W. and Cafruny, E. J. (eds.), pp. 211–240 (New York: Appleton–Century–Crofts)

McGiff, J. C., Crowshaw, K., Terragno, N. A., Lonigro, A. J., Strand, J. C., Williamson, M. A., Lee, J. B. and Ng, K. K. F. (1970). Prostaglandin-like substances appearing ir canine renal venous blood during renal ischemia. Their partial characterization by pharmacologic and chromatographic procedures. *Circulation Res.*, **27**, 765

McGiff, J. C., Crowshaw, K., Terragno, N. A., Malik, K. U. and Lonigro, A. J. (1972). Differential effect of noradrenaline and renal nerve stimulation on vascular resistance in the dog kidney and the release of a prostaglandin E-like substance. *Clin. Sci.*, **42**, 223

McGiff, J. C. and Itskovitz, H. D. (1973). Prostaglandins and the kidney. *Circulation Res.*, **33**, 479

McGiff, J. C., Itskovitz, H. D. and Terragno, N. A. (1975). The actions of bradykinin and eledoisin in the canine isolated kidney: relationships to prostaglandins. *Cl. Sci. Mol. Med.* In press

McGiff, J. C. and Nasjletti, A. (1973). Renal prostaglandins and the regulation of blood pressure. In *Prostaglandins and cyclic AMP*, Lands, W. E. M. and Kahn, J. R. (eds.), pp. 119–149 (New York and London: Academic Press)

McGiff, J. C., Terragno, D. A., Terragno, N. A., Colina, J. and Nasjletti, A. (1975). Prostaglandins and their relationships to the kallikrein–kinin system. *In Chemistry and Biology of the Kallikrein–Kinin system in Health and Disease*, Pisano, J. J. (ed.) In press

McGiff, J. C., Terragno, N. A., Malik, K. U. and Lonigro, A. J. (1972). Release of prostaglandin E-like substance from canine kidney by bradykinin. Comparison with eledoisin. *Circulation Res.*, **31**, 36

McGiff, J. C., Terragno, N. A., Strand, J. C., Lee, J. B., Lonigro, A. J. and Ng, K. K. F. (1969). Selective passage of prostaglandins across the lung. *Nature (Lond.)*, **223**, 742

McNay, J. L. and Miyazaki, M. (1973). Effect of indomethacin on the renal circulation. *Proc. VI Am. Soc. Nephrol.*

Mills, I. H., MacFarlane, N. A. A. and Ward, P. (1974). Increase in kallikrein excretion during the natriuresis produced by arterial infusion of substance P. *Nature (Lond.)*, **247**, 108

Muirhead, E. E., Germain, G., Leach, B. E., Pitcock, J. A., Stephenson, P., Brooks, B., Brosius, W. L., Daniels, E. G. and Hinman, J. W. (1972). Production of renomedullary prostaglandins by renomedullary interstitial cells grown in tissue culture. *Circulation Res.*, **31**, (Suppl. II) 161

Muirhead, E. E., Jones, F. and Stirman, J. A. (1960). Antihypertensive property in renoprival hypertension of extract from renal medulla. *J. Lab. Clin. Med.*, **56**, 167

Mujovic, V. M. and Fisher, J. W. (1974). The effects of indomethacin on erythropoietin production in dogs following renal artery constriction. I. The possible role of prostaglandins in the generation of erythropoietin by the kidney. *J. Pharmacol. Exp. Ther.*, **191**, 575

Nanra, R. S., Chirawong, P. and Kincaid-Smith, P. (1973). Medullary ischemia in experimental analgesic nephropathy—the pathogenesis of renal papillary necrosis. *Aust. N.Z. Med.*, **3**, 580

Nasjletti, A., Colina-Chourio, J. and McGiff, J. C. (1975). Disappearance of bradykinin in the renal circulation of dogs: effects of kininase inhibition. *Circulation Res.* In press

Needleman, P., Douglas, J. R., Jakschik, B., Stoecklein, P. B. and Johnson, E. M. (1974). Release of renal prostaglandin by catecholamines: relationship to renal endocrine function. *J. Pharmacol. Exp. Ther.*, **188**, 453

Needleman, P., Kauffman, A. H., Douglas, J. R., Johnson, E. M. and Marshall, G. R. (1973). Specific stimulation and inhibition of renal prostaglandin release by angiotensin analogs. *Am. J. Physiol.*, **244**, 1415

Needleman, P., Minkes, M. S. and Douglas, J. R. (1974). Stimulation of prostaglandin biosynthesis by adenine nucleotides. *Circulation Res.*, **34**, 455

Nissen, H. M. and Andersen, H. (1968). On the localization of a prostaglandin-dehydrogenase activity in the kidney. *Histochemie*, **14**, 189

Nissen, H. M. and Bojesen, I. (1969). On lipid droplets in renal interstitial cells. IV. Isolation and identification. *Z. Zellforsch.*, **97**, 274

Rasmussen, H. (1970). Cell communication, calcium ion, and cyclic adenonine monophosphate. *Science*, **170**, 404

Samuelsson, B. (1963). Isolation and identification of prostaglandins from seminal plasma. *J. Biol. Chem.*, **238**, 3229

Samuelsson, B. (1973). Quantitative aspects of prostaglandin synthesis in Man. *Adv. Biosci.*, **9**, 7

Samuelsson, B., Granström, E. and Hamberg, M. (1967). On the mechanism of the biosynthesis of prostaglandins. *Prostaglandins, Proceedings of the second Nobel Symposium, Stockholm, June 1966.* Bergström, S. and Samuelsson, B. (eds.), pp. 31–44 (Stockholm: Almqvist and Wiksell)

Sinclair, R. J., Bell, R. D. and Keyl, M. J. (1974). Effects of prostaglandin E_2 (PGE$_2$) and histamine on renal fluid dynamics. *Am. J. Physiol.*, **5**, 1062

Smeby, R. R., Sen, S. and Bumpus, F. M. (1967). Naturally occurring renin inhibitor. *Circulation Res.*, **21**, 129

Smith, H. W., Rovenstine, E. A., Goldring, W., Chasis, H. and Ranges, H. A. (1939). The effects of spinal anaesthesia on the circulation in normal, unoperated man with reference to the autonomy of the arterioles, and especially those of the renal circulation. *J. Clin. Invest.*, **18**, 319

Stein, J. H., Boonjarern, S., Wilson, C. B. and Ferris, T. F. (1973). Alterations in intrarenal blood flow distribution: method of measurement and relationship to sodium balance. *Circulation Res.*, **21 (Suppl. I)**, 61

Stein, J. H., Boonjarern, S., Mauk, R. C. and Ferris, T. F. (1973). Mechanisms of the redistribution of renal cortical blood flow during haemorrhagic hypotension in the dog. *J. Clin. Invest.*, **52**, 39

Strandhoy, J. W., Ott, C. E., Schneider, E. G., Willis, L. R., Beck, N. P., Davis, B. B. and Knox, F. G. (1974). Effects of prostaglandins E_1 and E_2 on renal sodium reabsorption and Starling's forces. *Am. J. Physiol.*, **226**, 1015

Strong, J. C., Boucher, R., Nowaczyski, W. and Genest, J. (1966). Renal vasodepressor lipid. *Mayo Clinic Proc.*, **41**, 433

Sweet, C. S., Kadowitz, P. J. and Brody, M. J. (1971). A hypertensive response to infusion of prostaglandin $F_{2\alpha}$ into the vertebral artery of the conscious dog. *Eur. J. Pharmacol.*, **16**, 229

Tannenbaum, J., Splawinski, J. A., Oates, J. A. and Nies, A. S. (1975). Enhanced renal prostaglandin production in the dog. I. Effects on renal function. *Circulation Res.*, **36**, 197

Terragno, D. A., Crowshaw, K., Terragno, N. A. and McGiff, J. C. (1975). Prostaglandin synthesis by bovine mesenteric arteries and veins. *Circulation Res.*, **36 and 37**, (Suppl. 1), 76

Terragno, N. A., Lonigro, A. J., Malik, K. U. and McGiff, J. C. (1972). The relationship of the renal vasodilator action of bradykinin to the release of a prostaglandin E-like substance. *Experientia*, **28**, 437

Terragno, N. A., Nasjletti, A., Malik, K. U., Terragno, D. A. and McGiff, J. C. (1976). Renal prostaglandins. In Advances in Prostaglandin and Thromboxane Research, **Vol. 2**, Samuelsson, B. and Paoleth, R. (eds.) pp. 561–571 (New York: Raven Press)

Terragno, N. A., Terragno, D. A., Pacholczyk, D. and McGiff, J. C. (1974). Prostaglandins and the regulation of uterine blood flow in pregnancy. *Nature (Lond.)*, **249**, 57

Thurau, K. (1964). Renal hemodynamics. *Am. J. Med.*, **36**, 698

Thurston, H. and Laragh, J. H. (1975). Prior receptor occupancy as a determinant of the pressor activity of infused angiotensin II in the rat. *Circulation Res.*, **36**, 113

Tobian, L., O'Donnell, M. and Smith, P. (1974). Intrarenal prostaglandin levels during normal and high sodium intake. *Circulation Res.*, **34 and 35 (Suppl. I)**, 83

Van Dorp, D. A. (1971). Recent developments in the biosynthesis and the analyses of prostaglandins. *Prostaglandins symposium of the New York Academy of Sciences*, Ramwell, P. W. and Shaw, J. E. (eds.), 181

Vander, A. J. (1968). Direct effects of prostaglandin on renal function and renin release in anesthetized dogs. *Am. J. Physiol.*, **214**, 218

Vane, J. R. (1969). The release and fate of vasoactive hormones in the circulation. *Br. J. Pharmacol.*, **35**, 209

Vane, J. R. (1971). Inhibition of prostaglandin synthesis as a mechanism of action for aspirin-like drugs. *Nature New Biology*, **231**, 232

Vargaftig, B. B. and Dao Hai, N. (1972). Selective inhibition by mepacrine of the release of 'rabbit aorta contracting substance' evoked by the administration of bradykinin. *J. Pharm. Pharmacol.*, **24**, 159

Venuto, R. C., O'Dorisio, T., Stein, J. H. and Ferris, T. F. (1975). Uterine prostaglandin E secretion and uterine blood flow. *J. Clin. Invest.*, **55**, 193

Webster, M. E. and Gilmore, J. P. (1964). Influence of kallidin-10 on renal function. *Am. J. Physiol.*, **206**, 714

Wennmalm, Å. and Hedqvist, P. (1971). Inhibition of prostaglandin E_1 of parasympathetic neurotransmission in the rabbit heart. *Life Sci. (I)*, **10**, 465

Williamson, H. E., Bourland, W. A. and Marchand, G. R. (1974). Inhibition of ethacrynic acid induced increase in renal blood flow by indomethacin. *Prostaglandins*, **8**, 297

Zins, G. R. (1975). Renal prostaglandins. *Am. J. Med.*, **58**, 14

Zusman, R. M., Caldwell, B. V. and Speroff, L. (1972). Radioimmunoassay of the A prostaglandins. *Prostaglandins*, **2**, 41

Zusman, R. M. Spector, D., Caldwell, B. V., Speroff, L., Schneider, G. and Mulrow, P. J. (1973). Effect of chronic sodium loading and sodium restriction on plasma prostaglandin A, E and F concentrations in normal humans. *J. Clin. Invest.*, **52**, 1093

7
Prostaglandins and the Alimentary Tract

ALAN BENNETT

7.1 DISTRIBUTION, RELEASE AND METABOLISM OF PROSTAGLANDINS
     IN THE GUT   248

7.2 ACTIONS ON GUT MUSCLE   250

7.3 PERISTALSIS *in vitro*   252

7.4 MOTILITY *in vivo*   253

7.5 GASTRIC SECRETION   254
     7.5.1 *Rats*   254
     7.5.2 *Dogs*   256
     7.5.3 *Other laboratory animals*   257
     7.5.4 *Man*   258

7.6 GASTRIC BLEEDING WITH ASPIRIN-LIKE DRUGS   260

7.7 INTESTINAL ULCERATION   260

7.8 INTESTINAL SECRETION   261

7.9 INTESTINAL ABSORPTION   262

7.10 SALIVARY SECRETION   262

7.11 PANCREAS   262
     7.11.1 *Exocrine secretion and blood flow*   262
     7.11.2 *Insulin secretion*   263

7.12 THE BILIARY TRACT   264

7.13 PROSTAGLANDINS AS FACTORS IN DISEASE   265
     7.13.1 *Diarrhea*   265

7.13.2 *Cancer*   268
7.13.3 *Inflammation*   269
7.13.4 *The mouth*   269

ACKNOWLEDGEMENTS   269

REFERENCES   269

Since the chapter in the first edition of *The Prostaglandins: Progress in Research* was published (Bennett, 1972) there have been several other reviews of prostaglandins (PGs) and the gut (Wilson, 1972; Bennett, 1973; Main, 1973; Robert, 1973, 1974a; Waller, 1973; Karim and Ganesan, 1974a). These are in addition to the earlier surveys by Bass and D. R. Bennett (1968) and Bennett (1970), so it is unnecessary to discuss again all the work to date on the alimentary tract. Where appropriate in the present chapter, the basic information available up to 1972 is merely restated in general terms.

7.1 DISTRIBUTION, RELEASE AND METABOLISM OF PROSTAGLANDINS IN THE GUT

There has still been no formal characterization of the PG-like material extracted from the gut and it should therefore be referred to as 'PG-like'. E and F prostaglandins are the main types reported to occur in the gut, but PGA_2-like material has been found in human saliva and gastric juice (Peskar *et al.*, 1974). It is not known whether gut tissues (or indeed other tissues) form PGs only 'on demand' or if stores are present. This is a difficult point to answer, because regardless of the precautions taken, PG formation may occur during preparation or extraction procedures. Pretreating animals with inhibitors of PG synthesis may not solve the problem because inhibition may not be complete, and stores of PG might be used up prior to extraction. Evidence favouring the possibility that PGs are present in gut tissue is the presence of PG-like material in extracts of rat and guinea pig intestine frozen in liquid nitrogen immediately on removal (Stamford and Bennett, unpublished).

Information about the distribution of PGs in the gut has now increased. It was known in 1968 (Bennett, Murray and Wyllie) that the PGE_2-like material extracted from human stomach occurs mostly in the mucosa and submucosa, with less in the muscle layers. This was confirmed by Bennett *et al.* (1973) who assessed 'basal levels' of PGE_2 and the capacity to synthesize PG in all layers of the stomach. Sections of stomach wall cut parallel to the mucosa on a freezing microtome were homogenized in the presence of indomethacin or acid ethanol (to give 'basal' levels), or in Krebs solution alone to give 'basal' plus 'synthesized' amounts of PG. Relatively high 'basal' levels' and synthetic ability occurred throughout the mucosa and submucosa, with much less in the muscle layers. PG inactivation during the procedures was not measured and might have distorted these findings.

The presence of PG-like material in gastric juice and saliva has been confirmed, and this is discussed in Section 7.5.4. Nevertheless, it is still not clear whether the PG is secreted and/or whether it is released from dead or dying cells.

The PG distribution and type in human colon is different from that in the stomach. Extracts of colonic muscle contain more activity/g than the mucosa and submucosa, as judged by bioassay on the rat gastric fundus (Bennett *et al.*, unpublished). Furthermore, various PG-like compounds occur in the colon and the types sometimes differ between specimens. Most commonly found were substances resembling prostaglandins E_1, E_2, $F_{1\alpha}$, and material which runs slowly on chromatography in the AII system of Gréen and Samuelsson (1964). Prostaglandin $F_{2\alpha}$-like material occurred in the mucosa and submucosa of some specimens. Other tissues of the human alimentary tract which contain PGE-like material include pancreas and salivary glands (PGE$_2$ and PGF$_{2\alpha}$; Karim *et al.*, 1967) and ileum (PGE and/or PGF; Bennett and Stamford, unpublished).

In guinea pig and rat gut there are regional differences in the PG content and synthetic ability. The rat stomach, especially the antrum, can synthesize more PG-like material than the other regions, as judged by comparing activity in samples homogenized in Krebs solution and acid ethanol. In guinea pig gut the greatest amounts are found in the pyloric and ileal regions, but the content and synthetic ability seem less than in rat gut (Stamford and Bennett, unpublished). Rat isolated stomach and segments of hamster colon or guinea pig isolated ileum appear capable of synthesizing PGs from arachidonic acid, since contractions induced by this substance are inhibited by blocking PG synthesis (Vargaftig and Dao Hai, 1972; Tsai *et al.*, 1972).

There is now evidence in several papers that PG is released from isolated gut, and may contribute to the maintenance of muscle tone. Release of PGs probably indicates their formation (Piper and Vane, 1971), but since there is some evidence for 'basal' PG in the tissue, this might not be entirely true. The preparations studied include the longitudinal muscle of rabbit jejunum (Ferreira *et al.*, 1972), rat fundus (Eckenfels and Vane, 1972; Herman *et al.*, 1972; Bennett and Posner, 1971), guinea pig ileum and colon (Botting and Saltzmann, 1974; Gandini *et al.*, 1971; Herman *et al.*, 1972; Bennett *et al.*, 1975a), and human small intestine (Ganesan and Karim, 1973; Stockley and Bennett, 1976). In the circular muscle of guinea pig isolated ileum and colon, and in human gut, PGE release might keep the muscle relaxed (Bennett *et al.*, 1975a, and unpublished). Further indirect evidence that rat isolated gastric fundus releases PG comes from finding that polyphloretin phosphate 20–100 μg/ml caused dose-dependent contractions of the tissue (Bennett and Posner, 1971). Although this substance is a PG antagonist (Eakins *et al.*, 1970), it has little blocking effect on the rat fundus (Bennett and Posner, 1971): by contrast, it potentiates responses to PGs, apparently by inhibiting PG 15-hydroxy-dehydrogenase (Ganesan and Karim, 1973). Contraction of the tissue might therefore be due to potentiation of PG released in the tissue. Several of these *in vitro* experiments do not show the source of the PGs (they might be released within the muscle or the mucosa), but in the experiments with human tissue the mucosa and submucosa were removed. Some *in vivo* evidence favours a role for PGs in human cardiac sphincter tone. Indomethacin raised the pressure within the lower esophageal sphincter, and this is consistent with the possibility that synthesis of an inhibitory PGE compound was being prevented (Dilawari *et al.*, 1973, 1975). Aspects relevant to this will be discussed later (Section 7.4).

Human colonic cancer cells in tissue culture release more PGE-like material than normal mucosa, as shown by radioimmunoassay (see Jaffe, 1974, for references). Extraction experiments indicate that human colonic and rectal tumours contain and can synthesize more PG-like material than normal mucosa and submucosa from the same specimens (Bennett and del Tacca, 1975). However, PG inactivation was not studied in any of these experiments, and another (less likely) explanation might be greater inactivation of released PGs in normal tissue. Another interesting development on the formation of PGs within the gut and its relation to pathology, is the finding by Herman and Vane (1975) that intravenous injection of *Escherichia coli* endotoxin in rabbits increases the release of PG-like material from the isolated jejunum (see Section 7.13.1).

PGs seem to be metabolized rapidly in the gut, as previously shown in the rat by Parkinson and Schneider (1969). In the anaesthetized dog, absorption of PGE_1 can be demonstrated only after administering large amounts intraduodenally. 3 mg PGE_1/kg intraduodenally caused a fall in blood pressure and a four-fold rise in blood PGE_1 content coinciding with the maximal hypotension. 1 mg/kg PGE_1 did not lower the blood pressure (Barac *et al.*, 1972). Only small amounts of $PGF_{2\alpha}$ administered into the canine intestine reach the blood stream, although there are appreciable blood levels of 15(S)-methyl-$PGF_{2\alpha}$ given in this way. The methyl ester of this analogue is de-esterified in the mucosa (Robert *et al.*, 1974). It is also possible that certain analogues are metabolized in the human intestine (Nylander *et al.*, 1974).

7.2 ACTIONS ON GUT MUSCLE

Some 'new' gut muscle preparations have been suggested for bioassay and to aid identification. The hamster stomach seems to work on a 3 minute cycle, to have a low error, high precision and a sensitivity of about 1 ng/ml PGE_1 or PGE_2. Sensitivity to $PGF_{1\alpha}$ or PGA_1 was much lower (Ubatuba, 1973). Frog upper small intestine is inhibited by PGE_1 or PGE_2 but the suggestion that this could aid identification of PG-like material is hampered by the relatively high concentration needed (50 ng/ml) (Hudson, 1972). The circular muscle of guinea pig colon is inhibited by substantially lower concentrations (Fleshler and Bennett, 1969). The ability of PGE compounds to inhibit the circular muscle of the gut, but to contract the longitudinal muscle, has also been shown in rabbit (McKirdy, 1972), in addition to the previous demonstrations in various other species. The responses of the longitudinal muscle of the human fetal intestine to PGE_2 or $PGF_{2\alpha}$ generally resemble those in adult tissue. Contraction always occurred in the colon, and usually in the ileum. The sensitivities to PGE_2 and $PGF_{2\alpha}$ were usually: ileum 0.1 and 0.4 μg/ml respectively; colon 1 and 7 μg/ml respectively (Hart, 1974). Polyphloretin phosphate antagonized the responses at concentrations (80–160 μg/ml), lower than those required on adult intestine (Bennett and Posner, 1971).

Several new developments have occurred in our understanding of the effects of PGs on gut muscle. The similar pA_2 values (measurements of antagonism) obtained with the antagonist SC-19220 against PGE_2 and $PGF_{2\alpha}$ in the *longitudinal* muscle of guinea pig ileum had previously led to suggestion that both might act as the same receptors. Earlier studies also suggested that PGE_1 and PGE_2 were capable of stimulating both the longitudinal muscle and its cholinergic nerves within the ileal wall. It is now clear that $PGF_{1\alpha}$ and $PGF_{2\alpha}$ act similarly in this tissue, since responses to it are reduced by the neuron-blocking drug tetrodotoxin and by the cholinergic antagonist hyoscine (Bennett *et al.*, 1975a). The similar mode of action of PGE and PGF compounds supports the possibility that they act on the same receptors. Although this may not seem surprising, it should be remembered that there is strong evidence that more than one type of PG receptor exists in other tissues. For example, in the *circular* muscle of the gut it is usual for PGF compounds to cause contraction, whereas PGE compounds induce relaxation; antagonists of PG action block the excitatory effects of the PGE and PGF compounds but not the inhibitory responses to PGE compounds on the circular muscle (Bennett and Posner, 1971).

In the longitudinal muscle of guinea pig colon an even more complicated picture emerges. The contractions to prostaglandins E_1, E_2, $F_{1\alpha}$ and $F_{2\alpha}$ were reduced, but not prevented, by tetrodotoxin, suggesting both direct stimulation of the muscle and indirect stimulation of excitatory nerves. However, only the responses to the PGF compounds were significantly reduced by hyoscine (to about the same extent as with tetrodotoxin). It therefore appears that the nerves stimulated by the PGF compounds are cholinergic, but those stimulated by the E-type PGs are mainly non-cholinergic. Furthermore, PGE_1 seems more potent than PGE_2 in stimulating these non-cholinergic nerves, since tetrodotoxin reduced the response to PGE_1 more than to PGE_2 (Bennett *et al.*, 1975a).

PGs have been suggested as modulators of responses in various tissues, and this may be so with the cholinergic nerve supply to the longitudinal muscle of guinea pig ileum. Ehrenpreis *et al.* (1973) found that morphine, PG antagonists, or PG synthetase inhibitors reduced contractions of this tissue to electrical nerve stimulation: the effect was reversed by low concentrations of PGE_1 or PGE_2. They concluded that a PGE compound couples 'cholinergic nerve terminal excitation with acetylcholine release'. The argument seems logical with regard to morphine which acts in this tissue by inhibiting acetylcholine release at low frequencies of stimulation. However, the experiments with the PG antagonists are not so easy to understand. The doses of SC-19220 and polyphloretin phosphate used were more than sufficient to antagonize the excitatory effects of PGs (Bennett and Posner, 1971). Perhaps the antagonists caused non-selective depression, and the PGs stimulated receptors insensitive to these antagonists. The fact that PGs reversed the depressant effect of indomethacin on electrically mediated contractions, is also not sufficient evidence to support Ehrenpreis' conclusion. The high concentration (40 μg/ml) of indomethacin used inhibits responses of the tissue to various agonists, including histamine and acetylcholine which act directly on the muscle (Sorrentino *et al.*, 1972; Bennett *et al.*, 1975b). It therefore seems unlikely that PGE_2 only couples nerve excitation and acetylcholine release, although the indomethacin-induced depression was greater with nicotine or nerve stimulation at 0.1 to 4 H2 than with histamine or acetylcholine (Bennett *et al.*, 1975b). Chong and Downing (1974) reached a differently phrased conclusion from somewhat similar experiments with angiotensin in guinea pig ileum. Since low concentrations of PGE_2 reversed the inhibition of angiotensin-induced contractions by indomethacin (20 μg/ml), they suggested tentatively 'that some component of the contractile action of angiotensin II on the guinea pig ileum involves the release of prostaglandins'. Kadlec *et al.* (1974) showed in elegant experiments that low concentrations of indomethacin (0.36 μg/ml) reduced contractions due to indirectly acting stimuli (electrical nerve stimulation or angiotensin) but not to direct stimulation of the muscle by acetylcholine. A low concentration of PGE_2 (2.1 μg/ml) restored or (with electrical stimulation) increased the contractions. The effectiveness of this lower concentration of indomethacin favours the view that PGs are involved in the response to nerve stimulation in guinea pig ileum. Using Krebs solution as the bathing fluid, Bennett *et al.* (1975b) were unable to repeat their observations; only small reductions of responses occurred with 3.5 μg/ml indomethacin, 10 times the concentration used by Kadlec *et al.* (1974). However, with bathing solution used by Kadlec *et al.* (1974) which was modified in various ways (e.g. it lacked phosphate), Bennett *et al.* (1975b) reproduced their findings. These experiments may throw more light on the mechanism by which indomethacin inhibits PG synthesis than on the question of a PG link in nerve-mediated responses, but Bennett *et al.* (1975b) consider that PGs might modulate responses to various agonists. Since the effect of indomethacin is greater on nerve-mediated responses than on directly acting stimulants, PGs might be involved in nerve transmission.

7.3 PERISTALSIS *IN VITRO*

The initial finding that serosally applied PGE_1 or PGE_2 inhibits peristalsis in guinea pig isolated ileum (Bennett *et al.*, 1968a) was mainly confirmed by Radmanović (1972). However, he found an additional effect with low concentrations of PGE_1: 10–50 ng/ml first stimulated peristalsis and then inhibited it on washout. Only inhibition occurred with higher concentrations of PGE_1 (0.5–1 μg/ml). Perhaps the initial augmentation with low doses is due to potentiation of neurogenic contractions of the longitudinal muscle as suggested in Section 7.2, but the inhibitory effect on the circular muscle is dominant at higher concentrations. Radmanović also suggested that since the inhibition was less in reserpinized intestine, PGE_1 might act partly by releasing catecholamines. This does not fit in with the conclusion of Bennett *et al.* (1968b), although on re-examination of their Fig. 6 there might be a slightly reduced effect of PGE_2 on the circular muscle in the presence of α- and β-adrenoceptor blockers. Khairallah *et al.* (1967) suggested that PGE_1-induced relaxation of rat duodenum involves catecholamine release.

Both PGE and PGF compounds have been studied on peristalsis in guinea pig isolated ileum and colon, thus extending the observations of Bennett *et al.* (1968a). Their effects were not always consistent, but $PGF_{1\alpha}$

and $PGF_{2\alpha}$ applied serosally tended to increase peristaltic contractions of the circular muscle in the ileum and colon. Serosally applied PGE_1 or PGE_2 stimulated colonic circular muscle peristaltic contractions, in contrast to the inhibition obtained previously in the ileum (Bennett, Eley and Stockley, unpublished). Aspirin 20–$100\ \mu g/ml$ or indomethacin 1–$4\ \mu g/ml$ (but not polyphloretin phosphate or SC-19220) appear suitable for studying the role of PGs in the peristaltic reflex, because they have relatively little effect on responses to direct stimulation of the longitudinal muscle of guinea pig ileum or of its post-ganglionic cholinergic innervation. These inhibitors of PG synthesis applied serosally to guinea pig ileum or colon inhibited the peristalsis induced by raising the intraluminal pressure, and their effect was reversed by adding PGE_2. PGs might therefore contribute to peristaltic activity (Bennett, Eley and Stockley, unpublished).

In cat isolated intestine PGE_1 usually increased the intra-ileal pressure on the first dose, but subsequent doses produced only inhibition which was not affected by dehydroergotamine or reserpine (Türker and Onur, 1971). By contrast, they obtained only inhibition when E_1 was infused into the intestine *in situ*.

7.4 MOTILITY *IN VIVO*

In *dogs* PGE_1 0.01–$1\ \mu g/min$ infused intra-arterially decreased ongoing jejunal motility (Burns *et al.*, 1972). This agrees with the finding of Shehadeh *et al.* (1969), whereas $PGF_{2\alpha}$ increased jejunal motility (Shehadeh *et al.*, 1969). Chawla and Eisenberg (1969) found that PGE_1 inhibited antral motility. In cats too, PGE_1 $1\ \mu g/min$ infused intra-arterially inhibited motility in 80% of experiments and its effect was unaltered by dihydroergotamine, guanethidine, atropine, mepyramine, phentolamine, propranolol or methysergide (Türker and Onur, 1971). By contrast, Villanueva *et al.* (1972) found that PGE_2 $30\ \mu g/kg$ or $PGF_{2\alpha}$ 15–$30\ \mu g/kg$ given intravenously in cats stimulated intestinal motility. Perhaps this is because of differences in the PG used (E_2 versus E_1), its route of administration, or dose. These authors also obtained initial stimulation of intestinal motility with polyphloretin phosphate $200\ mg/kg$ intravenously. Perhaps this was due to inhibition of PG-15-hydroxy-dehydrogenase before PG receptors were blocked.

In rats $PGF_{2\alpha}$ 2 or $4\ mg/kg$ subcutaneously retarded gastric emptying, reduced small bowel propulsion and increased duodenal reflux (Nilsson and Ohrn, 1974). The effects of intravenously administered PGA_2, PGE_1 and $PGF_{2\alpha}$ 0.15–$8\ \mu g/kg$ have been studied on the lower esophageal sphincter of the lightly anaesthetized opossum. PGA_2 had little effect, PGE_1 always caused dose-dependent relaxations of the sphincter (maximal response to $2\ \mu g/kg$), and $PGF_{2\alpha}$ usually caused dose-dependent contractions of the sphincter (maximal response to $4\ \mu g/kg$), but sometimes relaxation or a biphasic response occurred (Goyal *et al.*, 1972; Rattan *et al.*, 1972). The response to PGE_1 was unaffected by phentolamine, propranolol, atropine or hexamethonium, but it was antagonized by nicotinic acid (which inhibits adenylate cyclase) or imidazole (which stimulates phosphodiesterase) (Goyal and Rattan, 1973). In man intravenous infusion of PGE_2 0.01–$0.08\ \mu g/kg$

per min did not affect the resting pressure of the cardiac (lower esophageal) sphincter, but it tended to inhibit the sphincter contracted by pentagastrin. In contrast, intravenous $PGF_{2\alpha}$ 0.05–0.8 $\mu g/kg$ per min (but not bolus injections of up to 40 $\mu g/kg$) caused dose-dependent increases in cardiac sphincter pressure. This did not seem to be mediated by gastrin release. $PGF_{2\alpha}$ did not impair the relaxation of the sphincter during swallowing, and no changes in gastric fundal pressure were recorded. Rectal administration of 200 mg indomethacin also raised the sphincter pressure, suggesting that formation of an inhibitory (E-type) PG had been inhibited. The authors suggested that release of an E-type PG in esophagitis might increase esophageal reflux and worsen the condition, and that analogues of PGF compounds might be useful in preventing reflux (Dilawari et al., 1973, 1975). $PGF_{2\alpha}$ infused intravenously in man (0.28–0.85 $\mu g/kg$ per min) inhibited the frequency of segmenting pressure waves in the jejunum, but the slowing of transit along the jejunum was not statistically significant. At the highest dose the pressure activity in the ileum was profoundly reduced, but there was no significant change in transit time. Nevertheless, jejunal and ileal flow rates increased. Most of the subjects experienced mild abdominal colic and passed copious watery stools due to stimulation of intestinal secretion (Cummings et al., 1973; Milton-Thompson et al., 1974). Intravenous infusions of PGE_2 0.08 $\mu g/kg$ per min for 20 min into human subjects inhibited motility of the sigmoid colon, whereas $PGF_{2\alpha}$ 0.8 $\mu g/kg$ per min had no significant effect. Nevertheless $PGF_{2\alpha}$ sometimes caused abdominal cramps (Hunt et al., 1975), and since it inhibits the small bowel and sigmoid colon, perhaps the colic arises from muscle contraction in the ileocaecal sphincter or colon proximal to the sigmoid region. The authors also suggested that inhibition of segmental contractions might facilitate onward propulsion and contribute to diarrhea.

The ability of PGs to produce diarrhea in man is well established. Indirect support that in man release of PGs within the gut can produce diarrhea comes from the finding that oral administration of 4 g polyphloretin phosphate caused diarrhea, possibly due to inhibition of PG-15-hydroxy-dehydrogenase (Karim, 1974; Karim and Ganesan 1974b). This effect either overrides any inhibition of PG action by polyphloretin phosphate, or the PG receptors involved are not reached by the drug or are insensitive to its action, since 2 g polyphloretin phosphate did not prevent the diarrhea induced by PGE_2 or $PGF_{2\alpha}$.

7.5 GASTRIC SECRETION

PGs have continued to be studied in a variety of species, and recent developments are of particular therapeutic interest.

7.5.1 Rats

In rats, like guinea pigs and cats, but unlike man and the dog, PGE_1 or PGE_2 applied to the gastric mucosa were previously shown to inhibit gastric acid secretion. This has been confirmed by Banerjee *et al.* (1972) who found in addition that PGE_2 bathing the mucosa was longer-acting than PGE_1. The drugs were equipotent intravenously but the inhibition of pentagastrin-stimulated acid secretion by PGE_1, but not PGE_2, was preceded by a rise.

PGE_2 0.05–5 mg given orally in an iso-osmotic buffer (Na_2HPO_4, pH 7.4) to pylorus-ligated rats decreased the acidity and acid output in the gastric juice but did not affect the volume secreted or protease activity. It inhibited ulcer formation in rats following pylorus ligation (0.05 mg/rat and above) or administration of reserpine (0.5 mg/rat) but doses up to 1 mg/rat did not affect steroid-induced ulcers (Lee *et al.*, 1973). These results differ from the findings of Robert *et al.* (1968) in two ways: these authors had found that PGE_1 administered subcutaneously inhibited the volume, H^+ concentration, pepsin output and fucose secretion (a measure of mucus secretion), and it inhibited prednisolone-induced ulcers.

Earlier reports that in the rat PGs do not act primarily by reducing mucosal blood flow have been confirmed. The ratio of mucosal blood flow (^{14}C-aniline clearance) to acid secretion always rose when PGE_1 or PGE_2 (1–2 $\mu g/kg$ per min) and PGA_1 or PGA_2 (4 $\mu g/kg$ per min) were infused intravenously (Main and Whittle, 1972a, b; Whittle, 1972). In some experiments where acid output was low, PGs increased clearance at a time when acid secretion was being inhibited.

Cyclic nucleotides have been increasingly implicated as the mechanism involved in rat gastric acid secretion and the response to PGs. Ramwell and Shaw (1968) found that cyclic AMP 10^{-4} M bathing the mucosa increased acid output and this effect was inhibited by PGE_1. Jawaharlal and Berti (1972) considered that since stimulation of acid secretion by dibutyryl cAMP (DBcAMP) in the rat was reduced by PGE_1 (1 $\mu g/ml$ per min in the gastric perfusate), this prostaglandin acts elsewhere than just on the adenylate cyclase. These authors reported also that cAMP and DBcGMP were ineffective on rat gastric acid secretion. Whittle (1972) found that the secretory effect of DBcAMP was greater when the stomach was made to secrete with pentagastrin or histamine, and intravenous or intraluminal PGE_2 only partly reduced the DBcAMP stimulation of gastric acid secretion. He considered that PGE_2 non-selectively lowered acid secretion by antagonizing cAMP formation and did not selectively block the action of DBcAMP. More recently Hohnke (1974) has shown that DBcAMP produces graded increases in acid secretion, and that inhibition of pentagastrin-stimulated acid secretion by PGE_2 can be almost completely prevented by administering DBcAMP. The inhibiting effect of PGE_1 in unanaesthetized rats was not due to inactivation of either histidine decarboxylase or histamine release in the stomach. In fact, repeated administration of PGE_1 elevated levels of histidine decarboxylase, but this may have been due to gastrin release when the gastric pH was lowered, since the effect was prevented by antrectomy (Liedberg and Håkanson, 1972; Håkanson *et al.*, 1973).

The importance of reducing acid secretion lies in gastric ulcer therapy, and inhibition of gastric and duodenal ulcer formation in rats by natural PGs is well established (Robert *et al.*, 1968). Recently, Usardi *et al.*, (1974) found that PGE_2, and to a lesser extent $PGF_{2\alpha}$, administered subcutaneously protects rats against stress-induced gastric ulcers. Indomethacin 5 mg/kg orally increased the severity of these ulcers and this effect was prevented by PGE_2. The mechanism by which indomethacin causes ulceration is not clear, but reduction of mucosal blood flow might be involved, and in the unanaesthetized rat this substance increases the acid secretion stimulated by pentagastrin or DBcAMP (Main and Whittle, 1973a, b). Usardi *et al.* (1974) found no increase in acid secretion during stress, but perhaps this was because of back-diffusion of H^+ through the mucosa (Davenport, 1965).

The search for anti-secretory PG analogues has expanded. Grossman and Doležal (1972) reported in an abstract that some substituted ω-cyclopentyl-straight chain fatty acids diminished acid and pepsin secretion in rats. Dol 7-ω(2-hydroxypentyl) hexanoic acid (dose not stated) reduced ulcer formation. Lee and Bianchi (1972) found that $\Delta^{8(12)13}$-PGE_1 inhibited ulcers in Shay rats (ED50 = 0.32 mg/kg p.o.) and exertion-induced ulcers (ED100 = 50 mg/kg p.o.), presumably by inhibiting acid secretion. Carter *et al.* (1974) studied the analogue 15-(R)-15-methyl-PGE_2 methyl ester (first found to inhibit acid secretion in human studies; Karim *et al.*, 1973a, b). Doses of 25 or 50 μg/kg in the gastric lumen of Shay rats reduced gastric and esophageal ulceration measured 21 h after pyloric ligation. The compounds may therefore be effective over many hours.

7.5.2 Dogs

Earlier work showing that intravenous PGE and A compounds in dogs inhibit gastric acid secretion has been verified by a number of workers. They have used various preparations and secretory stimuli, and have also studied the mechanism of action. More recently Reeder *et al.* (1972) found that PGE_1 15 μg/kg per hour infused intravenously for 90 min after eating, potentiated the rise in serum gastrin but inhibited acid output. They concluded that PGE_1 blocked the action of gastrin on the parietal cell, but it is clear that the antagonism could involve a variety of mechanisms. As in rats, the evidence again points to a primary effect on acid secretion rather than on blood flow (Wilson and Levine, 1972). PGE_1 1 or 2 μg/kg per min intravenously in conscious dogs caused a biphasic response in clearance of aminopyrine into the gastric juice, suggesting an initial shunting of blood from the mucosa, but clearance increased as inhibition of secretion became maximal. Intravenous PGE_2 in dogs reduced both acid and pepsin output but not acid concentration (Robert and Magerlein, 1973; Robert *et al.*, 1972). Nakano and Prancan (1972) measured total gastric blood flow in anaesthetized dogs. Intravenous PGE_1 or PGA_1 (1 μg/kg) decreased systemic arterial pressure, gastric artery perfusion pressure and peripheral resistance without causing alteration of the gastric venous pressure. By contrast, Wilson and Levine (1969) and Jacobson (1970) had obtained gastric mucosal vasoconstriction (probably as a result of reduced acid secretion). In an attempt to explain the difference, Nakano and Prancan (1972) pointed out that the other authors had studied a vasodilated system due to secretory stimulation, and that PGE_1 might redistribute blood from the mucosa to the other layers. A further difference is that the other authors used conscious dogs. In the dog isolated stomach PGE_2 5–100 μg/ml added to the perfusing blood caused an increase in total gastric blood flow but inhibited the secretory response to histamine, pentagastrin or vagal stimulation (Urquhart and Shaw, 1973).

As in man, PGE_2 in the dog gastric lumen does not affect gastric acid secretion (Shaw and Urquhart, 1972; Robert and Magerlein, 1973). This may be due to lack of absorption from the mucosal surface, as shown by studies with radiolabelled PGE_2 (Shaw and Urquhart, 1972). Nor is PGE_2 400 μg/kg (as the methyl ester) active by the intrajejunal route in dogs (Robert and Magerlein, 1973). However, the analogues 15(S)-methyl-PGE_2 methyl ester or 16,16-dimethyl-PGE_2 methyl ester inhibit histamine-induced acid secretion when given orally, intrajejunally or intravenously. The ED50 values for the methyl esters of PGE_2, 15(S)-15-methyl-PGE_2, and 16,16-dimethyl-PGE_2 were 10, 0.3 and 0.1 μg/kg with single intravenous injections. With oral administration of the 16,16-dimethyl analogue (20 μg/kg), inhibition of acid secretion started after 30 min and lasted several hours. It was 2.8 times as potent as the 15-methyl analogue given orally but caused vomiting; this did not occur with intrajejunal administration. Not only were the analogues more potent than intravenous PGE_2 but their effect was long-lasting by all routes of administration. Pepsin secretion was also inhibited by all three PGs (Robert and Magerlein, 1973). Vomiting with oral administration of 20 μg/kg 16,16-dimethyl-PGE_2 methyl ester in dogs was also observed by P. E. O'Brien and D. C. Carter (personal communication) and they found in addition that mild transient vomiting was common with 7.5 μg bolus intravenous injection. Furthermore, oral, but not intravenous, administration of the analogue damaged the mucosal barrier and caused a moderate but significant back-diffusion of H^+ and secretion of Na^+. The mechanisms for this undesirable action and for the inhibition of acid secretion seem likely to be different.

7.5.3 Other laboratory animals

Before discussing man we should first mention other species in which gastric secretion has been studied to some extent. Koch *et al.* (1972) concluded that in the cat intravenous PGE_2 first reduces mucosal blood flow, and reduction of acid secretion then follows. This differs from results in other species, but the authors accept that there might also be an effect directly on the parietal cell. Oral PGE_2 2.5 mg/kg or $\Delta^{8(12)13}$-PGE_1 (ED50 = 7.5 mg/kg) inhibited pentagastrin-induced ulcers in cats (Lee *et al.*, 1973; Lee and Bianchi, 1972). In the conscious gastric-fistula ferret PGE_1, 0.5 mg/kg subcutaneously inhibited *basal* acid secretion, but there was little effect on pentagastrin-stimulated secretion (Pfeiffer and Lewandowski, 1972). Perhaps this was because a maximal pentagastrin stimulus was used—clearly an inhibitory effect would be more obvious on a submaximal stimulus. In guinea pigs PGE_2 orally inhibited histamine- or pentagastrin-induced duodenal ulcers (0.2 and 0.5 mg/guinea pig respectively although doses of 0.8 or 1 mg were fatal in histamine-stimulated animals). (Lee *et al.*, 1973). Oral $\Delta^{8(12)13}$-PGE_1 inhibited duodenal ulcer formation with histamine or pentagastrin (ED50 = 3.2 and 75 mg/kg respectively, doses which are 10–230 times those effective in pylorus-ligated rats (Lee and Bianchi, 1972).

7.5.4 Man

Human gastric juice contains small amounts of bioassayable PGE-like material (2.4 ± 0.85 ng PGE_2 equivalents/ml in basal juice, 1.19 ± 0.28 ng/ml in secretion stimulated by pentagastrin or histamine), but it is not clear whether this is secreted and/or comes from dead or dying cells sloughed off from the mucosa (Bennett *et al.*, 1973). During stimulation with pentagastrin the concentration of PGE-like material fell, apparently due to dilution in a greater volume of secretion. This fact, together with the finding that indomethacin (200 mg rectally) did not increase acid secretion, was taken as tentative evidence that PGE_2 in human gastric mucosa does not have an inhibitory role in acid secretion. The conclusion depends on several assumptions, including the accessibility and sensitivity to indomethacin *in vivo*. Radioimmunoassay of PGs in gastric juice has produced rather similar results in three recent studies. Hinsdale *et al.* (1974) found that PGE-like activity was higher in the basal gastric juice of normal subjects than in asymptomatic duodenal ulcer patients, but the concentration in betazol-stimulated juice was not significantly different from normal in duodenal ulcer patients. The concentration of PGE-like material was higher in the venous plasma of normal subjects under basal or betazol-stimulated conditions. The total activity in the juice rose slightly during stimulation of acid secretion, but the concentration fell because of the greater volume of secretion. Tonnesen *et al.* (1974) found levels of 1.6 ± 0.19 ng/ml in normal basal gastric juice and again the concentration fell during secretion. The concentration tended to be lower than normal in the gastric juice of patients with duodenal ulcer (probably because of the greater volume), but this was not statistically significant. They considered it unlikely that PG deficiency plays a role in peptic ulcer disease. Interestingly, Tonnesen *et al.* (1974) observed a circadian fluctuation in PG output. In normal people peaks occurred at midday and midnight with a low output in the early morning, but no significant peaks occurred in duodenal ulcer patients. They raised the possibilities that the 'desynchronization' either contributes to the disease or occurs just because of ageing (the ulcer patients were older). Peskar *et al.* (1974) found PGA_2- and PGE_2-like material in human gastric juice, but little or no $PGF_{2\alpha}$. They thought that the PGA_2 was secreted as PGE_2 and converted in the gastric juice. A pH-dependent conversion of $^3H\text{-}PGE_2$ to PGA occurred in gastric juice, although Bennett *et al.* (1973) had found no loss of biological activity of PGE_2 incubated with 0.2M HCl at 37 °C for 45 min, and Lee *et al.* (1973) found that only 50% of PGE_2 in HCl pH 2 was destroyed in 48 h. Perhaps another factor besides HCl in the gastric juice aids the conversion. However, some of the PGA_2 might have come from the saliva which they found to be quite rich in this PG. Their basal levels of PGE_2- and PGA_2-like material in gastric juice were approximately 0.44 ± 0.05 and 0.15 ± 0.02 ng/ml respectively. The total output of PG increased during stimulation with pentagastrin but the concentration did not change. Unlike intravenous administration, oral PGE_1 or PGE_2 do not inhibit acid secretion in man (Horton *et al.*, 1968; Karim *et al.*, 1973a). However PGA_2 5–20 mg orally in man regularly inhibited gastric acid secretion, but PGA_1 10–50 mg or 15-epi-PGA_2

5–20 mg did not have any consistent effect (Bhana *et al.*, 1973). $PGF_{2\alpha}$ administered intravenously does not inhibit acid secretion (Newman *et al.*, 1975).

Karim *et al.* (1973a, b, c) showed that 16,16-dimethyl-PGE_2 methyl ester and both the R and the S configurations of 15-methyl-PGE_2 methyl ester given orally in man reduce basal gastric secretion; they also thought that mucus secretion was stimulated. The S derivative was a potent (25–50 μg dose) inhibitor of acid secretion but it sometimes produced nausea, whereas the R derivative (100–200 μg) and the 16-16-dimethyl analogue (200 μg) were free from side effects. The potency of the R derivative was surprising since it is thought to have low biological activity. It seems that the R form is converted in the stomach to the S form (A. Robert, personal communication), but perhaps no side effects occur since the conversion takes place in small amounts near to the site of action. It remains to be seen whether the analogues cause back-diffusion of H^+ as in the dog. Robert *et al.* (1974) confirmed that inhibition of gastric acid secretion occurred with 15(S)-15-methyl-PGE_2 methyl ester and 16,16-dimethyl-PGE_2 given orally to human subjects. Nylander and Andersson (1974) obtained similar results with these two compounds and with the 16,16-dimethyl PGE_2 methyl ester. All analogues produced a dose-dependent inhibition with an ED50 of about 40 μg/subject. The reduction was mainly due to inhibition of the volume secreted, but there was also a reduction in acid concentration. The analogues also tended to cause duodenal regurgitation, but this was not responsible for the decreased amount of acid. None of the analogues caused changes in blood pressure, heart rate or body temperature, but with 80 μg they sometimes caused slight abdominal discomfort. The authors suggested that Karim obtained no side effects with the 16,16-dimethyl analogue because he aspirated some of the dose after the 30 min contact with the gastric mucosa. Also in contrast to Karim *et al.* (1974a, c), they obtained a reduction of gastric juice volume. Experiments of Nylander *et al.* (1974) suggest that the analogues act locally on the human stomach. 16,16-dimethyl PGE_2 and its methyl ester (200 μg) given into the proximal small intestine were almost ineffective in man (in contrast to dogs), although 12.5 μg of the methyl ester is effective intravenously (Karim *et al.*, 1973c). The 15(S) compound administered intra-intestinally was less effective than after intragastric administration, and its effectiveness decreased with more distal administration. The authors suggested that rapid inactivation might occur in the intestine (supported by the onset of subjective side effects with 80 μg in the stomach but not with 200 μg in the duodenum, and by Karim's demonstration of activity with intravenous administration), and that the main site of absorption might be proximal to the lower duodenum. 15(R)15-methyl-PGE_2 methyl ester does not seem to act by inhibiting gastrin release. Indeed, blood levels of immunoreactive gastrin (heptadecapeptide antibody) usually rose, probably as a result of decreased gastric pH (Ganesan *et al.*, 1974).

The possible therapeutic value of 15(R)15-methyl PGE_2 methyl ester in peptic ulcer disease has been studied in man. Single oral doses in peptic ulcer patients elevated gastric pH and relieved epigastric pain and tenderness for more than 3 h (Fung and Karim, 1974). Furthermore, oral doses (150 μg) of this analogue every 6 h in Chinese patients with proven gastric ulceration was associated with substantial healing compared to controls given antacid (Fung, Karim and Tye, 1974; Fung, Lee and Karim, 1974).

7.6 GASTRIC BLEEDING WITH ASPIRIN-LIKE DRUGS

Aspirin-like drugs in contact with the gastric mucosa cause back-diffusion of H^+, and this might explain why gastric bleeding occurs (Davenport, 1965). An additional explanation was postulated by Bennett *et al.* (1973). They suggested that PG released within blood vessels walls or reaching them through the blood stream might help maintain vasodilatation, and that PG synthetase inhibitors might cause gastric mucosal vasoconstriction. Indomethacin is known to cause vasoconstriction in certain vascular beds, and there is accumulating evidence favouring a vasodilator role of PGE or PGA compounds present in blood. If the ensuing vasoconstriction were severe enough there could be local tissue ischaemia, tissue breakdown and bleeding, although fairly intense ischaemia does not break the gastric mucosal barrier in dogs (Davenport and Barr, 1973). Severe haemorrhage might occur with aspirin-like drugs only in tissues with a pre-existing tendency to ischaemia where a vasodilator effect of PGs is particularly important. This could explain why aspirin only rarely causes massive bleeding—more than one factor would have to be in operation for such a serious event to occur. Work in the dog (O'Brien and Silen, 1973) has shown that perfusion of 20 mM aspirin through denervated fundic pouches reduced mucosal blood flow (aminopyrine clearance) to $57 \pm 12\%$ of control. This might represent almost complete ischaemia in some regions, particularly since instillation of aspirin without perfusion reduced values to $29 \pm 9.6\%$. Although there was also back-diffusion of H^+, this did not seem responsible for the reduction in blood flow. Application of aspirin to denervated gastric pouches in dogs stimulated submaximally with pentagastrin may reduce mucosal blood flow, although to a lesser extent (Bennett, Curwain and Holton, unpublished). It may be that only non-steroidal anti-inflammatory drugs absorbed by the stomach cause gastric bleeding: aspirin particles in contact with the mucosa cause bleeding, but aspirin given in an alkaline solution (Alka Seltzer) which ensures absorption only in the small intestine does not do so (Bouchier and Williams, 1969; Leonards and Levy, 1969). Nor does paracetamol which is basic and virtually unabsorbed in the stomach. Perhaps the acidic compounds (aspirin, indomethacin, phenylbutazone, etc.) which are absorbed in an acid environment might diffuse to the mucosal blood vessels in high concentrations when particles of the drug are in contact with the gastric mucosa. Might a small amount of a PGE analogue added to unbuffered aspirin-like drugs counteract the gastric bleeding?

7.7. INTESTINAL ULCERATION

In rats, administration of indomethacin (10 mg/kg orally for 2 days or 4 mg/kg subcutaneously for 4 days) or flufenamic acid (100 mg/kg subcutaneously twice daily for 4 days) caused severe intestinal ulceration. Administration of various PGs or their analogues subcutaneously caused dose-related inhibition of the ulceration with the following ED50 values against indomethacin-induced ulcers: $PGE_2 = 0.3$; $PGF_{2\alpha} = 5$; $PGB_2 = 7.5$ $\mu g/kg$ per min); 16,16-dimethyl analogues of $PGA_2 = 1$; $E_2 = 0.4$; $PGF_{2\alpha} = 0.5$ mg (twice daily) (Robert, 1974b). Robert suggested that the ulcers were caused by inhibition of PG synthesis.

7.8 INTESTINAL SECRETION

It is well established that PGs stimulate intestinal secretion. This contrasts with their inhibition of gastric acid secretion. In anaesthetized dogs, the accumulation of fluid in the jejunum following PGE_1 0.01–1 $\mu g/min$ intra-arterially was accompanied by vasodilatation in the arteries and small blood vessels. There was also a decrease in ongoing jejunal motility which is discussed in Section 7.4 (Burns *et al.*, 1972). The effect of PGE_1 and PGE_2 on electrical activity has been studied in the rat and hamster jejunum and colon (Eggenton *et al.*, 1974). PGE_1 or PGE_2 0.05–6 μg intravenously caused a dose-dependent transient increase in the potential difference in the jejunum and colon. In the rat, theophylline did not affect the jejunal response to PG but it increased the maximal response of the colon. In everted isolated sacs of rat and hamster intestine with muscle layers removed, 'submucosally' applied PGs caused an increase in potential difference without altering the resistance, but the sensitivity was 20–60 times lower than *in vivo*. PGE_1 or PGE_2 10 μg in the fluid bathing the serosal surface of everted hamster jejunum reduced fluid transfer, suggesting that the potential difference increased due to electrogenic anion secretion rather than enhanced cation absorption.

Intrajejunal PGE_1 0.9 $\mu g/kg$ per min in human subjects reversed the net absorption of water and electrolytes into profuse secretion (Matuchansky *et al.*, 1972; Matuchansky and Bernier, 1973). This might explain the diarrhea obtained with oral PGE_1 (Horton *et al.*, 1968; Misiewicz *et al.*, 1969), but Matuchansky and Bernier (1972) found no increase in jejunal transit time. When they used mannitol instead of glucose in the perfusate, the PGE_1-induced secretion of water and sodium was decreased. No studies have been reported with intrajejunal PGE_2 but a similar effect would be expected since PGE_2 given orally can cause diarrhea (Karim, 1971), and both PGE_1 and PGE_2 stimulate rabbit intestinal adenylate cyclase (Kimberg *et al.*, 1971). These authors also obtained a modest stimulation with prostaglandins A_1, B_1, $F_{1\beta}$ and $F_{2\beta}$, but $F_{1\alpha}$ and $F_{2\alpha}$ had little or no effect. However, Kantor *et al.* (1974) reported that PGA_1 inhibits rabbit intestinal adenylate cyclase, whereas PGE_1 causes activation.

Studies in man have shown stimulation of secretion with $PGF_{2\alpha}$ in the small intestine, but colon function was not significantly affected. Net secretion of Na^+, Cl^- and water occurred in the jejunum and ileum respectively when $PGF_{2\alpha}$ 0.81–0.85 or 0.65–0.86 $\mu g/kg$ per min was infused intravenously. The ileum thus appeared a little more sensitive than the jejunum, but in neither case was the effect observed until 30–40 min after the start of the infusion. The intraluminal flow rate increased in both regions, and bicarbonate was secreted into the ileum in 3 out of 4 subjects (Cummings *et al.*, 1973; Milton-Thompson *et al.*, 1975). Measurements of motility recorded in these studies are discussed in Section 7.4. In later studies $PGF_{2\alpha}$ (0.4 μg/kg per min) increased the ileal flow rate, as did PGE_2 (0.08 and 0.1 μg/kg per min) in both patients studied. Since there was no significant change in colonic absorptive function with either PG, the diarrhea was presumably of small intestinal origin (Milton-Thompson *et al.*, 1974; Milton-Thompson *et al.*, 1975).

7.9 INTESTINAL ABSORPTION

Prostaglandins E_1, E_2 or $F_{2\alpha}$ perfused for 20 min through rat small intestine at an initial concentration of 1.4×10^{-4} M reduced the absorption of glucose. A tenth of this concentration was without effect (Coupar and McColl, 1972). These levels are high and may have no physiological or even pathological significance, but perhaps they were rapidly reduced by metabolism. A lower concentration of PGE_1 infused into the human jejunum (0.9 μg/kg per min) reduced glucose absorption by 25% (Matuchansky and Bernier, 1973). The effects of intravenous PGs on absorption of this and other substances remain to be determined.

7.10 SALIVARY SECRETION

In the anaesthetized dog, $PGF_{2\alpha}$ 1–16 μg/kg caused a dose-related salivation. PGE_1 by contrast was without effect. $PGF_{2\alpha}$ seemed to be stimulating post-ganglionic parasympathetic nerves since its effect was potentiated by eserine, prevented by atropine and unaffected by ganglion blockade (Hahn and Patil, 1972, 1974).

7.11 PANCREAS

Studies have been made on both the exocrine and endocrine secretion from the pancreas.

7.11.1 Exocrine secretion and blood flow

In conscious dogs PGE_1 0.5–50 μg/kg as single intravenous injections (ED50 = 23 μg/kg) or infusions of 0.5–5 μg/kg per min (ED50 = 1.8 μg/kg per min) inhibited volume and bicarbonate secretion from the gland at rest or during stimulation with secretin or secretin and pancreozymin. In contrast, enzyme output was stimulated, but PGE_1 was less effective than pancreozymin (Rudick *et al.*, 1971). The same picture emerged in anaesthetized dogs with PGE_2 0.05–0.4 μg/kg per min during submaximal pancreatic stimulation with secretin (G. Glazer, personal communication). $PGF_{2\alpha}$ 0.4 μg/kg per min however, slightly increased the volume of juice and stimulated enzyme secretion, but the bicarbonate output varied only with juice volume. Pancreatic blood flow measured by ^{133}Xe, was depressed by PGE_2 or $PGF_{2\alpha}$ 0.2 µg/kg per min given intra-aortically. Blood flow changes might therefore explain the depression of juice volume by PGE_2 but not the slight increase with $PGF_{2\alpha}$ (G. Glazer, personal communication). The situation in anaesthetized cats differs in some respects from dogs, and furthermore, different results occur *in vivo* and *in vitro*. As in dogs, PGE_1 or PGE_2 (0.5–10 µg intra-arterially) *in vivo* during stimulation with secretin, usually reduced both pancreatic blood flow (probably reflexly due to a fall in systemic blood pressure) and secretion. However, this was sometimes preceded by a transient increase in blood flow and secretion. In the saline-perfused cat isolated pancreas prostaglandins E_1, E_2, $F_{1\alpha}$ or $F_{2\alpha}$ 1–10 µg intra-arterially as single injections or 0.12 µg/min always stimulated water and electrolyte secretion ($E_1 = E_2 \gg F_{1\alpha} = F_{2\alpha}$). Theophylline potentiated these responses, indicating the involvement of cyclic AMP. There was no increase of enzyme (amylase) secretion (Case and Scratcherd, 1972). Enzyme release was increased in guinea pig pancreatic slices by PGE_1 0.1 µg/ml and from the rat pancreas *in vivo* by PGE_1 1 µg/kg. The response was greater and qualitatively different *in vivo* when pancreozymin was also given, but the hormone had no further effect *in vitro* (Gabryelewicz et al., 1974). PGs might affect pancreatic blood flow in the rat since PGE_2 reduced and $PGF_{2\alpha}$, PGB_1 and PGB_2 increased vascular resistance in the rat isolated perfused pancreas (Saunders and Moser, 1972a, b).

In man (three patients) the trypsin concentration in the ileal contents during small intestinal perfusion fell by roughly a third when $PGF_{2\alpha}$ was infused intravenously (0.4 or 0.8 µg/kg per min), but there was almost a 3-fold increase in the volume of fluid secreted by the small intestine (Milton-Thompson et al., 1975).

7.11.2 Insulin secretion

The effect of PGs on insulin is far from clear—they have been reported to increase, decrease or have no effect on its secretion *in vitro* or *in vivo*. In anaesthetized dogs PGE_1 0.5 or 1 µg/kg per min lowered both the systemic blood pressure and the pancreatico–duodenal vein haematocrit. Total insulin output was unchanged during the PGE_1 infusion but increased when the infusion was stopped (Lefebvre and Luyckx, 1973). In contrast, Robertson (1974) found that insulin secretion, stimulated by glucose administration, was lowered (together with the blood pressure) by PGE_1 or PGE_2 10 µg/min infused intravenously. This did not seem to involve α-adrenoceptors since intravenous phentolamine 0.2 mg/kg per min did not alter the effect. Lastly, in dogs, PGA_1 0.25 µg/kg per min intravenously did not alter basal insulin secretion but it impaired the secretory response to glucose. Since there was no change in superior mesenteric artery blood flow this did not seem to explain the effect of PGA_1 but a change in pancreatic microcirculation could not be excluded (Sacca et al., 1973).

In rat isolated pancreatic islet cells, the increased release of insulin by PGE_1 1 µg/ml was not statistically significant (Vance et al., 1971), and PGE_1

or PGA_1 10^{-4} M were also ineffective (Rossini et al., 1971). By contrast, Johnson et al. (1973) showed that E_1, 10^{-8} to 10^{-5} M increased the release of insulin during stimulation with glucose and theophylline, and increased the content of cAMP. PGE_2 and $PGF_{2\alpha}$ also approximately doubled insulin release, but high concentrations (10^{-4} M) were needed. PGA_1 10^{-4} M was ineffective, and none of the PGs stimulated basal insulin release. The authors explain the difference between their results and those of Vance et al. (1971) and Rossini et al. (1971) on the basis of (a) the glucose concentration used (PGs stimulated at 3 mg/ml glucose but not at 0.3 mg/ml), (b) the presence of theophylline, and (c) the lower effectiveness of PGE_1 above 10^{-5} M than at this concentration. Since then the situation has become even more complex. Burr and Sharp (1974) found that PGE_1 0.3 ng/ml stimulated release of insulin from rat islets in vitro in the presence of 0.5 mg/ml glucose, but it reduced the release by glucose 3 mg/ml. However, the inhibition by epinephrine of glucose-induced insulin secretion was reversed by PGE_1. In anaesthetized rats intracardiac injection of 5 μg PGE_1 had no significant effect on plasma insulin levels (Hertelendy et al., 1972). Johnson et al. (1974) went on to show that in homogenates or membrane preparations of rat isolated pancreatic islets 10 μM PGE_1 or guanosine 5'-triphosphate slightly stimulated adenylate cyclase, but had no effect on phosphodiesterase. Adenylate cyclase activity doubled when both substances were given together. In the presence of 20 μM guanosine 5'-triphosphate the effect of PGE_1 was evident at 0.2 μM, and PGE_2 or PGA_1 10 μM slightly increased adenylate cyclase activity.

In mice 2.5 and 5 μg PGE_1 intraperitoneally raised plasma insulin levels, and since this was reduced by β-receptor blockade (0.5 mg MJ 1999 intraperitoneally) the authors suggested that β-adrenoceptors were involved in the action of PGE_1 (Bressler et al., 1968). In conscious sheep, E_1 20 μg/kg intravenously had no effect on plasma insulin levels (Hertelendy et al., 1972) and in women in the last month of pregnancy there was no change with PGE_2 or $PGF_{2\alpha}$ infused intravenously at rates up to 2.4 and 20 μg/min respectively (Spellacy et al., 1971).

7.12 THE BILIARY TRACT

Extracts of human gallbladders, removed at cholecystectomy for cholelithiasis, contain PGE- and PGF-like material in both mucosa and muscle (Wood and Stamford, 1974). Similar PG-like fractions have been isolated from guinea pig gallbladder (Wood and Stamford, personal communication). Isolated gallbladder strips from the cat and guinea pig were contracted by prostaglandins E_1, E_2 or $F_{2\alpha}$. This was associated in the guinea pig with increased phosphodiesterase activity and decreased cyclic AMP levels (Andersson et al., 1973). In the anaesthetized cat, PGE_2 3–5 μg/kg intravenously increased the gallbladder pressure (Anderson et al., 1973), and PGE and PGF compounds increased the intravesicular pressure in guinea pig isolated gallbladder (Morton et al., 1974). In contrast, the cat isolated sphincter of Oddi was relaxed by PGE_1 or PGE_2 whereas $PGF_{2\alpha}$ relaxed some preparations and contracted others. PGE_2-induced relaxation of the sphincter

was associated with an increase in tissue cAMP content, but since phosphodiesterase activity also increases, the change in cAMP presumably reflects an
activation of adenylate cyclase (Andersson *et al.*, 1973). Electromyographic
and pressure studies on the rabbit sphincter demonstrate contractile effects
with $PGF_{2\alpha}$ and inconsistent relaxant effects with PGE_1 or PGE_2 (Sakaki
et al., 1974).

Since PGE_2 can mimic the effects of cholecystokinin on the gallbladder
and sphincter of Oddi, experiments were done with the C-terminal octapeptide of cholecystokinin (C8-CCK) and arachidonic acid, indomethacin,
SC-19220 and polyphloretin phosphate. These indicate that local synthesis
and release of PGs play no essential role in the contractile effect of C8-CCK
in guinea pig gallbladder (Andersson *et al.*, 1974). It is therefore not known
whether PGs play a physiological role in the biliary tract. Nevertheless, direct
actions of PGs on this region might contribute to the presence of large
amounts of bile in gastric aspirates following oral administration of PGE_1
(Horton *et al.*, 1968). This PG relaxes the circular muscle of the human
stomach *in vitro* (Bennett, Murray and Wyllie, 1968) and inhibits the motility
of the pyloric antrum of the dog *in vivo* (Chawla and Eisenberg, 1969).
PGE_1-induced evacuation of the gallbladder and relaxation of the pylorus
might both play a part in bile reflux. The importance of pyloric relaxation
is not clear since PGE_2 analogues and $PGF_{2\alpha}$ cause gastric reflux in the rat,
(a species which has no gallbladder, Main and Whittle, 1974; Nilsson and
Ohrn, 1974); pyloric relaxation might be expected with the PGE analogues
but probably not with $PGF_{2\alpha}$.

In the guinea pig isolated gallbladder, serosally applied prostaglandins
E_1, E_2 or $F_{2\alpha}$ produced a dose-dependent inhibition of net fluid absorption,
PGE_1 and PGE_2 being more potent than $PGF_{2\alpha}$ (Morton *et al.*, 1974;
Heintze *et al.*, 1974). PGA compounds and arachidonic acid also caused a
dose-dependent inhibition of gallbladder fluid transport, and all the PGs
tested inhibited transport when applied mucosally (Wood, Saverymuttu and
Morton, personal communication). Thus, endogenous PG-like substances in
the gallbladder might influence the rate at which fluid is transported across its
epithelium. Human gallbladders which fail to visualize radiologically have
raised mucosal PG levels, and this non-visualization may reflect a pathological inhibitory effect of PGs on gallbladder fluid transport (Wood and
Stamford, 1974).

7.13 PROSTAGLANDINS AS FACTORS IN DISEASE

PGs have been implicated in various gut diseases including diarrhea, carcinoma and inflammation.

7.13.1 Diarrhea

The mediation of PGs in various types of diarrhea has still not been firmly
established. Several reports have suggested the involvement of PGs in
medullary carcinoma of the thyroid, since blood levels of PG-like activity

were raised (Williams *et al.*, 1968; Kaplan *et al.*, 1973; Jaffe *et al.*, 1973; Jaffe, 1974) but others have not confirmed this (Van Dorp, 1971; Melvin *et al.*, 1972; Feldman and Plonk, 1974). However, 2 of the 12 patients in the latter study did show a modest elevation of blood $PGF_{2\alpha}$-like material, and in the work of Melvin *et al.* (1972) the sensitivity of the assay may have been too low. The finding of raised PG levels in peripheral blood is surprising in view of the expected metabolism in the lungs and elsewhere. Barrowman *et al.* (1975) found that blood PG-like activity was higher than normal in a patient with pulmonary metastases, but it could be argued that here the PG-like material was released distally to its site of inactivation in the lung. This patient's diarrhea responded to nutmeg (which among other things seems to be a potent inhibitor of PG synthesis (Bennett *et al.*, 1974). In another case of medullary carcinoma of the thyroid reported recently, the plasma PG concentration was elevated (to 3.6 ng/ml E_2 equivalents) on only one of 4 occasions. The patient's jejunal electrolyte transport was normal, but the ileum was unable to absorb Na^+ and Cl^- against a concentration gradient. Indomethacin 50 mg three times daily for 8 weeks or aspirin 600 mg three times daily for 4 weeks had no effect on the frequency or volume of the stools, although indomethacin returned the ileal transit time to normal (Isaacs *et al.*, 1974). Again, a raised blood PG level would only be expected if the released PG were not broken down by the lungs, and even then only if the tumour secreted constantly. Measurements of PG metabolites in blood (Feldman and Plonk, 1974) or urine would therefore be a better indication of PG secretion by tumours.

Other tumours associated with changed bowel activity in which PG release has been implicated include neural crest and carcinoid tumours (Sandler *et al.*, 1968; Jaffe, 1974).

Work in the rat and cat (Jacoby and Marshall, 1972; Finck and Katz, 1972) support the possibility of PG involvement in the diarrhea of cholera. Some studies in other species contradict this view, but in many cases the arguments have not been completely water-tight, and sometimes there is a great tendency to extrapolate from one tissue to another. *In vitro* studies on rabbit intestine (Kimberg *et al.*, 1974) showed that maximal stimulation of cyclic AMP levels by cholera enterotoxin was not significantly inhibited by indomethacin under conditions where mucosal PG synthesis was inhibited. Their conclusion that PG does not provide an essential link in the action of the toxin on rabbit isolated intestine seems justified, but do these results rule out a *contribution* by PGs which might be released? Indomethacin tended to reduce cyclic AMP formation in some tests (their Table IV) and might this have been more evident with submaximal stimulation by cholera toxin? Perhaps not, since PGE_1 still produced an effect after maximal stimulation of cAMP formation by cholera toxin, even though both PG and the toxin activate adenylate cyclase. However, does this apply to PGE_2 or $PGF_{2\alpha}$ (thought to occur in rabbit intestine) (Ambache *et al.*, 1966), their precursors or metabolites? Evidence from several sources indicates that precursors or metabolites are sometimes more active than the respective PGs. Overall there was an increased release of PG-like material when cholera toxin was incubated *in vitro* with rabbit intestine but there were only four tests and the results were clearly not significant (Kimberg *et al.*, 1974). The rate of inactivation of

PG by the tissue might be important, but the possibility that cholera toxin alters this was not investigated. The toxin seemed to have a variable effect on PG inactivation by human and guinea pig ileum, but when this was taken into account, it seemed unlikely that cholera toxin released PGs from the isolated tissues (Bennett and Charlier, unpublished). Nevertheless, it still remains possible that the toxin can release PGs from other parts of the gut (e.g. proximal small intestine) of man or other species, either *in vivo* or *in vitro*. The importance of *in vivo* studies is shown by Herman and Vane (1975) who injected *E. coli* endotoxin intravenously in rabbits and then removed the intestine. This treatment increased the release of PG from the isolated intestine but there was no effect with normal intestine incubated *in vitro* with the toxin. They considered that combination with a blood component, possibly complement, was essential for the PG-releasing action. Since cholera toxin or a choleragenic agent may be absorbed from the intestine (Vaughan-Williams *et al.*, 1969) *in vivo* studies are essential.

It seems likely that cholera toxin can stimulate cyclic AMP formation without the mediation of PGs, as shown in some of the papers referred to above and elsewhere (Bourne, 1973; unpublished work of Field, using turkey erythrocytes which contain little if any PG, cited in Kimberg *et al.*, 1974). But this does not exclude the possibility that in some tissues cholera toxin stimulates cAMP formation at least in part by the release of PG. Indeed, some work *in vivo* with cholera toxin, besides that cited earlier, supports this view. Valiules and Long (1973) found that indomethacin 2.5 mg/kg caused a 20% inhibition of intestinal fluid secretion induced in guinea pigs and rabbits by crude cholera toxin. Dlugolecka (1974) states that indomethacin did not affect cholera-induced secretion in rabbits, but re-calculation of her graphical data shows a statistically significant reduction at 2 h. Gots *et al.* (1974) found that indomethacin (3×10 mg/kg doses subcutaneously) in rabbits significantly reduced (by 40–63%) the secretion induced by pure or crude cholera toxin or live *Vibrio cholerae*. Moroever, the last injection of indomethacin was made 10 h before killing the animals, so that little may have been present in the last few hours. However, having made this observation they argue from the data of Bourne (1973) and Kimberg *et al.* (1974) that indomethacin must have acted by a non-PG pathway. Indomethacin undoubtedly has many other actions besides inhibition of PG synthesis, but the evidence certainly does not exclude a possible role for PGs in cholera in the rabbit. Gots *et al.* (1974) also studied other toxins which are discussed later. Lastly, in man, De *et al.* (1974) showed only a small reduction of fluid output in cholera patients treated with the anti-inflammatory drug ibuprofen. Although they did not give any statistical data, the effect was obviously not significant. This is probably good indirect evidence against a major role of PGs in cholera in man, but a serious short-coming is that ibuprofen has not been shown to inhibit PG synthesis in human gut. Inhibition is likely, but it is by no means certain; PG synthetases differ markedly in their sensitivities to inhibitory drugs (Flower and Vane, 1972). Furthermore, it is not known how much of the ibuprofen was vomited.

The situation with endotoxins seems much clearer: it seems likely that they release PGs in other regions (e.g. brain in fever), and several studies have shown elevated blood levels of PG-like material in endotoxin shock (e.g.

Anderson et al., 1972). The endotoxin-induced diarrhea in mice might have been due to $PGF_{2\alpha}$; it was prevented by indomethacin 2 mg/kg, and also by cyproheptadine 5 μg/kg which the authors suggest inhibits PG release (Harper and Skarnes, 1972; Skarnes and Harper, 1972). Indomethacin 10 mg/kg given to rabbits 3 h before inoculating intestinal loops with *Salmonella typhimurium*, and then twice more at 7 h intervals (last indomethacin injection 10 h before killing the animal), almost prevented intestinal fluid secretion. The effect of *Shigella flexneri* (and *Vibrio cholerae*) was reduced by about 60 % (Gots et al., 1974). Of particular interest is the observation that the greatest reduction occurred with the organism (*S. typhimurium*) that invaded the mucosa and caused local inflammation. Herman and Vane (1975) injected *E. coli* endotoxin (100 μg/kg intravenously) into rabbits and found that release of PG-like material from the isolated jejunum removed 2 h later was significantly increased compared to non-injected controls (37.6 ± 3.7 ng PGE_2 equivalents/g wet weight released in 30 min compared to 7.2 ± 1.5 ng/g). Pretreatment with indomethacin (2 mg/kg intravenously 30 min before, simultaneously with, and 60 min after the endotoxin injection) reduced the PG release (from 44.8 ± 12.6 ng PGE_2 equivalents/g wet weight to 7.6 ± 1.5 ng/g). However, addition of *E. coli* endotoxin to the organ bath (100 μg/ml) did not release PGs from control jejuna (including everted preparations where the mucosa was more exposed). The authors considered that PG release by endotoxin required interaction with a blood component, possibly complement.

Diarrhea due to X-irradiation of the bowel might also involve PGs, since normal therapeutic doses of aspirin often markedly improved the condition which was resistant to usual antidiarrheal agents such as codeine (Mennie and Dalley, 1973). Perhaps PGs are released due to X-ray damage of cells. Because of these data, it would seem preferable for De et al. (1974) to have used aspirin rather than ibuprofen in their cholera trial.

Before leaving the subject of diarrhea, it should be pointed out that PGs are not the only fatty acids which have this effect. Ricinoleic and 10-hydroxystearic acids are C18 compounds which act on human jejunum and colon in concentrations of 2 mM (Ammon and Phillips, 1972). PG precursors or metabolites might also have important physiological or pathological roles.

7.13.2 Cancer

PGs have also been implicated in cancer, and raised levels have been found in various tumours, some of which were discussed in Section 7.13.1 (Jaffe, 1974) found that human colonic cancer cells in tissue culture released more PG-like material than normal. Confirmatory evidence of a different type was provided by Bennett and del Tacca (1975) who extracted tumours and found that those from human colon and rectum contained and could synthesize more PG-like material than normal mucosa and submucosa from the same specimens. The significance of the raised levels of PGs is not known, but may be important in the rate of cell proliferation (Jaffe, 1974).

7.13.3 Inflammation

In view of the role suggested for PGs in many inflammatory conditions, it is not surprising that evidence has been obtained for a similar involvement in the alimentary tract. Pancreatitis in dogs (caused by injecting a bile-salt/ trypsin mixture into the pancreatic duct) significantly increased the PG-like material in the pancreatic venous blood and peritoneal exudate. No change occurred in the control dogs undergoing just pancreatic duct ligation (Glazer and Bennett, 1974, 1975). It therefore seems likely that PGs contribute to the signs and symptoms of pancreatitis. Ulcerative colitis is an inflammatory condition of the large bowel which responds to sulphasalazine. This substance inhibits seminal vesicle and rat fundus PG synthetase (Butt *et al.*, 1974). Its metabolites (5-aminosalicylic acid and sulphapyridine formed in the colon) usually inhibited the synthesis of PG-like material by colonic mucosa and submucosa from human descending and sigmoid colon (concentrations of 1 to 1000 μg/ml used; Bennett, Eastwood and Stamford, unpublished).

7.13.4 The Mouth

In a discussion of the pathology of the alimentary tract, it is relevant to mention the possible roles of PGs in peridontal disease and in formation of dental cysts. The gingiva have raised levels of PGE_2-like material when they are inflamed in peridontal disease (Goodson *et al.*, 1974), and systemic indomethacin improves the condition (Ota *et al.*, 1969). Dental cysts seem to grow by dissolving bone: several PGs resorb bone in low concentrations, cyst wall resorbs bone in tissue culture and releases substantial amounts of PG-like material, and the resorption is inhibited by indomethacin or poly-phloretin phosphate (Harris *et al.*, 1973).

Acknowledgements

I thank John R. Wood for help with the section on the biliary tract.

References

Ambache, N., Brummer, H. C., Rose, J. G. and Whiting, J. (1966). Thin-layer chromato-graphy of spasmogenic unsaturated hydroxy-acids from various tissues. *J. Physiol. (Lond.)*, **185**, 77P

Ammon, H. V. and Phillips, S. F. (1972). Fatty acids inhibit intestinal water absorption in man: fatty acid diarrhoea? *Gastroenterology*, **62**, 717

Anderson, F. L., Jubiz, W., Kralios, A. C., Tsagaris, T. J. and Kuida, H. (1972). Plasma prostaglandin levels during endotoxin shock in dogs. *Circulation (Suppl. II)*, **46**, 124

Andersson, K. E., Andersson, R., Hedner, P. and Persson, C. G. A. (1973). Parallelism between mechanical and metabolic responses to cholecystokinin and prostaglandin E_2 in extrahepatic biliary tract. *Acta Physiol. Scand.*, **89**, 571

Andersson, K. E., Hedner, P. and Persson, C. G. A. (1974). Differentiation of the contractile effects of prostaglandin E_2 and the C-terminal octapeptide of cholecystokinin in isolated guinea-pig gallbladder. *Acta Physiol. Scand.*, **90**, 657

Banerjee, A. K., Phillips, J. and Winning, W. W. (1972). E-type prostaglandins and gastric acid secretion in the rat. *Nature New Biology*, **238**, 177

Barac, G., Deby, C. and Neuray, J. (1972). Essais sur l'absorption intestinale de la prostaglandine PGE₁ chez le chien. *J. Physiol. (Paris)*, **65**, 194

Barrowman, J. A., Bennett, A., Hillenbrand, P., Rolles, K., Pollock, D. J. and Wright, J. T. (1975). Diarrhoea in medullary carcinoma of the thyroid: evidence for the role of prostaglandins and the therapeutic effect of nutmeg. *Br. Med. J.* In press

Bass, P. and Bennett, D. R. (1968). Local chemical regulation of motor action of the bowel—substance P and lipid-soluble acids. In *Handbook of Physiology, Sect. 6, Alimentary canal, C.F. Code*, pp. 2193–2212 (Washington: Am. Physiol. Soc.)

Bennett, A. (1970). Control of gastrointestinal motility by substances occurring in the gut wall. *Rend. Rom. Gastroenterol.*, **2**, 133

Bennett, A. (1972). Effects of prostaglandins on the gastrointestinal tract. In *The Prostaglandins Progress in Research*, Karim, S. M. M. (ed.) pp. 205–221 (Lancaster: MTP)

Bennett, A. (1973). Prostaglandins and the gut. In *Topics in Gastroenterology*, Truelove, S. C. and Jewell, D. P. (eds.), pp. 281–293 (Oxford: Blackwell Scientific Publications)

Bennett, A., Bucknell, A. and Dean, A. C. B. (1966). The release of 5-hydroxytryptamine from the rat stomach *in vitro*. *J. Physiol. (Lond.)*, **182**, 57

Bennett, A. and Del Tacca, M. (1975). Prostaglandins in human colonic carcinoma. *Gut*. In press

Bennett, A., Eley, K. G. and Scholes, G. B. (1968a). Effect of prostaglandins E₁ and E₂ on intestinal motility in the guinea-pig and rat. *Br. J. Pharmacol.*, **34**, 639

Bennett, A., Eley, K. G. and Scholes, G. B. (1968b). Effects of prostaglandins E₁ and E₂ on human, guinea-pig and rat isolated small intestine. *Br. J. Pharmacol.*, **34**, 630

Bennett, A., Eley, K. G. and Stockley, H. L. (1975a). The effects of prostaglandins on guinea-pig isolated intestine and their possible contribution to muscle activity and tone. *Br. J. Pharmacol.* **54**, 197

Bennett, A., Eley, K. G. and Stockley, H. L. (1975b). Modulation by prostaglandins of contractions in guinea-pig ileum. *Prostaglandins*. In press

Bennett, A., Gradidge, C. F. and Stamford, I. F. (1974). Prostaglandins, nutmeg and diarrhoea. *New Engl. J. Med.*, **290**, 110

Bennett, A., Murray, J. G. and Wyllie, J. H. (1968). Occurrence of prostaglandin E₂ in the human stomach, and a study of its effects on human isolated gastric muscle. *Br. J. Pharmacol.*, **32**, 339

Bennett, A. and Posner, J. (1971). Studies on prostaglandin antagonists. *Br. J. Pharmacol.*, **42**, 584

Bennett, A., Stamford, I. F. and Unger, W. G. (1973). Prostaglandin E₂ and gastric acid secretion in man. *J. Physiol. (Lond.)*, **229**, 349

Bhana, D., Karim, S. M. M., Carter, D. C. and Ganesan, P. A. (1973). The effect of orally administered prostaglandins A₁, A₂ and 15-epi-A₂ on human gastric secretion. *Prostaglandins*, **3**, 307

Botting, J. H. and Salzmann, R. (1974). The effect of indomethacin on the release of prostaglandins E₂ and acetylcholine from guinea-pig isolated ileum at rest and during field stimulation. *Br. J. Pharmacol.*, **50**, 119

Bouchier, I. A. D. and Williams, H. S. (1969). Determination of faecal blood loss after combined alcohol and sodium acetylsalicylate intake. *Lancet*, **i**, 178

Bourne, H. R. (1973). Cholera enterotoxin: failure of anti-inflammatory agents to prevent cyclic AMP accumulation. *Nature (Lond.)*, **241**, 399

Bressler, R., Vargas-Condon, M. and Lebovitz, H. E. (1968). Tranylcypromine: a potent insulin secretagogue and hypoglycemic agent. *Diabetes*, **17**, 617

Burns, T., Radawski, D., Underwood, R. and Daughterty, R. (1972). Effects of prostaglandin E₁ (PGE₁) on vascular resistances and weight of the jejunum. *Abstr. 5th Int. Cong. Pharmacol. 23–28th July, 1972*, p. 34 (San Francisco)

Burr, I. M. and Sharp, R. (1974). Effects of prostaglandin E₁ and of epinephrine on the dynamics of insulin release *in vitro*. *Endocrinology*, **94**, 835

Butt, A. A., Collier, H. O. J., Gardiner, P. J. and Saeed, S. A. (1974). Effects on prostaglandin biosynthesis of drugs affecting gastrointestinal function. *Gut*, **15**, 344

Carter, D. C., Ganesan, P. A., Bhana, D. and Karim, S. M. M. (1974). Effect of locally administered 15-(R)-15-methyl prostaglandin E₂ methyl ester on gastric ulcer formation in the Shay rat preparation. *Prostaglandins*, **5**, 455

Case, R. M. and Scratcherd, T. (1972). Prostaglandin action on pancreatic blood flow and on electrolyte and enzyme secretion by exocrine pancreas *in vivo* and *in vitro*. *J. Physiol. (Lond.)*, **226**, 393

Chawla, R. C. and Eisenberg, M. M. (1969). Effect of prostaglandin E_1 on the motility of innervated antral pouches in dogs. *Clin. Res.*, **17**, 299

Chong, E. K. S. and Downing, O. A. (1974). Reversal by prostaglandin E_2 of the inhibitory effect of indomethacin on contractions of guinea-pig ileum induced by angiotensin. *J. Pharm. Pharmacol.*, **26**, 729

Collier, H. O. J. (1974). Prostaglandin synthetase inhibitors and the gut. In *Prostaglandin synthetase inhibitors*. Robinson, H. J. and Vane, J. R. (eds.), pp. 121–133. (New York: Raven Press)

Coupar, I. M. and McColl, I. (1972). Inhibition of glucose absorption by prostaglandins E_1, E_2 and $F_{2\alpha}$. *J. Pharm. Pharmacol.*, **24**, 254

Cummings, J. H., Newman, A., Misiewicz, J. J., Milton-Thompson, G. J. and Billings, J. A. (1973). Effect of intravenous prostaglandin $F_{2\alpha}$ on small intestinal function in man. *Nature (Lond.)*, **243**, 169

Davenport, H. W. (1965). Damage to the gastric mucosa: effects of salicylates and stimulation. *Gastroenterology*, **49**, 189

Davenport, H. W. and Ball, L. L. (1973). Failure of ischemia to break the dog's gastric mucosal barrier. *Gastroenterology*, **65**, 619

De, S., Sicar, B. K., Sasmal, D., De, S. P. and Mondal, A. (1974), Ibuprofen (Brufen) in cholera and other diarrhoeas. *Indian J. Med. Res.*, **62**, 756

Dilawari, J. B., Newman, A., Poleo, J. and Misiewicz, J. J. (1973). Prostaglandins and the cardiac sphincter in man. *Proc. 4th Int. Symposium on Gastrointestinal Motility, Banff, Canada*, Daniel, E. E. (ed.), pp. 281–286 (Vancouver: Mitchell Press)

Dilawari, J. B., Newman, A., Poleo, J. and Misiewicz, J. J. (1975). Response of the human cardiac sphincter to circulating prostaglandins $F_{2\alpha}$ and E_2 and to anti-inflammatory drugs. *Gut*, **16**, 137

Dlugolecka, M. J. (1974). The failure of indomethacin to modify the response of cat intestine to cholera enterotoxin. *Pol. J. Pharmacol. Pharm.*, **26**, 93

Dorp, D. A. Van (1971). In discussion of 'Recent Developments in the biosynthesis and the analyses of prostaglandins'. *Ann. N.Y. Acad. Sci.*, **180**, 181

Eakins, K. E., Karim, S. M. M. and Miller, J. D. (1970). Antagonism of some smooth muscle actions of prostaglandins by polyphloretin phosphate. *Br. J. Pharmacol.*, **39**, 556

Eckenfels, A. and Vane, J. R. (1972). Prostaglandins, oxygen tension and smooth muscle tone. *Br. J. Pharmacol.*, **45**, 451

Eggenton, J., Flower, R. J., Hardcastle, P. T., Sanford, P. A. and Smyth, D. H. (1974). Prostaglandins and intestinal function. *J. Physiol. (Lond.)*, **238**, 79P

Ehrenpreis, S., Greenberg, J. and Belman, S. (1973). Prostaglandins reverse inhibition of electrically-induced contractions of guinea-pig ileum by morphine, indomethacin and acetylsalicylic acid. *Nature New Biology*, **245**, 280

Feldman, J. M. and Plonk, J. W. (1974). Serum prostaglandin F_2 alpha concentration in the carcinoid syndrome. *Prostaglandins*, **7**, 501

Ferreira, S. H., Herman, A. and Vane, J. R. (1972). Prostaglandin generation maintains the smooth muscle tone of the rabbit jejunum. *Br. J. Pharmacol.*, **44**, 328P

Finck, A. D. and Katz, R. L. (1972). Prevention of cholera-induced intestinal secretion in the cat by aspirin. *Nature (Lond.)*, **238**, 273

Fleshler, B. and Bennett, A. (1969). Responses of human, guinea-pig and rat colonic circular muscle to prostaglandins. *J. Lab. Clin. Med.*, **74**, 872

Flower, R. J. and Vane, J. R. (1972). Inhbition of prostaglandin synthetase in brain explains the anti-pyretic activity of paracetamol (4-acetamidophenol). *Nature (Lond.)*, **240**, 410

Fung, W. P. and Karim, S. M. M. (1974). Treatment of peptic ulcer pain with prostaglandin 15(R)-15-methyl E_2 methyl ester. *Int. Res. Commun. System*, **2**, 1001

Fung, W. P., Karim, S. M. M. and Tye, C. Y. (1974). Effect of 15(R)-15-methyl prostaglandin E_2 methyl ester on the healing of gastric ulcers. Controlled endoscopic study. *Lancet*, **ii**, 10

Fung, W. P., Lee, S. K. and Karim, S. M. M. (1974). Effect of prostaglandin 15(R)15-methyl-E_2-methyl ester on the gastric mucosa in patients with peptic ulceration—an endoscopic and histological study. *Prostaglandins*, **5**, 465

Gabryelewicz, A., Szalaj, W., Kinalska, I., Stasiewicz, J. and Langiewicz, J. (1974). Effect of prostaglandin E_1 on exocrine pancreatic secretion (*in vivo* and *in vitro*). *Pol. J. Pharmacol. Pharm.*, **26**, 263

Gandini, A., Lualdi, P. and Della Bella, D. (1971). Release of prostaglandins and its effects on the colon responses to transmural stimulation. *Arch. Exp. Path. Pharmacol.*, **269**, 388

Ganesan, P. A. and Karim, S. M. M. (1973). Polyphloretin phosphate temporarily potentiates prostaglandin E_2 on the rat fundus, probably by inhibiting PG 15-hydroxydehydrogenase. *J. Pharm. Pharmacol.*, **25**, 229

Ganesan, P. A., Salmon, J. A., Ng, B. K. and Karim, S. M. M. (1974). The effect of 15(R)15-methyl-PGE_2-methyl ester on serum gastrin levels in man. *Int. Res. Commun. System*, **2**, 1587

Glazer, G. and Bennett, A. (1974). Elevation of prostaglandin-like activity in the blood and peritoneal exudate of dogs with acute pancreatitis. *Br. J. Surg.*, **61**, 922

Glazer, G. and Bennett., A (1975).

Goodson, J. M., Dewhirst, F. E. and Brunetti, A. (1974). Prostaglandin E_2 levels and human peridontal disease. *Prostaglandins*, **6**, 81

Gots, R. E., Formal, S. B. and Giannella, R. A. (1974). Indomethacin inhibition of *Salmonella typhimurium*, *Shigella flexneri*, and cholera-mediated rabbit ileal secretion. *J. Infect. Dis.*, **130**, 280

Goyal, R. K. and Rattan, S. (1973). Mechanism of the lower esophageal sphincter relaxation action of prostaglandin E_1 and theophylline. *J. Clin. Invest.*, **52**, 337

Goyal, R. K., Rattan, S. and Hersh, T. (1972). Dose-response curves of the effects of the different prostaglandins on the lower esophageal sphincter. *Clin. Res.*, **20**, 454

Gréen, K. and Samuelsson, B. (1964). Thin layer chromatography of the prostaglandins. *J. Lipid Res.*, **5**, 117

Grossman, V. and Dolezal, S. (1972). The effect of some prostaglandin derivatives on gastric secretion and their therapeutic values as antiulcers. *Abstr. 5th Int. Congr. Pharmacol.*, *23–28th July*, *1112*, p. 89 (San Francisco)

Hahn, R. A. and Patil, P. N. (1972). Salivation induced by prostaglandin $F_{2\alpha}$ and modification of the response by atropine and physostigmine. *Br. J. Pharmacol.*, **44**, 527

Hahn, R. A. and Patil, P. N. (1974). Further observations on the interaction of prostaglandin $F_{2\alpha}$ with cholinergic mechanisms in canine salivary glands. *Eur. J. Pharmacol.*, **25**, 279

Håkanson, R., Leidberg, G. and Oscarson, J. (1973). Effects of prostaglandin E_1 on acid secretion, mucosal histamine content and histidine decarboxylase activity in rat stomach. *Br. J. Pharmacol.*, **47**, 498

Harper, M. J. K. and Skarnes, R. C. (1972). Inhibition of abortion and fetal death produced by endotoxin and prostaglandin $F_{2\alpha}$. *Prostaglandins*, **2**, 295

Harris, M., Jenkins, M. V., Bennett, A. and Wills, M. R. (1973). Prostaglandin production and bone resorption by dental cysts. *Nature* (*Lond.*), **245**, 213

Hart, S. L. (1974). The actions of prostaglandins E_2 and $F_{2\alpha}$ on human foetal small intestine. *Br. J. Pharmacol.*, **50**, 159

Heintz, K., Leinesser, W. and Heidenreich, O. (1974). Biphasic action of prostaglandins $F_{2\alpha}$, E_1 and E_2 on fluid transport of the isolated gallbladder. *Naunyn-Schmiedeberg's Arch. Pharmacol.*, **284**, R30

Herman, A. G., Eckenfels, A., Ferreira, S. H. and Vane, J. R. (1972). Relationship between tone of isolated smooth muscle preparations and production of prostaglandins. *Abstr. 5th Int. Congr. Pharmacol.*, *23–28th July*, *1972*, p. 100 (San Francisco)

Herman, A. G. and Vane, J. R. (1975). Endotoxin and production of prostaglandins by the isolated rabbit jejunum. Influence of indomethacin. *Archs: int. Pharmacodyn. Ther.*, **213**, 238

Hertelendy, F., Todd, H., Ehrhart, K. and Blute, R. (1972). Studies on growth hormone secretion: IV. *In vivo* effects of prostaglandin E_1. *Prostaglandins*, **2**, 79

Hinsdale, J. G., Engel, J. J. and Wilson, D. E. (1974). Prostaglandin E in peptic ulcer disease. *Prostaglandins*, **6**, 495

Hohnke, L. A. (1974). Interaction of dibutryl cyclic AMP and PGE_2 on stimulated gastric acid secretion in rats. *Fed. Proc.*, **33**, 329

Horton, E. W., Main, I. H. M., Thompson, C. J. and Wright, P. M. (1968). Effect of orally administered prostaglandin E_1 on gastric secretion and gastrointestinal motility in man. *Gut*, **9**, 655

Hudson, D. G. (1972). The effect of prostaglandin E_1 and E_2 on isolated frog intestine. *J. Physiol. (Lond.)*, **221**, 3P

Hunt, R. H., Dilawari, J. B. and Misiewicz, J. J. (1975). The effect of intravenous prostaglandin $F_{2\alpha}$ and E_2 on the motility of the sigmoid colon. *Gut*, **16**, 47

Isaacs, P., Whittaker, S. M. and Turnberg, L. A. (1974). Diarrhoea associated with medullary carcinoma of the thyroid. *Gastroenterology*, **67**, 521

Jacobson, E. D. (1970). Comparison of prostaglandin E_1 and norepinephrine on the gastric mucosal circulation. *Proc. Soc. Exp. Biol. Med.*, **133**, 516

Jacoby, H. I. and Marshall, C. H. (1972). Antagonism of cholera enterotoxin by antiinflammatory agents in the rat. *Nature (Lond.)*, **235**, 163

Jaffe, B. M. (1974). Prostaglandins and cancer: an update. *Prostaglandins*, **6**, 453

Jaffe, B. M., Behrman, H. R. and Parker, C. W. (1973). Radio-immunoassay measurement of prostaglandins E, A and F in human plasma. *J. Clin. Invest.*, **52**, 398

Jawaharlal, K. and Berti, F. (1972). Effects of dibutyryl cyclic AMP and a new cyclic nucleotide on gastric acid secretion in the rat. *Pharmacol. Res. Commun.*, **4**, 143

Johnson, D. G., Fujimoto, W. Y. and Williams, R. H. (1973). Enhanced release of insulin by prostaglandins in isolated pancreatic islets. *Diabetes*, **22**, 658

Johnson, D. G., Thompson, W. J. and Williams, R. H. (1974). Regulation of adenylyl cyclase from isolated, pancreatic islet cells by prostaglandins and guanosine 5'-triphosphate. *Biochemistry*, **13**, 1920

Kadlec, O., Mašek, K. and Šeferna, I. (1974). A modulating role of prostaglandins in contractions of the guinea-pig ileum. *Br. J. Pharmacol.*, **51**, 565

Kantor, H. S., Tao, P. and Kiefer, H. C. (1974). Kinetic evidence for the presence of two prostaglandin receptor sites regulating the activity of intestinal adenylate cyclase sensitive to *Escherichia coli* enterotoxin. *Proc. Nat. Acad. Sci. (USA)*, **71**, 1317

Kaplan, E. L., Sizemore, G. W., Peskin, G. W. and Jaffe, B. M. (1973). Humoral similarities of carcinoid tumours and medullary carcinomas of the thyroid. *Surgery*, **74**, 21

Karim, S. M. M. (1971). Effects of oral administration of prostaglandins E_2 and $F_{2\alpha}$ on the human uterus. *J. Obstet. Gynaec. Br. Commonwealth*, **28**, 289

Karim, S. M. M. (1974). The effect of polyphloretin phosphate and other compounds on prostaglandin-induced diarrhoea in man. *Ann. Acad. Med. (Singapore)*, **3**, 201

Karim, S. M. M. and Ganesan, P. A. (1974). The effect of polyphloretin phosphate on prostaglandin-induced diarrhoea. *Int. Res. Comm. System*, **2**, 1585

Karim, S. M. M., Carter, D. C., Bhana, D. and Ganesan, P. A. (1973a). Effect of orally administered prostaglandin E_2 and its 15-methyl analogues on gastric secretion. *Br. Med. J.*, **1**, 143

Karim, S. M. M., Carter, D. C., Bhana, D. and Ganesan, P. A. (1973b). Effect of orally and intravenously administered prostaglandin 15(R)15-methyl E_2 on gastric secretion in man. *Adv. Biosci.*, **9**, 255

Karim, S. M. M., Carter, D. C., Bhana, D. and Ganesan, P. A. (1973c). The effect of orally and intravenously administered prostaglandin 16:16 dimethyl E_2 methyl ester on human gastric acid secretion. *Prostaglandins*, **4**, 71

Karim, S. M. M. and Ganesan, P. A. (1974a). Prostaglandins and the digestive system. *Ann. Acad. Med. (Singapore)*, **3**, 286

Karim, S. M. M., Sandler, M. and Williams, E. D. (1967). Distribution of prostaglandins in human tissues. *Br. J. Pharmac. Chemother.*, **31**, 340

Khairallah, P. A., Page, I. H. and Turker, R. K. (1967). Some properties of prostaglandin E_1 action on smooth muscle. *Archs. int. Pharmacodyn. Ther.*, **169**, 328

Kimberg, D. V., Field, M., Gershon, E. and Henderson, A. (1974). Effects of prostaglandins and cholera enterotoxin on intestinal mucosal cyclic AMP accumulation. Evidence against an essential role for prostaglandins in the action of toxin. *J. Clin. Invest.*, **53**, 941

Kimberg, D. V., Field, M., Johnson, J., Henderson, A. and Gershon, E. (1971). Stimulation of intestinal mucosal adenyl cyclase by cholera enterotoxin and prostaglandins. *J. Clin. Invest.*, **50**, 1218

Koch, H., Demling, L. and Classen, M. (1972). The influence of prostaglandin E_2 on the blood flow and secretion of the stomach stimulated with pentagastrin in the anaesthetized cat. *Arch. Fr. Mal. App. Dig.*, **61**, 268C

Lee, Y. H. and Bianchi, R. G. (1972). The antisecretory and anti-ulcer activity of a prostaglandin analogue, SC-24665, in experimental animals. *Abstr. 5th Int. Congr. Pharmacol., 23–28th July, 1972*, p. 136 (San Francisco)

Lee, Y. H., Cheng, W. D., Bianchi, R. G., Mollison, K. and Hansen, J. (1973). Effects of oral administration of PGE_2 on gastric secretion and experimental peptic ulcerations. *Prostaglandins*, **3**, 29

Lefebvre, P. J. and Luyckx, A. S. (1973). Stimulation of insulin secretion after prostaglandin PGE_1 in the anaesthetized dog. *Biochem. Pharm.*, **22**, 1773

Leonards, J. R. and Levy, G. (1969). Reduction or prevention of aspirin-induced occult gastrointestinal blood loss in man. *Clin. Pharm. Therap.*, **10**, 571

Liedberg, G. and Håkanson, R. (1972). Effect of prostaglandin E_1 on acid secretion, histidine decarboxylase activity and histamine content in rat gastric mucosa. *Acta Pharmacol. Toxicol. (Kbh).*, **31**, 108

Main, I. H. M. (1973). Prostaglandins and the gastrointestinal tract. In *The Prostaglandins, Pharmacological and Therapeutic Advances*, Cuthbert, M. F. (ed.), pp. 287–323 (London: Heinemann)

Main, I. H. M. and Whittle, B. J. R. (1972a). Effects of prostaglandin E_2 on rat gastric mucosal blood flow, as determined by ^{14}C-aniline clearance. *Br. J. Pharmacol.*, **44**, 331P

Main, I. H. M. and Whittle, B. J. R. (1972b). Effects of prostaglandins of the E and A series on rat gastric mucosal blood flow as determined by ^{14}C-aniline clearance. *Abstr. 5th Int. Congr. Pharmacol. 23–28th July*, p. 145 (San Francisco)

Main, I. H. M. and Whittle, B. J. R. (1973a). Effects of indomethacin on rat gastric acid secretion and mucosal blood flow. *Br. J. Pharmac.*, **47**, 666P

Main, I. H. M. and Whittle, B. J. R. (1973b). Potentiation of dibutyryl cyclic 3'5'-AMP induced gastric acid secretion in rats by non-steroidal anti-inflammatory drugs. *Br. J. Pharmacol.*, **49**, 162P

Main, I. H. M. and Whittle, B. J. R. (1974). Methyl analogues of prostaglandin E_2 and gastrointestinal function in the rat. *Br. J. Pharmacol.*, **52**, 113P

Matuchansky, C. and Bernier, J. J. (1973). Effect of prostaglandin E_1 on glucose, water and electrolyte absorption in the human jejunum. *Gastroenterology*, **64**, 1111

Matuchansky, C., Mary, J. Y. and Bernier, J. J. (1972). Effets de la prostaglandine E_1 sur le temps de transit et les mouvements nets et unidirectionnels de l'eau et des électrolytes dans le jéjenum humain. *Biol. Gastroenterol.*, **5**, 175

McKirdy, H. C. (1972). Functional relationship of longitudinal and circular layers of the muscularis externa of the rabbit large intestine. *J. Physiol. (Lond.)*, **227**, 839

Melvin, K. E. W., Tashjian, A. H. and Miller, H. H. (1972). Studies in familial (medullary) thyroid carcinoma. *Rec. Progr. Horm. Res.*, **28**, 399

Mennie, A. T. and Dalley, V. (1973). Aspirin in radiation-induced diarrhoea. *Lancet*, **i**, 1131

Milton-Thompson, G. J., Billings, J. A., Cummings, J. H., Newman, A. and Misiewicz, J. J. (1974). Motor and secretory responses of the human small intestine to circulating prostaglandin $F_{2\alpha}$. In *Proceedings of the Fourth Internat. Symposium on Gastrointestinal Motility*. Daniel, E. E. (ed.), pp. 271–280 (Vancouver: Mitchell Press)

Milton-Thompson, G. J., Cummings, J. H., Newman, A., Billings, J. A. and Misiewicz, J. J. (1975). Colonic and small intestinal response to intravenous prostaglandin $F_{2\alpha}$ and E_2 in man. *Gut*, **16**, 42

Misiewicz, J. J., Waller, S. L., Kiley, N. and Horton, E. W. (1969). Effect of oral prostaglandin E_1 on intestinal transit in man. *Lancet*, **i**, 648

Morton, I. K. M., Saverymuttu, S. H. and Wood, J. R. (1974). Inhibition by prostaglandins of fluid transport in the isolated gallbladder of the guinea-pig. *Br. J. Pharmacol.*, **50**, 460P

Nakano, J. and Prancan, A. V. (1972). Effect of prostaglandins E_1 and A_1 on the gastric circulation in dogs. *Proc. Soc. Exp. Biol. Med.*, **139**, 1151

Newman, A., Prado, J., Philippakos, D. and Misiewicz, J. J. (1975). Effects of prostaglandin E_2 and $F_{2\alpha}$ on human gastric function. *Gut*. In press

Nilsson, F. and Öhrn, P. G. (1974). Duodeno-gastric reflux after administration of prostaglandin $F_{2\alpha}$. Studies of gastrointestinal propulsion in the rat. *Int. Res. Commun. System*, **2**, 1558

Nylander, B. and Andersson, S. (1974). Gastric secretory inhibition induced by three methyl analogues of prostaglandin E_2 administered intragastrically to man. *Scand. J. Gastroenterol.*, **9**, 751

Nylander, B., Robert, A. and Andersson, S. (1974). Gastric secretory inhibition by certain methyl analogs of prostaglandin E_2 following intestinal administration in man. *Scand. J. Gastroenterol.*, **9**, 759

O'Brien, P. and Silen, W. (1973). Effect of bile salts and aspirin on the gastric mucosal blood flow. *Gastroenterology*, **64**, 246

Ota, N., Mizuno, K. and Akita, Y. (1969). A clinical evaluation of 'Indacin' in peridontal disease. *Aichi. Gakuin J. Dent. Sci.*, **7**, 187 (in Japanese; cited in Goodson *et al.*, 1974)

Parkinson, T. M. and Schneider, J. C. (1969). Absorption and metabolism of prostaglandin E_1 by perfused rat jejunum *in vitro*. *Biochim. Biophys. Acta*, **176**, 78

Peskar, B. M., Holland, A. and Peskar, B. A. (1974). Quantitative determination of prostaglandins in human gastric juice by radioimmunoassay. *Clin. Chem. Acta*, **55**, 21

Pfeiffer, C. J. and Lewandowski, L. G. (1972). Wirkung von Prostaglandin und Aspirin auf die Magensekretion des Laborfrettchens. *Leber Magen Darm*, **2**, 142

Piper, P. and Vane, J. (1971). The release of prostaglandins from lung and other tissues. *Ann. N.Y. Acad. Sci.*, **180**, 363

Radmanović, B. Z. (1972). Effect of prostaglandin E_1 on the peristaltic activity of the guinea-pig isolated ileum. *Archs. Int. Pharmacodyn. Ther.*, **200**, 396

Ramwell, P. W. and Shaw, J. E. (1968). Prostaglandin inhibition of gastric secretion. *J. Physiol. (Lond.)*, **195**, 34P

Rattan, S., Hersh, T. and Goyal, R. K. (1972). Effect of prostaglandin $F_{2\alpha}$ and gastrin pentapeptide on the lower esophageal sphincter. *Proc. Soc. Exp. Biol. Med.*, **141**, 573

Reeder, D. D., Becker, H. D. and Thompson, J. C. (1972). Effect of prostaglandin E_1 on food stimulated gastrin and gastric secretion in dogs. *Physiologist*, **15**, 246

Robert, A. (1973). Prostaglandins and gastric secretion. *Res. Prostaglandins*, **2**, 1

Robert, A. (1974a). Effects of prostaglandins on the stomach and the intestine. *Prostaglandins*, **6**, 523

Robert, A. (1974b). An intestinal disease in the rat probably caused by a prostaglandin deficiency. *Gastroenterology*, **66**, 765

Robert, A., Magee, W. E., Miller, O. V. and Nezamis, J. E. (1974). Intestinal absorption of prostaglandin $F_{2\alpha}$ 15(S)-15-methyl prostaglandin $F_{2\alpha}$ and their methyl esters in the dog. *Biochim. Biophys. Acta*, **348**, 269

Robert, A. and Magerlein, B. J. (1973). 15-methyl PGE_2 and 16,16-dimethyl PGE_2: potent inhibitors of gastric secretion. *Adv. Biosci.*, **9**, 247

Robert, A., Nezamis, J. E. and Lancaster, C. (1972). 15-methyl-prostaglandin E_2: a potent inhibitor of gastric secretion. *Adv. Biosci. (Suppl.)*, **9**, 42

Robert, A., Nezamis, J. E. and Phillips, J. P. (1968). Effect of prostaglandin E_1 on gastric secretion and ulcer formation in the rat. *Gastroenterology*, **55**, 481

Robert, A., Nylander, B. and Andersson, S. (1974). Marked inhibition of gastric secretion by two prostaglandin analogs given orally to man. *Life Sci.*, **14**, 533

Robertson, R. P. (1974). *In vivo* insulin secretion: prostaglandin and adrenergic inter-relations. *Prostaglandins*, **6**, 501

Rossini, A. A., Lee, J. B. and Frawley, T. F. (1971). An unpredictable lack of effect of prostaglandins on insulin release in isolated rat islets. *Diabetes*, **20**, 374

Rudick, J., Gonda, M., Dreiling, D. A. and Janowitz, H. D. (1971). Effects of prostaglandin E_1 on pancreatic exocrine function. *Gastroenterology*, **60**, 272

Sacca, L., Rengo, F., Chairiello, M. and Condorelli, M. (1973). Glucose intolerance and impaired insulin secretion by prostaglandin A_1 in fasting anaesthetized dogs. *Endocrinology*, **92**, 31

Sandler, M., Karim, S. M. M. and Williams, E. D. (1968). Prostaglandins in amine and peptide-secreting tumours. *Lancet*, **ii**, 1053

Sakaki, H., Teraki, Y. and Tsunoo, S. (1974). Effect of prostaglandins on the sphincter of Oddi and the duodenal muscle of rabbits. *Jap. J. Pharm.*, **24**, 30

Saunders, R. N., and Moser, C. A. (1972a). Changes in vascular resistance induced by prostaglandins E_1 and E_2 in the isolated rat pancreas. *Archs. int. Pharmacodyn. Ther.*, **197**, 86

Saunders, R. N. and Moser, Ca. (1972b). Increased vascular resistance by prostaglandins B_1 and B_2 in the isolated rat pancreas. *Nature New Biology*, **237**, 285

Shaw, J. E. and Urquhart, J. (1972). Parameters of the control of acid secretion in the isolated blood-perfused stomach. *J. Physiol. (Lond.)*, **226**, 107P

Shehadeh, Z., Price, W. E. and Jacobson, E. D. (1969). Effects of vasoactive agents on intestinal blood flow and motility in the dog. *Am. J. Physiol.*, **216**, 386

Skarnes, R. C. and Harper, M. J. K. (1972). Relationship between endotoxin-induced abortion and the synthesis of prostaglandin F. *Prostaglandins*, **1**, 191

Sorrentino, L., Capasso, F. and Di Rosa, M. (1972). Indomethacin and prostaglandins. *Eur. J. Pharmacol.*, **17**, 306

Spellacy, W. N., Buhi, W. C. and Holsinger, K. K. (1971). The effect of prostaglandin $F_{2\alpha}$ and E_2 on blood glucose and plasma insulin levels during pregnancy. *Am. J. Obstet. Gynecol.*, **111**, 239

Stockley, H. L. and Bennett, A. (1976). Modulation of activity by prostaglandins in human gastrointestinal muscle. *Proceedings of the Fifth International Symposium on Gastrointestinal Motility, Leuven, Belgium.* In press

Tonnesen, M. G., Jubiz, W., Moore, J. G. and Frailey, J. (1974). Circadian variation of prostaglandin E (PGE) production in human gastric juice. *Am. J. Dig. Dis.*, **19**, 644

Tsai, T. H., Parmeter, L., White, H. L. and Maxwell, R. A. (1972). Effect of indomethacin and aspirin on the response of isolated guinea-pig ileum to arachidonic acid, a precursor of prostaglandin E_2. *Abstr. 5th Int. Congr. Pharmacol. 23–28th July*, p. 237 (San Francisco)

Türker, R. K. and Onur, R. (1971). Effect of prostaglandin E_1 on intestinal motility of the cat. *Archs. int. Physiol. Biochim.*, **79**, 535

Ubtatuba, F. B. (1973). The use of the hamster stomach *in vitro* as an assay preparation for prostaglandins. *Br. J. Pharmac.*, **49**, 662

Urquhart, J. and Shaw, J. E. (1973). Effect of prostaglandin E_2 on the isolated perfused stomach of the dog. *Gastroenterology*, **64**, 872

Usardi, M. M., Franceschini, J., Mandelli, V., Daturi, S. and Mizzotti, B. (1974). Prostaglandins VIII: a proposed role for PGE_2 in the genesis of stress-induced gastric ulcers. *Prostaglandins*, **8**, 43

Valiulis, E. and Long, J. F. (1973). Effects of drugs on intestinal water secretion following cholera toxin in guinea-pigs and rabbits. *Physiologist*, **16**, 475

Vance, J. E., Buchanan, K. D. and Williams, R. H. (1971). Glucagon and insulin release. Influence of drugs affecting the autonomic nervous system. *Diabetes*, **20**, 78

Vargaftig, B. B. and Dao Hai, (1972). Inhibition of the rat stomach contractions due to arachidonic acid: a simple procedure for detection of inhibitors of prostaglandin synthesis. *Adv. Biosci. (Suppl.)*, **9**, 74

Vaughan-Williams, E. M., Dohadwalla, A. N. and Dutta, N. K. (1969). Diarrhoea and accumulation of intestinal fluid in infant rabbits infected with *Vibrio cholerae* in an isolated jejunal segment. *J. Infect. Dis.*, **120**, 645

Villanueva, R., Hinds, L., Katz, R. L. and Eakins, K. E. (1972). The effect of polyphloretin phosphate on some smooth muscle actions of prostaglandins in the cat. *J. Pharmac. exp. Ther.*, **180**, 78

Waller, S. L. (1973). Prostaglandins and the gastrointestinal tract. *Gut*, **14**, 402

Whittle, B. J. R. (1972). Studies on the mode of action of cyclic 3′5′-AMP and prostaglandin E_2 on rat gastric acid secretion and mucosal blood flow. *Br. J. Pharmac.*, **46**, 546P

Williams, E. D., Karim, S. M. M. and Sandler, M. (1968). Prostaglandin secretion by medullary carcinoma of the thyroid. *Lancet*, **i**, 22

Willis, A. L., Davison, P. and Ramwell, P. W. (1974). Inhibition of intestinal tone, motility and prostaglandin biosynthesis by 5,8,11,14-eicosatetraynoic acid (TYA). *Prostaglandins*, **5**, 355

Wilson, D. E. (1972). Prostaglandins and the gastrointestinal tract. *Prostaglandins*, **1**, 281

Wilson, D. E. and Levine, R. A. (1972). The effect of prostaglandin E_1 on canine gastric acid secretion and gastric mucosal blood flow. *Am. J. Dig. Dis.*, **17**, 527

Wood, J. R. and Stamford, I. F. (1974). Prostaglandins and non-visualization at cholecystography. *Br. J. Radiol.* **47**, 825

8
Prostaglandins and Blood Coagulation

PETER W. HOWIE

8.1 INTRODUCTION 277

8.2 PLATELETS IN HAEMOSTASIS 278

8.3 PROSTAGLANDINS AND PLATELET AGGREGATION/ADHESION 279
8.3.1 *Effect of PGE$_1$ on platelet aggregation/adhesion* in vitro 279
8.3.2 *Effect of PGE$_1$ on platelet aggregation/adhesion* in vivo 280
8.3.3 *PGE$_1$ and platelets in humans* 281
8.3.4 *Effect of PGE$_2$ on platelet aggregation/adhesion* in vitro 281
8.3.5 *Effect of PGE$_2$ on platelet aggregation/adhesion* in vivo 282
8.3.6 *Effect of other prostaglandins on platelet aggregation/adhesion* 282

8.4 EFFECT OF PROSTAGLANDINS ON BLOOD COAGULATION 284

8.5 MECHANISM OF ACTION 284
8.5.1 *Mechanism of action of PGE$_1$ on platelet aggregation* 284
8.5.2 *Mechanism of action of PGE$_2$ and PGF$_{2\alpha}$ on platelet aggregation* 286

8.6 CLINICAL IMPLICATIONS OF PROSTAGLANDINS AND PLATELET AGGREGATION 286

8.7 CONCLUSION 287
REFERENCES 287

8.1 INTRODUCTION

During recent years there has been an explosive increase in the understanding of the mechanisms responsible for normal haemostasis and thrombus formation, and it is now well established that platelets play a central role in both processes. Since the demonstration by Kloeze (1967) that prostaglandin E_1 (PGE_1) could inhibit platelet aggregation, the relationship between platelets and prostaglandins has been studied with increasing interest. These investigations have been stimulated not only because prostaglandins may prove to have a role as therapeutic agents, but also because prostaglandins may play a fundamental part in normal platelet aggregation. Recent developments in this field are discussed in the present chapter.

8.2 PLATELETS IN HAEMOSTASIS

In the first edition of this book, Mody (1972) discussed the normal mechanisms of platelet aggregation/adhesion and the commonly used methods of studying platelet function. There have been other detailed reviews of these subjects (Mustard and Packham, 1970; Turpie et al., 1972; Born, 1972) and the part played by platelets in normal haemostasis will only be summarized here.

When a blood vessel is injured, haemostasis is brought about by the formation of a platelet plug (Zucker, 1947; Jorgensen and Borchgrevink, 1963; Hovig, et al., 1967) which is subsequently stabilized by the formation of fibrin (see Figure 8.1). Within two to three seconds of injury, platelets adhere to the subendothelial collagen fibres which have been exposed (Hugues, 1960; Hovig et al., 1967), but the mechanism of adhesion of platelets to collagen is unknown. When collagen is added to platelets in vitro, it stimulates platelet aggregation only after a lag phase of some minutes so that it is likely that some other factors play a part in this initial phase of adhesion (Zucker and Borrelli, 1962). Very rapidly after the injury, the platelets change

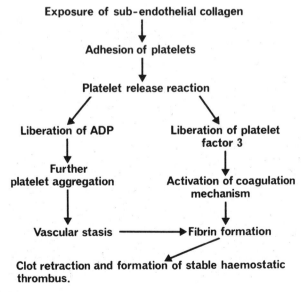

Figure 8.1 Mechanisms in the formation of haemostatic thrombus

from their disc-like shape to spheroids with pseudopodia projecting from their surface (Macmillan and Oliver, 1965). This initial shape-change can be induced by ADP which may contribute to the initial phase of platelet adhesion to the vessel wall. The first phase of platelet adhesion to collagen stimulates the platelet release reaction and ADP is released (Zucker and Borelli, 1962; Spaet and Zucker, 1964) to cause the second phase of platelet aggregation (Gaarder et al., 1961; Born, 1962). Many compounds can cause platelet aggregation but they seem to act by the common pathway of stimulating ADP release so that present evidence suggests that ADP plays a major role in this second phase of platelet aggregation (Haslam, 1968). The action of ADP in platelet aggregation is not fully understood but it has been suggested that ADP is associated with binding sites on the platelet surface (Born, 1962; Hellem and Owren, 1964). Platelets carry a mutually repulsive negative charge (Hampton and Mitchell, 1966) and a complex formed by ADP, Ca^{++}, and a protein, probably the von Willeband factor, may neutralize that charge and permit binding among the platelets (Hellem and Owren, 1964; Mitchell, 1968).

In addition to ADP, several other compounds are liberated from platelets during the release reaction including serotonin (5-HT) and catecholamines which may augment the action of ADP. The platelet release reaction also liberates platelet factor 3 which is a lipoprotein with the capacity to accelerate the intrinsic coagulation mechanism to produce thrombin (see Figure 8.1). (Mustard et al., 1964; Castaldi et al., 1965; Hardisty and Hutton, 1966). Thrombin will induce fibrin formation to stabilize the platelet plug but may also contribute to further platelet aggregation by stimulating ADP release (Mustard et al., 1967).

After haemostasis has been secured, the stabilized platelet plug or thrombus will undergo retraction in response to the action of thrombasthenin, a contractile protein which is present in platelets (Bettex-Galland and Luscher, 1961). Finally the thrombus is dissolved by the action of the fibrinolytic system to restore vascular patency. As will be discussed in the later sections of this chapter, prostaglandins of the E group exert a major effect on the platelet release reaction, ADP-induced platelet aggregation, clot retraction and thrombus formation in vivo and these findings may have important implications in understanding the normal mechanisms of platelet aggregation.

8.3 PROSTAGLANDINS AND PLATELET AGGREGATION/ADHESION

8.3.1 Effect of PGE₁ on platelet aggregation/adhesion *in vitro*

Kloeze (1967) was the first to report the strong inhibitory action of PGE_1, on ADP-induced platelet aggregation in rat, pig and human platelet-rich plasma. Other workers confirmed this and showed that PGE_1 also inhibited the aggregation of platelets by a large number of different compounds including thrombin, collagen, norepinephrine, ATP, 5-HT, antigen–antibody complexes and gamma-globulin coated polystyrene particles (Emmons et al., 1967; Chandrasekhar, 1967; Irion and Blomback, 1969;

Kinlough-Rathbone et al., 1970; Ball et al., 1970; Boullin et al., 1972). In addition, PGE₁ inhibited platelet to glass adhesiveness, the electrokinetic response of platelets to ADP and norepinephrine (Emmons et al., 1967) and the normal rate of clot retraction (Sekhar, 1970; Murer, 1971). Platelet aggregation was inhibited when PGE₁ was mixed with platelet-rich plasma before the addition of ADP, but PGE₁ also broke up ADP-induced platelet aggregates when added after the nucleotide (Chandrasekhar, 1967; Emmons et al., 1967; Boullin et al., 1972). Collagen-induced platelet aggregation proved to be less reversible than ADP-induced aggregation because PGE₁ like most other inhibitors of platelet aggregation, was unable to break up platelet aggregates already formed in response to collagen (Chandrasekhar, 1967; Murakami et al., 1972).

PGE₁ also inhibited the platelet release reaction since ADP, ATP and 5-HT were not liberated in response to collagen and thrombin from platelets exposed to PGE₁ (Kinlough-Rathbone et al., 1970; Ball et al., 1970). PGE₁ inhibited ADP-induced swelling of platelets and stimulated their recovery from the swollen state without affecting the metabolism of added ADP (Shio et al., 1970). The inhibitory effect of PGE₁ depended both on the concentration of PGE₁ and of the aggregating agent (Emmons et al., 1967; Irion and Blomback, 1969; Kinlough-Rathbone et al., 1970) but the concentration of PGE₁ required to inhibit ADP-induced aggregation was much lower (50–100 nM) than that required to prevent the initial change in platelet shape (100 μM) (Kinlough-Rathbone et al., 1970). When platelets, which had been incubated with PGE₁, were washed and resuspended in fresh medium they aggregated normally in response to ADP (Kinlough-Rathbone et al., 1970; Mody, 1972) and, since PGE₁ was not taken up by the platelets, Kinlough-Rathbone et al. (1970) suggested that PGE₁ must be in the ambient fluid to exert its effect. These several observations have established that PGE₁ is one of the most potent inhibitors of platelet adhesion/aggregation in vitro which has yet been identified.

8.3.2 Effect of PGE₁ on platelet aggregation/adhesion *in vivo*

Several reports have described an inhibitory effect on both platelet aggregation and thrombus formation when PGE₁ has been administered to experimental animals. When PGE₁ was applied topically or administered intravenously, platelet thrombus formation was suppressed in injured rabbit-brain arteries (Emmons et al., 1967; Kinlough-Rathbone et al., 1970). A single intra-arterial injection of PGE₁ in rabbits had a short-lived action, normal platelet aggregation having returned in 5 min, but a continuous intravenous infusion (10 μg/kg per min) prolonged bleeding times and effectively inhibited haemostasis at the site of injury in rabbit blood vessels.

The duration of action of PGE₁ may be dose-related because a large single intravenous injection of PGE₁ in the rat (2 mg/kg) prevented platelet aggregation for at least 30 min after the infusion (Chandrasekhar, 1967). The route of administration of PGE₁ also influenced the duration of its effect because subcutaneous, intramuscular and intraperitoneal injections of 50 μg of PGE₁ in the rat inhibited platelet aggregation for 10–20, 30–40 and over 90 min respectively (Hornstra, 1971). An intravenous injection of PGE_1 in rats inhibited the thrombocytopenia and increased the LD50 of an ADP injection, the PGE_1 having inhibited the platelet thrombi which are normally associated with an animal's death following an ADP injection (Kloeze, 1970a). In further animal studies, PGE_1 has been shown to inhibit platelet aggregation induced by electric stimuli (Kloeze, 1970b) and to reduce platelet aggregation in haemorrhagic shock (Hissen et al., 1969).

Bousser (1973) noted in her studies that the dose of PGE_1 required to inhibit thrombus formation was less than the dose required to inhibit platelet aggregation. This suggested that the influence of PGE_1 on thrombus formation was not mediated solely through its effect on platelet aggregation but that its effects on vasodilatation and the vessel wall might also be important.

One study found that a single intravenous injection of PGE_1 had no effect upon platelet aggregation at the site of laser-induced trauma (Arfors et al., 1968) but the generally held view is that PGE_1 is able to inhibit platelet aggregation and thrombus formation in vivo when given in sufficient doses.

8.3.3 PGE_1 and platelets in humans

The inhibitory effect of PGE_1 on platelet aggregation both in vitro and in vivo led to the speculation that PGE_1 might have potential therapeutic value in man (Emmons et al., 1967; Hornstra, 1971; Lancet, leading article, 1971). Carlsson et al. (1968) infused PGE_1 into three male volunteers at a rate of 0.1 μg/kg per min and demonstrated no effect on ADP-induced aggregation. Elkeles et al. (1969) infused PGE_1 at 0.2 μg/kg per min into eight volunteers and found a variable response in their subjects. PGE_1 in this dosage had no effect on ADP-induced aggregation, inhibited platelet to glass adhesiveness in only 50% of their subjects but inhibited the platelet electrophoretic response to ADP in all patients. Troublesome side-effects were encountered, however, such as facial flushing, chest discomfort, hypotension, giddiness and nausea. It was concluded that, because of its side-effects, PGE_1 would have limited use as an antithrombotic agent in man. The small effect of PGE_1 upon platelet function in man was probably related to the dose because similar concentrations in animals had little inhibitory effect on platelets (Bousser, 1973).

8.3.4 Effect of PGE_2 on platelet aggregation/adhesion in vitro

While there has been unanimity about the inhibitory effect of PGE_1 upon platelets, there has been much less agreement about the effect of PGE_2 upon platelet aggregation. Kloeze (1967) found that PGE_2 potentiated ADP-induced platelet aggregation in pig and rat platelets but had little effect on human platelets. Irion and Blomback (1969) reported that PGE_2 inhibited ADP-induced platelet aggregation but that it had only one-fifth of the activity of PGE_1 while Weeks et al. (1969) found PGE_2 to be such a weak inhibitor of platelet aggregation that its effect was barely measureable. In contrast, Shio and Ramwell (1972a) demonstrated that PGE_2 weakly inhibited the first phase of ADP-induced platelet aggregation but strongly potentiated the secondary phase. Salzman *et al.* (1973) also found that PGE_2 augmented platelet aggregation. The discrepancy in results may be explained by some of the preparations of PGE_2 being contaminated with small concentrations of PGE_1 (Kloeze, 1969) since it is very difficult to purify the preparations of PGE_2 completely. As increasingly purified preparations of PGE_2 have been prepared, the weight of evidence now favours PGE_2 having a stimulatory effect on platelet aggregation rather than the reverse.

An interesting observation was made by van Crevald and Pascha (1968) that the excessively rapid platelet disaggregation in some patients with von Willebrand's disease was corrected by PGE_2.

8.3.5 Effect of PGE₂ on platelet aggregation/adhesion *in vivo*

Very few reports have described the effect of PGE_2 upon platelets *in vivo* but from their *in vitro* observations, Shio and Ramwell (1972a) warned that PGE_2 therapy might carry a risk of thrombosis, particularly in patients with a history of vascular and thrombotic disease. Karim and Filshie (1972) found no effect on platelet to glass adhesiveness during PGE_2 infusions given for the purpose of inducing therapeutic abortion. In contrast, Howie *et al.* (1973) found that PGE_2 accelerated disaggregation following ADP-induced platelet aggregation and inhibited platelet adhesiveness to a cellophane membrane in a test-cell system (Lindsay *et al.*, 1973) but had no effect on platelet adhesiveness to glass beads as measured by Hellem's method (Hellem, 1960, as modified by Hirsh *et al.*, 1966) (see Figure 8.2). The differing results between the two methods of measuring platelet adhesiveness was of interest. In the glass bead column method, whole blood was driven through a column of glass beads causing disruption of red cells with release of ADP and other nucleotides. Since prostaglandins may exert their effect by inhibiting the release of ADP from platelets, this effect would be swamped by the ADP from the red cells. Since there was no red cell destruction in the test-cell method, this may have provided a more sensitive index of the effect of PGE_2 upon platelet behaviour. The results from this study suggested that intravenous PGE_2 would be more likely to inhibit than to promote thrombus formation *in vivo*. This *in vivo* effect of PGE_2 appears to contradict some of the *in vitro* observations but, since PGE_2 disappears from the circulation very rapidly (Ferreira and Vane, 1967) a metabolite of PGE_2 may be responsible for this inhibitory effect rather than PGE_2 itself. PGE_2 has fewer toxic effects than PGE_1, so that further *in vivo* studies to investigate the potential of PGE_2 as an anti-thrombotic agent would be of interest.

8.3.6 Effect of other prostaglandins upon platelet aggregation/adhesion

Most investigations have found the prostaglandins of the A, B and F groups to be only very weak inhibitors of platelet adhesion and aggregation (Kloeze,

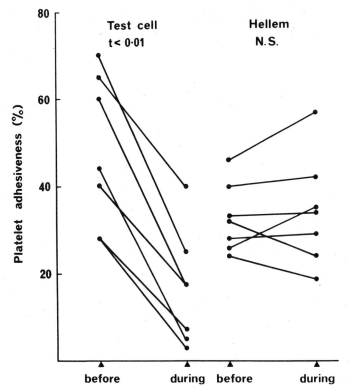

Figure 8.2 The *in vivo* effect of PGE_2 upon platelet adhesiveness in humans (reproduced from *J. Clin. Path.* (1973) **26**, 354, by kind permission of the Editor)

1969; Weeks *et al.*, 1969; Irion and Blomback, 1969; Sekhar, 1970). The exception to this was the report that ω-homo-E_1 had about four times the inhibitory capacity of PGE_1 (Kloeze, 1969).

Kloeze (1969) has related the activity of prostaglandins on platelet aggregation to their chemical structure. The E type structure of the cyclopentane ring was required for either an inhibiting or stimulating effect on platelet aggregation, the keto group at C-9 being essential. The hydroxyl group at C-15 was also important since oxidation of this group inactivated the prostaglandin. The length of the ω-side chain with one C atom influenced the activity of the prostaglandin on platelet aggregation, a longer chain being associated with greater activity. Finally, all prostaglandins with a stimulating activity on platelets had a *cis* double bond in the side chain between C-5 and C-6. It would be of great importance if new prostaglandins could be synthesized with a specific action on platelet aggregation and lacking the other undesirable effects of PGE_1. The powerful inhibitory action of ω-homo PGE_1 on platelet aggregation is of great interest and deserves further study.

8.4 EFFECT OF PROSTAGLANDINS UPON BLOOD COAGULATION

In contrast to their action upon platelets, prostaglandins exert little effect on the factors responsible for fibrin formation and fibrinolysis. In their detailed study, Duboff et al. (1974) have reported PGE_1, PGE_2 and $PGF_{2\alpha}$ to have no effect on factors V, VII, VIII, IX, X, XI and XII confirming the findings of other investigators (Kloeze, 1970c; Karim and Filshie, 1972; Howie et al., 1973; Phillips, 1973). The only exceptions to this have been a lengthening of the partial thromboplastin time in plastic (Phillips, 1973) and an increase in euglobulin lysis activity and antithrombin activity following PGE_2 infusion (Howie et al., 1973). These observations would suggest that PGE_2 has an antithrombotic activity rather than the reverse. Badraoui et al. (1973 a and b) found that $PGF_{2\alpha}$, whether used intravenously, extra-amniotically or intra-amniotically, induced a transient intravascular coagulation when used to terminate mid-trimester pregnancy, though the changes were less marked than those associated with saline-induced pregnancy termination. Sekhar (1970) found that PGE_1 had no effect on fibrinolysis in the rat. These observations suggest that prostaglandins exert only a minor effect on blood coagulation and fibrinolysis and that their main influence on haemostasis and thrombosis will be mediated through their effects on platelets.

8.5 MECHANISM OF ACTION

8.5.1 Mechanism of action of PGE_1 on platelet aggregation

The mechanism whereby PGE_1 inhibits ADP-induced aggregation is not yet fully understood but the most widely-held hypothesis is that PGE_1 mediates its influence on platelet aggregation by increasing levels of cAMP. In this system cAMP is formed from ATP by the action of adenylate cyclase, an enzyme located in the cell membrane, which is sensitive to various platelet aggregating agents. The enzyme phosphodiesterase can destroy cAMP so that agents which inhibit or potentiate phosphodiesterase can influence levels of cAMP within the platelet (Salzman, 1972). Four main pieces of evidence have been advanced to support the hypothesis that PGE_1 inhibits platelet aggregation through an action on cAMP (Robison, 1971; Bousser, 1973) and these are summarized below.

1. PGE_1 stimulates adenylate cyclase activity both in platelet membrane fractions and in intact platelets (Marquis et al., 1969; Wolfe and Shulman, 1969; Zieve and Greenough, 1969; Moskowitz et al., 1970; Scott, 1970). Furthermore, calcium ions inhibit the effect of PGE_1 on platelets (Emmons et al., 1967) and also inhibit the stimulatory effect of PGE_1 upon adenylate cyclase (Vigdahl et al., 1969)
2. PGE_1 has been shown to increase cAMP in intact platelets (Marquis et al., 1969; Robison et al., 1969; Ball et al., 1970; Scott, 1970; Wolfe et al., 1970). Using adenosine ^{14}C, Vigdahl et al. (1969) demonstrated

that the conversion of ATP to intracellular cAMP was increased by PGE_1 and that the level of cAMP was related in time to the degree of platelet inhibition effected by PGE_1

3. Various compounds which inhibit phosphodiesterase, such as caffeine and theophylline, had a synergistic effect with PGE_1 both on the inhibition of platelet aggregation and the synthesis of cAMP (Marquis et al., 1969; Vigdahl and Marquis, 1969; Ball et al., 1970; Wolfe and Shulman, 1969; Mills and Smith, 1971), suggesting that the levels of cAMP were related to the inhibition of aggregation

4. The inhibitory effect of PGE_1 on platelet aggregation was reproduced by cAMP (Marquis et al., 1969; Wolfe and Shulman, 1970). Dibutyryl cAMP was more active in this respect than cAMP itself and this effect probably lay in the ability of dibutyryl cAMP to enter the cell where it functioned like cAMP (Abdulla, 1969; Salzman and Levine, 1971)

This evidence has led to the hypothesis that substances which inhibit platelet aggregation initiate a rise in cAMP and that those which cause platelet aggregation stimulate a fall in cAMP (Salzman and Levine, 1971). Some observations have been made by Haslam and Taylor (1971a, b and c) which are at variance with this hypothesis. They found that some substances which caused platelet aggregation, such as ADP and epinephrine, did not cause a significant decrease in cAMP. They have also found that considerable platelet aggregation took place in the presence of PGE_1 with platelet cAMP levels above the resting value. In addition to this, Marquis et al. (1969) have found that PGA_1 and $F_{1\alpha}$ stimulated cAMP levels but that they were poor inhibitors of platelet aggregation. Mody (1972) argued that if PGE_1 inhibited platelet aggregation solely through its stimulating effect on adenylate cyclase then the degree of inhibition should be temperature dependent, but he found this not to be so. It is possible that the rise in platelet cAMP in response to PGE_1 is a secondary effect rather than the primary mechanism responsible for the inhibition of platelet aggregation.

An alternative explanation for the inhibitory effect of PGE_1 on platelet aggregation is that it may interfere with the binding of ADP to receptors on the platelet membrane (Boullin et al., 1972). In support of this they have shown, using ^{14}C-ADP, that platelet aggregation was linearly related to the log platelet bound ADP, and that nearly all the platelet radioactivity was unmetabolized ADP. If PGE_1 was added before ADP, the inhibition of platelet aggregation was related to the decrease in ADP uptake and when PGE_1 was added after ADP, platelet aggregation was reversed with an accompanying decrease in platelet bound ADP. Platelet aggregation by ADP and its inhibition by PGE_1 are both reversible phenomena and these are consistent with a hypothesis of drug association and dissociation with receptors. When rats have been fed on a fatty-acid deficient diet, the inhibitory effect of PGE_1 on their platelets is much reduced and Vincent et al. (1974) suggested that this may be due to an induced deficiency in the platelet cell membrane. These data do not, however, exclude the possibility that accumulation of cAMP has a role in the inhibition of platelet aggregation and the action of PGE_1 upon platelets may be due to the interaction of several factors.

8.5.2 Mechanism of action of PGE$_2$ and PGF$_{2\alpha}$ on platelet aggregation

Recent studies have shown that PGE$_2$ and PGF$_{2\alpha}$ are formed during blood clotting and platelet aggregation and that these prostaglandins are released by the platelets (Smith and Willis, 1970; Silver *et al.*, 1972; Salzman *et al.*, 1973; Smith *et al.*, 1973). These observations, coupled with the stimulatory effect that PGE$_2$ may have on platelet aggregation *in vitro* (Kloeze, 1967; Shio and Ramwell, 1972a; Salzman *et al.*, 1973) raise the possibility that PGE$_2$ and PGF$_{2\alpha}$ may play a part in normal platelet aggregation. Alternatively, precursors of these prostaglandins may be important because arachidonic acid is capable of stimulating platelet aggregation (Smith *et al.*, 1974). Two groups of workers have concurrently shown that an intermediate of prostaglandin biosynthesis, which is readily converted to PGE$_2$ or PGF$_{2\alpha}$, is released during platelet aggregation (Willis and Kuhn, 1973; Smith *et al.*, 1974). This endoperoxide intermediate was released from platelets in response to arachidonic acid, collagen and L-epinephrine and was closely related to the release of adenine nucleotides and 5-HT. Furthermore, it appeared outside the platelet before collagen-induced platelet aggregation had occurred and its maximal concentration preceded that of PGE$_2$ and PGF$_{2\alpha}$ (Smith *et al.*, 1974). Willis (1974) described the intermediate compound as labile-aggregation stimulating substance (LASS) and reported that aspirin, which inhibited the conversion of arachidonic acid to LASS and PGE$_2$, also inhibited the trigger to platelet aggregation. Similarly 5,8,11,14 eicosatetraynoic acid (TYA) inhibited the conversion of arachidonic acid to LASS and PGE$_2$ and suppressed irreversible platelet aggregation (Willis *et al.*, 1974). These workers speculate that this prostaglandin intermediate might be the trigger to the platelet release reaction. These observations suggest that prostaglandins may have an important role in platelet aggregation and further developments can be expected in this interesting field.

8.6 CLINICAL IMPLICATIONS OF PROSTAGLANDINS AND PLATELET AGGREGATION

One valuable implication of the inhibitory effect of PGE$_1$ upon platelet aggregation is that it can be used to greatly improve the harvesting of platelets for transfusion from refrigerated whole blood (Becker *et al.*, 1972; Shio and Ramwell, 1972b; Valeri *et al.*, 1972; Becker *et al.*, 1974). When blood is stored, platelets readily aggregate and within 6 h are not available for the purpose of preparing a platelet transfusion. If a small concentration of PGE$_1$ (3 μg per unit) is added to the blood, this prevents platelet aggregation so that 75% of platelets remain therapeutically viable three days after storage at 4 °C (Becker *et al.*, 1974). When the blood is infused, the PGE$_1$ is present in such a low concentration that it causes no side effects. After infusion, the PGE$_1$ is inactivated in the lungs, and the platelets become available for haemostatic purposes. It has also been suggested that the PGE$_1$ could be used to prevent the formation of platelet aggregates within heart–lung machines

(Stibbe *et al.*, 1973). This platelet aggregation is not prevented by heparin and Stibbe *et al.* (1973) have shown that the fall in platelet count in the heart–lung machine can be inhibited by PGE_1. The continued use of PGE_2 and $PGF_{2\alpha}$ for the purpose of pregnancy termination is supported by the reports that PGE_2 inhibits platelet adhesiveness when infused in humans (Howie *et al.*, 1973) and that $PGF_{2\alpha}$ causes less disturbance of the coagulation mechanism than intra-amniotic saline (Bradaoui *et al.*, 1973).

Prostaglandin E_1, by virtue of its inhibitory effect on platelet aggregation, has potential value as an antithrombotic agent, but the factors preventing its use are the transient nature of its effect and the toxic side-effects. As more information is gained about the chemical characteristics which are responsible for the various actions of prostaglandins, it may be possible to prepare a prostaglandin analogue with a selective action on platelet aggregation.

8.7 CONCLUSION

PGE_1 has a powerful inhibitory action on ADP-induced platelet aggregation and the platelet-release reaction both *in vitro* and *in vivo*. When given intravenously the effect of PGE_1 on platelets *in vivo* is transient and the unpleasant side-effects of PGE_1 will limit its use as a therapeutic agent in man. The effect of PGE_2 on platelets *in vitro* is disputed, having been reported by different investigators to inhibit and to stimulate platelet aggregation. The *in vivo* effect of PGE_2 has been studied only to a limited extent but PGE_2 has been reported to inhibit human platelet adhesiveness to a cellophane membrane. Prostaglandins of the A, B and F groups have little effect on platelet aggregation and prostaglandins have only minor effects on blood coagulation and fibrinolysis.

The mechanism whereby PGE_1 inhibits platelet aggregation is not known, but PGE_1 may act by stimulating adenylate cyclase to convert ATP to cAMP or by competing with ADP for receptor sites on the platelet membrane. PGE_2 and $PGF_{2\alpha}$ are formed and released by platelets during aggregation and may play an important part in the physiology of platelet aggregation. A precursor of PGE_2 and $PGF_{2\alpha}$ named labile aggregation stimulating substance, is also formed during platelet aggregation and has been proposed as a possible trigger to the platelet release reaction.

PGE_1 may have practical value in the preparation of platelet transfusions and in the inhibition of platelet aggregation in heart–lung machines. Future studies may throw further light on the mechanisms responsible for platelet aggregation and indicate new uses for prostaglandins as therapeutic agents.

References

Abdulla, Y. H. (1969). α-Adrenergic receptors in human platelets. *J. Atheroscler. Res.*, **9**, 171

Arfors, K. E., Hint, H. C., Dhall, D. P. and Matheson, N. A. (1968). Counteraction of platelet activity at sites of laser induced endothelial trauma. *Br. Med. J.*, **4**, 430

Badraoui, M. H. H., Bonnar, J., Hillier, K. and Embrey, M. P. (1973a). Coagulation changes during termination of pregnancy by prostaglandins and by vacuum aspiration. *Br. Med. J.*, **1**, 19

Badraoui, M. H. H., Bonnar, J., Hillier, K. and Embrey, M. P. (1973b). Blood coagulation changes during mid-trimester abortion induced by prostaglandin $F_{2\alpha}$. Br. Med. J., 4, 375

Ball, G., Brereton, G. G., Fulwood, M., Ireland, D. M. and Yates, P. (1970). Effect of prostaglandin E_1 alone and in combination with theophylline or aspirin on collagene-induced platelet aggregation and on platelet nucleotides including adenosine 3'5' cyclic monophosphate. Biochem. J., 120, 709

Becker, G. A., Chalos, M. K., Tuccelli, M. and Aster, R. H. (1972). Prostaglandin E_1 in preparation and storage of platelet concentrates. Science, 175, 538

Becker, G. A., Kunicki, T. and Aster, R. H. (1974). Effect of prostaglandin E_1 on harvesting of platelets from refrigerated whole blood. J. Lab. Clin. Med., 83, 304

Bettex-Galland, M. and Luscher, E. F. (1961). Thrombasthenin—a contractile protein from thrombocytes. Extraction from human blood platelets and some of its properties. Biochem. Biophys. Acta, 49, 536

Born, G. V. R. (1962). Aggregation of blood platelets by adenosine diphosphate and its reversal. Nature (Lond.), 194, 927

Born, G. V. R. (1972). Platelets. Functional Physiology. In Human Blood Coagulation, Haemostasis and Thrombosis, Biggs, R. (ed.), p. 159, (Oxford: Blackwell Scientific Publications)

Boullin, D. J., Green, A. R. and Price, K. S. (1972). The mechanism of ADP-induced platelet aggregation: binding to platelet receptors and inhibition of binding and aggregation by prostaglandin E_1. J. Physiol. (Lond.), 221, 415

Bousser, M. G. (1973). Prostaglandin E_1 and platelets. Biomedicine, 18, 95

Carlsson, L. A., Irion, E. and Orö, L. (1968). Effect of infusion of prostaglandin E_1 on the aggregation of platelets in man. Life Sci., 7, 85

Castaldi, P. A., Larrieu, M. J. and Caen, J. (1965). Availability of platelet factor 3 and activation of factor XII in thrombasthenia. Nature (Lond.), 207, 422

Chandrasekhar, N. (1967). Inhibition of platelet aggregation by prostaglandins. Blood, 30, 554

Crevald, S. van and Pascha, C. N. (1968). Influence of prostaglandins E_1 and E_2 on aggregation of blood platelets. Nature (Lond.), 218, 361

Duboff, G. S., Penner, J. A. and Rohwedder, J. (1974). Effect of prostaglandins E_1, E_2 and $F_{2\alpha}$ on human blood coagulation. Nature (Lond.), 251, 430

Ekeles, R. S., Hampton, J. R., Harrison, M. J. G. and Mitchell, J. R. A. (1969). Prosta-glandin E_1 and human platelets. Lancet, ii, 111

Emmons, P. R., Hampton, J. R., Harrison, M. J. G., Honour, A. J. and Mitchell, J. R. A. (1967). Effect of prostaglandin E_1 on platelet behaviour in vitro and in vivo. Br. Med. J., 2, 468

Ferriera, S. H. and Vane, J. R. (1967). Prostaglandins: their disappearance from and release into the circulation. Nature, 216, 868

Gaarder, A., Jonsen, J., Laland, S., Hellem, A. and Owren, P. A. (1961). Adenosine diphosphate in red cells as a factor in the adhesiveness of human blood platelets. Nature (Lond.), 192, 531

Hampton, J. R. and Mitchell, J. R. A. (1966). Effect of aggregating agents on the electro-phoretic mobility of human platelets. Br. Med. J., 1, 1074

Hardisty, R. M. and Hutton, R. A. (1966). Platelet aggregation and the availability of platelet factor 3. Br. J. Haemat., 12, 764

Haslam, R. J. (1968). Biochemical aspects of platelet function. In Proc. XIIth Congr. Int. Soc. Haematol., p. 198 (N.Y.)

Haslam, R. J. and Taylor, A. (1970a). Effects of aggregating agents on platelet cyclic AMP levels. In 2nd Int. Cong. on Thrombosis and Haemothasis, p. 210 (Oslo)

Haslam, R. J. and Taylor, A. (1971b). Role of cyclic 3'5' adenosine monophosphate in platelet aggregation. In Platelet Aggregation, p. 85 (Paris: Masson et Cie)

Haslam, R. J. and Taylor, A. (1971c). Effects of catecholamines on the formation of cAMP in human blood platelets. Biochem. J., 125, 377

Hellem, A. J. (1960). The adhesiveness of human blood platelets in vitro. Scand. J. Clin. Lab. Invest., 12, Suppl. 51, 1

Hellem, A. and Owren, P. A. (1964). The mechanism of the hemostatic function of blood platelets. Acta Haemat., 31, 230

Hirsh, J., McBride, J. A. and Dacie, J. V. (1966). Thrombo-embolism and increased platelet adhesiveness in post-splenectomy thrombocytosis. Aust. Ann. Med., 15, 122

Hissen, W., Fleming, J. S., Bierwagen, M. E. and Pindell, M. H. (1969). Effect of prostaglandin E_1 on platelet aggregation *in vitro* and in hemorrhagic shock. *Microvasc.-Res.*, **1**, 374

Hornstra, G. (1971). Degree and duration of prostaglandin E_1-induced inhibition of platelet aggregation in the rat. *Eur. J. Pharmacol.*, **15**, 343

Hovig, T., Rowsell, H. C., Dodds, W. J., Jorgensen, L. and Mustard, J. F. (1967). Experimental hemostasis in normal dogs and in dogs with congenital disorders of blood coagulation. *Blood*, **30**, 636

Howie, P. W., Calder, A. A., Forbes, C. D. and Prentice, C. R. M. (1973). Effect of intravenous prostaglandin E_2 on platelet function, coagulation and fibrinolysis. *J. Clin. Pathol.*, **26**, 354

Hugues, J. (1960). Accolement des plaquettes aux collagene. *Soc. Biol. (Paris)*, **154**, 866

Irion, E. and Blomback, M. (1969). Prostaglandins in platelet aggregation. *Scand. J. Clin. Lab. Invest.*, **24**, 141

Jorgenson, L. and Borchgrevink, C. F. (1963). The platelet plug in normal persons. *Acta Path. Microbiol. Scand.*, **57**, 40

Karim, S. M. M. and Filshie, G. M. (1972). The use of prostaglandin E_2 for therapeutic abortion. *J. Obstet. Gynaec. Br. Commonwealth*, **79**, 1

Kinlough-Rathbone, R. L., Packham, M. A. and Mustard, J. F. (1970). The effect of prostaglandin E_1 on platelet function *in vitro* and *in vivo*. *Br. J. Haemat.*, **19**, 559

Kloeze, J. (1967). Influence of prostaglandins on platelet adhesiveness and platelet aggregation. In *Prostaglandins, 2nd Nobel Symposium*, Bergström, S. and Samuelsson, B. (eds.), pp. 241–252 (Stockholm: Almqvist and Wiksell)

Kloeze, J. (1969). Relationship between chemical structure and platelet aggregation activity of prostaglandins. *Biochem. Biophys. Acta*, **187**, 285

Kloeze, J. (1970a). Prostaglandins and platelet aggregation *in vivo*. 1. Influence of prostaglandin E_1 and ω-homo-prostaglandin E_1 on transient thrombocytopenia and of prostaglandin E_1 on the LD50 of ADP. *Thromb. Diath. Haemorrh.*, **23**, 286

Kloeze, J. (1970b). Prostaglandins and platelet aggregation *in vivo*. II. Influence of prostaglandin E_1 and prostaglandin $F_{2\alpha}$ on platelet thrombus formation induced by an electric stimulus in veins on the rat brain surface. *Thromb. Diath. Haemorrh.*, **23**, 293

Kloeze, J. (1970c). Influence of prostaglandins E_1 and E_2 on coagulation of rat blood. *Experientia*, **26**, 307

Lancet (Leading article), (1971). Management of thrombosis. *Lancet*, **ii**, 361

Lindsay, R. M., Prentice, C. R. M., Ferguson, D., Muir, W. M. and McNicol, G. P. (1973). A method for the measurement of platelet adhesiveness by use of dialysis membranes in a test-cell. *Br. J. Haemat.*, **24**, 377

MacMillan, D. C. and Oliver, M. F. (1965). The initial changes in platelet morphology following the addition of adenosine diphosphate. *J. Atheroscler. Res.*, **5**, 440

Marquis, N. R., Vigdahl, R. L. and Tavormina, P. A. (1969). Platelet aggregation II. Regulation by cyclic AMP and prostaglandin E_1. *Biochem. Biophys. Res. Commun.*, **36**, 965

Mills, D. C. B. and Smith, J. B. (1971). The influence on platelet aggregation of drugs that affect the accumulation of adenosine 3'5' monophosphate in platelets. *Biochem. J.*, **121**, 185

Mitchell, J. R. A. (1968). Platelets and Thrombosis. *Sci. Basis Med., Ann. Rev.*, 266

Mody, N. J. (1972). Effects of prostaglandins on platelet function. In *The Prostaglandins, Progress in Research*, Karim, S. M. M. (ed.), 1st Ed., pp. 239–262 (Oxford: MTP)

Moskowitz, J., Harwood, J. P., Reid, W. D. and Krishna, G. (1970). Interaction between nor-epinephrine and prostaglandin E_1 on adenyl cyclase in blood platelets. *Fed. Proc.*, **29**, 602

Murakami, M., Odake, K., Takase, M. and Yoshino, K. (1972). Potentiating effect of adenosine on other inhibitors of platelet aggregation. *Thromb. Diath. Haemorrh.*, **27**, 252

Murer, E. H. (1971). Effect of prostaglandin E_1 on clot retraction. *Nature (Lond.)*, **229**, 112

Mustard, J. F., Glynn, M. F., Nishizawa, E. E. and Packham, M. A. (1967). Platelet surface interactions: relationship to thrombosis and hemostasis. *Fed. Proc.*, **26**, 106

Mustard, J. F., Hegardt, B., Rowsell, H. C. and MacMillan, R. L. (1964). Effect of adenosine nucleotides on platelet aggregation and clotting time. *J. Lab. Clin. Med.*, **64**, 548

Mustard, J. F. and Packham, M. A. (1970). Factors influencing platelet function; adhesion, release and aggregation. *Pharmacol. Rev.*, **22**, 97

Phillips, L. L. (1973). Effect of prostaglandins on the coagulation mechanism of the pregnant rat. *Am. J. Obstet. Gynecol.*, **115**, 227

Robison, G. A. (1971). Effects of prostaglandins on functions and cyclic AMP levels of human blood platelets. *Ann. N.Y. Acad. Sci.*, **180**, 324

Robison, G. A., Arnold, A. and Hartmann, R. C. (1969). Divergent effects of epinephrine and prostaglandin E_1 on the level of cyclic AMP in human blood platelets. *Pharmacol. Res. Commun.*, **1**, 325

Salzman, E. W. (1972). Cyclic AMP and platelet function. *New Engl. J. Med.*, **286**, 358

Salzman, E. W. and Levine, L. (1971). Cyclic 3'5' adenosine monophosphate in human platelets. 2. Effect of N.0. 2'-0-dibutryl cyclic 3'5' adenosine monophosphate on platelet function. *J. Clin. Invest.*, **50**, 131

Salzman, E. W., Stead, N. and Deykin, D. (1973). Interrelations of platelet prostaglandin synthesis and cyclic AMP metabolism. In *IVth Int. Cong. on Thrombosis and Haemostasis*, Abst., p. 78 (Vienna)

Scott, R. E. (1970). Effects of prostaglandins, epinephrine and NaF on human leukocyte, platelet and liver adenyl cyclase. *Blood*, **35**, 514

Sekhar, N. C. (1970). Effect of eight prostaglandins on platelet aggregation. *J. Med. Chem.*, **13**, 39

Shio, H., Plasse, A. M. and Ramwell, P. W. (1970). Platelet swelling and prostaglandins. *Microvasc. Res.*, **2**, 294

Shio, H. and Ramwell, P. (1972a). Effect of prostaglandin E_2 and aspirin on the secondary aggregation of human platelets. *Nature New Biology*, **236**, 45

Shio, H. and Ramwell, P. W. (1972b). Prostaglandin E_1 in platelet harvesting: an *in vitro* study. *Science*, **175**, 536

Silver, M. J., Smith, J. B., Ingerman, C. and Kocsis, J. J. (1972). Human blood prostaglandins: formation during clotting. *Prostaglandins*, **1**, 429

Smith, J. B., Ingerman, C., Kocsis, J. J. and Silver, M. J. (1973). Formation of prostaglandins during the aggregation of human blood platelets. *J. Clin. Invest.*, **52**, 965

Smith, J. B., Ingerman, C., Kocsis, J. J. and Silver, M. J. (1974). Formation of an intermediate in prostaglandin biosynthesis and its association with the platelet release reaction. *J. Clin. Invest.*, **53**, 1468

Smith, J. B. and Willis, A. L. (1970). Formation and release of prostaglandins by platelets in response to thrombin. *Br. J. Pharmac.*, **40**, 545

Spaet, T. H. and Zucker, M. B. (1964). Mechanism of platelet plug formation and role of adenosine diphosphate. *Am. J. Physiol.*, **206**, 1267

Stibbe, J., Ong, G. L., ten Hoor, F. and Nauta, J. (1973). The influence of PGE_1 on platelet decrease in the heart-lung machine. In *IVth Int. Cong. on Thrombosis and Haemostasis*, Abst., p. 412 (Vienna)

Turpie, A. G. G., McNichol, G. P. and Douglas, A. S. (1971). Platelets: Haemostasis and Thrombosis. In *Recent Advances in Haematology*, Goldbert, A. and Brain, M. C. (eds.), p. 249 (Edinburgh: Livingstone)

Valeri, C. R., Zaroulis, C. G., Rogers, J. C., Handin, R. I. and Marchionni, L. D. (1972). Prostaglandins in the preparation of blood components. *Science*, **175**, 539

Vigdahl, R. C. and Marquis, N. R. (1969). Cyclic AMP mediated inhibition of platelet aggregation by vasodilation. *Circulation*, **42, Suppl. 1, 111**, 50

Vigdahl, R. C., Marquis, N. R. and Tavormina, P. A. (1969). Platelet aggregation II: adenyl cyclase, prostaglandin E_1 and calcium. *Biochem. Biophys. Res. Commun.*, **37**, 409

Vincent, J. E., Melai, A., Bonta, I. L. (1974). Comparison of the effects of prostaglandin E_1 on platelet aggregation in normal and essential fatty-acid deficient rats. *Prostaglandins*, **5**, 369

Weeks, J. R., Sekhar, N. C. and DuCharme, D. W. (1969). Relative activity of prostaglandins E_1, A_1, E_2 and A_2 on lipolysis, platelet aggregation, smooth muscle and the cardiovascular system. *J. Pharm. Pharmacol.*, **21**, 103

Willis, A. L. and Kuhn, D. C. (1973). A new potential mediator of arterial thrombosis whose biosynthesis is inhibited by aspirin. *Prostaglandins*, **4**, 127

Willis, A. L. (1974). An enzymatic mechanism for the antithrombotic and antihaemostatic actions of aspirin. *Science*, **183**, 325

Willis, A. L., Kuhn, D. C. and Weiss, H. J. (1974). Acetylenic analog of arachidonate that acts like aspirin on platelets. *Science*, **183**, 327

Wolfe, S. M., Muenzer, J. and Shulman, N. R. (1970). Role of cyclic adenosine 3'5' monophosphate and prostaglandins in platelet aggregation. *J. Clin. Invest.*, **49**, 104

Wolfe, S. M. and Shulman, N. R. (1969). Adenyl cyclase activity in human platelets. *Biochem. Biophys. Res. Commun.*, **35,** 265

Zieve, P. D. and Greenough, W. B. (1969). Adenyl cyclase in human platelets: activity and responsiveness. *Biochem. Biophys. Res. Commun.*, **35,** 462

Zucker, M. B. (1947). Platelet agglutination and vasoconstriction as factors in spontaneous hemostasis in normal, thrombocytopenic, heparinised and hypoprothrombinemic rats. *Am. J. Physiol.*, **148,** 275

Zucker, M. B. and Borrelli, J. (1962). Platelet clumping produced by connective tissue suspensions and by collagen. *Proc. Soc. Exp. Biol. (N.Y.)*, **109,** 779

9
Prostaglandins and Inflammation

M. W. GREAVES

9.1 INTRODUCTION   293

9.2 INFLAMMATORY ACTIONS OF PROSTAGLANDINS   293

9.3 PRESENCE OF PROSTAGLANDINS IN INFLAMMATORY REACTIONS   295

9.4 SYNTHESIS OF PROSTAGLANDINS IN INFLAMMATION AND ITS
    INHIBITION BY ANTI-INFLAMMATORY DRUGS   298

    REFERENCES   300

9.1 INTRODUCTION

The view that prostaglandins are important mediators of inflammation in man is now widely held. The supporting evidence, most of which has appeared over the last three or four years, derives from studies of a wide variety or organs, tissues and species from very many laboratories throughout the world. The involvement of prostaglandins in inflammation in different systems is discussed in the various chapters in this book. The purpose of this review is an appraisal of reports which are representative of the more significant milestones in progress towards clarification of the role of prostaglandins in inflammation.

9.2 INFLAMMATORY ACTIONS OF PROSTAGLANDINS

That some prostaglandins possess pro-inflammatory activity was recognized in 1963 by Horton who showed that PGE_1 increased blood flow in the hind limb of the cat. Horton also demonstrated increased vascular permeability in guinea pig skin due to PGE_1, maximum effect being obtained with 1 μg.

Vasodilatation due to PGE_1 in man is characteristically a long-lasting, erythema due to a single intradermal injection persisting for up to 10 h (Solomon *et al.*, 1968). Subsequent studies in the rat by Crunkhorn and Willis (1969) established that both PGE_1 and PGE_2 increase skin vascular permeability, the threshold dose for PGE_2 in this tissue being 1 ng. By contrast $PGF_{1\alpha}$ and $PGF_{2\alpha}$ were without effect even at μg dosage. In man Crunkhorn and Willis (1969) noted that intradermal injection of 50–100 ng PGE_1 or PGE_2 caused maximum local edema and redness within 15–30 min of injection. They also proposed that the vasoactivity of PGs E_1 and E_2 might be due, at least in part, to local histamine release since the vascular responses to PGE_2 in the rat could be reduced by prior administration of the antihistamine, mepyramine, or the chemical histamine liberator, compound 48/80 (Crunkhorn and Willis, 1971a). The same conclusion was reached in man by Sondergaard and Greaves (1971a) who found that the whealing, but not the erythematous response to prostaglandin E_1 could be reduced but not completely blocked by prior administration of the potent antihistamine chlorpheniramine and by local depletion of histamine stores in skin using the histamine liberator polymyxin B. Thus it seems probable that PGs E_1 and E_2 have both a direct permeability action and an indirect one due to histamine release.

Another indirect permeability action of PGs E_1 and E_2 of possible importance in the pathology of inflammation has recently attracted great interest. Moncada *et al.*, (1973) showed that PGs E_1 and E_2 potentiate rat paw swelling induced by bradykinin, histamine and carageenin. Similar potentiation was demonstrated by Thomas and West (1974) between PGE_2 and bradykinin in rat skin. The possibility arises that a lowering of the threshold of the blood vasculature to the permeability actions of other mediators may be an important role of the E prostaglandins in inflammation. Similar studies of the interactions of the E prostaglandins and other vasoactive agents in human tissues would clearly be of great interest.

The leukotactic action of the prostaglandins has excited considerable interest. Using a modified Boyden chamber, Kaley and Weiner (1971) showed a highly significant chemotactic action of PGE_1 (1 μg/ml) on rabbit polymorphonuclear leukocytes. That this action of PGE_1 may also occur in man *in vivo* is suggested by studies of the cellular exudate in human skin using a skin window technique. Sondergaard and Wolf-Jorgensen (1972) observed an initial migration of polymorphonuclear leukocytes of 12 h duration, followed by a predominantly mononuclear invasion lasting 24 h, and a final second wave of polymorphonuclear leukocytes. The pattern of immigration was identical in the presence of PGE_1 or $PGF_{1\alpha}$. However, it cannot be assumed that Sondergaard's findings represent the chemotactic response demonstrated *in vitro* by Kaley and Weiner since accumulation of different cell types in inflammatory lesions depends on factors additional to chemotaxis.

Evaluation of the inflammatory actions of prostaglandins would be incomplete without considering their ability to mediate the symptoms of inflammation—pain and (in skin) itch. Horton (1963) could not demonstrate a pain-producing action of PGE_1 following application to a blister base and subsequent studies have confirmed the low potency of the E prostaglandins in respect of pain production (Kingston and Greaves, 1975). However,

PGE_1 causes marked hyperalgesia and infusions of PGE_1 sub-dermally potentiate the pain-producing action of histamine or bradykinin (Ferreira, 1972). Ferreira also noted that a combined intradermal infusion of PGE_1 and histamine produced itching. This finding was confirmed and extended recently by Greaves and McDonald-Gibson (1973a) who showed that PGE_1 lowers the threshold of human skin to histamine-evoked itching. Thus it seems that alteration of threshold responses of components of inflammation to other mediators may be an important general role of PGs.

The ability of PGs to evoke fever in experimental situations has stimulated great interest. In 1970 Milton and Wenlandt identified a prostaglandin-like substance from the cerebrospinal fluid of a febrile cat. Subsequent experiments showed that $PGF_{1\alpha}$, PGA_1, PGE_1 but not $PGF_{2\alpha}$ produced a pyrexial response when injected into the cat lateral ventricle.

These results were later confirmed and extended by Feldberg and Saxena (1971) who found that nanogram amounts of PGE_1 produced fever when injected into the cerebral ventricles of several laboratory species. It seems possible that antipyretic drugs may owe their action at least in part to reduced formation of prostaglandins by the anterior hypothalamus (see also Chapter 1).

In this discussion emphasis has been placed on the pro-inflammatory properties of prostaglandins. However, the relationship of prostaglandin to the inflammatory response is more complex. Prostaglandins also possess anti-inflammatory properties and the development and regression of inflammation probably depends partly upon relative concentrations of pro- and anti-inflammatory prostaglandin activity and possibly also on a feedback inhibition by prostaglandins. Hillier and Karim drew attention in 1968 to the opposing actions of E and F prostaglandins on human blood vessels. In skin Crunkhorn and Willis (1971b) demonstrated the antagonistic action of $PGF_{2\alpha}$ on increased vascular permeability due to PGE_1 or PGE_2. This work, as well as their own findings on relative concentrations of PGE and PGF in inflammatory exudates at different stages of the inflammation response, has led Willoughby and his colleagues (Velo et al., 1973) to suggest that the acuteness of an inflammatory reaction at a particular moment may depend on the ratio of PGE to PGF. Looking at the same problem from a different angle, Lichtenstein et al. (1972) have demonstrated inhibition of in vitro models of immediate and delayed hypersensitivity by PGE_1. Because of PGE_1's stimulatory action on adenylate cyclase it is of particular interest that in both instances increase in cellular cAMP concentrations paralleled the degree of inhibition of the immune response. In view of the theory of Goldberg (1972) that some mechanisms involving the intermediary cAMP may be opposed by cGMP, determination of the relative concentrations of the two nucleotides in the target cells of these two immune reactions in the presence and absence of PGE_1 would be of great interest.

9.3 PRESENCE OF PROSTAGLANDINS IN INFLAMMATORY REACTIONS

Credit for the first evidence implicating prostaglandins as mediators of inflammation should go to Ambache et al. who in 1965 reported experiments in which they obtained perfusates from the anterior chamber of the rabbit eye. After irritation of the iris they detected the presence in the perfusates of a smooth muscle contracting agent, which was distinct from other known smooth muscle contracting agents and which was termed 'Irin' and later identified as a mixture of PGE_2- and $PGF_{2\alpha}$-like substances. Subsequent work has confirmed the presence of increased prostaglandin activity in anterior uveitis both in the rabbit and in man (Eakins, Whitelocke, Bennett and Martenet, 1972; Eakins, Whitelocke, Perkins, Bennett and Ungar, 1972). Much work, initiated by Willis (1969) has been done on characterizing prostaglandin in activity in inflammatory exudate due to carrageenan in laboratory animals. However the significance of carrageenan edema as a model of human inflammation is uncertain. The presence of increased prostaglandin activity in human inflammation has been firmly established by studies in inflamed skin due to thermal injury (Änggård et al., 1970; Arturson et al., 1973) allergic contact eczema (Greaves et al., 1971; Goldyne et al., 1973) primary irritant contact eczema (Sondergaard and Greaves, 1974) and ultraviolet irradiation (Greaves and Sondergaard, 1970; Mathur and Gandhi, 1972).

In the experiments of Greaves et al. (1971) human forearm skin was perfused by a physiological solution for periods of up to 8 h. The perfusates were then analysed for smooth muscle contracting activity by physicochemical and pharmacological methods. The value and limitation of the perfusion technique used by these workers has been evaluated by them elsewhere (Sondergaard and Greaves, 1971a). In inflamed skin due to allergic contact eczema the perfusates contained pharmacological activity distinct from known vasoactive agents (Figure 9.1). This activity, which could be demonstrated against a wide range of smooth muscle preparations, was acidic lipid in nature since on solvent partition of perfusate solution between ethyl

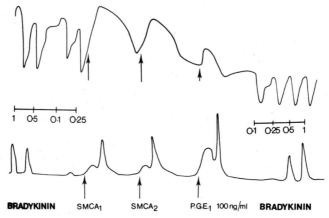

Figure 9.1 Responses of 2 isolated organ preparations to perfusates from inflamed skin of human allergic contact eczema. Upper tracing: rat duodenum. Lower preparation: rat uterus. Perfusing solution: Tyrode. Doses of standard bradykinin ranging from 0.025–1 μg caused relaxation of the duodenum and contraction of the uterus. Two additions of perfusates from inflamed skin ($SMCA_1$ and $SMCA_2$) caused contraction of both preparations. A standard dose of prostaglandin E_1 1 μg also caused contraction of the two preparations qualitatively similar to that caused by $SMCA_1$ and $SMCA_2$.

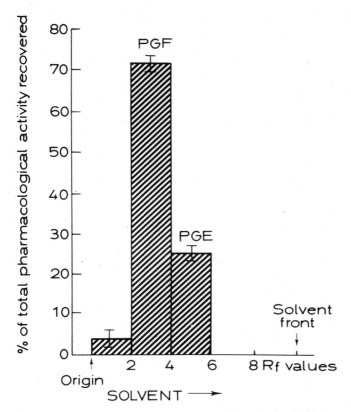

Figure 9.2 Thin layer chromatogram distribution of prostaglandin-like material recovered by ethyl acetate extraction from perfusates of inflamed skin due to allergic contact eczema using the A1 solvent system of Gréen and Samuelsson. Pharmacological activity, in terms of prostaglandin E_1-equivalents, is expressed as a % of total activity present. Mean values shown ±S.E.M.

acetate and water at pH 3 the smooth muscle contracting activity appeared in the organic phase. Thin-layer chromatography revealed that the acidic lipid activity co-chromatographed with PGF and PGE (Figure 9.2). The concentration of prostaglandin-like activity in perfusates from inflamed skin of contact eczema was about 10 times higher than in control perfusates from non-inflamed skin of contact eczema which contained little or no activity. Confirmatory evidence on the identity of the prostaglandins in the perfusate was obtained from further chromatographic separation into PGs E_1, E_2, $F_{1\alpha}$ and $F_{2\alpha}$ and by parallel bioassay using the method of Chang and Gaddum (1933). Identical results in allergic contact eczema perfusates have been obtained subsequently by Goldyne *et al.* (1973). These workers used a radioimmunoassay method to identify and quantitate prostaglandin activity.

That increased prostaglandin activity is a feature not only of the integument but also of deep tissues is suggested by the presence of prostaglandin activity in synovial fluid of patients with rheumatoid arthritis (Velo *et al.*, 1973). However, at least in skin, prostaglandin activity does not seem to be a feature of immediate wheal and flare reactions (Sondergaard and Greaves, 1971b).

It is most improbable that prostaglandins are the sole mediators of inflammatory reactions in which they are found. Most studies of inflammatory exudates and perfusates have revealed the presence of other mediators including histamine and serotonin (characteristically early on in the reaction) and bradykinin (Sondergaard and Greaves, 1970; DiRosa *et al.*, 1971). No doubt others, hitherto unidentified, play a part. The possibility of synergism between different mediators as an important factor in the pharmacogenesis of inflammatory reactions has already been alluded to.

Recently a new group of prostaglandin endoperoxide derivatives has been described (Hamberg *et al.*, 1975) called thromboxanes. These agents, although unstable, are highly active pharmacologically. Their role in response to tissue injury remains to be elucidated.

9.4 SYNTHESIS OF PROSTAGLANDINS IN INFLAMMATION AND ITS INHIBITION BY ANTI-INFLAMMATORY DRUGS

With the exception of semen, most body fluids and tissues contain little or no free prostaglandin activity under basal conditions. In inflammation prostaglandins are synthesized locally in response to the injurious stimulus. At a subcellular level the prostaglandin-synthesizing activity is located mainly in the microsomal fraction. In addition to local synthesis, local degradation also occurs since prostaglandin-degrading enzymes are also widely distributed in the body tissues and thus the concentration of prostaglandins in a tissue at a given time is the net result of the difference between rates of synthesis and degradation. The cellular localization of prostaglandin synthetase activity in inflamed tissues is a matter of some debate. That the increased enzyme activity in inflammation may not be derived from the 'native' cellular constituents of the healthy tissue is suggested by Whitelocke *et al.* (1973) who noted marked differences in the ratio of PGE to PGF in aqueous humour of inflamed eyes compared with healthy eyes. They attributed increased prostaglandin formation to invading polymorphonuclear cells which are found in large numbers in the aqueous in anterior uveitis and it is of interest that prostaglandin synthesis by bacterially stimulated rabbit polymorphonuclear leukocytes has been demonstrated (Higgs and Youlten, 1972). However, the role of contaminating platelets in the observed prostaglandin formation in these experiments is difficult to evaluate since platelets are also rich in prostaglandin synthetase (Smith and Willis, 1970). Platelets could also provide a significant source of prostaglandin synthetase in delayed inflammation since platelet thrombi in the microvasculature are a feature of many delayed inflammatory reactions, and it is of interest that aspirin is a potent inhibitor of prostaglandin synthesis by human platelets.

The importance of prostaglandin synthesis inhibition as a basic mode of action of non-steroid anti-inflammatory drugs has been highlighted by the work of Vane and his colleagues (Vane, 1971; Smith and Willis, 1971; Ferreira *et al.*, 1971). Vane used a prostaglandin synthetase preparation contained in the cell-free supernatant of homogenates of guinea pig lung and demonstrated dose-related inhibition of prostaglandin synthesis by the non-steroid anti-inflammatory and antipyretic drugs indomethacin, aspirin and salicylate. By contrast hydrocortisone had little or no inhibitory action on prostaglandin synthesis. Similar effects of non-steroid anti-inflammatory drugs were observed on prostaglandin formation in platelet suspensions and the spleen. Aspirin was shown to inhibit thrombin-evoked prostaglandin synthesis from human platelets *in vitro*, and platelets obtained from volunteers who had previously ingested aspirin showed reduced ability to synthesize prostaglandin on subsequent *in vitro* testing. Aspirin and indomethacin also inhibited adrenergically stimulated prostaglandin synthesis from the isolated dog spleen. The results thus suggested that inhibition of prostaglandin synthesis might be an important therapeutic mode of action of this group of drugs. This suggestion is strengthened by the rough correlation of the ID50 of the drugs on inhibition of prostaglandin synthesis with their rank order of anti-inflammatory activity (Flower *et al.*, 1972). Prostaglandin synthetase preparations from different tissues show differing sensitivities to the inhibitory action of anti-inflammatory drugs. Flower and Vane (1972) compared the inhibitory action of indomethacin and 4-acetamidophenol (paracetamol) on synthetase preparations from dog spleen and rabbit brain. Indomethacin was about 20 times more potent as an inhibitor on spleen synthetase than on brain synthetase, whereas 4-acetamidophenol had 7 times greater inhibitory activity on brain synthetase than on spleen synthetase. The effect of corticosteroids on PG activity is complex. Greaves and his colleagues (Greaves and McDonald-Gibson, 1973b; Greaves, Kingston and Pretty, 1975) have shown that the potent glucocorticoid fluocinolone acetonide inhibits PG formation in crude homogenates of skin, but does not inhibit synthesis by the microsomal fraction of skin. Other recent work suggests that corticosteroids may act on release of preformed PGs or on availability of lipid substrate (Lewis and Piper, 1975; Gryglewski *et al.*, 1975). In skin, non-steroid anti-inflammatory drugs show inhibitory activity on prostaglandin synthesis which resembles that reported in other tissues although skin synthetase seems generally less sensitive than preparations from other tissues (Greaves and McDonald-Gibson, 1973b). Thus the relationship of anti-inflammatory drugs to prostaglandin biosynthesis still requires further elucidation and it may be significant that most anti-inflammatory drugs inhibit other enzyme systems in addition to prostaglandin synthetase.

The evidence for implication of prostaglandins in the pathogenesis of inflammation both as mediators and possibly as regulators through a feedback inhibition mechansim is thus strong, if not overwhelming. Further support is likely to come from detailed quantitative studies of prostaglandin formation in inflammation and correlation of rate of formation with the evolution and involution of model inflammatory reactions. Confirmation may well have to await the advent of specific inhibitors or antagonists of the pro-inflammatory E prostaglandins.

The sequence of events linking the injurious stimulus with local prostaglandin synthesis at the site of injury is the subject of some debate. It has been suggested (Anderson *et al.*, 1971) that the initial step involves release of the enzyme phospholipase A which is present in lysosomes and in plasma membrane. Phospholipase A then releases the fatty acid substrates for prostaglandin synthesis (20-carbon unsaturated fatty acids) from the phospholipid of the plasma membrane. In support of this, Anderson showed that there was a positive correlation between appearance of prostaglandins and lysosomal enzymes in the carrageenin inflammatory reaction in the rat. Injection of phospholipase A into isolated perfused lungs results in prompt appearance of prostaglandins in the perfusate, and the rate of spontaneous synthesis of prostaglandins by homogenates of sheep vesicular glands is greatly enhanced by inclusion of phospholipase A in the incubation medium (Kunze and Vogt, 1971). It is also of interest that intradermal injection of phospholipase A into a skin air bleb in the rat results in local prostaglandin formation (Whelan 1974). The available evidence is thus compatible with an important role for phospholipase activity in increasing fatty acid substrate concentration for prostaglandin synthesis in the inflammatory reaction. However, the important question which remains to be answered is whether increased local substrate concentration alone is the only prerequisite for triggering prostaglandin synthesis. Since intradermal injection of arachidonic acid does not evoke an inflammatory reaction (Greaves, M. W., unpublished results) it appears that, at least in skin, additional factors are necessary for initiation of prostaglandin synthesis. Such factors may include direct activation of synthetase enzymes, or neutralization of an inhibitor, or supply of an essential enzyme cofactor.

References

Ambache, N., Kavanagh, L. and Whiting, J. (1965). Effect of mechanical stimulation on rabbits eyes: release of active substances in anterior chamber perfusates. *J. Physiol. (Lond.)*, **176**, 378

Anderson, A. J., Brocklehurst, W. E. and Willis, A. L. (1971). Evidence for the role of lysosomes in the formation of prostaglandins during carageenin-induced inflammation in the rat. *Pharmac. Res. Comm.*, **3**, 13

Änggård, E., Arturson, G. and Jonsson, C. -E. (1970). Efflux of prostaglandins in lymph from scalded tissues. *Acta Physiol. Scand.*, **80**, 46A

Arturson, G., Hamberg, M. and Jonsson, C.-E. (1973). Prostaglandins in human burn blister fluid. *Acta Physiol. Scand.*, **87**, 270

Chang, C. H. and Gaddum, J. H. (1933). Choline esters in disease extracts. *J. Physiol. (Lond.)*, **79**, 255

Crunkhorn, P. and Willis, A. L. (1969). Actions and interactions of prostaglandin administered intradermally in rat and in man. *Br. J. Pharmacol.*, **36**, 216P

Crunkhorn, P. and Willis, A. L. (1971a). Cutaneous reactions to intradermal prostaglandins. *Br. J. Pharmacol.*, **41**, 49

Crunkhorn, P. and Willis, A. L. (1971b). Interaction between prostaglandins E and F given intradermally in the rat. *Br. J. Pharmacol.*, **41**, 507

Di Rosa, M., Giroud, J. P. and Willoughby, D. A. (1971). Studies of the mediators of the acute inflammatory response induced in rats in different sites by carageenan and turpentine. *J. Pathol.*, **104**, 15

Eakins, K. E., Whitelocke, R. A. F., Bennett, A. and Martenet, A. C. (1972). Prostaglandin-like activity in ocular inflammation. *Br. Med. J.*, **3**, 452

Eakins, K. E., Whitelocke, R. A. F., Perkins, E. S., Bennett, A. and Ungar, W. G. (1972). Release of prostaglandins in ocular-inflammation in the rabbit. *Nature New Biology*, **239**, 248

Feldberg, W. and Saxena, P. N. (1971). Fever produced by prostaglandin E_1. *J. Physiol. (Lond.)*, **317**, 547

Ferreira, S. H. (1972). Prostaglandins, aspirin-like drugs and analgesia. *Nature New Biology*, **240**, 200

Ferreira, S. H., Moncada, S. and Vane, J. R. (1971). Indomethacin and aspirin abolish prostaglandin release from the spleen. *Nature New Biology*, **231**, 237

Flower, R., Gryglewski, R., Herbaczynska-Cedro, K. and Vane, J. R. (1972). Effects of anti-inflammatory drugs on prostaglandin biosynthesis. *Nature New Biology*, **238**, 104

Flower, R. and Vane, J. R. (1972). Inhibition of prostaglandin synthetase in brain explains the antipyretic activity of paracetamol (4-acetamidophenol). *Nature (Lond.)*, **240**, 410

Goldberg, N. D. (1972). Possible role(s) of cyclic 3, '5'-guanosine monophosphate (cyclic GMP). In *Symposium: Pharmacological implications of cyclic nucleotides*. 5th International Congress on Pharmacology (San Francisco)

Goldyne, M. E., Winkelmann, R. K. and Ryan, R. J. (1973). Prostaglandin activity in human cutaneous inflammation: detection by radioimmunoassay. *Prostaglandins*, **4**, 737

Greaves, M. W., Kingston, W. P. and Pretty, K. M. (1975). Action of a series of non-steroid and steroid anti-inflammatory drugs on prostaglandin synthesis by the microsomal fraction of rat skin. *Br. J. Pharmacol.*, **53**, 470P

Greaves, M. W. and McDonald-Gibson, W. (1972). Prostaglandin biosynthesis by human skin and its inhibition by corticosteroids. *Br. J. Pharmac.*, **46**, 172

Greaves, M. W. and McDonald-Gibson, W. (1973a). Itch: role of prostaglandins. *Br. Med. J.*, **3**, 608

Greaves, M. W. and McDonald-Gibson, W. (1973b). Effect of non-steroid anti-inflammatory and anti-pyretic drugs on prostaglandin biosynthesis by human skin. *J. Invest. Derm.*, **61**, 127

Greaves, M. W. and Sondergaard, J. S. (1970). Pharmacological agents released in ultraviolet inflammation studied by continuous skin perfusion. *J. Invest. Derm.*, **54**, 365

Greaves, M. W., Sondergaard, J. and McDonald-Gibson, W. (1971). Recovery of prostaglandins in human cutaneous inflammation. *Br. Med. J.*, **2**, 258

Gryglewski, R. J., Panczenko, B., Korbut, R., Grodzinska, L. and Ocetkiewicz, A. (1975). Corticosteroids inhibit prostaglandin release from perfused mesenteric blood vessels of rabbit and from perfused lungs of sensitized guinea pig. *Prostaglandins*, **10**, 343

Hamberg, M., Svensson, J. and Samuelsson, B. (1975). Thromboxanes: a new group of biologically active compounds derived from prostaglandin endoperoxides. *Proc. Nat. Acad. Sci. (USA)*, **72**, 2994

Higgs, G. A. and Youlten, L. J. F. (1972). Prostaglandin production by rabbit peritoneal polymorphonuclear leucocytes *in vitro*. *Br. J. Pharmac.*, **44**, 330P

Hillier, K. and Karim, S. M. M. (1968). Effects of prostaglandins E_1, E_2, $F_{1\alpha}$ and $F_{2\alpha}$ on isolated human umbilical and placental blood vessels. *J. Obstet. Gynaec. Br. Commonwealth*, **75**, 667

Horton, E. (1963). Action of prostaglandin E_1 on tissues which respond to bradykinin. *Nature (Lond.)*, **200**, 892

Kaley, G. and Weiner, R. (1971). Effect of prostaglandin E on leucocyte migration. *Nature New Biology*, **234**, 114

Kingston, W. P. and Greaves, M. W. (1975). In preparation.

Kunze, H. and Vogt, W. (1971). Significance of phospholipase A for prostaglandin formation. *Ann. N.Y. Acad. Sci.*, **180**, 123

Lewis, G. P. and Piper, P. J. (1975). Inhibition of release of prostaglandins as an explanation of some of the actions of anti-inflammatory corticosteroids. *Nature (Lond.)*, **254**, 308

Lichtenstein, L. M., Gillespie, E., Bourne, H. R. and Henney, C. S. (1972). The effects of a series of prostaglandins on *in vitro* models of the allergic response and cellular immunity. *Prostaglandins*, **2**, 519

Mathur, G. P. and Gandhi, V. M. (1972). Prostaglandin in human and albino rat skin. *J. Invest. Derm.*, **58**, 291

Milton, A. S. and Wendlandt, S. (1970). A possible role for prostaglandin E_1 as a modulator for temperature regulation in the central nervous system in the cat. *J. Physiol. (Lond.)*, **207**, 76P

Moncada, S., Ferreira, S. H. and Vane, J. R. (1973). Prostaglandins, aspirin-like drugs and the oedema of inflammation. *Nature (Lond.)*, **246**, 217

Smith, J. B. and Willis, A. L. (1970). Formation and release of prostaglandins by platelets in response to thrombin. *Br. J. Pharmac.*, **40**, 545P

Smith, J. B. and Willis, A. L. (1971). Aspirin selectively inhibits prostaglandin production in human platelets. *Nature New Biology*, **231**, 235

Solomon, L. M., Juhlin, L. and Kirschenbaum, M. B. (1968). Prostaglandin on cutaneous vasculature. *J. Invest. Derm.*, **51**, 280

Sondergaard, J. S. and Greaves, M. W. (1970). Pharmacological studies in inflammation due to exposure to ultraviolet irradiation. *J. Pathol.*, **101,** 93

Sondergaard, J. S. and Greaves, M. W. (1971a). Continuous skin perfusion *in vitro* as a method for study of pharmacological agents in human skin. *Acta Dermatovener.*, **51,** 50

Sondergaard, J. S. and Greaves, M. W. (1971b). Director recovery of histamine from cutaneous anaphylaxis in man. *Acta Dermatovener.*, **51,** 98

Sondergaard, J. S. and Greaves, M. W. (1974). Recovery of prostaglandins in human primary irritant dermatitis. *Arch. Derm.* In press

Sondergaard, J. S. and Wolf-Jorgensen, P. (1972). The cellular exudate of human cutaneous inflammation induced by prostaglandins E_1 and $F_{1\alpha}$. *Acta Dermatovener.*, **52,** 361

Thomas, G. and West, G. B. (1974). Prostaglandins, kinin and inflammation in the rat. *Br. J. Pharmac.*, **50,** 231

Vane, J. R. (1971). Inhibition of prostaglandin synthesis as a mechanism of action for aspirin-like drugs. *Nature New Biology*, **231,** 232

Velo, G. P., Dunn, C. J., Giroud, J. P., Timsit, J. and Willoughby, D. A. (1973). Distribution of prostaglandins in inflammatory exudate. *J. Pathol.*, **111,** 149

Whelan, C. J. (1974). Production of an inflammatory exudate containing prostaglandins. *J. Pharm. Pharmac.*, **26,** 355

Whitelocke, R. A. F., Eakins, K. E. and Bennett, A. (1973). Acute anterior uveitis and prostaglandins. *Proc. Roy. Soc. Med.*, **66,** 429

Willis, A. L. (1969). Parallel assay of prostaglandin-like activity in rat inflammatory exudate by means of cascade superfusion. *J. Pharm. Pharmac.*, **21,** 126

10
Prostaglandins and Tumours

SULTAN M. M. KARIM and BHASHINI RAO

10.1 INTRODUCTION   304

10.2 HUMAN STUDIES   307
    10.2.1 *Medullary carcinoma of the thyroid*   307
    10.2.2 *Carcinoid tumour*   309
    10.2.3 *Renal cell carcinoma*   311
    10.2.4 *Phaeochromocytoma*   311
    10.2.5 *Kaposis sarcoma*   311
    10.2.6 *Ganglioneuroma*   312
    10.2.7 *Neuroblastoma*   312
    10.2.8 *Breast cancer*   312
    10.2.9 *Dental cyst and bone resorption*   313

10.3 ANIMAL STUDIES   314
    10.3.1 *Mouse fibrosarcoma*   314
    10.3.2 *Moloney sarcoma*   315
    10.3.3 *B.P. 8/P_1 tumours*   316
    10.3.4 *Sarcoma 180*   317
    10.3.5 *Chondrosarcoma*   317

10.4 TISSUE CULTURE STUDIES   317
    10.4.1 *Prostaglandin synthesis in normal and tumour cell lines*   317
    10.4.2 *Effects of prostaglandins on cellular growth and differentiation*   318

10.5 PROSTAGLANDINS AND CYCLIC AMP INTERACTION   321

10.6 COMMENTS   322

    REFERENCES   323

10.1 INTRODUCTION

After more than half a century of systematic research by many scientists, the question as to how and why a normal body cell changes into a tumour cell has remained essentially unanswered. While the search for the answer goes on, an immediate need for the clinician is to identify changes or symptoms associated with tumour growth and to find means to counteract these changes and symptoms and suppress tumour growth.

In recent years prostaglandins have added another dimension to the physiology of tumours. They have been implicated in various aspects of tumour growth including cell replication, morphological alterations, hypercalcaemia and bone resorption. In several instances, symptoms associated with tumours are thought to be due to an over-production of prostaglandins. Indeed, it is interesting to note that many of the changes associated with prostaglandins are in fact diametrically opposite to those that take place during tumour growth. For example:

(a) while PGEs promote morphological differentiation of malignant cells, dedifferentiation is a characteristic feature of malignant transformation

(b) PGEs inhibit growth of tumour cells *in vitro* whereas unrestrained growth of cells is the main feature of tumour condition

(c) PGEs increase cellular adhesiveness while tumour cells have diminished adhesiveness

(d) platelet aggregation is inhibited by PGEs; in contrast platelet aggregation seems to increase in neoplasia and

(e) while PGEs elevate cellular cAMP levels, increase of cAMP levels suppresses growth of transformed cells and enhances anti-tumour immunity.

Williams *et al.* (1968) were the first to report elevated levels of prostaglandins in tumour tissues and in plasma of patients with medullary carcinoma of the thyroid. Since then a large number of investigators have not only confirmed their findings but have also shown the presence of appreciable amounts of prostaglandins in a variety of other human and animal carcinomas (see Tables 10.1 and 10.2). Several investigators have measured prostaglandin levels in blood from patients with different types of tumours. Whereas in some patients the blood levels of prostaglandins are high this is not so in every case. The failure to detect prostaglandins could be due either to the absence of prostaglandin in some tumours or to the lack of sensitivity of the assay method used.

Recently sufficient evidence has accumulated to show that human dental cyst synthesizes and secretes prostaglandins. Since it is known that dental cysts actively resorb bone within the jaw, the above observation becomes especially relevant to the study of the role of prostaglandins in bone resorption and hypercalcaemia—conditions often associated with many carcinomas.

Modern methods of experimental cancer research are being used increasingly to study the role of prostaglandins in tumour physiology. Instead of relying

Table 10.1   Prostaglandins in human tumours

Tumour	Prostaglandins		References
	Tumour tissue	Blood	
Medullary carcinoma of thyroid	E_2, $F_{2\alpha}$	E_2, $F_{2\alpha}$	Williams, Karim and Sandler (1968)
		E	Jaffe, Behrman and Parker (1973)
		E	Kaplan, Sizemore, Peskin and Jaffe (1973)
Papillary carcinoma of thyroid	E_2, $F_{2\alpha}$		Williams, Karim and Sandler (1968)
Anaplastic carcinoma of thyroid	$F_{2\alpha}$		Williams, Karim and Sandler (1968)
Neuroblastoma		E_2	Williams, Karim and Sandler (1968)
		E	Jaffe, Behrman and Parker (1973a)
Carcinoma of bronchus	E_2, $F_{2\alpha}$		Sandler, Williams and Karim (1969)
Islet cell tumour	E_2, $F_{2\alpha}$		Sandler, Williams and Karim (1969)
Exocrine carcinoma of pancreas	E_2		Sandler, Williams and Karim (1969)
Phaechromocytoma	E_1, E_2, $F_{2\alpha}$		Sandler, Williams and Karim (1969)
		E	Jaffe (1974)
Ileal, carcinoid		E	Kaplan, Sizemore, Peskin and Jaffe (1973)
Jejunum carcinoid		E	Kaplan, Sizemore, Peskin and Jaffe (1973)
		E	Jaffe, Behrman and Parker (1973a)
Rectal carcinoid		E	Jaffe, Behrman and Parker (1973a)
		E	Kaplan, Sizemore, Peskin and Jaffe (1973)
	E		Bennett and Tacca (1975)
Breast tumour	E, F		Bennett, MacDonald, Simpson and Stamford (1975)
Descending colon	E		Bennett and Tacca (1975)
Kaposis sarcoma		E_2, $F_{2\alpha}$	Bhana, Hillier and Karim (1971)
Liver metastasis	E		Brereton, Halushka, Alexander, Mason, Keiser and Devita (1974)
Lung metastasis	E		Brereton, Halushka, Alexander, Mason, Keiser and Devita (1974)
Renal cell carcinoma	E, F	A	Zusman, Snider, Cline, Caldwell and Speroff (1974)

on the spontaneous appearance of tumours in humans or laboratory animals it is now possible to experimentally induce various types of tumours in laboratory animals especially in 'pure line mice'. Many investigators have made use of these experimentally induced tumours to study the importance of prostaglandins in tumour growth and bone resorption. Both *in vitro* and *in vivo* experiments have provided interesting results.

Experiments with mouse fibrosarcoma and Walker carcinoma have contributed significantly to the understanding of the role of prostaglandins in hypercalcaemia of neoplastic disease. Results from these animal models have important clinical bearing.

A different experimental approach to the problem has been the use of tissue culture methods which provide an excellent tool for the study of the

Table 10.2   Prostaglandins in animal tumours

Tumour	Prostaglandins		References
	Tumour tissue	Blood	
Mouse fibrosarcoma	E_2	E_2	Tashjian, Voelkel, Goldhaber and Levine (1972, 1973)
Moloney sarcoma	E_2, F		Humes and Strausser (1974)
BP8/P_1 tumour	E_2		Sykes and Maddox (1972)
Sarcoma 180	E_2		Sykes and Maddox (1972)
Rat mammary tumour	E_2		Tan, Privett and Goldyne (1974)

role of prostaglandins in cellular growth and differentiation. This area of research received a special impetus with the discovery that prostaglandins stimulate adenylate cyclase activity in many tissues and thereby modify their cAMP levels. Since it has been known for quite some time that cAMP plays a principal role in biological regulation, the fact that prostaglandins can modify the levels of this cyclic nucleotide gave prostaglandins an added importance.

A number of cell lines from normal and neoplastic tissues have been studied. The effect of exogenous prostaglandins on the growth and morphology of these cells has been explored. From the studies reported to date one could perhaps make one important generalization that under *in vitro* conditions the increase in prostaglandin concentration inhibits cell growth.

As is perhaps to be expected, however, the data generated by the implication of prostaglandins in tumour physiology have raised a number of basic questions:

1. Are prostaglandins an essential feature of tumour growth?
2. Are all neoplastic tissues capable of synthesizing prostaglandins *in vitro*?
3. Are different prostaglandins associated with different tumours or is this role confined to one specific prostaglandin?
4. Is the elevated level of prostaglandins in tumour cells the result of the transformation of the normal cell to the neoplastic cell or does a disturbance in the synthesis of prostaglandins in some way contribute to this transformation?
5. Are all the effects of prostaglandins in the tumour tissue mediated through cAMP or do prostaglandins exert their influence through other agents?
6. What is the role of prostaglandins in hypercalcaemia and bone resorption?
7. What are the biochemical mechanisms underlying prostaglandin-induced cellular differentiation?
8. Are clinical symptoms associated with different tumours the result of overproduction and release of prostaglandins?

It is against the background of such questions that an attempt is made to review the literature pertaining to the relationship between prostaglandins and tumours.

10.2 HUMAN STUDIES

10.2.1 Medullary carcinoma of the thyroid

The medullary carcinoma of the thyroid arises from the thyroid parafollicular cells. These cells bear some morphological relationship to the intestinal argentaffin cells which are responsible for the carcinoid syndrome, and to the islet of Langerhans which are responsible for hypoglycaemic syndrome and also for the Zollinger–Ellison syndrome. The functions of the normal parafollicular cells of the thyroid are not fully understood but they are known to contain 5-hydroxytryptamine, kallikrein and are also the site of production of calcitonin (Flack et al., 1964; Foster et al., 1966; Williams, 1966).

Clinical manifestations include severe diarrhea and occasional flushing. The association between medullary carcinoma of the thyroid and diarrhea was first reported by Williams (1966). The frequencies of the finding of chronic diarrhea associated with medullary carcinoma of the thyroid was 29.3% in Williams's (1966) series and 28.3% in the series of Ibanez et al. (1967) which included 41 and 51 cases respectively. Williams produced evidence that the link between diarrhea and medullary carcinoma of the thyroid was humoral. Diarrhea is usually worse when the tumour is widespread and it improves after resection of large amounts of tumour but recurs when the tumour becomes widespread again.

Excessive secretion of calcitonin is a consistent feature of medullary carcinoma of the thyroid (see Baylin, 1974 for refs.). However, calcitonin is devoid of effect on gastrointestinal motility and is unlikely to be the cause of diarrhea.

5-Hydroxytryptamine (5-HT) has been implicated as the humoral agent causing diarrhea and indeed in several patients increased excretion of urinary 5-hydroxyindoleacetic acid (5-HIAA) has been found and abnormally large amounts of 5-HT have been shown to be present in the metastases (Williams 1970). In several other patients, however, 5-HIAA excretion has been normal, implying that some other humoral agent may also be responsible for diarrhea.

It is now well recognized that cells which give rise to one pharmacologically active substance often synthesize others. Rat mast cells produce histamine, 5-HT and heparin, some pancreatic islet cells of the new-born guinea pigs contain both dopamine and 5-HT, carcinoid tumour tissue elaborates 5-HT, kallikrein and sometimes histamine. There is also evidence that some of these agents may act synergistically (Gozsy and Kalo, 1966; Weiner and Altura, 1967).

Williams et al. (1968) first reported the presence of prostaglandins E_2 and $F_{2\alpha}$ in tumour tissue and plasma of patients with medullary carcinoma of the thyroid and suggested that the associated diarrhea could be due to these substances. Tumour tissues obtained from four out of seven patients with medullary carcinoma of the thyroid contained 36–674 ng/g of PGE_2 and 15–844 ng/g of $PGF_{2\alpha}$. Raised blood levels were detected in two patients, concentrations being considerably higher in blood draining the tumour than in peripheral blood. Both patients had diarrhea. As a control Williams *et al.* (1968) investigated prostaglandin levels in blood of patients with other forms of diarrhea. Prostaglandins levels in these patients were not raised. Profuse watery diarrhea has been encountered when PGE and PGF compounds are administered orally or intravenously to normal human subjects (Karim, 1972). Occasional flushing associated with medullary carcinoma of the thyroid may also be due to raised levels of prostaglandins produced and released by the tumour. Intravenous infusion of PGE compounds in man cause flushing.

Kaplan *et al.* (1973) using radioimmunoassay found raised plasma levels of PGE in three patients with medullary carcinoma of the thyroid. The values were 2375, 1000 and 1000 pg/ml respectively. Normal plasma PGE values using the same radioimmunoassay were 385 to 30 pg/ml.

In a case of medullary carcinoma of the thyroid with associated diarrhea, Isaacs *et al.* (1974) found raised plasma prostaglandin levels in only one out of four samples taken at different times. This suggests that prostaglandin secretion by the tumour may be intermittent despite the fact that diarrhea was persistent.

Melvin and colleagues (1972) also using a radioimmunoassay did not detect any PGA, PGB or PGE in sera of 10 out of 11 patients with medullary carcinoma of the thyroid and were unable to detect $PGF_{2\alpha}$ in the sera of six. However, the sensitivity of their assay may have been too low.

Prostaglandin production in continuous monolayer cultures of a medullary carcinoma of the thyroid has been reported by Grimley *et al.* (1969). Prostaglandin E_2 (11.7 ng/ml) and $PGF_{2\alpha}$ (58.4 ng/ml of medium) corresponding to 1100 ng PGE_2 and 5000 ng of $PGF_{2\alpha}$ per gram of tissue per 24 h were recovered.

Isaacs *et al.* (1974) attempted to inhibit prostaglandin production by treating medullary carcinoma of the thyroid with associated diarrhea in one patient with indomethacin, a known inhibitor of prostaglandin synthesis. This 'caused the mean ileal transit time to revert to normal although it had no effect on permeability'. However repeated administration of 50 mg indomethacin three times a day for 8 weeks failed to influence the frequency and volume of diarrhea. A 4-week course of aspirin (also a prostaglandin synthesis inhibitor) in a dose of 600 mg three times daily was also without effect. However, although both indomethacin and aspirin are known to inhibit prostaglandin synthesis in several systems, it must also be recognized that prostaglandin synthetases in different tissues differ markedly in their sensitivity to inhibitory drugs (Flower and Vane, 1974). It is possible that both aspirin and indomethacin are weak inhibitors of prostaglandin synthetase present in medullary carcinoma of the thyroid.

Barrowman *et al.* (1975) have reported a case of a female patient with medullary carcinoma of the thyroid with lung secondary and associated diarrhea. Elevated levels of prostaglandin-like activity was present in peripheral (arm) vein blood ($\equiv$ 5.4 ng assayed as PGE_2 in plasma). Diarrhea persisted after thyroidectomy but responded to oral administration of nutmeg which has previously been shown to be an inhibitor of prostaglandin synthesis (Bennett *et al.*, 1974).

Comments

Medullary carcinoma of the thyroid contains high amounts of prostaglandin E_2 and $F_{2\alpha}$. These tumours are also able to synthesize prostaglandins *in vitro* in monolayer tissue culture. Several investigators have reported elevated blood levels of prostaglandins in patients with medullary carcinoma of the thyroid. Others have failed to confirm these findings. The failure to detect increased blood levels could be either due to the absence of prostaglandins in some tumours (see Williams *et al.*, 1968) or due to lack of sensitivity of the assay method. Whereas in some patients there is an association between symptoms and high levels of prostaglandins in the tumour, this is not so in every case. Diarrhea is usually present in 25–30% of the patients with medullary carcinoma of the thyroid. In one patient Williams *et al.* (1968) found very high amounts of prostaglandins in the tumour but there was no associated diarrhea. Similarly in some patients who had diarrhea, tumour tissue contained little or no prostaglandins. Absence of diarrhea in the presence of elevated blood levels of prostaglandins could be due to differing sensitivity of the gastrointestinal tract to prostaglandins. When used clinically oral doses of as little as 0.5 mg PGE_2 produce diarrhea in the occasional patient, while in other patients a dose as high as 5 mg given orally is without any effect (Karim, 1972). The humoral agent responsible for diarrhea associated with medullary carcinoma of the thyroid may be different in different patients, i.e. other substances such as 5-HT, or kinins may be involved. Two or more of these substances may act synergistically to produce diarrhea. Aspirin and indomethacin failed to prevent diarrhea whereas nutmeg has been effective. The implication is that nutmeg acts selectively on tumour prostaglandin synthetase or acts by some other as yet unknown mechanism.

10.2.2 Carcinoid tumour

The typical carcinoid tumour producing the carcinoid syndrome is a compact collection of argentaffin cells which is found nowhere else in mammals and only in such sites and species as the venom sac of the toad (*Bufo marinus*) and the posterior salivary gland of the octopus (Grahame-Smith, 1973). Some similarities have been noted between medullary carcinoma of the thyroid and carcinoid tumour, such as origin from a cell related to the Kuttschintzncy cells and production and release of certain local hormones.

The main manifestations of the carcinoid syndrome are flushing, diarrhea and a distinctive form of valvular heart disease which may produce cardiac failure, edema and paroxysmal asthma. Other minor features are pellagra-like skin lesions due to nicotinic acid deficiency, a possible increased incidence of peptic ulcers and joint pains. Patients with carcinoid tumour present with one or more of the above symptoms and the difference in the presentation may be the result of the capacity of the tumour to produce different quantities and types of hormones and the patient's reaction to the hormones. The carcinoid syndrome has been attributed to elevated concentrations of serum serotonin, histamine, bradykinin, calcitonin and prostaglandins.

Sandler *et al.* (1968) first reported the presence of prostaglandins in a carcinoid tumour. A bronchial carcinoid tumour tissue contained 32.3 ng/g PGE_2 and 420 ng/g $PGF_{2\alpha}$. However, in two cases of ileal carcinoid with associated diarrhea no E or F prostaglandins were detected in the tumour tissue. Blood and tumour tissues from these two patients contained appreciable amounts of an unknown hydroxy fatty acid with smooth muscle stimulating property.

Smith and Greaves (1974) have reported a case of carcinoid syndrome with unusual skin lesions and a rise in blood prostaglandin activity associated with norepinephrine-induced flushing. Blood samples were taken both before norepinephrine injection and during the subsequent flushing, and whole blood prostaglandin estimated by bioassay. Before the injection of norepinephrine the whole blood prostaglandin activity was 0.35 ng/ml rising to 2.0 ng/ml after norepinephrine. The total prostaglandin activity before norepinephrine was 2/3 E prostaglandin and 1/3 F prostaglandin while after norepinephrine the recovered activity was due almost entirely to E prostaglandins.

Kaplan *et al.* (1973) (see also Jaffe, 1974) have measured plasma PGE concentrations in four patients with ovarian, ileal, jejunal and rectal carcinoid. The plasma concentration in one patient with jejunal carcinoid associated with flushing was 3300 pg/ml and in another patient with rectal carcinoid PGE concentration was 967 pg/ml.

In a series of 12 patients Feldman *et al.* (1974) measured $PGF_{2\alpha}$ 13,14-dihydro-15-keto $PGF_{2\alpha}$ (a metabolite of $PGF_{2\alpha}$), serum 5-HT and urinary 5-HIAA. Nine of the patients had a primary tumour originating in the small intestine, one had a rectal carcinoid and in two the tumour originated in the lungs. All had hepatic metastases. Two of the patients had elevated serum $PGF_{2\alpha}$ levels and two had elevated serum levels of $PGF_{2\alpha}$ metabolite. The authors concluded that there was a poor correlation between levels of $PGF_{2\alpha}$ or $PGF_{2\alpha}$ metabolite and carcinoid symptoms. These results however do not rule out the possibility that other prostaglandins (A, B and E) play a role in carcinoid syndrome or the possibility that $PGF_{2\alpha}$ is produced in selected patients only during the acute carcinoid symptom complex.

Comments

Elevated levels of prostaglandins have been found in some but not all carcinoid tumour tissue. Similarly increased blood levels have been reported in some cases. However, before any link between the prostaglandins and carcinoid syndrome can be firmly established it would be essential to measure levels of several prostaglandins simultaneously in the same sample, i.e. Es, Fs, As and Bs. It is also important to measure prostaglandins in several samples from the same patient in case the release is intermittent. In order to establish a link between prostaglandins and flushing, samples of blood should be taken before and during an attack of flush. Elevated levels of prostaglandins during flush produced by other substances do not necessarily mean that prostaglandins are released from the tumour, e.g. norepinephrine has an α-adrenergic fat mobilising effect which leads to the formation and release of prostaglandins from tissue. Prostaglandins may be involved in some but not all of the symptoms associated with carcinoid tumour.

10.2.3 Renal cell carcinoma

Zusman *et al.* (1974) have reported one case of renal cell carcinoma with elevated plasma PGA concentration. The patient was a 49-year-old female who 20 years previously was found to be hypertensive with a maximum recorded blood pressure of 240/140 mm Hg and was treated with various antihypertensives for $18\frac{1}{2}$ years. After this period her blood pressure stabilized at normotensive level and all antihypertensive treatment was discontinued. The patient was found to have a carcinoma in the lower pole of the left kidney and the left kidney was resected with segmental resection of the descending colon. The blood pressure before operation was 130/70 but three hours later it was 160/90 and remained elevated for several months after the operation (range 150/100 to 180/115). The plasma concentration of PGA before the operation was 8.05 ng/ml, falling to 2.05 and 1.18 ng/ml 5 days and 1 year after operation respectively. The prostaglandin content of the tumour was 3.86, 10.38, 8.93 ng/g for PGA, E and F respectively. The authors suggested that the elevated PGA levels reduced blood pressure in this previously hypertensive patient. After the removal of the tumour tissues the PGA level fell precipitously with simultaneous elevation of blood pressure.

Indirect evidence to support the above is provided by a case reported by Brereton *et al.* (1974). A 54-year-old male patient with a renal cell adenocarcinoma had persistent hypercalcaemia and was successfully treated with indomethacin. The authors suggest that hypercalcaemia could have been due to increased production of prostaglandin-like material by the tumour. They only measured PGE- and PGF-like material in the patient's plasma after treatment with indomethacin was commenced and the levels of these prostaglandins were within normal limits. Whether the patient's hypercalcaemia was the result of overproduction of prostaglandins by tumour tissue is not clear. In the case reported by Zusman (discussed above) the patient's serum calcium was within normal limits in spite of elevated plasma prostaglandin levels.

10.2.4 Phaeochromocytoma

In four out of seven phaeochromocytomas high amounts of prostaglandins E_2 and/or $F_{2\alpha}$ were reported by Sandler *et al.* (1968). Prostaglandins were also assayed in blood draining the tumour in two of these patients but could not be detected in either. Peripheral plasma PGE concentrations in patients with phaeochromocytoma were measured in five subjects by Jaffe (1974). One patient had elevated levels while in two patients the levels were within the upper limits of normal.

10.2.5 Kaposis sarcoma

Clinical features associated with Kaposis sarcoma include pricking pains, itching, increased local sweating and edema of the affected limb. In addition, a small percentage of patients develop gastrointestinal symptoms such as abdominal pain and diarrhea. Bhana *et al.* (1971) examined tumour tissue, blood and urine for the presence of 5-HT, histamine, catecholamines and prostaglandins to determine if an overproduction of any of these substances might be associated with some of the clinical features of the tumour. In these patients 5-HT, histamine and catecholamine concentrations were within normal limits. However, prostaglandin-like materials (PGE_2 and $F_{2\alpha}$) were found in all Kaposis sarcoma tissue tested. Incubation of tumour tissue homogenate with arachidonic acid showed that the amount of PGE-like material increased 13.5 fold and PGF 6.6 fold when compared with tumour tissue without added arachidonic acid. Raised blood levels of PGE_2 and $PGF_{2\alpha}$ were also found in some patients.

10.2.6 Ganglioneuroma

Diarrhea also occurs with ganglioneuroma (Rosenstein and Engelman, 1963). High prostaglandin levels were reported in tumour tissue from one child with the syndrome of catecholamine-secreting ganglioneuroma with diarrhea (Sandler, Karim and Williams, 1968). The amount of PGE_2 was 34.5 ng and $F_{2\alpha}$ 480 ng/g of tumour tissue.

10.2.7 Neuroblastoma

Sandler *et al.* (1968) measured PGE and PGF levels in tumours from three cases of catecholamine-secreting neuroblastoma. Only in one tumour tissue was an elevated level (120 ng/g) of $PGF_{2\alpha}$ encountered. None of the patients had diarrhea. Jaffe (1974) has reported elevated plasma PGE levels in two patients with neuroblastoma. In both cases, the levels were extremely high, 12 000 and 5875 pg/ml respectively (control values 385 to 30 pg/ml). However no details of the patients' symptoms were reported.

10.2.8 Breast cancer

Osteolytic bone metastases and bone resorption often develop in patients with breast cancer. Powles *et al.* (1973) first showed that osteolysis produced *in vitro* by some human breast tumours may be inhibited by aspirin and that in the rat, osteolytic bone deposits and hypercalcaemia produced by Walker carcinosarcoma can be prevented by aspirin and indomethacin. Since both these drugs are potent inhibitors of prostaglandin synthesis, the above findings imply a role for prostaglandins in breast cancer.

Bennett *et al.* (1975) in a study of 23 patients with breast cancer showed that malignant tumour tissue contained and synthesized more prostaglandins than normal breast tissue from the same patient. Levels of prostaglandins in the benign tumours were not elevated. The basal levels (expressed as ng PGE_2 equivalents per g moist tissue) were 8 (1.7–62) $n = 23$ in malignant tumours; 0 (0–2.5) $n = 5$ in benign tumours; and 0 (0–1.4) $n = 19$ in normal breast tissue. Tumour tissues from patients with bone metastases contained and synthesized more prostaglandin-like material than tumour tissues from patients without metastases. Furthermore, when breast tumour was associated with metastases, mainly F prostaglandins were present whereas in the absence of metastases predominantly E prostaglandins were found in tumour tissues. Thus, both the amounts and the type of prostaglandins may be important in evaluating the tumour condition.

Elevated levels of PGE_2 in breast tumour induced by intravenous injection of 7,12-dimethylbenz(a) anthracine in mice have been previously reported by Tan *et al.* (1974). Tumour tissues also contained higher amounts of arachidonic acid than normal tissues.

10.2.9 Bone resorption by dental cyst

Dental cysts seem to grow by dissolving bone, and resorption of bone by dental cysts has been shown to be due to material released from the cyst wall (Harris and Goldhaber, 1973). Klein and Raisz (1970) have shown that prostaglandins E_1 and E_2 are potent stimulators of bone resorption *in vitro*. Prostaglandin production in human periodontal disease has been suggested as a possible cause of bone resorption by dental cysts (Harris *et al.*, 1973; Goodson *et al.*, 1974).

Harris *et al.* (1973) showed that extracts of dental cyst tissue contained basal levels of 0–60 ng/g PGE_2-like material. After incubation of the tissue with Krebs' solution 23–233 ng/g PGE_2-like activity was recovered suggesting the ability of the dental cyst to synthesize prostaglandins. Dental cysts in tissue culture also synthesized prostaglandin-like material and this synthesis was inhibited by indomethacin, a known inhibitor of prostaglandin biosynthesis. Substantial bone resorption by dental cysts in tissue culture was also demonstrated by Harris *et al.* (1973). This effect could be prevented by the prostaglandin antagonist polyphloretin phosphate. The authors suggested that if prostaglandins play a role in bone resorption by dental cyst then they are presumably released at a site accessible to the bone. Bone resorption was not significantly less when the calvaria were incubated with cyst capsule rather than with the full thickness of cyst wall (Harris and Goldhaber, 1973). The bone resorbing factor therefore seems to be released by the outer capsule adjacent to the bone rather than by the lining epithelium. The authors concluded that the findings support the possibility that prostaglandins produced by the dental cyst capsule are responsible for bone resorption by cysts within the jaws.

Goodson *et al.* (1974) have also measured levels of PGE_2 in tissue and exudate from human periodontal disease and in normal tissue. Inflamed gingival tissue from four subjects contained 29, 230, 330 and 390 ng/g (wet weight) of PGE_2 measured by radioimmunoassay. In 6 samples of healthy gingiva PGE_2 levels were 5, 7, 7, 8, 31 and 160 ng/g respectively. Prostaglandin E_2 in gingival exudate obtained from a case of acute necrotizing gingivitis was 230 ng/g. An exudate from a draining tooth abscess which had perforated the alveolar bone contained 440 ng/g PGE_2. They concluded that the findings are consistent with the hypothesis that PGE_2 synthesized in periodontal disease contributes to the clinical manifestation of inflammation and stimulates bone resorption.

Drugs which interfere with prostaglandin synthesis or action may prove useful in the treatment of periodontal disease. Indomethacin has been reported effective for this purpose (Ota *et al.*, 1969).

10.3 ANIMAL STUDIES

10.3.1 Mouse fibrosarcoma

Goldhaber in 1960 described the induction of a transplantable fibrosarcoma, $HSDM_1$, in a Swiss albino mouse by subcutaneous implantation of a Millipore filter. This tumour was found to synthesize and to secrete a potent bone resorption-stimulating factor. When fragments of this tumour were placed in a culture vessel together with mouse calvaria, marked resorption of the bone was observed. Furthermore, the culture medium in which the tumour tissue was cultured could, on its own, stimulate bone resorption when added to mouse calvaria maintained in organ culture.

It is also possible to grow $HSDM_1$ tumour cells in monolayer cultures (Voelkel *et al.*, 1972). Various clonal strains of $HSDM_1$ have been established. Cells from these strains when injected into mice can induce fibrosarcoma. Moreover, *in vitro* all strains synthesize bone resorption-stimulating factor. Therefore, by retaining their specialized function *in vitro* these cells provide a very useful system for the study of biochemical mechanisms underlying bone resorption.

What is the nature of the $HSDM_1$ bone resorption-stimulating factor? To answer this, Voelkel and his associates (Voelkel *et al.*, 1972) extracted this humoral factor, both from the tumour tissue and from the medium of $HSDM_1$ cells grown in tissue culture. They found that $HSDM_1$ factor was heat stable, resistant to enzymatic proteolysis and extractable in organic solvents. These characteristics of the $HSDM_1$ factor, combined with the observations of Klein and Raisz (1970) that prostaglandins stimulate bone resorption *in vitro* led these investigators to postulate that $HSDM_1$ factor might very well be a prostaglandin.

This suggestion stimulated Levine *et al.* (1972) to look for the presence of prostaglandins in $HSDM_1$ cells in tissue culture. Their findings showed that several strains of $HSDM_1$ cells grown in tissue culture do indeed synthesize and secrete large quantities (0.7–2.0 μg/mg cell protein per 24 h) of prostaglandins. The authors tentatively designated this material as PGE_2 although the presence of PGA and PGB was not ruled out. In contrast, when culture medium from certain other mouse cell lines (mouse fibroblasts, mouse neuroblastoma, mouse adrenal) were assayed for the presence of prostaglandins the amount present was relatively insignificant (< 0.03 μg/mg protein per day).

$HSDM_1$ cells produce PGE_2 both in the logarithmic and stationary phase of growth cycle. The amount of intracellular prostaglandin was only 0.3 μg/mg cell protein which indicates that most of the prostaglandins synthesized are secreted into the medium and are not retained by the cells. When the effect of aspirin, sodium salicylate and indomethacin on the production of prostaglandins was examined it was found that all three agents caused a marked reduction in the synthesis of PGE_2, indomethacin, being the most potent. At a dose level of 1 ng/ml indomethacin caused 50% inhibition of prostaglandin synthesis while for the same level of inhibition 10 μg/ml of aspirin and 50 μg/ml of sodium salicylate were required. However, reduction of prostaglandin synthesis did not affect cell growth.

Having established that $HSDM_1$ cells synthesize prostaglandins, Tashjian and his colleagues (Tashjian *et al.*, 1972) undertook further studies to substantiate the evidence that the bone resorption-stimulating factor, produced by mouse fibrosarcoma cells, is prostaglandin E_2. Using a highly efficient and quantitative assay in which bone resorption-stimulating activity is measured in terms of ^{45}Ca-release from mice calvaria these authors were able to furnish an impressive set of results to support the above hypothesis.

(1) The aqueous and the ether extracts of $HSDM_1$ tissue which contained bone resorption-stimulating activity also contained PGE_2.
(2) This was also true for extracts of medium from cultures of $HSDM_1$ cells.
(3) The specific biological activity of the $HSDM_1$ bone resorption-stimulating factor was comparable to that of the parathyroid hormone and PGE_2.
(4) When $HSDM_1$ cells were grown in the presence of indomethacin (500 ng/ml) the medium was found to lack any bone resorption-stimulating activity. However, this activity was completely restored with the addition of 100 ng/ml of PGE_2.

The *in vitro* results have been supported by the *in vivo* findings. It has been shown, again by the same group of researchers (Tashjian *et al.*, 1973) that mice bearing $HSDM_1$ fibrosarcoma have significantly higher concentrations of both serum calcium (10.8 ng/100 ml versus control 9.9 ng/100 ml) and PGE_2 (475 pg/ml versus control 250 pg/ml). Administration of indomethacin orally to these mice at an average dose of 100–125 μg/mouse per day reduced the concentrations of both serum calcium and serum PGE_2 to control levels. At these dose levels indomethacin was not toxic. There was, in addition, a marked reduction in the indomethacin-treated mice of tumour PGE_2 content and of bone resorption-stimulating activity.

It is interesting to note that contrary to the *in vitro* results indomethacin in the *in vivo* situation did affect the growth of tumours. Tumours from indomethacin-treated mice were significantly smaller than those from the control mice.

So far it has not been possible to show the calcium releasing effect of PGE_1 or PGE_2 in intact or parathyroidectomized rats. This could perhaps be due to the rapid metabolism of PGEs when injected into the animal. On the other hand, the constant high secretory rate of the $HSDM_1$ tumour might keep the level of PGE_2 in plasma sufficiently high to stimulate bone resorption (see also Section 10.2.8).

10.3.2. Moloney sarcoma

Moloney sarcoma virus (MSV) preparation when injected into hind limbs of male BALB/CJ mice gives rise to palpable tumours in more than 80% of the injected limbs (Moloney, 1960). The tumour mass is at a maximum between days 10–14 after the virus injection. Humes and Strausser (1974) using radio-immunoassay were able to show that the virus-induced Moloney sarcoma tumours contain 53 times more PGE (15.9 ± 9.3 pmol/mg protein) than the amounts found in normal leg muscles (0.3 ± 0.09 pmol/mg protein). The increase in the amount of prostaglandin F was only 7-fold (0.89 ± 0.17 versus 0.13 ± 0.04 pmol/mg protein). Thus the ratio of PGE to PGF in the tumour tissue is much higher than that in the control. Using thin-layer chromatography the prostaglandin of the E series associated with the tumour was identified as PGE_2. Humes and Strausser (1974) also measured the levels of cyclic nucleotides in the control and tumour tissues. The concentration of cAMP in the tumour tissue was about twice that in the control. No significant change in the level of cGMP was observed. Chronic administration of indomethacin (Humes *et al.*, 1974) 5 mg/kg administered subcutaneously on alternate days beginning on the day after the MSV injection, resulted in 67% inhibition of $PGF_{2\alpha}$. Concentrations of cAMP and cGMP were not affected. In the indomethacin-treated mice not only was the onset of tumour delayed but the growth was also suppressed.

Effects of indomethacin in mice whose immune response system is suppressed by administering anti-lymphocyte serum at the time of MSV inoculation were also evaluated. Since the induction and regression of virus-induced tumours depends on the immune system of the host, rapidly growing tumours appeared in the anti-lymphocyte serum treated mice earlier than in the control mice. Administration of indomethacin to immunosuppressed MSV-inoculated mice resulted in significant suppression of tumour growth. The levels of prostaglandins or cyclic nucleotides in the tumours from anti-lymphocyte serum treated mice were not reported.

Under *in vitro* conditions, tissues from MSV-induced tumours continue to synthesize large quantities of PGE_2 from endogenous substrates (Humes and Strausser, 1974). Most of the prostaglandin was recovered in the incubation medium and was not retained by the tumour tissue. When the tumour tissues were incubated in the presence of 0.1 mM indomethacin prostaglandin synthesis was completely blocked.

10.3.3 BP8/P₁ tumours

Diarrhea is often present in mice bearing BP8/P$_1$ tumours. Preliminary investigation of the ascitic fluid of the mice with these tumours showed a very low level of prostaglandin activity (Sykes, 1970). However, further investigation of BP8/P$_1$ tumours (Sykes and Maddox, 1972) revealed that in contrast to the ascitic fluid the prostaglandin E_2 content of the tumour cells is very high ($2.5–25$ μg/g cells). These concentrations of PGE_2 in the tumour cells are exceeded only by those found in the seminal fluid. $PGF_{2\alpha}$ was not detected in these tumours.

Daily intraperitoneal injections of indomethacin (5 mg/kg) to mice bearing solid BP8/P$_1$ tumours reduced the prostaglandin levels to an average of 66%. However, indomethacin treatment had no significant effect on tumour growth.

In vitro homogenates of BP8/P$_1$ tumours, when tested for prostaglandin synthetase activity, showed a 10% conversion of arachidonic acid, increasing PGE_2 levels to 125 $\mu g/g$ cells. The presence of both reduced glutathione and hydroquinone in the incubation medium was required for the conversion of arachidonic acid to PGE_2. Hydroquinone, however, could be replaced by epinephrine or 5-hydroxytryptamine. It is interesting to note here that although no $PGF_{2\alpha}$ is found associated with these tumours *in vivo* the tumour homogenates *in vitro* can synthesize both PGE and $PGF_{2\alpha}$. In $BP8/P_1$ ascites cell system, in the presence of glutathione and hydroquinone, indomethacin (15 μM) caused 80% inhibition of prostaglandin synthesis.

10.3.4 Sarcoma 180

Sykes and Maddox (1972) studied the concentration of prostaglandin in sarcoma 180 (S180) tumour. The tumour was implanted subcutaneously into male Schneider mice. Fourteen days after implantation the solid tumour was removed, and the prostaglandin content of the tissue determined by using both the superfusion bioassay and gas chromatography–mass spectroscopy techniques. Sarcoma 180 was estimated to contain 1 μg prostaglandin E_2/g of tissue. Prostaglandin $F_{2\alpha}$ could not be detected.

Homogenates of S180 exhibited prostaglandin synthetase activity by converting exogenous arachidonic acid to prostaglandin E_2 *in vitro*. The conversion rate was 0.7% with final PGE_2 level of 8 $\mu g/g$ tissue.

10.3.5 Chondrosarcoma

Eisenbarth *et al.* (1974a) studied the effect of prostaglandins on normal cartilage. Their results showed that prostaglandins A and B, but not E or F, inhibit macromolecular synthesis in the cartilage. To determine if malignant transformation of the cartilage cells alters their response to prostaglandins, Eisenbarth and his associates (1974b) studied the effect of various prostaglandins on macromolecule synthesis in two chondrosarcomas—one a well differentiated rat chondrosarcoma, the other a poorly differentiated murine chondrosarcoma. *In vitro* synthesis of proteins RNA and DNA was followed by incubation of tumour tissue with radioactive precursors of these molecules. It was found that neither PGE_1 nor $PGF_{2\alpha}$ at 25 $\mu g/ml$ had any effect on protein synthesis. In contrast PGA_1 at the same concentration drastically inhibited protein, RNA and DNA synthesis in both the tumours. These effects of PGA_1 were shown to be irreversible. Thus the effects of prostaglandins on macromolecular synthesis in neoplastic cartilage tissue were similar to the effects previously observed in normal cartilage.

10.4 TISSUE CULTURE STUDIES

10.4.1 Prostaglandin synthesis in normal and tumour cell lines

Several tumour cell lines have been known to secrete prostaglandins *in vitro*. We have already discussed prostaglandin production by clonal strains of mouse fibrosarcoma (Section 10.3.1).

Hammerström *et al.* (1973) using mass spectroscopic techniques determined the prostaglandin levels in normal and virus transformed fibroblasts maintained in cell culture. The three cell lines investigated were BHKC113 a Syrian hamster fibroblast which retains a normal cell response to growth controls effective in culture, BHKWtC12A the same cell line transformed by a wild type polyoma virus which no longer responds to growth restraints, and BHKts-3C17C, a line obtained from the control BHKC113 line through transformation by a thermosensitive mutant of polyoma virus. Compared with cells from the control line BHKC113 the polyoma transformed cells of BHKts-3C17C contained ten times more PGE_2 (mean 285.2 versus control 33.5 ng/100 μg cellular DNA). Cultures of BHKWtC12A cells produced 30–115 times more PGE_2 (1989 ng/100 μg cellular DNA) than the untransformed controls. Ninety-seven per cent of PGE_2 was found in the medium. $PGF_{2\alpha}$ production also increased in the transformed cells but only to a very slight extent. These results show clearly that polyoma virus transformation of baby hamster kidney fibroblasts leads to a considerable increase in their PGE_2 production. Using radioimmunoassay techniques Jaffe and his associates (Jaffe *et al.*, 1973b) and Hamprecht *et al.* (1973) measured concentrations of PGA, PGE and PGF in three clonal cell lines *in vitro*. The three cell lines were N4, a mouse neuroblastoma clone, B82, a mutant cell line and C_6 a rat glioma clone. All three cell lines synthesized prostaglandins. The main prostaglandin produced by these cells was PGE. No PGA or PGF could be detected in the media from the three cell lines. However, low amounts of PGA and PGF were found in the cells, the concentrations of PGA being 8% and PGF 2% respectively of the PGE concentration. Most of the PGE produced by the three cell lines was found in the medium and only 8–23% was retained by the cells.

Addition of dibutyryl cAMP to the growth medium enhanced the synthesis of PGE. Dibutyryl cAMP also inhibited cell growth in all three cell lines, implying an inverse relation between cell proliferation and prostaglandin concentration. It is also interesting to note that when NUTG3 cells entered the stationary phase of contact inhibition, there was a spurt of PG production.

10.4.2 Effects of exogenous prostaglandins on cellular growth and differentiation

Mouse neuroblastoma cells

Mouse neuroblastoma C-1300 cells when cultured in monolayers display a number of physical and chemical properties characteristic of the neurons. They resemble neurons in morphology, contain enzymes involved in neurotransmitter synthesis and respond to neurohormones (see Hamprecht and Schultz, 1973 for references).

These characteristics make this cell line a very useful experimental system in which neuronal functions can be studied. Gilman and Nirenberg (1971) were the first to study the effect of different prostaglandins on growth and cAMP production in these cells. Their work showed that PGE_1 markedly stimulated cAMP in four clonal cell lines derived from mouse neuroblastoma

C-1300. In one of the cell lines (N10) the increase in cAMP due to PGE_1 stimulation was about five times that of control (210 pmol/mg protein). Other prostaglandins $PGF_{2\alpha}$, PGA, PGB had no effect on cAMP production while PGE_2 caused slight stimulation. Theophylline (an inhibitor of cyclic nucleotide phosphodiesterase) potentiated the effect of PGE_1 on cAMP production.

As compared to the control cells the growth of PGE_1 $(1.5 \times 10^{-5} M)$ treated cells was inhibited. Only one-third as many cells were present on day 5 as in control plates. While theophylline alone had no effect on cell multiplication the combination of PGE_1 and theophylline virtually prevented any multiplication of the cells.

Hamprecht and Schultz (1973) studied five cell lines derived from mouse neuroblastoma C-1300. They investigated the effect of PGE_1 on the concentration of cAMP in these cell lines. In all the five cell lines PGE_1 increased the levels of cAMP several hundredfold above the control levels. However, this increase was different for different cell lines. The authors suggest that the differential response to PGE_1 is perhaps due to the different genetic constitution of the cells. Although all the cell lines studied are derived from the same tumour nevertheless they differ in their morphology, size and karyotype (Amano *et al.*, 1972). The cellular content of cAMP was considerably increased when phosphodiesterase inhibitors were used. Hamprecht *et al.* (1973) have also shown that in the mouse neuroblastoma cell lines the presence of dibutyryl cyclic AMP markedly decreased the growth rate of the cells.

Prasad (1972a, 1972b) in an elegant series of experiments studied the prostaglandin-induced morphological differentiation in mouse neuroblastoma cells in culture. Although an uncloned neuroblastoma cell line was the principal line used in the study, the effects of PGE_1 on two other neuroblastoma clones (NBA_5 and $NBA_2(1)$) were also studied. Amongst the many interesting points that emerged from this study the following seem to be of particular interest:

(a) PGE_1 and PGE_2 induce irreversible morphological differentiation of mouse neuroblastoma cells in culture as shown by the formation of axon-like processes

(b) $PGF_{2\alpha}$ does not induce any morphological differentiation

(c) The differentiated cells show morphological maturation as shown by an increase in nuclear and cellular size

(d) The degree of differentiation depends both on the concentration and the length of time the cells are in contact with the prostaglandin. The optimum concentration of PGE was 10 μg/ml and the optimum time about 3–5 days

(e) The presence of PG in the media markedly reduced cell growth

(f) Actinomycin-D (5 μg/ml) which reduced RNA synthesis by 95% in these cells did not block the PGE_1-induced axon formation, thereby indicating that the synthesis of new RNA was not required for the differentiation process

(g) However, when cycloheximide, a potent inhibitor of protein synthesis, was used, at a level when 90% of the protein synthesis is inhibited the PG-induced axon formation was completely blocked. Thus it seems that axon formation is controlled more at the translational rather than at the transcriptional level

(h) PGE treated cells attach to the cell surface more firmly than the control cells. This is interesting since it has been shown that malignant cells have diminished cellular adhesiveness (Abercombie and Ambrose, 1962)

(i) Dibutyryl cAMP and certain inhibitors of phosphodiesterase also induce morphological differentiation of mouse neuroblastoma cells

(j) In a clone of neuroblastoma cells NBDB, insenstitive to dibutyryl cAMP, differentiation can be induced by PGE_1. As expected, inhibitors of phosphodiesterase are also ineffective in inducing differentiation in cells from this clone. The last observation would imply that at least in this clone prostaglandin action is not mediated through cAMP.

Fibroblasts

The relationship between prostaglandins and adenylate cyclase in normal and transformed fibroblasts from a variety of sources, has been studied by Peery et al. (1971) and Johnson et al. (1972). PGE_1 stimulated the production of cAMP in various lines of mouse, hamster and rat fibroblasts maintained in culture. However, there are some exceptions. Two cell lines, derived from mouse embryo fibroblasts by transformation with polyoma or SV40 virus, were unresponsive to all the prostaglandins tested so far. It is interesting to note that the original untransformed Balb 3T3 cells from which these lines are derived show very low levels of adenylate cyclase activity and are also unresponsive to prostaglandins. Furthermore, PGE_1 does not affect the morphology, growth or adhesion characteristics of the transformed or untransformed Balb 3T3 cells. On the other hand, in the responsive cell lines, PGE_1 not only stimulates cAMP production but produces the same changes in growth rate, morphology, motility and adhesiveness as are observed in cells incubated with dibutyryl cAMP or cAMP alone, that is, slower growth rate, slower cell motion, altered cell morphology and increased adhesion to the substratum.

In order to further evaluate the role of prostaglandins as modulators of growth Thomas et al. (1974) examined the relationship between concentrations of PGE and rates of cell proliferation in vitro in three established cell lines Hep-2, L and HeLa. PGE_1 concentrations were increased either exogenously by adding PGE_1 to the medium or endogenously by adding dibutyryl cAMP. On the other hand, concentrations of PGE were decreased with indomethacin, a potent inhibitor of prostaglandin synthesis. Under control conditions cells from all these three lines produce measurable quantities of intracellular and extracellular PGE and the mean PGE production per million cells per day is characteristic for each cell line. The rate of cell proliferation under all experimental conditions, was inversely related to prostaglandin concentration. Addition of dibutyryl cAMP (1 mM) to the media resulted in about 54 % increase in PGE synthesis and a similar decrease in cell replication. Addition of exogenous PGE_1 to the culture media (1 $\mu g/ml$) also inhibited cell proliferation by 41 %. On the other hand when PGE concentration was reduced by adding indomethacin (10^{-8} M) to the medium, cell replication was significantly stimulated. Addition of PGE_1 to indomethacin-containing media restored growth rate to that observed in the absence of indomethacin. These results demonstrate beautifully an inverse relationship between cell growth and prostaglandin concentrations.

10.5 PROSTAGLANDINS—CYCLIC AMP

The role of cAMP in the regulation of cell processes is well established. A number of studies suggest that cAMP inhibits cell proliferation, induces differentiation, increases cell generation time, causes malignant morphology to revert back to normal and increases cell adhesion in many normal and tumour cell lines. In general there seems to be a mutual antagonism between the effects of cAMP and tumour condition. It has also been shown that prostaglandins, especially those of the E series, have an ability to increase the levels of cAMP in many tissues. This prompted many workers to explore the action of prostaglandins in cellular processes and to determine whether these effects were mediated through cAMP.

Animal tumours have been shown to contain high amounts of prostaglandins and cAMP, implying a link between cAMP and prostaglandins. However, chronic administration of indomethacin in mice bearing Moloney sarcoma tumours, while reducing the level of PGE_2, had no effect on the cAMP levels of the tumour tissue (see Section 10.3.2).

In vitro studies, in general support the suggestion that the action of prostaglandins is mediated through cAMP. Prostaglandins increase adenylate cyclase activity in many tumour cell lines. Relative abilities of different prostaglandins in stimulating the adenylate cyclase system in L929 cells have been studied by Peery *et al.* (1971). PGE_1 was the most effective followed by PGE_2, $PGF_{2\alpha}$, and PGB_1. PGA_2 produced only a slight response. Makman (1971) showed that PGE_1 stimulated adenylate cyclase activity in HeLa, HTC and L cells. Gilman and Nirenberg (1971) studied the effect of different prostaglandins on cAMP production in mouse neuroblastoma. Their results showed that PGE_1 markedly stimulated cAMP in these cells. $PGF_{2\alpha}$, PGA and PGB were without any effect while PGE_2 caused slight stimulation. In another study on mouse neuroblastoma cell lines Hamprecht and Schultz (1973) found that the concentration of cAMP was increased several hundredfold in cells exposed to prostaglandin E_1 (see Section 10.4.2).

What seems significant is that in addition to stimulating adenylate cyclase activity prostaglandins also induce differentiation, reduce growth rate and increase cell adhesion. These cellular alterations are similar to those affected by dibutyryl cAMP. This strongly suggests the possibility that prostaglandins act via increased cAMP. However, there are some exceptions. Prasad (1972b) while studying prostaglandin-induced morphological differentiation in mouse neuroblastoma cells describes a clone ($NBDB^-$) which, while being insensitive to the action of dibutyryl cAMP, responded well to PGE_1. In this clone inhibitors of phosphodiesterase are also ineffective in inducing cellular differentiation. Thus is seems that at least in these cells prostaglandin action is not mediated via cAMP.

The interrelation between the action of prostaglandin and cAMP is further complicated by the fact that in certain cell lines addition of dibutyryl cAMP increases PGE synthesis (Hamprecht *et al.*, 1973; Thomas *et al.*, 1974).

Finally it seems that much more work is required to elucidate the exact nature of the link between the action of prostaglandins and cAMP.

10.6 COMMENTS

Although with the present state of our knowledge the implication of prostaglandins in tumour physiology is not very clear, nevertheless, it is possible to draw certain general conclusions and attempt to answer some of the questions raised in the introduction to this chapter.

A wide range of human and animal tumours are able to synthesize and release prostaglandins both *in vitro* and *in vivo* and increased prostaglandin activity is associated with a variety of tumours. PGE_2 is most frequently encountered in tumour tissues although elevated amounts of PGA and PGF compounds in tumour tissues have also been reported.

The elevated levels of prostaglandins in tumour cells could be the result of the transformation of the normal cell to the neoplastic cell. Alternatively, this transformation could result from overproduction of prostaglandins. The results of most *in vitro* studies show that exogenous prostaglandins inhibit cell growth and stimulate cell differentiation. It is thus tempting to postulate that overproduction of prostaglandins by tumour cells is one of the mechanisms to counteract the abnormal state of growth and other chemical processes associated with the neoplastic condition. However, results from some studies in which administration of indomethacin (a prostaglandin synthetase inhibitor) *in vivo* reduces the growth of tumour argue against this hypothesis. This apparent paradox can perhaps be explained by the possibility that *in vivo* indomethacin apart from inhibiting prostaglandin synthetase system has also an inhibitory effect on other biochemical processes important in tumour growth.

Prostaglandins increase adenylate cyclase activity in many tumour tissues, and *in vitro* their effects on cellular growth and morphology are in many ways similar to those of cAMP. These facts strongly argue for the hypothesis that the action of prostaglandins in tumour tissue is mediated through cAMP. However, the exact nature of the relationship between cAMP and prostaglandins is still far from clear.

Hypercalcaemia, a common syndrome of many carcinomas, is often attributed to the secretion of parathyroid-hormone-like peptide. However, in man this immuno-reactive parathyroid hormone is not always found either in the plasma or in the tumour tissue from patients with hypercalcaemia syndrome. It has been suggested that humoral substances other than parathyroid hormone (perhaps prostaglandins) are responsible for hypercalcaemia in these patients.

Although the role of prostaglandins in hypercalcaemia and bone resorption is well established in the laboratory animal the relationship of prostaglandins to the bone-resorbing factor in the human remains to be clarified. High plasma-prostaglandin concentrations have not been found in patients with hypercalcaemia and non-metastatic tumours. However, in one patient with renal carcinoma, calcium levels were successfully lowered by the use of indomethacin. Osteolysis produced by some human tumours *in vitro* can also be inhibited by aspirin. The latter findings imply that prostaglandins may also be involved in hypercalcaemia and bone resorption in the human.

References

Abercombie, M. and Ambrose, E. J. (1962). The surface properties of cancer cells: a review: *Cancer Research*, **22**, 525

Amano, T., Richelson, E. and Nirenberg, M. (1972). Neurotransmitter synthesis by neuroblastoma clones. *Proc. Nat. Acad. Sci. (USA)*, **69**, 258

Barrowman, J. A., Bennett, A., Hillebrand, P., Rolles, K., Pollock, D. J. and Wright, J. T. (1975). Diarrhoea in medullary carcinoma of the thyroid: evidence for the role of prostaglandins and the therapeutic effect of nutmeg. *Br. Med. J.* In press.

Baylin, S. B. (1974). Medullary carcinoma of the thyroid gland. Use of biochemical parameters in detection and surgical management of the tumour. *Surgical Clinics of North America*, **54**, 309

Bennett, A. and Tacca, M. (1975). Prostaglandins in human colonic carcinoma. (Meetings Abstr.). *Gut*, **16(5)**, 409

Bennett, A., Gradidge, C. F. and Stamford, I. F. (1974). Prostaglandins, nutmeg and diarrhoea. *New Engl. J. Med.*, **290**, 110

Bennett, A., McDonald, A. M., Simpson, J. S. and Stamford, I. F. (1975). Breast cancer, prostaglandins and bone metastases. *Lancet*, **i**, 1218

Bhana, D., Hillier, K. and Karim, S. M. M. (1971). Vasoactive substance in Kaposi's sarcoma. *Cancer*, **27**, 233

Brereton, H. D., Halushka, P. V., Alexander, R. W., Mason, D. M., Keiser, H. R. and Devita, V. (1974). Indomethacin-responsive hypercalcemia in a patient with renal-cell adenocarcinoma. *New Engl. J. Med.*, **291**, 83

Eisenbarth, G. S., Beuttel, S. C. and Lebovitz, H. E. (1974a). Inhibition of cartilage macromolecular synthesis by prostaglandin. *J. Pharmac. exp. Ther.*, **189**, 213

Eisenbarth, G. S., Wellman, D. K. and Lebovitz, H. E. (1974b). Prostaglandin A_1 inhibition of chondrosarcoma growth. *Biochem. Biophys. Res. Commun.*, **60**, 1302

Feldman, J. M., Plonk, J. W. and Cornette, J. C. (1974). Serum prostaglandin $F_{2\alpha}$ concentration in the carcinoid syndrome. *Prostaglandins*, **7**, 501

Flack, B., Larson, B., Mecklenberg, C. V., Rosengren, E. and Svenaeus, K. (1964). On the presence of a second specific cell system in mammalian thyroid gland. *Acta Physiol. Scand.*, **62**, 491

Flower, R. J. and Vane, J. R. (1974). Inhibition of prostaglandin biosynthesis. *Biochem. Pharmacol.*, **23**, 1439

Foster, G. V., Joplin, G. F., MacIntyre, I., Melvin, K. E. W. and Slack, E. (1966). Effect of thyrocalcitonin in man. *Lancet*, **i**, 107

Gilman, A. G. and Nirenberg, M. (1971). Regulation of adenosine 3', 5'-cyclic monophosphate metabolism in cultured neuroblastoma cells. *Nature (Lond.)*, **234**, 356

Goldhaber, P. (1960). Enhancement of bone resorption in tissue culture by mouse fibrosarcoma. *Proc. Am. Assoc. Cancer Res.*, **3**, 113

Goodson, J. M., Dewhurst, F. E. and Brunetti, A. (1974). Prostaglandin E_2 levels and human disease. *Prostaglandins*, **6**, 81

Grahame-Smith, D. G. (1973). Endocrine tumours producing gastrointestinal symptoms. In *Pharmacology of gastrointestinal motility and secretion. Vol. II.* Holton, P. (ed.), pp. 639–665 (Oxford: Pergamon Press)

Gozsy, B. and Kalo, L. (1966). Role of histamine serotonin and catecholamines in the vascular tonus and permeability in the skin. *Dermatologica*, **133**, 262

Grimley, P. M., Dettos, L. J., Weeks, J. R. and Robson, A. S. (1969). Growth *in vitro* and ultrastructure of cells from medullary carcinoma of the human thyroid gland: Transformation by Simian virus 40 and evidence of thyrocalcitonin and prostaglandins. *J. Nat. Cancer Inst.*, **42**, 663

Hammerström, S., Samuelsson, B. and Bjursell, G. (1973). Prostaglandin levels in normal and transformed baby-hamster kidney fibroblasts. *Nature New Biology*, **243**, 50

Hamprecht, B., Jaffe, B. M. and Philpott, G. W. (1973). Prostaglandin production by neuroblastoma, glioma and fibroblast cell lines; stimulation by N^6, $O^{2'}$-dibutyryl adenosine 3′, 5′-cyclic monophosphate. *FEBS Lett.*, **36**, 193

Hamprecht, B. and Schultz, J. (1973). Stimulation by prostaglandin E_1 of adenosine 3′, 5′-cyclic monophosphate formation in neuroblastoma cells in the presence of phosphodiesterase inhibitors. *FEBS Lett.*, **34**, 85

Harris, M. and Goldhaber, P. (1973). The production of a bone resorbing factor by dental cysts *in vitro. Br. J. Oral Surgery*, **10**, 334

Harris, M., Jenkins, M. V., Bennett, A. and Wills, M. R. (1973). Prostaglandin production and bone resorption by dental cysts. *Nature (Lond.)*, **245**, 213

Humes, J. L., Cupo, J. J. and Strausser, H. R. (1974). Effects of indomethacin on Moloney sarcoma virus-induced tumours. *Prostaglandins*, **6**, 463

Humes, J. L. and Strausser, H. R. (1974). Prostaglandins and cyclic nucleotides in Moloney sarcoma tumours. *Prostaglandins*, **5**, 183

Ibanez, M. L., Cole, V. W., Russel, W. O. and Clark, R. L. (1967). Solid carcinoma of the thyroid. Analysis of 53 cases. *Cancer (Philad.)*, **20**, 706

Isaacs, P., Whittaker, S. M. and Turnberg, L. A. (1974). Diarrhoea associated with medullary carcinoma of the thyroid. *Gastroenterology*, **67**, 521

Jaffe, B. M. (1974). Prostaglandins and cancer. *Prostaglandins*, **6**, 453

Jaffe, B. M., Behrman, H. R. and Parker, C. W. (1973a). Radioimmunoassay measurement of prostaglandins E, A and F in human plasma. *J. Clin. Invest.*, **52**, 398

Jaffe, B. M., Philpott, G. W., Hamprecht, B. and Parker, C. W. (1973b). Prostaglandin production by cells *in vitro. Adv. Biosci.*, **9**, 179

Johnson, G. S., Pastan, I., Oyer, D. S. and D'Armiento, M. (1972). Prostaglandins, cyclic AMP and transformed fibroblasts. *Adv. Biosci.*, **9**, 173

Kaplan, E. L., Sizemore, G. W., Peskin, G. W. and Jaffe, B. M. (1973). Humoral similarities of carcinoid tumours and medullary carcinomas of the thyroid. *Surgery*, **74**, 21

Karim, S. M. M. (1972). Prostaglandins and reproduction. Physiological roles and clinical uses of prostaglandins in relation to human reproduction. In *The Prostaglandins— Progress in Research*, Karim, S. M. M. (ed.), pp. 71–164 (Oxford and Lancaster: MTP)

Klein, D. C. and Raisz, L. G. (1970). Prostaglandins: stimulation of bone resorption in tissue culture. *Endocrinology*, **86**, 1436

Levine, L., Hinkle, P. M., Voelkel, E. F. and Tashjian, A. H. (1972). Prostaglandin production by mouse fibrosarcoma cells in culture: inhibition by indomethacin and aspirin. *Biochem. Biophys. Res. Commun.*, **47**, 888

Makman, M. H. (1971). Conditions leading to enhanced response to glucagon, epinephrine, or prostaglandins by adenylate cyclase of normal and cultured cells. *Proc. Nat. Acad. Sci. (USA)*, **68**, 2127

Melvin, K. E. W., Tashjian, A. H. and Miller, H. H. (1972). Studies in familial (medullary) thyroid carcinoma. *Rec. Prog. Horm. Res.*, **28**, 399

Moloney, J. B. (1960). Biological studies on a lymphoid-leukemia virus extracted from sarcoma 37.1. Origin and introductory investigations. *J. Nat. Cancer Inst.*, **24**, 933

Ota, N., Mizuno, K. and Akita, Y. (1969). A clinical evaluation of 'Indacin' in periodontal disease. *Aichi. Gakuin. J. Dental Sci.*, **7**, 154

Peery, C., Johnson, G. S. and Pastan, I. (1971). Adenyl cyclase in normal and transformed fibroblasts in tissue culture. *J. Biol. Chem.*, **246**, 5785

Powles, T. J., Clark, S. A., Easty, D. M., Easty, G. C. and Munro, N. A. (1973). The inhibition by aspirin and indomethacin of osteolytic tumour deposits and hypercalcaemia in rats with Walker tumour and its possible application to human breast cancer. *Br. J. Cancer*, **28**, 316

Prasad, K. N. (1972a). Morphological differentiation induced by prostaglandin in mouse neuroblastoma cells in culture. *Nature New Biology*, **236**, 49

Prasad, K. N. (1972b). Neuroblastoma clones: prostaglandin versus dibutyryl cyclic AMP, 8-benzylthio-cyclic AMP, phosphodiesterase inhibitors and X-rays. *Proc. Soc. Exp. Biol. Med.*, **140**, 126

Rosenstein, B. J. and Engelman, K. (1963). Diarrhoea in a child with a catecholamine-secreting ganglioneuroma. *J. Pediatr.*, **63**, 217

Sandler, M., Karim, S. M. M. and Williams, E. D. (1968). Prostaglandins in amine-peptide-secreting tumours. *Lancet*, 1053

Sandler, M., Williams, E. D. and Karim, S. M. M. (1969). The occurrence of prostaglandins in amine- peptide-secreting tumours. In *Prostaglandins, Peptides and Amines*, Mantegazza, P. and Horton, E. W. (eds.), pp. 3–7, (London and New York: Academic Press)

Smith, A. G. and Greaves, M. W. (1974). Blood prostaglandin activity with noradrenaline-provoked flush in the carcinoid syndrome. *Br. J. Dermatology*, **90**, 547

Sykes, J. A. C. (1970). Pharmacologically active substances in malignant ascites fluid. *Br. J. Pharmac.*, **40**, 595

Sykes, J. A. C. and Maddox, I. S. (1972). Prostaglandin production by experimental tumours and effects of anti-inflammatory compounds. *Nature New Biology*, **237**, 59

Tan, W. C., Privett, O. S. and Goldyne, M. E. (1974). Studies of prostaglandins in rat mammary tumours induced by 7,12-dimethyl-benz (a) anthracene. *Cancer Res.*, **34**, 3229

Tashjian, A. H., Voelkel, E. F., Levine, L. and Goldhaber, P. (1972). Evidence that the bone-resorption-stimulating factor produced by mouse fibrosarcoma cells is prostaglandin E_2. *J. Exp. Med.*, **136**, 1329

Tashjian, A. H., Voelkel, E. F., Goldhaber, P. and Levine, L. (1973). Successful treatment of hypercalcemia by indomethacin in mice bearing a prostaglandin producing fibrosarcoma. *Prostaglandins*, **3**, 515

Thomas, D. R., Philpott, G. W. and Jaffe, B. M. (1974). The relationship between concentration of prostaglandin E and rates of cell replication. *Exp. Cell Res.*, **84**, 40

Voelkel, E. F., Tashjian, A. H. and Goldhaber, P. (1972). A non-peptide factor produced by fibrosarcoma cells that stimulates bone resorption in organ culture. In *Calcium Parathyroid and Calcitonins, Proceedings 4th Parathyroid Conference*. Talmage, R. V. and Munson, P. L. (eds.), pp. 478–480 (Amsterdam: Excerpta Medica)

Weiner, R. and Altura, B. M. (1967). Serotonin–beadykinin synergism in the mammalian capillary bed. *Proc. Soc. Exp. Biol. Med.*, **124**, 494

Williams, E. D. (1966). Diarrhoea and thyroid carcinoma. *Proc. Roy. Soc. Med.*, **59**, 602

Williams, E. D. (1970). The origin and association of medullary carcinoma of the thyroid. In *Tumours of the thyroid gland, Vol. IV (Monographs on Neoplastic Disease)*, Smithers, D. (ed.), pp. 130–140. (London: Livingstone)

Williams, E. D., Karim, S. M. M. and Sandler, M. (1968). Prostaglandin secretion by medullary carcinoma of the thyroid. *Lancet*, **i**, 22

Zusman, R. M., Snider, J. J., Cline, A., Caldwell, B. V. and Speroff, L. (1974). Antihypertensive function of renal-cell carcinoma. *New Eng. J. Med.*, **290**, 843

11
Pharmacology of some Prostaglandins Analogues

SULTAN M. M. KARIM and P. GANESAN ADAIKAN*

11.1 INTRODUCTION		328
11.2 GASTROINTESTINAL TRACT		329
11.2.1 *Gastric secretion*		329
	11.2.1.1 Animal studies	329
	11.2.1.2 Human studies	333
11.2.2 *Antiulcer effect*		334
	11.2.2.1 Animal studies	334
	11.2.2.2 Human studies	335
11.2.3 *Mucosal blood flow*		338
11.2.4 *Pancreatic secretion*		338
11.2.5 *Bile*		338
11.2.6 *Pepsin*		338
11.2.7 *Gastrin*		339
11.2.8 *Effect on gut motility*		339
	11.2.8.1 *In vitro* studies	339
	11.2.8.2 *In vivo* studies	339
11.3 CARDIOVASCULAR EFFECTS		340
11.3.1 *Animal studies*		340
	11.3.1.1 15 (S) PGA$_2$ and 15 (R) PGA$_2$	340
	11.3.1.2 15 (S) 15-Methyl PGA$_1$ methyl ester and 15 (S) 15-methyl PGA$_2$ methyl ester	340
	11.3.1.3 8-iso PGE$_1$	341
	11.3.1.4 15 (S) 15-Methyl PGE$_2$ methyl ester and 15 (S) 15-methyl PGF$_{2\alpha}$ methyl ester	341
	11.3.1.5 PGE$_2$ Methyl ester and PGF$_{2\alpha}$ methyl ester	342

* Formerly P. A. Ganesan

11.3.1.6   15 (R) Prostaglandins   343
11.3.1.7   15-Methyl ether methyl ester   343
11.3.1.8   17-Phenyl prostaglandins   343
11.3.1.9   16, 16-Dimethyl PGE_2 and methyl ester   344
11.3.1.10 16 (R) Methyl-13, 14-dihydro-PGE_2 methyl
           ester: ONO-464   344
11.3.1.11 Other compounds   344
11.3.2 *Human studies*   345
11.3.3 *Antithrombotic effect*   345

11.4 SMOOTH MUSCLE STIMULATING ACTIVITY   348
11.4.1   *11, 15-Epi-prostaglandins E_1, A_1 and E_2*   348
11.4.2   *8-Iso PGE_1*   348
11.4.3   *7-Oxa prostaglandin derivatives*   348
11.4.4   *3, 5- and 13-oxa prostaglandins*   349
11.4.5   *17-Oxa compound*   349
11.4.6   *15-Methyl analogues of PGE_2 and $PGF_{2\alpha}$*   350
11.4.7   *16-Methyl analogues*   350
11.4.8   *16-Fluoro analogues*   350
11.4.9   *17-Phenyl analogues*   351
11.4.10 *2a, 2b-Dihomo-(15S)-15-methyl $PGF_{2\alpha}$ and its methyl
          ester*   351

11.5 PROSTAGLANDINS ANALOGUES AS ANTAGONISTS AND SYNTHESIS
INHIBITORS   351
11.5.1   *Prostaglandin analogues as antagonists*   351
11.5.2   *Prostaglandin analogues as inhibitors of PG synthetase*   353

11.6 EFFECT OF POLYPHLORETIN PHOSPHATE ON 15-METHYL
PROSTAGLANDINS   353

11.7 RESPIRATORY SYSTEM   353
11.7.1   *Animal studies*   353
11.7.2   *Human studies*   354

11.8 REPRODUCTIVE SYSTEM   355
11.8.1   *Animal studies*   355
11.8.2   *Human studies*   355

11.9 COMMENTS   355

11.1 INTRODUCTION

Several notable advances in prostaglandin research have been made since the pharmacological effects of human seminal fluid were discovered in the early 1930s. These include:

1. The elucidation of chemical structures of prostaglandins.
2. Demonstration of widespread distribution of prostaglandins in mammalian tissues and their wide range of pharmacological actions.

3. Elucidation of the biosynthetic pathways and total synthesis of prostaglandins.
4. Studies on the metabolism and degradation of prostaglandins.
5. Drug-induced inhibition of prostaglandin biosynthesis.

The above mentioned advances have led to a better understanding of the involvement of prostaglandins in various physiological and pathological processes. This has led to therapeutic applications of prostaglandins and their synthesis inhibitors in several areas. However, because of a wide spectrum of pharmacological actions of naturally occurring prostaglandins attention has been focussed in recent years on prostaglandin analogues with the hope of discovering more potent compounds with selective and specific effects on the target organ. A large number of analogues have been synthesized (see Schneider, 1976) but pharmacological effects of only a small number have so far been studied. In this Chapter the biological properties of some prostaglandins analogues are reviewed.

11.2 GASTROINTESTINAL TRACT

11.2.1 Gastric secretion

11.2.1.1 Animal studies

The gastric antisecretory and ulcer healing effects of several naturally occurring prostaglandins in laboratory animals are discussed in Chapter 7. In human studies, however, most of these compounds inhibited acid secretion only when given by continuous intravenous infusion and at effective doses side effects were present. Because of the potential therapeutic application of prostaglandins in the treatment of gastrointestinal ulcers a number of analogues have been studied with the aim of developing compounds that would selectively inhibit gastric secretion when given orally.

Lippman studied a series of prostaglandins analogues (shown in Figures 11.1 and 11.2) for their effect on gastric secretion in the Shay rat preparation (Lippman, 1969, 1970, 1971, 1974; Lippman and Seethaler, 1973). Although most of these compounds inhibited acid secretion when given subcutaneously, they were less potent than prostaglandin E_1.

An analogue of prostaglandin E_1 ($\Delta^8(12)13$-PGE or SC-24665) was reported by Lee and Bianchi (1972) to inhibit gastric secretion in the rat when given orally. The potency of this analogue relative to natural prostaglandin is not known.

Naturally occurring prostaglandins are very susceptible to enzymatic inactivation in the body. Of the several enzyme systems acting on different parts of the prostaglandin molecule, the enzyme 15-hydroxy dehydrogenase which oxidizes the hydroxyl group in the 15 position appears very important. An additional methyl group in the 15 position of the prostaglandin molecule has provided analogues which are not substrates for the enzyme 15-OH dehydrogenase. Several 15-methyl analogues of prostaglandins have been synthesized and shown to be biologically more active than the parent prostaglandins and

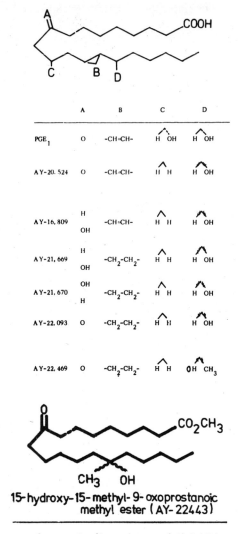

Figure 11.1   Structures of prostaglandin analogues which inhibit gastric secretion in rat (After Lippman, 1969, 1970, 1971, 1974 and Lippman and Seethaler, 1973).

have a significantly longer duration of action (see Figure 11.3). Two such compounds, 15(S)15-methyl PGE_2 and 15(R)15-methyl PGE_2 (both as free acid and methyl esters), have been extensively evaluated for their effects on gastric secretion and ulcer healing in laboratory animals and in man. 15(S)15-methyl PGE_2 methyl ester is 30–100 times more potent than PGE_2 in inhibiting gastric acid secretion stimulated by histamine or pentagastrin in dogs with denervated (Heidenhain) gastric pouch (Robert and Magerlein, 1973; Robert, Lancaster, Nezamis and Badalamenti, 1973) and in rats (Whittle, 1975). The analogue inhibits acid secretion by the oral, intravenous and intrajejunal routes (Robert and Magerlein, 1973).

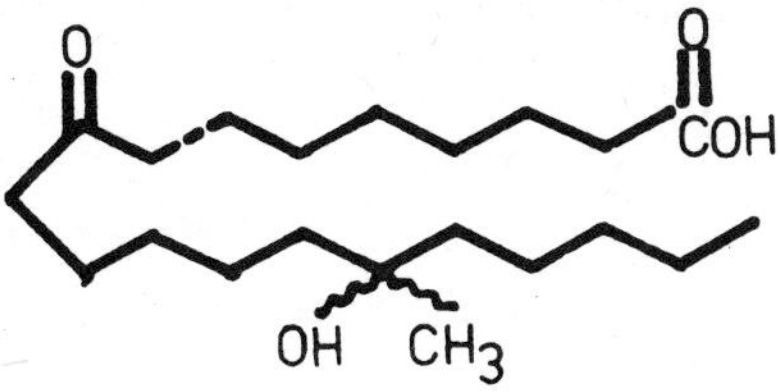

[±], rac- AY- 22469

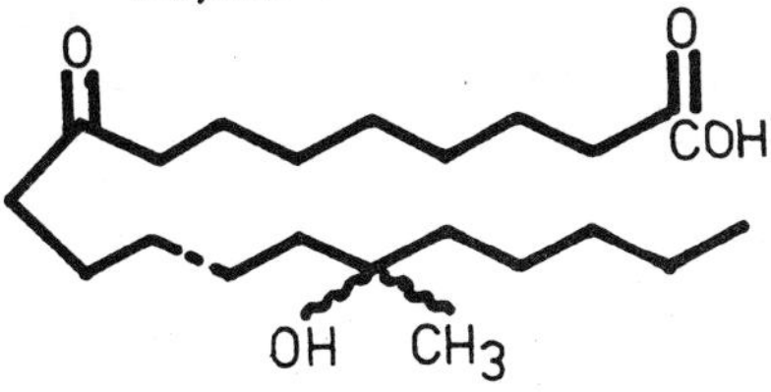

[±], ent- AY- 22469

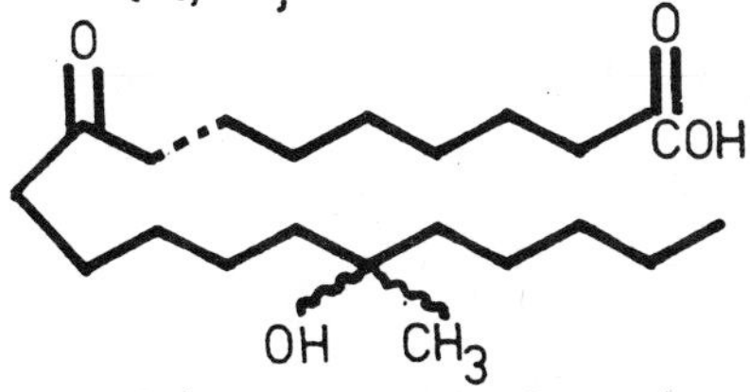

[-], nat- AY- 22469

Enantiomorphs of 15-hydroxy 15-methyl 9-oxoprostanoic acid (AY-22469)

Figure 11.2   As Figure 11.1

15(R)15-methyl PGE$_2$ methyl ester (an epimer of 15(S)15-methyl PGE$_2$ methyl ester) also inhibits gastric acid secretion in animals and man but is only active by the oral route (Karim *et al.*, 1973a; Robert and Yankee, 1975). There is some evidence to suggest that in the acid environment of the stomach some of the 15(R)15-methyl PGE$_2$ methyl ester is converted to 15(S)15-methyl PGE$_2$ methyl ester. When incubated at 37 °C in acid medium the 15R analogue epimerizes at C-15 to give a 1:1 mixture of 15(S)15-methyl PGE$_2$ methyl ester and 15(R)15-methyl PGE$_2$ methyl ester. Intrajejunal administration of 15(R)15-methyl PGE$_2$ methyl ester is without any effect on gastric acid secretion in the dog whereas 15(S)15-methyl E$_2$ methyl ester inhibits acid secretion. However, when diluted in acid, 15(R)15-methyl E$_2$ methyl ester inhibits gastric secretion by the jejunal route (Robert and Yankee, 1975).

The alkylated compound, 16,16-dimethyl PGE$_2$ (Figure 11.3) is also a potent inhibitor of basal or pentagastrin stimulated gastric acid secretion when given orally (Nylander and Andersson, 1975a) and intravaginally (Robert, Lancaster and Nezamis, 1975) to dogs. When adminstered intravenously to chronic fistula rats, 16,16-dimethyl PGE$_2$ is 100 times more active than PGE$_2$ in inhibiting resting secretion (Whittle, 1975).

A new analogue 16(S)methyl-13-dehydro PGE$_2$ (K 10134) given intravenously to dogs showed marked inhibition of gastric secretion provoked

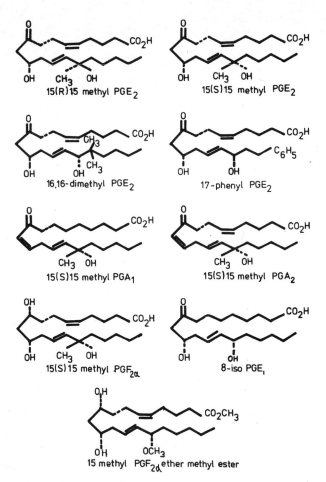

Figure 11.3 Structures of some prostaglandin analogues which have been studied in man

by different secretagogues. The threshold dose of this analogue ranged from 0.1 to 1.0 μg/kg (Impicciatore, Bertaccini and Usardi, 1975).

Another PGE_1 analogue SC-29333 produced a prolonged inhibition of stimulated acid secretion in Heidenhain pouch dog. The lowest effective intravenous and intragastric bolus doses were 0.3 and 10 μg/kg respectively. This compound is approximately 30 times more potent than PGE_1 methyl ester. Administered intragastrically in Shay rat SC-29333 inhibited gastric secretion at a dose of 300 μg/kg (Dajani *et al.*, 1975).

Recently, two 17-phenyl compounds (*rac*-17-phenyl-trinor-PGE_2 methyl ester and 17-phenyl-trinor-PGE_2) (Figure 11.3) were tested for antisecretory effects in dogs. Both compounds reduced gastric secretion when given by the intravenous route but were less active than prostaglandins E_2 (Miller, Weeks, Lauderdale and Kirton, 1975).

11.2.1.2 Human studies

Although naturally occurring prostaglandins of the E and A series have been shown to inhibit gastric secretion in man when given by the intravenous route, these compounds are either inactive or exhibit only a transient effect when given by mouth (Classen *et al.*, 1970; Wada and Ishizawa, 1970; Wilson *et al.*, 1971; Bhana *et al.*, 1973; Karim *et al.*, 1973a; Horton *et al.*, 1968). In contrast several of the synthetic analogues of prostaglandin E_2 have been shown to inhibit gastric secretion in man when given orally.

Karim and collaborators (1973a–d; Carter *et al.*, 1973) first demonstrated the gastric anti-secretory effect of 15(R)15-methyl PGE_2 methyl ester, 15(S)15-methyl PGE_2 methyl ester and 16,16-dimethyl PGE_2 methyl ester in healthy human volunteers. 15(R)15-methyl PGE_2 methyl ester was active only by the oral route whereas the other two analogues were active both by the oral and intravenous routes (Figure 11.4). The inhibition of gastric acid

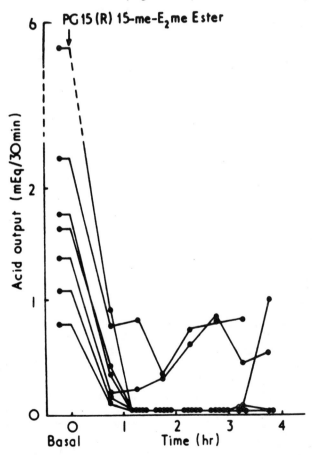

Figure 11.4   Effect of single oral dose of 200 µg of 15 (R) 15-methyl prostaglandin E_2 methyl ester on the basal acid output in adult healthy male subjects. (After Karim *et al.*, 1973b)

secretion produced by a single dose of these compounds was both marked and sustained for several hours and was due mainly to an increase in pH without a significant change in the volume of gastric juice. The three prostaglandin analogues when given orally were also shown to inhibit pentagastrin stimulated gastric acid secretion.

Robert et al. (1974) studied the effect of 15(R)15-methyl PGE_2 methyl ester and 16,16-dimethyl PGE_2 on pentagastrin stimulated gastric acid secretion in healthy human volunteers. Both prostaglandin analogues inhibited gastric acid secretion and the oral dose inhibiting acid output by 50% ranged from 60 to 70 μg per subject. The pH of gastric juice rose from 1.1 to around 7.0 but in contrast to the results reported by Karim et al. (1973b, c, d) the volume of gastric secretion was significantly reduced. This difference is possibly due to the fact that Karim et al. studied the effect of prostaglandin analogues on basal acid output whereas Robert et al. studied the effect on pentagastrin stimulated secretion. When given intraduodenally 15(S)15-methyl PGE_2 methyl ester was more active in inhibiting gastric secretion than 16,16-dimethyl PGE_2.

Nylander and Andersson (1975a) studied the effects of 16,16-dimethyl PGE_2 and its methyl ester on gastric acid and pepsin secretion in five patients with duodenal ulcer. Both analogues produced significant dose dependent inhibition of acid secretion. The dose required for 50% inhibition of acid output was 140 μg compared with 60–70 μg in non-ulcer subjects (see also Nylander and Andersson, 1975b, Florence).

Dose dependent inhibition of pentagastrin stimulated acid secretion in healthy subjects with orally administered 15(R)15-methyl PGE_2 methyl ester and 15(S)15-methyl PGE_2 methyl ester has also been confirmed by Konturek et al. (1975).

Bhana et al. (1973) studied the effect of orally administered 15-epi-PGA_2 on human gastric acid secretion. Unlike the 15-methyl analogues described above, this compound did not consistently affect gastric secretion.

11.2.2 Antiulcer effect

11.2.2.1 Animal studies

Prostaglandin of the E series have been studied for antiulcer effect in rats. Prostaglandin E_1 inhibited ulcers in Shay rats produced by pylorus ligation (Robert, 1968; Robert, Nezamis and Phillips, 1967). Prostaglandin E_2 was shown to inhibit duodenal ulcers produced in rats by infusion of secretagogues or a high dose of histamine (Robert, Stowe and Nezamis, 1971; Robert and Standish, 1973).

Lee and Bianchi (1972) showed that when given orally to rats ^{8}(12)13-PGE or SC-24665 (a synthetic analogue of PGE_1) prevented ulcer formation induced by pylorus ligation, exertion, restraint or reserpine treatment. 9-Oxoprostanoic acid (AY-22469) which reduced gastric acid secretion in rats when given orally has also been shown to have an anti-ulcer effect in the Shay rat (Lippman and Seethaler, 1973). This analogue is effective in preventing indomethacin induced ulcer formation in the rat (Lippman, 1974).

15(R)15-methyl PGE_2 methyl ester prevented ulcer formation in 21-hour pyloric ligated (Shay) rat (Carter *et al.*, 1974). Intraluminal administration of 25 or 50 $\mu g/kg$ body weight of the analogue at the time of ligation reduced the incidence and severity of gastric and esophageal ulceration. The ulcer healing effect of 15(R)15-methyl PGE_2 and its methyl ester has since been confirmed in man (Fung *et al.*, 1974a; Fung and Karim, 1976a; Karim and Fung, 1975a; Karim and Fung, 1976). Robert (1973) showed that 16,16-dimethyl PGE_2 is capable of preventing gastric (Shay and steroid induced) and duodenal (secretagogue-induced) ulcers when given orally or subcutaneously. In addition Robert (1974) has reported that indomethacin and flufenamic acid when given in high doses to rats produce severe syndrome of intestinal (jejunum and ileum) perforating ulcers that cause death by peritonitis. Administration of PGE_2, $PGF_{2\alpha}$ and 16,16-dimethyl analogues of PGA_2, PGE_2 or $PGF_{2\alpha}$ prevented the intestinal lesions induced by indomethacin and flufenamic acid. Robert (1974) has suggested that indomethacin and flufenamic acid produce intestinal ulcers by depleting the body tissues of endogenous prostaglandins. In this connection it is interesting to note that increased gastric mucosal permeability caused by aspirin and indomethacin can be prevented by 15(S)15-methyl PGE_2 methyl ester in dogs with Heidenhain pouch (Cohen, 1975). This analogue also prevents indomethacin induced mucosal erosion in the rat (Whittle, 1975). It is likely that gastrointestinal mucosal prostaglandins normally maintain the integrity of mucosal barrier and inhibition of prostaglandin synthesis may be one of the factors in aspirin and indomethacin induced gastric mucosal injury. In contrast, 16,16-dimethyl PGE_2 methyl ester instilled into the Heidenhain dog pouch (but not when given intravenously) caused a significant change in the ionic permeability of the mucosa (O'Brien and Carter, 1975). The possible link between prostaglandin deficiency and gastrointestinal ulcers has been discussed by Karim and Fung, 1976.

11.2.2.2 Human studies

In preliminary studies the following prostaglandin analogues have been shown to be potent inhibitors of gastric acid secretion when given orally to man (see Section 11.2.1.2)

15(R)15-methyl PGE_2 and its methyl ester
15(S)15-methyl PGE_2 and its methyl ester
16,16-dimethyl PGE_2 and its methyl ester

Theoretically all these compounds should be useful in the treatment of peptic ulcers. However, repeated administration of 15(S)15-methyl and 16,16-dimethyl compounds produces nausea, vomiting and diarrhea. In addition, the 16,16-dimethyl analogues given orally have a marked stimulant action on the human uterus (Karim and Amy, 1973). In contrast, 15(R)15-methyl PGE_2 and its methyl ester, when administered orally to normal human subjects, are well tolerated and so far clinical studies in ulcer healing have been restricted to these two compounds.

In ten patients with proven peptic ulceration, 15(R)15-methyl PGE_2

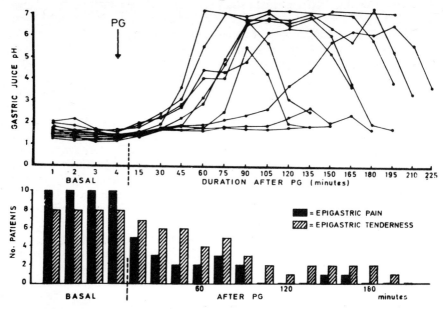

Figure 11.5   Effects of single oral dose of 150 μg of 15 (R) 15-methyl prostaglandin E_2 methyl ester on the gastric pH, epigastric pain and tenderness in 10 ulcer patients. (After Fung and Karim, 1974)

methyl ester in a single dose of 150 μg resulted in an elevation of gastric pH from around 1.5 to 7.0. Epigastric pain and tenderness were relieved when the gastric pH was raised above to 3.0 (Figure 11.5). The effect of a single dose of prostaglandin lasted for over 3 hours (Fung and Karim, 1974). Subsequently, a double blind study to compare the effects of 15(R)15-methyl PGE_2 methyl ester and an antacid, in the relief of epigastric pain and tenderness, was carried out. The mean duration of peptic ulcer pain relief following a single dose of 150 μg of the prostaglandin analogue was 81.32 min and for epigastric tenderness was 93.16 min. The mean duration of relief following a single dose of a standard antacid was 70.31 min for epigastric pain and 82.05 min for epigastric tenderness. Although the analogue appeared to be superior to antacid, the difference was not statistically significant (Fung, Karim and Tye, 1974a, b).

In a controlled endoscopic study, ten subjects with proven gastric ulcers were given 15 (R) 15-methyl PGE_2 methyl ester in oral doses of 150 μg 6-hourly for a period of 2 weeks. Control group of nine subjects, also with proven gastric ulcers received no prostaglandin. Gastric ulcer healing was assessed endoscopically with a duodenofiberscope. Endoscopic visualization and colour photography of the ulcer craters were undertaken before and 2 weeks after treatment. Patients in the control group were given antacid when they complained of pain. In the prostaglandin group, complete healing was seen in three cases, considerable healing in six cases and slight healing in one case (Table 11.1). In the control group complete healing was seen in none, considerable healing in two cases, slight healing in four cases and no healing in

Table 11.1   Effect of 15 (R) 15-methyl prostaglandin E$_2$ on ulcer healing in a double blind endoscopic study in man (After Karim and Fung, 1976)

15 (R) 15-Methyl Prostaglandin E$_2$				Control			
Age (yrs)	Sex	Initial ulcer size (cm)	Percentage healing	Age (yrs)	Sex	Initial ulcer size (cm)	Percentage healing
78	M	3.8	6	45	M	1.0	0
67	M	0.5	100	44	F	1.7	0
64	F	1.1	0	42	M	0.5	70
62	F	1.9	100	52	F	1.0	8
71	M	0.9	50	43	M	1.8	10
50	M	2.8	54	42	M	0.6	33
54	M	0.8	75	44	M	0.8	0
53	F	0.9	78	74	F	2.3	40
40	M	3.5	70	66	M	0.6	10
44	M	2.5	100	55	M	0.6	0

	Mean	S.D.	PG versus control	
			t	p
Gastric-ulcer healing (%)				
Prostaglandin (PG) control	63.3	34.62	3.39	< 0.005
	17.1	22.09		
Initial ulcer size (cm)				
Prostaglandin (PG) control	1.87	1.15	1.75	< 0.05
	1.09	0.59		
Age (years)				
Prostaglandin (PG) control	58.3	11.5	1.46	N.S.
	50.7	10.63		

three cases. The difference in the results of the two groups was highly significant. There was no significant difference between the two groups, in the severity of ulcer, or in age and sex distribution (Fung, Karim and Tye, 1974a).

The above findings have been recently confirmed in a double blind study using 15(R)15-methyl PGE$_2$ (free acid) (Karim and Fung, 1975; Fung and Karim, 1976a; Karim and Fung, 1976b).

An endoscopic and histological study of the effect of 15(R)15-methyl PGE$_2$ methyl ester on gastric mucosa in patients with peptic ulceration was reported by Fung, Lee and Karim (1974). 150 μg of this analogue had a powerful stimulant effect on the mucus secreting cells of gastric mucosa. The mucus secreting cells were bulging with increased amount of intracellular mucus and the lumina of the gastric pits were filled with mucus. Liberation of this substance may aid healing of gastric ulceration but whether this effect is attributed to the elevated pH noted after administration of the prostaglandin analogue is not clear. Light microscopy did not show significant changes in parietal or chief cells.

11.2.3 Mucosal blood flow

Robert (1973) has discussed evidence against the possibility that the inhibition of gastric secretion produced by PGE_1 in the dog is secondary to gastric mucosal ischaemia. Main and Whittle (1974) have shown that prostaglandin analogues which inhibit gastric secretion cause an increase in mucosal blood flow. In the urethane anaesthetized rat, during secretory stimulation with pentagastrin or histamine, intravenous infusion of 15(S)15-methyl PGE_2 methyl ester or 16,16-dimethyl PGE_2 (2 μg/kg for 20 min) caused maximal inhibition of acid output. Both analogues produced an increase in mean blood flow per unit acid output during inhibition of gastric secretion.

11.2.4 Pancreatic secretion

16,16-Dimethyl PGE_2 is more potent than PGE_1 in its action on pancreatic secretion. In dogs with chronic duodenal fistula, PGE_1 reduced the volume and bicarbonate concentration of basal and secretin stimulated pancreatic secretion but increased the concentration of enzymes as measured by protein content (Rudick et al., 1971). Rosenberg et al. (1974) have shown that in dogs with chronic duodenal fistula, 16,16-dimethyl PGE_2 produced a marked and prolonged inhibition of volume and bicarbonate concentration in the resting pancreas and pancreas stimulated with (a) secretin (b) secretin with cholecystokinin–pancreozymin.

11.2.5 Bile

Bile was noted in the aspirated sample of gastric juice after oral (Horton et al., 1968) and intravenous (Classen et al., 1970; Classen, Koch, Bickhardt, Topf and Demling, 1971) administrations of PGE_1 in man. The presence of bile was also noted in the gastric fistula dogs during parenteral administration of PGE_1 (Main, 1973). PGE_2, however, did not seem to share this effect in the dog (Sokoloff and Berk, 1973) and in man (Karim et al., 1973b).

After administration of single oral doses of 15-methyl and 16,16-dimethyl analogues of PGE_2, no appreciable amount of bile was noted in the gastric juice of man (Karim et al., 1973 a–d).

In the unanaesthetized chronic fistula rat, however, subcutaneous administration of 1.25–2.5 μg/kg 15-methyl analogues of PGE_2 caused reflux of bile into the gastric lumen (Main and Whittle, 1974). It is not clear whether the presence of bile in the gastric juice is due to duodenal reflux, direct stimulation of bile secretion or effect on gall bladder.

11.2.6 Pepsin

Salmon et al. (1975) studied the effect of 15(R)15-methyl PGE_2 methyl ester on basal and pentagastrin stimulated pepsin secretion in four adult healthy male volunteers. Inhibition of pepsin paralleled inhibition of acid output in three out of four subjects after oral administration of 200 μg of the prostaglandin analogue. Inhibition of pentagastrin stimulated pepsin secretion with 15(S)15-methyl PGE_2 methyl ester and 15(R)15-methyl PGE_2 methyl ester administered orally in healthy young human volunteers has also been reported by Konturek *et al.* (1975). The results are in agreement with those reported in dogs (Robert and Yankee, 1975).

16,16-Dimethyl PGE_2 and its methyl ester have also been shown to inhibit pepsin secretion in dogs and man (Robert, Lancaster and Nezamis, 1975; Nylander and Andersson, 1975a).

11.2.7 Gastrin

Prostaglandin E_1 inhibits gastrin induced gastric acid secretion in man (Classen *et al.*, 1971) and in dogs (Robert, 1968). The possibility therefore exists that prostaglandins inhibit gastric secretion by interfering with the release of gastrin. However, inhibition of gastric secretion by prostaglandins is not specific to gastrin but extends to pentagastrin, histamine, food, carbachol and reserpine (Robert, 1973). PGE_1 inhibits acid secretion and increases gastrin release (as determined by serum gastrin levels) in Heidenhain pouch dogs stimulated with food. Increased serum gastrin levels after oral administration of 200 μg 15(R)15-methyl PGE_2 methyl ester in healthy human subjects has also been demonstrated (Adaikan *et al.*, 1974). The increase in serum gastrin level paralleled the increase in pH of gastric juice (Figure 11.6). It was concluded that the increased gastrin release was the result of diminished acid inhibition of antrum due to prostaglandin induced raised pH of gastric juice. Therefore prostaglandins do not appear to inhibit gastric acid secretion by preventing the release of gastrin.

11.2.8 Effect on gut motility

11.2.8.1 *In vitro* studies

The actions of synthetic analogues on various gastrointenstinal smooth muscle preparation *in vitro* are discussed in Section 11.4.

11.2.8.2 *In vivo* studies

The effect of 15(S)15-methyl PGE_2 methyl ester and 16,16-dimethyl PGE_2 on gastrointestinal motility in rat, has been studied by Main and Whittle, 1974. Intraluminal pressure was recorded in the duodenum, jejunum and ileum of the anaesthetized rat. Both analogues (0.5–5 μg/kg intravenously) showed increase in intestinal tone and motility and were about 20 times more potent than PGE_2 (*in vitro*, these analogues are weaker than PGE_2 in stimulating gastrointestinal smooth muscle).

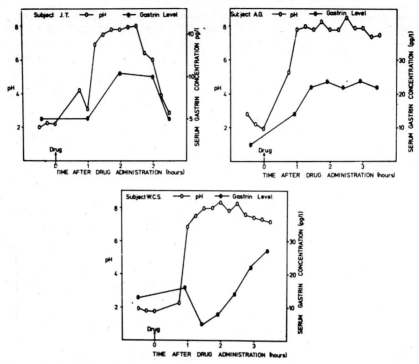

Figure 11.6 Action of 15 (R) 15-methyl PGE_2 methyl ester on pH of gastric juice and serum gastrin levels in three subjects. (After Adaikan *et al.*, 1975)

11.3 CARDIOVASCULAR EFFECTS

11.3.1 Animal studies

11.3.1.1 15(S)PGA₂ and 15(R)PGA₂

The sea animal, gorgonian (*Plexaura homomalla*) is a rich source of 15(R)-PGA_2, a 15 epimer of naturally occurring prostaglandin A_2 (15(S)PGA_2). Intravenous injections of 2.5–256 µg/kg of 15(R)PGA_2 had no effect on the cardiovascular system in dogs. In contrast 15(S)PGA_2 (PGA_2) increased heart rate, myocardial contraction and reduced mean systemic arterial blood pressure in dogs (Nakano, 1969). 15(R)PGA_2 did not modify the cardiovascular effects of 15(S)PGA_2 (Nakano and Kessinger, 1970a).

11.3.1.2 15(S)15-Methyl PGA₁ methyl ester and 15(S)15-methyl PGA₂ methyl ester

Both 15(S)15-methyl PGA_1 methyl ester and 15(S)15-methyl PGA_2 methyl ester (Figure 11.3) lowered arterial blood pressure in the rat when injected intravenously. The threshold dose for both was between 1 and 3.2 µg/kg. At

higher doses (100–320 μg/kg), 15(S)15-methyl PGA_2 methyl ester showed a biphasic effect—an increase followed by a decrease in blood pressure (Bundy *et al.*, 1973).

11.3.1.3 8-Iso PGE_1

8-Iso PGE_1 (Figure 11.3) lowered arterial blood pressure in the rat, cat and dog when injected intravenously but was one-tenth to one-hundredth as active as PGE_1 (Shekhar, Weeks and Kupieki, 1968). In open-chest pentobarbital anaesthetized dogs, intravenous injections of 8-iso PGE_1 increased heart rate, myocardial contractile force and pulmonary arterial pressure. Dogs in which pulmonary arterial blood flow was kept constant by means of a pump, pulmonary arterial injection of 2 μg/kg PGE_1 decreased pulmonary arterial pressure while the same dose of 8-iso PGE_1 and $PGF_{2\alpha}$ increased the pulmonary arterial pressure. Prostaglandin $F_{2\alpha}$ was twice as potent as 8-iso PGE_1. This analogue of PGE_1 is therefore a unique compound which has a mild hypotensive action in systemic circulation and a marked hypertensive action in the pulmonary circulation in dogs (Nakano and Kessinger, 1970b).

11.3.1.4 15(S)15-Methyl PGE_2 methyl ester and 15(S)15-methyl $PGF_{2\alpha}$ methyl ester

The cardiovascular effects of the 15-methyl analogues of PGE_2 and $PGF_{2\alpha}$ (methyl esters) have been studied in rats (Weeks *et al.*, 1973; Bundy *et al.*, 1973; Strand, Miller and McGiff, 1974; Karim and Adaikan, 1974); dogs (Weeks *et al.*, 1973; Strand, Miller and McGiff, 1974; Weir *et al.*, 1975a) and baboons (Adaikan and Karim, 1974).

In anaesthetized dogs Weeks *et al.* (1973) compared the effects of PGE_2 methyl ester and 15(S)15-methyl PGE_2 methyl ester on mean arterial blood pressure, cardiac output, total peripheral resistance and left ventricular dp/dt. Both compounds caused a dose-dependent decrease in mean arterial blood pressure over the range 0.032–3.2 μg/kg injected intravenously. The dose–response curves for the two compounds were similar and there was no significant difference in the hypotensive effects of the two compounds at any dose. The effects of these two compounds on other cardiovascular parameters were in marked contrast. PGE_2 methyl ester caused a dose-related increase in cardiac output and decrease in calculated total peripheral resistance, while left ventricular dp/dt and cardiac rate remained essentially unchanged. The effects of 15(S)15-methyl PGE_2 methyl ester followed those of the parent compound up to 0.32 μg/kg but at 1 and 3.2 μg/kg cardiac output, left ventricular dp/dt and cardiac rate dropped sharply and calculated total peripheral resistance increased. Pulmonary arterial pressure increased in a dose-related manner after both agents.

Comparison was also made between the cardiovascular effects of $PGF_{2\alpha}$ methyl ester and 15(S)15-methyl $PGF_{2\alpha}$ methyl ester (Figure 11.1) in anaesthetized dogs (Weeks *et al.*, 1973). Both compounds caused dose-related increases in mean arterial blood pressure and pulmonary artery pressure.

The difference in relative potency of the two compounds was not statistically significant. However, 15(S)15-methyl $PGF_{2\alpha}$ methyl ester had a longer duration of action on pulmonary arterial pressure.

Weir et al. (1975a), compared cardiovascular effects of $PGF_{2\alpha}$ and 15(S)15-methyl $PGF_{2\alpha}$ in anaesthetized dogs. The two prostaglandins were given by the intramuscular and intravenous routes. By both routes 15(S)15-methyl $PGF_{2\alpha}$ produced a greater and more sustained rise in pulmonary arterial pressure than $PGF_{2\alpha}$. Intramuscular injection of the analogue also elicited a more prolonged increase in pulmonary vascular resistance than prostaglandin $F_{2\alpha}$ given intramuscularly or intravenously. The 15-methyl analogue also caused a greater initial fall in systemic arterial oxygen tension and cardiac output and a greater increase in systemic resistance than $PGF_{2\alpha}$.

Both 15-methyl PGE_2 and 15-methyl $PGF_{2\alpha}$ produced an increase in lobar arterial perfusion pressure in intact dogs which was accompanied by an increase in pressure in lobar small veins. The compounds were able to increase pulmonary vascular resistance by over 100% when pulmonary flow was maintained at a constant level. These results indicate that the 15-methyl analogues increase pulmonary vascular resistance in the dog by constricting lobar veins and upstream vessels (Kadowitz and Hyman, 1974). Strand et al. (1974) found 15(S)15-methyl PGE_2 methyl ester to be 2.6 times less active than PGE_2 methyl ester and 77.3 times less active than PGE_2 (free acid) in its renal vasodilator action in the dog. In contrast 15(S)15-methyl PGE_2 methyl ester was slightly more potent than PGE_2 methyl ester in femoral vasodilator activity.

The lack of significant increase in potency and duration of action of 15-methyl analogues of PGE_2 and $PGF_{2\alpha}$ on various cardiovascular parameters is in contrast both to the marked increase in potency on the pregnant human and primate uterus (Bygdeman et al., 1972; Karim and Sharma, 1972; Karim and Amy, 1975; Kirton and Forbes, 1972; Adaikan and Karim, 1974) and in inhibition of gastric secretion. The increased potency and duration of action of the 15-methyl analogues on these parameters are thought to be related to the fact that these compounds are not substrates for prostaglandin 15-OH dehydrogenase. It is possible that in areas where the analogues are not more potent than the parent compound, increased inactivation by enzymes other than 15-OH dehydrogenase is taking place.

11.3.1.5 PGE_2 methyl ester and $PGF_{2\alpha}$ methyl ester

PGE_2 methyl ester was shown to be five times more potent than PGE_2 (free acid) in stimulating pregnant human uterus in vivo (Karim et al., 1973). However, on the isolated jird colon, guinea pig ileum and rat stomach strips the methyl ester was less active than the free acid (Karim et al., 1973; Strand et al., 1974). Similarly PGE_2 methyl ester showed less vasodepressor activity than PGE_2 in the baboon (Karim et al., 1973) (Table 11.2) but the two compounds were equipotent in lowering rat blood pressure (Strand et al., 1974). In the dog PGE_2 methyl ester was 29.6 times less active in renal vasodilator activity and 6.2 times less active in increasing femoral blood flow than PGE_2.

Table 11.2   Comparative values of biological activities of some prostaglandin analogues relative to respective parent compounds (PGE$_2$ or PGF$_{2\alpha}$ taken as one)

Prostaglandin	Jird colon	Guinea-pig ileum	Rat uterus	Baboon blood pressure (arterial)
17-phenyl PGE$_2$ (free acid)	1.5	0.74	0.88	0.33 ↓
15 (R) 15-methyl PGE$_2$ methyl ester	0.008	0.005	0.006	0.043 ↓
15 (S) 15-methyl PGE$_2$ methyl ester	0.40	0.22	0.56	0.7 ↓
PGE$_2$ methyl ester	0.065	0.031	0.04	0.35 ↓
15 (S) 15-methyl PGF$_{2\alpha}$ methyl ester	0.79	1.0	0.57	1.6 ↑
PGF$_{2\alpha}$ methyl ester	0.72	0.11	0.5	1.0 ↑

Karim and Adaikan (1974)

Prostaglandin F$_{2\alpha}$ and its methyl ester were equipotent in raising blood pressure in the baboon and stimulating pregnant human uterus *in vivo* when given by bolus intravenous injections (Karim *et al.*, 1973).

11.3.1.6   15(R)Prostaglandins

15(R) PGF$_{2\alpha}$, 15(R)15-methyl PGE$_2$ (and methyl ester), 15(R)15-methyl PGF$_{2\alpha}$ (and methyl ester) were less active than PGE$_2$ or PGF$_{2\alpha}$ on the blood pressure of rat and baboon (Table 11.2) (Bundy *et al.*, 1973; Karim and Adaikan, 1974). 15(R)15-methyl PGF$_{2\alpha}$ was twice as active as 15(R)F$_{2\alpha}$ in raising blood pressure in the rat (Bundy *et al.*, 1973).

11.3.1.7   15-Methyl ether methyl ester

The synthesis and biological effects of PGF$_{2\alpha}$ 15-methyl ether methyl ester was reported by Youngdale and Lincoln (1974) (Figure 11.1). When administered intravenously to rat, this compound exhibited similar vasodepressor potency to PGF$_{2\alpha}$.

11.3.1.8.   17-Phenyl prostaglandins

17-Phenyl trinor PGE$_2$ given intravenously was three times less active than PGE$_2$ in lowering blood pressure in the cat and baboon. In the rat and rabbit this analogue was between 18 and 80 times weaker than PGE$_2$ in its vasodepressor effect but tachyphylaxis made accurate comparison difficult (Karim and Adaikan, 1974).

17-Phenyl trinor PGF$_{2\alpha}$ was five times more potent than PGF$_{2\alpha}$ in raising blood pressure in the rat whereas 17-phenyl trinor PGE$_2$ produced a biphasic response—a brief depressor effect followed by a prolonged pressor effect (Miller et al., 1975).

11.3.1.9 16, 16-Dimethyl PGE₂ and methyl ester

Unlike other PGE analogues, 16,16-dimethyl PGE_2 given as bolus intravenous injection produced a depressor followed by a pressor effect. In the perfused hind limb of the rat, 16,16-dimethyl PGE_2 showed vasoconstriction in contrast to the vasodilator effect of PGE_2 (Weeks and DuCharme, 1975). In the anaesthetized dog (Weeks and DuCharme, 1975) and baboon (Karim and Adaikan, 1975) 16,16-dimethyl PGE_2 lowered arterial blood pressure (Table 11.3). Total peripheral resistance decreased followed by an increase in the dog (Weeks and DuCharme, 1975).

Table 11.3 Comparative values of blood pressure effect (pressor ↑ or depressor ↓) and guinea-pig ileum stimulating effects of some prostaglandin analogues relative to respective parent compounds (PGE_2 or $PGF_{2\alpha}$ taken as one)

Prostaglandin	Baboon blood pressure (arterial)	Guinea-pig ileum
15 (R) 15-Methyl $PGF_{2\alpha}$ methyl ester	0.5 ↑	0.55
2a, 2b-Dihomo 15 (S) 15-methyl $PGF_{2\alpha}$ methyl ester	0.05 ↑	0.01
5-Oxa $F_{1\alpha}$ ($F_{2\alpha}$ as 1)	0.7 ↑	0.006
Ent-13 dehydro-15-epi-$PGF_{2\alpha}$	0.132 ↑	negligible
An isomer of ent-13 dehydro-15-epi-$PGF_{2\alpha}$	0.72 ↑	0.65
I.C.I. 81008 (F compound)	3.84 ↑	0.02
11-Epi-15-epi-ent PGE₂ methyl ester	0.42 ↓	0.034
16, 16-Dimethyl PGE₂	1.53 ↓	0.23
16, 16-Dimethyl PGE₂ methyl ester	0.3 ↓	0.27
16, 16-Difluoro PGE₂	2.0 ↓	0.77
15 (S) 15-Methyl-17-phenyl-18-19-20 trinor PGE₂	0.07 ↓	0.88

Karim and Adaikan (1975)

11.3.1.10 16(R)Methyl-13, 14-dihydro PGE₂ methyl ester: ONO-464

By the oral route ONO-464 is 100 times more potent than PGE_2 in lowering arterial blood pressure in anaesthetized dogs whereas by the intravenous route it is 11 times more potent than PGE_2. In spontaneously hypertensive rats this prostaglandin analogue when given orally is 5–10 times more effective than PGE_2 in lowering blood pressure (Kawasaki et al., 1975).

11.3.1.11 Other compounds

Recently some newly synthesized analogues of prostaglandins have been studied for their effects on arterial blood pressure in baboon and smooth muscle stimulating action on guinea pig ileum *in vitro* (Table 11.3). In both parameters most of these compounds were shown to be less active than their respective parent compound (Karim and Adaikan, 1975). Of these 2a,2b-dihomo-15(S)15-methyl $PGF_{2\alpha}$ methyl ester is the least effective in elevating baboon blood pressure (20 times weaker than $PGF_{2\alpha}$) and stimulating guinea pig ileum (100 times weaker than $PGF_{2\alpha}$). The abortifacient use of this compound has been reported by Karim and Ratnam (1976).

11.3.2 Human studies

Several prostaglandin analogues have been clinically evaluated for the termination of human pregnancy. These include the 15-methyl, 16,16-dimethyl and 17-phenyl analogues of PGE_2 and $PGF_{2\alpha}$. At abortifacient doses (by various routes) these compounds are thought not to affect the cardiovascular system in man although few specific studies to confirm this have been carried out.

Karim and Adaikan (1975) have studied the effects of bolus intravenous injections of several analogues of PGE_2 on blood pressure in man from a cannulated brachial artery. The results of these studies are shown in Table 11.4.

Weir *et al.* (1975b) showed that 15(S)15-methyl $PGF_{2\alpha}$ administered intramuscularly to pregnant women in doses of 400 μg showed increases in pulmonary arterial pressure and pulmonary wedge pressure. With intramuscular doses of 800 μg of this analogue there was in addition a significant rise in systemic arterial pressure.

11.3.3 Antithrombotic effect

A comparative study was carried out for antithrombotic effects of 8-iso PGE_1 and PGE_1 (Weeks, Sekhar and Kupiecki, 1968; Sekhar *et al.*, 1968). Both 8-iso PGE_1 and PGE_1 inhibited aggregation of platelet in rat and human platelet rich plasma. They lysed ADP induced human platelet thrombin *in vitro* at 50 ng/ml and higher. In addition, platelet aggregation was inhibited in blood taken 10 minutes after intravenous administration of both prostaglandins at a dose of 3 mg/kg. In contrast, as a spasmogen on rabbit duodenum *in vitro*, cat intestine *in vivo* and as a vasodepressor in cat, rat and dog the potency of 8-iso PGE_1 was 1–10% of PGE_1. Furthermore, as an inhibitor of adrenaline-induced lipolysis in rat epididymal fat, its potency was 24% of PGE_1. These results suggest that 8-iso PGE_1 is a potent antithrombotic agent like PGE_1 but has less cardiovascular and smooth muscle stimulating actions (Sekhar, Weeks, Kupiecki, 1968).

Recently a PGE_1 analogue, ONO-747(17)(ξ)-ethyl-trans-Δ^2-PGE_1) was shown to be a potent inhibitor of platelet aggregation in human, rat and rabbit platelet rich plasma. This compound was 15.8, 12.0 and 2.1 times more potent than PGE_1 in human, rat and rabbit respectively (Ojima and Fujita, 1975).

Another ONO compound, 16-methylene PGE_2 methyl ester β-cyclodextrin clathrate (ONO-481CD) also inhibited ADP-induced human platelet aggregation *in vitro* but was 400 times less active than PGE_1 (Karim, Adaikan and Lo, 1976.)

Table 11.4 Cardiovascular effects of some prostaglandin analogues in man (After Karim and Adaikan, 1975)

Subject	PG	Dose	Control BP Syst.	Control BP Diast.	Control HR	Maximum Changes BP Syst.	Maximum Changes BP Diast.	Maximum Changes HR	Cardiovascular effects	Other effects
1	E₂	100 µg	133	72	65	−2	+5	+30	—	General weakness
	E₂ methyl ester	100 µg	128	75.5	85	−28	−17.5	+55	Tachycardia (returned to normal in 3 min) Hypotension	
	E₂ methyl ester	100 µg	110	65	75	+35	+30	+20	Tachycardia, hypertension	Shivering restlessness and shaking vigorously. Feeling cold (1 min after injection to 25 min). Dryness of mouth.
2	15(R)15-methyl E₂ methyl ester	100 µg	137	63	55	−6	0	+5	Mild tachycardia and hypotension	—
	15(R)15-methyl E₂ methyl ester	100 µg	125	68	55	−13	−6	+5	Mild tachycardia and hypotension	—
	15(S)15-methyl E₂ methyl ester	25 µg	121	62	57	−19	−3	+8	Tachycardia, hypotension	—
3	16,16-Di-methyl E₂ methyl ester	50 µg	108	63	50	+12	+11	+8	Tachycardia hypertension	Cold and slight shivering 18 min after injection.

4	16, 16-Di methyl E$_2$ methyl ester	50 μg	110	55	65	+16	+14	+5	Tachycardia, hypertension	Feverish and Cold —
5	16, 16-Di methyl E$_2$ methyl ester	50 μg	146	84	81	+18	+9	−7	Bradycardia, hypertension	—
6	17-Phenyl E$_2$	50 μg	131	79	68	+14 / −4	+11 / −7	+3 / −3	Hypertension in 1 min followed by hypotension in 5 min	—
7	17-Phenyl E$_2$	50 μg	133	84	75	−3	−2	−6	Bradycardia	
	17-Phenyl E$_2$	100 μg	125	65	64	+7	+10	−4		
	17-Phenyl E$_2$ 15(R)15-methyl E$_2$ methyl ester	100 μg	129	78	65	−5 / −11	+1 / −9	−1 / −4	Hypotension Tachycardia	3rd dose of Subject No. 5
		200 μg	134	84	69	−6	−6	+5		

11.4 SMOOTH MUSCLE STIMULATING ACTIVITY

11.4.1 11,15-Epi prostaglandins E_1, A_1, E_2

Ramwell *et al.* (1969) studied biological activities of some synthetic stereo-isomers of prostaglandins E_1 and A_1. The racemic compounds, *rac*-15-epi PGE_1, *rac*-11-epi PGE_1 and *rac*-11,15-epi PGE_1 were tested for activity on rat uterus, guinea pig ileum, rabbit jejunum and rat blood pressure. All the analogues were less active than the natural PGE_1 except *rac*-11,15-epi PGE_1 (8,12-diiso PGE_1) which was 5.4 times more potent than PGE_1 in stimulating rabbit jejunum. *Rac*-15-epi PGA_1 was twice as potent as natural PGA_1 on this preparation. *Ent*-PGE_1, which is a mirror image of PGE_1, had very little smooth muscle stimulating activity (one-thousandth of the activity of natural PGE_1). In various *in vitro* and *in vivo* biological preparations, 11,15-epi PGE_2 consistently showed effects similar to $PGF_{2\alpha}$ rather than PGE_1. It was suggested that this PGE_2 analogue may be acting at PGF receptors (Ceserani *et al.*, 1975a). The prostaglandin antagonistic effect of this compound is reported in Section 11.5.1.

11.4.2 8-Iso PGE_1

As a spasmogen on rabbit duodenum *in vitro* and cat intestine *in vivo*, this compound showed one tenth to one hundredth the activity of PGE_1 (Sekhar *et al.*, 1968).

11.4.3 7-Oxa prostaglandin derivatives

The smooth muscle stimulating activity of several 7-oxa prostaglandin derivatives of $PGF_{1\alpha}$ have been reported (Ford and Fried, 1969; Fried *et al.*, 1971). Although these compounds showed similar qualitative effects to natural prostaglandins, they were far less potent than $PGF_{1\alpha}$ in stimulating smooth muscle preparation of gerbil colon.

Derivatives possessing the same degree of hydroxylation as $PGF_{1\alpha}$ are more active than those lacking the 15-hydroxyl group. Likewise, compounds possessing the 13,14-*trans*-double bond or triple bond are more active than those analogues having a *cis*-double bond or no double bond. Thus, substitution of the 15-hydroxyl group by hydrogen and reduction of the 13,14-*trans*-double bond or its replacement by *cis*-double bond, lead to a progressive decrease in biological activity (Ford and Fried, 1969).

Some of the 7-oxa prostaglandins without the hydroxyl or keto groups in the carbocyclic ring were shown to antagonise smooth muscle contraction produced by PGE_1 and $PGF_{2\alpha}$ (Fried *et al.*, 1971).

Based on the structure activity relationships among the 7-oxa prostaglandins, Fried *et al.* (1971) concluded that smooth muscle activity is dependent on the degree of hydroxylation of these compounds. Thus pure agonism was noted in compounds with oxygen in the 9 and 11 positions, in the presence or absence of a 15-hydroxyl group. Pure antagonism was a feature of analogues without hydroxyl or keto groups. Agonism and antagonism were exhibited by substances possessing only a 15-hydroxyl group (Figure 11.7).

Apart from being agonists and antagonists of smooth muscle activity, some of the 7-oxa derivatives were shown to inhibit prostaglandin synthetase in bull testes (Fried et al., 1971) (see Section 11.5.2).

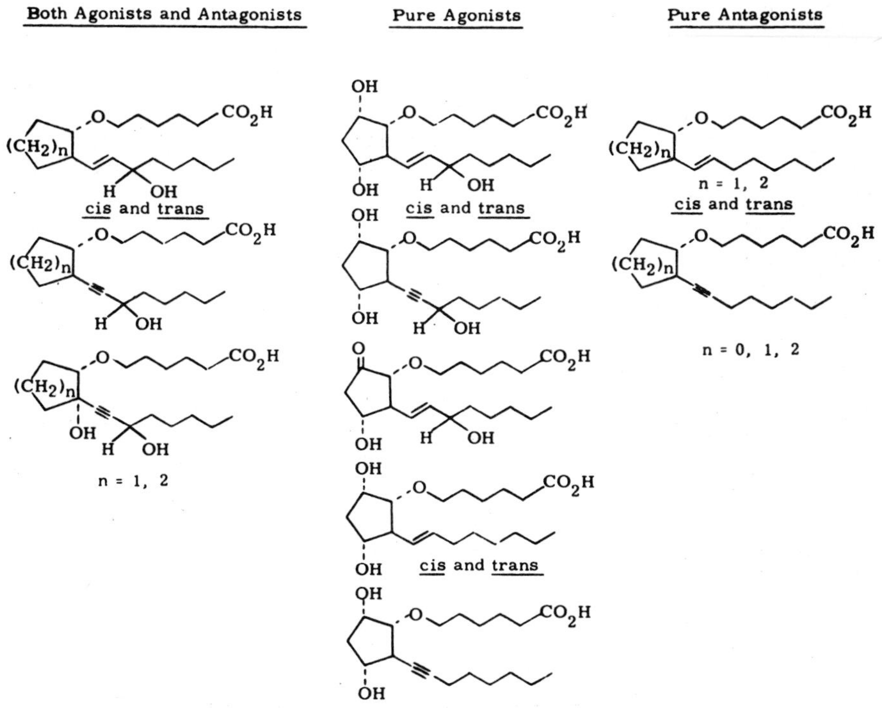

Figure 11.7 Structure–function relationship among 7-oxa prostaglandins. (After Fried et al., 1971)

11.4.4 3, 5 and 13-Oxa prostaglandins

The synthesis and smooth muscle stimulating effect of several 3,5- and 13-oxa derivatives of natural prostaglandins has been reported by Bundy et al. (1971). Oxa compounds which are less susceptible to β-oxidation of the carboxylic acid side chain, retained prostaglandin-like smooth muscle stimulating activity but were less potent than the parent prostaglandins. As an example dl-3-oxa PGE_1 had one twenty-fifth the activity of PGE_1 in stimulating isolated gerbil colon (Bundy et al., 1971).

11.4.5 17-Oxa compound

20-Ethyl-17-oxa $PGF_{2\alpha}$ is 10 times less active than $PGF_{2\alpha}$ in contracting guinea pig uterus in vitro (Bowler, Crossley and Dowell, 1975).

11.4.6 15-Methyl analogues of PGE_2 and $PGF_{2\alpha}$

The hydroxyl group at C-15 in the prostaglandin molecule is susceptible to oxidation by prostaglandin 15-hydroxydehydrogenase. The 15-methyl analogues of PGE_2 and $PGF_{2\alpha}$ are not substrates for the dehydrogenase and possibly as a result are several times more potent than the parent compounds in stimulating the human uterine and gastrointestinal smooth muscles *in vivo* (see Karim and Amy, 1975, for references). On the isolated rat uterus and gerbil colon preparations *in vitro* the 15(S)15-methyl analogues of PGE_2 and $PGF_{2\alpha}$ do not show an enhanced effect compared to the parent compounds probably because in *in vitro* situation enzymatic inactivation by 15-OH dehydrogenase is not important. The 15(R)15-methyl analogues of PGE_2 and $PGF_{2\alpha}$ are several times less active than the corresponding 15(S)15-methyl analogues both *in vivo* and *in vitro* (Weeks *et al.*, 1973; Karim and Adaikan, 1974; Bundy *et al.*, 1971; Bundy *et al.*, 1973; Youngdale and Lincoln, 1974) (see Tables 11.2 and 11.3).

11.4.7 16-Methyl analogues

The various 16-methyl analogues of prostaglandins E_2 and $F_{2\alpha}$ are poor substrates for 15-hydroxyprostaglandin dehydrogenase than the parent natural prostaglandins. For example, 16,16-dimethyl PGE_2 and 16,16-dimethyl $PGF_{2\alpha}$ were only 10% and 4% as efficient as PGE_1 as substrate for the dehydrogenase. This may partly account for the marked increase in potency and duration of action, of 16,16-dimethyl PGE_2 analogues in stimulating intact pregnant human uterus and the gastrointestinal tract. A single oral dose of 50 μg of 16,16-dimethyl PGE_2 or its methyl ester will produce diarrhea in human subjects whereas 20–30 times higher doses of PGE_2 or its methyl ester would be necessary for a similar effect. Similarly, 16,16-dimethyl PGE_2 and methyl esters are 20–50 times more potent than the parent compounds in stimulating the pregnant uterus *in vivo* (Karim and Amy, 1973; Karim, Sivasamboo and Ratnam, 1974) and in inhibiting gastric secretion (Karim *et al.*, 1973d).

In vitro the various 16-methyl analogues of PGE_2 and $PGF_{2\alpha}$ are more active than the parent prostaglandins in stimulating the gerbil colon (Magerlein *et al.*, 1973). However, on the guinea pig ileum, 16,16-dimethyl PGE_2 and its methyl ester were four times less active than PGE_2 (Karim and Adaikan, 1975–Table 11.3).

11.4.8 16-Fluoro analogues

16,16-Difluoro PGE_2 methyl ester and 16,16-difluoro $PGF_{2\alpha}$ methyl ester were synthesized by Yankee *et al.* (1975). The smooth muscle stimulating effects of these compounds were reported by Magerlein and Miller (1975) and Yankee *et al.* (1975). Both compounds were less active than the parent $PGF_{2\alpha}$ (Table 11.3).

11.4.9 17-Phenyl analogues

On the gerbil colon, rat uterus and guinea pig ileum *in vitro*, 17-phenyl trinor PGE_2 and $PGF_{2\alpha}$ have similar smooth muscle stimulating potencies to the corresponding parent prostaglandins (Miller *et al.*, 1975; Karim and Adaikan, 1974; Table 11.2).

Similarly 15(S)15-methyl 17-phenyl trinor $PGF_{2\alpha}$ methyl ester and 11α, 15(S)*ent*-17-phenyl-ω-trinor PGE_2 (both compounds are resistant to enzymatic inactivation at C-15 and ω and (ω − 1)) do not show an increase in gerbil colon stimulating potencies *in vitro* although both are several times more potent than their parent prostaglandins as antifertility agents in the hamster (Yankee *et al.*, 1975) (Table 11.5).

Table 11.5 Hamster antifertility and smooth muscle stimulating effects of some prostaglandin analogues

Analogue	Hamster antifertility potency	Smooth muscle stimulating potency
2a, 2b-Dihomo-15 (S)15-methyl $PGF_{2\alpha}$	5	< 1
15 (S)15-Methyl 17-phenyl-ω-trinor- $PGF_{2\alpha}$ methyl ester	20	1
11α, 15 (S)-*Ent*-17-phenyl-ω-trinor PGE_2	25	1
16, 16-Difluoro-$PGF_{2\alpha}$ methyl ester	5–10	1
16, 16-Difluoro-PGE_2 methyl ester	10–20	—

Yankee, Ayer, Bundy and Lincoln, 1975

On the pregnant human uterus 17-phenyl 18,19,20 trinor $PGF_{2\alpha}$ was 7 to 8 times more potent than $PGF_{2\alpha}$ when given as a bolus intravenous injection. In contrast 17-phenyl, 18,19,20 trinor PGE_2 was half as active as PGE_2 (Wiqvist *et al.*, 1975).

11.4.10 2a,2b-Dihomo 15 (S) 15-methyl $PGF_{2\alpha}$ methyl ester

This compound is several times less active than $PGF_{2\alpha}$ in stimulating various smooth muscles *in vitro* and in raising blood pressure in the rat and baboon (Karim and Adaikan, 1975; Yankee *et al.*, 1975; Table 11.5). *In vivo* 2a,-2b-dihomo 15(S)15-methyl $PGF_{2\alpha}$ methyl ester is at least ten times more potent than $PGF_{2\alpha}$ in stimulating pregnant human uterus and gastro-intestinal tract smooth muscle. The abortifacient effect of this compound has been reported by Karim and Ratnam (1976).

11.5 PROSTAGLANDIN ANALOGUES AS ANTAGONISTS AND SYNTHESIS INHIBITORS

11.5.1 Prostaglandin analogues as antagonists

Most of the 7-oxa prostaglandin analogues show affinity for prostaglandin receptors but lack smooth muscle stimulating activity. Several of these compounds have been tested for their prostaglandin antagonistic activity. The subject has been reviewed in this series of books by Sanner and Eakins, 1975.

11,15-Epi PGE_2 and *ent*-11,15-epi PGE_2 have both been shown to stimulate rat uterus and gerbil colon *in vitro*. After the drugs are washed out from the organ bath the responses to PGE_2 are reduced or abolished (Corey *et al.*, 1972). Karim and Adaikan (1975) have studied the prostaglandin antagonistic activity of 11-epi-15-epi-*ent* PGE_2 methyl ester on the guinea pig ileum *in vitro*. This compound is about 30 times less active than PGE_2 in stimulating the guinea pig ileum. As an antagonist 11-epi-15-epi-*ent* PGE_2 methyl ester (3.2 μg/ml) completely abolished the stimulant effect of PGE_2, reduced $PGF_{2\alpha}$ response by 60–80% while contractions induced with acetylcholine were unaffected. The prostaglandin blocking activity of this analogue was surmountable by increasing the doses of PGE_2 (Figure 11.8) or $PGF_{2\alpha}$.

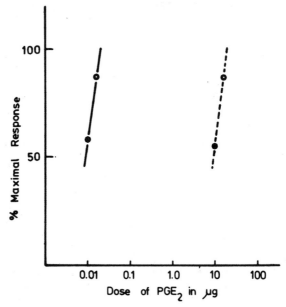

Figure 11.8   Antagonistic effect of 3.2 μg/ml 11-epi-15-epi-*ent* PGE_2 methyl ester on contraction produced by PGE_2 in guinea-pig ileum *in vitro*. Control doses: ——o——; in the presence of analogue – – o – –

An analogue of $PGF_{2\alpha}$, 13-dehydro 20ω $PGF_{2\alpha}$ (K 10136) showed a non-competitive inhibition of the stimulant action of $PGF_{2\alpha}$ but not of PGE_2 or other agonists on rat uterus (Ceserani *et al.*, 1975b).

A new prostaglandin analogue, 8-ethoxycarbonyl-10,11-dihydro-A prostaglandin, was reported to be a potent antagonist of prostaglandins on smooth muscle and has been claimed to be superior ro SC-19220 and 7-oxa-13-prostenoic acid (Schölkens and Babej, 1975). Adaikan *et al.* (1976) have shown that this compound produced complete inhibition of prostaglandin-induced smooth muscle contractions in gerbil colon (1 μg/ml), hamster fundus (2 μg/ml), rat fundus (4 μg/ml) and guinea pig ileum (4 μg/ml). In addition to antagonizing the effects of PGE_2 and $PGF_{2\alpha}$ the 8-ethoxycarbonyl-10,11-dihydro-A prostaglandin also produced complete inhibition of contractions produced by carbachol, acetylcholine, 5-HT and histamine.

11.5.2 Prostaglandin analogues as inhibitor of prostaglandin synthetase

The 7- and 5-oxa prostaglandin derivatives are inhibitors of prostaglandin synthetase of bull testes. 5-Oxa-13-prostenoic acid was most active causing complete inhibition of prostaglandin synthesis from arachidonic acid (Fried et al., 1971; McDonald-Gibson, Flack and Ramwell, 1973). However, some of these compounds also stimulated prostaglandin synthesis.

11.6 EFFECT OF POLYPHLORETIN PHOSPHATE ON 15-METHYL PROSTAGLANDINS

Polyphloretin phosphate (PPP) is an antagonist of smooth muscle actions of naturally occurring prostaglandins. The subject is discussed in detail by Sanner and Eakins (1976) in this series of books.

On the isolated guinea pig ileum and gerbil colon, PPP selectively antagonised the stimulant effects of 15(S)15-methyl PGE_2 methyl ester and 15(S)-15-methyl $PGF_{2\alpha}$ methyl ester. The two analogues were more readily blocked than PGE_2, possibly because in addition to prostaglandin blocking action, PPP is an inhibitor of enzyme 15-hydroxy dehydrogenase. Unlike PGE_2 or $PGF_{2\alpha}$ the 15-methyl analogues are not substrates of prostaglandin 15-hydroxydehydrogenase (Karim and Adaikan, 1975; Adaikan and Karim, 1973).

11.7 RESPIRATORY SYSTEM

11.7.1 Animal studies

In anaesthetized cats 8-iso-PGE_1 increased pulmonary vascular resistance while the arterial blood pressure was decreased (Nakano and Kessinger, 1970b). In open chest cats, 8,12-diiso-PGE_2 (ent-11-15-epi PGE_2) decreased pulmonary compliance and increased pulmonary vascular resistance. $PGF_{2\alpha}$ produced similar effects whereas PGE_2 did not alter the vascular or respiratory functions of the lungs (Ceserani et al., 1975a).

Brookes and Marshall (1974) studied respiratory effects of several natural and synthetic analogues of prostaglandins in rabbits. With the exception of 16,16-dimethyl $PGF_{2\alpha}$, all other prostaglandins elicited an increase (of up to ten times) in respiratory rate and respiratory minute volume in animals anaesthetized with pentobarbitone. The potency of the prostaglandins and analogues in decreasing order were as follows: 15(S)15-methyl PGE_2 methyl ester, 15(S)15-methyl $PGF_{2\alpha}$ methyl ester, 15(S)15-methyl $PGF_{2\alpha}$, PGE_1, 8-iso PGE_2, PGE_2, $PGF_{2\beta}$, $PGF_{2\alpha}$, $PGF_{1\beta}$, PGA_1, PGA_2, $PGF_{1\alpha}$, PBG_1, PGB_2, 5,6-trans $PGF_{2\alpha}$, 20-ethyl $PGF_{2\alpha}$ and 8-iso $PGF_{2\alpha}$.

As bronchodilators in guinea pigs dl-11-deoxy PGE_1, dl-15-deoxy PGE_1 and dl-11,15-bisdeoxy PGE_1 were less active than PGE_1 when injected itravenously (Dessy and Weiss, 1975).

Greenberg (1975) has evaluated the bronchodilator activity of 15-(nat)-hydroxy-9-oxoprost-13-enoic acid (AY 23578) and its 15-methyl analogue (AY 24559) in guinea pigs. The 15-methyl analogue was 72 and 32 times more potent than the non-methyl 11-deoxy prostaglandin when given as an aerosol and by the intravenous route respectively, in inhibiting histamine induced bronchoconstrictions. However, both compounds were equipotent

Table 11.6 Potencies of some prostaglandin analogues on circular muscle from guinea pig and human trachea _in vitro_ and guinea pig airway resistance (($\uparrow$) constrictor, $F_{2\alpha}$ as 1; ($\downarrow$) relevant, E_2* as 1).

Prostaglandins	Guinea pig trachea in vitro	Guinea pig lung resistance	Human trachea in vitro
2a,2b-Dihomo-15(S)15 methyl $PGF_{2\alpha}$ methyl ester	0.091 $\uparrow$	0.21 $\uparrow$	
16-Phenoxy-17,18,19,20-tetranor $PGF_{2\alpha}$	35.26 $\uparrow$	0.092 $\uparrow$	
15(S)15 methyl 17-phenyl 18,19,20-trinor $PGF_{2\alpha}$	20.26 $\uparrow$	13.02 $\uparrow$	
17-Phenyl $PGF_{2\alpha}$	4.98 $\uparrow$	5.45 $\uparrow$	
5-Oxa,17-phenyl 18,19,20-trinor $PGF_{2\alpha}$ methyl ester	0.74 $\uparrow$	0.84 $\uparrow$	
PGE_2			0.59 $\uparrow$
15(S)-15-Methyl-17-phenyl-18,19,20-trinor PGE_2	20.12 $\uparrow$	1.537 $\uparrow$	
11-Deoxy 16,16-dimethyl PGE_2	798.75 $\uparrow$	30.75 $\uparrow$	164.8 $\uparrow$
16-Phenoxy tetranor-prostaglandin E_2	15.95 $\uparrow$	22.96 $\uparrow$	8.9 $\uparrow$
9-Deoxy PGE_2	6.19 $\uparrow$	4.2 $\uparrow$	
15(S) 16,16-Dimethyl PGE_2	0.08 $\downarrow$	0.32 $\downarrow$	0.27 $\uparrow$
17-Phenyl PGE_2	30.95 $\uparrow$	0.104 $\downarrow$	
**(15R)15,16,16-Trimethyl $PGF_{2\alpha}$ methyl ester	3.10 $\uparrow$	2.25 $\uparrow$	
**(15S)15,16,16-Trimethyl $PGF_{2\alpha}$ methyl ester	1.37 $\uparrow$	0.85 $\uparrow$	
**(15S)15,16,16-Trimethyl PGE_2 methyl ester	2.478 $\uparrow$	0.187 $\uparrow$	0.19 $\uparrow$
**(15R)15,16,16-Trimethyl PGE_2 methyl ester	1.83 $\uparrow$	0.1189 $\uparrow$	0.19 $\uparrow$
Ent 15-epi-13-dehydro $PGF_{2\alpha}$	0.113 $\uparrow$	0.997 $\uparrow$	
13-dehydro-$PGF_{2\alpha}$	1.05 $\uparrow$	0.973 $\uparrow$	
I.C.I.81008 'Equimate' (F compound)	0.049 $\uparrow$	0.078 $\uparrow$	
16-Methylene-PGE_2 methyl ester β-cyclodextrin clathrate (ONO-481CD)	11.66 $\downarrow$	17.88 $\downarrow$	11.32 $\uparrow$

* In situations where PGE_2 and its analogues were constrictor, they were compared with $PGF_{2\alpha}$ as standard
** These compounds were synthesised by G. A. Youngdale (The Upjohn Co., Kalamazoo, Michigan, USA)

in relaxing isolated guinea pig tracheal chain _in vitro_. No comparison was made with a natural prostaglandin. In contrast, Lo, Karim and Adaikan (1976) have shown that 11-deoxy 16,16-dimethyl PGE_2 has a potent constrictor action on guinea pig tracheal and bronchial muscle _in vitro_ and _in vivo_. In fact several of the PGE_2 analogues studied (Table 11.6) have a constrictor effect on human and guinea pig respiratory muscle.

11.7.2 Human studies

Smith (1974) measured the forced expiratory volume and lung resistance with three analogues of prostaglandins in human subjects, namely 15-methyl

PGE_2, 15-epi-PGA_2 and 8-iso PGE_1. All three were non-irritant and did not show appreciable changes in forced expiratory volume and lung resistance in normal volunteers (six subjects). In asthmatic patients (six subjects) a minor bronchoconstriction was noted with 15-epi PGA_2. A weak bronchodilator effect with 15-methyl PGE_2 was seen in patients after histamine induced bronchoconstriction.

Serial pulmonary function tests were performed in four women undergoing second trimester abortion with intramuscular injections of 7.3 $\mu g/kg$ 15(S)-15-methyl $PGF_{2\alpha}$ (Weir et al., 1975b). This analogue caused considerable bronchoconstriction of the small airways. The authors concluded that 15-methyl $PGF_{2\alpha}$ should not be given to patients with a history of asthma.

Although prostaglandin E_2 usually produces bronchodilatation in guinea pig and man (Smith, 1976), PGE_2 and its analogues have a constrictor action on the circular muscle of human teachea in vitro (Lo, Karim and Adaikan, 1976).

11.8 REPRODUCTIVE SYSTEM

11.8.1 Animal studies

The effects of several prostaglandins analogues on the reproductive system of various animal species have been discussed in earlier chapters in this series (Kirton, 1975; Labhsetwar, 1975; Flint and Hillier, 1975; Cooper and Walpole, 1975).

11.8.2 Human studies

Several synthetic analogues of prostaglandins E_2 and $F_{2\alpha}$ have been evaluated for their abortifacient effects. These include the 15-methyl, 16,16-dimethyl and 17-phenyl analogues of PGE_2, $PGF_{2\alpha}$ and their methyl esters. Results of these studies have been reviewed in detail by Karim and Amy (1975) in an earlier chapter. Briefly the 15-methyl analogues of PGE_2 and $PGF_{2\alpha}$ given by the intrauterine and intramuscular routes are more effective and safer abortifacients than PGE_2 and $PGF_{2\alpha}$. However, analogues with a wider split in activity on the uterine and gastrointestinal tract smooth muscle are required in order to eliminate the side effects associated with the use of 15-methyl analogues of PGE_2 and $PGF_{2\alpha}$.

11.9 COMMENTS

Although pharmacological evaluation of prostaglandin analogues is at an early stage, some of the compounds are already finding useful clinical applications. For example, unlike PGE_2, orally administered 15-methyl and 16,16-dimethyl analogues of PGE_2 are potent inhibitors of gastric acid secretion in man. In preliminary studies 15(R)15-methyl PGE_2 and its methyl ester have been shown to have a marked healing effect on human gastric ulcers.

Similarly, 15(S)15-methyl analogues of PGE_2 and $PGF_{2\alpha}$ are more potent and selective stimulants of pregnant human uterus than parent natural prostaglandins. These analogues are now routinely used as abortifacients and offer advantages over PGE_2 and $PGF_{2\alpha}$.

Several analogues now being studied in laboratory animals promise to be of therapeutic use in different areas. Human studies with these compounds are needed to confirm data obtained in animals and to establish the relevance of various *in vitro* and animal models to man.

References

Adaikan, P. G. and Karim, S. M. M. (1973). Polyphloretin phosphate temporarily potentiates prostaglandin E_2 on rat fundus, probably by inhibiting PG-15 hydroxydehydrogenase. *J. Pharm. Pharmacol.*, **25**, 229

Adaikan, P. G. and Karim, S. M. M. (1974). Acute toxicity of prostaglandins E_2, $F_{2\alpha}$ and 15(S)15 methyl prostaglandin E_2 methyl ester in the baboon. *Prostaglandins*, **7**, 215

Adaikan, P. G., Lo, P. Y. and Karim, S. M. M. (1976). Antagonism of smooth muscle-stimulating activities of prostaglandins by a prostaglandin analogue—8-ethony-carbonyl-10,11-dihydro A prostaglandin. In press

Adaikan, P. G., Salmon, J. A., Ng, B. K. and Karim, S. M. M. (1974). The effect of 15 (R) 15 methyl PGE_2 methyl ester on serum gastrin level in man. *Int. Res. Commun. System*, **2**, 1587

Bhana, D., Karim, S. M. M., Carter, D. C. and Ganesan, P. A. (1973). The effect of orally administered prostaglandins A_1, A_2 and 15-epi-A_2 on human gastric acid secretion. *Prostaglandins*, **3**, 307

Bowler, J., Crossley, N. S. and Dowell, R. I. (1975). The synthesis and biological activity of alkyloxy prostaglandin analogues. *Prostaglandins*, **9**, 391–396

Brookes, L. G. and Marshall, R. C. (1974). The effect of some prostaglandins on respiration in the rabbit. *J. Pharm. Pharmacol.*, **26**, Suppl. 81P

Bundy, G., Lincoln, F., Nelson, N., Pike, J. and Schneider, W. (1971). Novel prostaglandin syntheses. *Ann. N.Y. Acad. Sci.*, **180**, 76

Bundy, G. L., Yankee, E. W., Weeks, J. R. and Miller, W. L. (1973). The synthesis and biological activity of a series of 15-methyl prostaglandins. *Adv. Biosci.*, **9**, 125

Bygdeman, M., Beguin, F., Toppozada, M. and Wiqvist, N. (1972). Further experience with intrauterine prostaglandin administration. *J. Reprod. Med.*, **9**, 392

Carter, D. C., Ganesan, P. A., Bhana, D. and Karim, S. M. M. (1974). The effect of locally administered prostaglandin 15 (R) 15 methyl E_2 methyl ester on gastric ulcer formation in the Shay rat preparation. *Prostaglandins*, **5**, 455

Carter, D. C., Karim, S. M. M., Bhana, D. and Ganesan, P. A. (1973). The effect of locally administered 15 (R) 15 methyl E_2 prostaglandin on basal and pentagastrin-induced acid secretion in man. *Br. J. Surg.*, **60**, 828

Cesearni, R., Gandolf, C., Usardi, M. M. and Bergamaschi, M. (1975a). Prostaglandins IX: 8, 12-diiso-PGE_2: Effect of steric configuration of side chains on biological activity. *Prostaglandins*, **9**, 97

Cesearni, R., Mandelli, V. and Orsini, G. (1975b). Antagonism of $PGF_{2\alpha}$ by 13 dehydro 20ω $PGF_{2\alpha}$. Abstract. *International Conference on Prostaglandins*, Florence, May 26–30, p. 136

Classen, M., Koch, H., Bickhardt, J., Topf, G. and Demling, L. (1971). The effect of prostaglandin E_1 on the pentagastrin-stimulated gastric secretion in man. *Digestion*, **4**, 333

Classen, M., Koch, H., Deyhle, P., Weidenhiller, S. and Demling, L. (1970). The effect of prostaglandin E_1 on basal gastric secretion in human. *Klin. Wochenschr.*, **48**, 876

Cohen, M. J. M. (1975). Prostaglandin E_2 protects gastric mucosal barrier. *International Conference on Prostaglandins*, Florence, May 26–30. Abstracts. p. 154.

Cooper, M. and Walpole, A. (1975). Practical applications of prostaglandins in animal husbandry. In: *Advances in prostaglandins Research*: *Prostaglandins and Reproduction*. Karim, S. M. M. (ed.), pp. 309–328 (Lancaster: Medical and Technical Publications).

Corey, E. J., Terashima, S., Ramwell, P. W., Jessup, R., Weishenker, N. M., Floyd, D. M. and Crosby, G. A. (1972). 11,15-epi prostaglandin E_2 and its enantiomer. Biological activity and synthesis. *J. Org. Chem.*, **37**, 3043

Dajani, E. Z., Driskill, D. R., Bianchi, R. G., Collins, P. W. and Pappo, R. (1975). Studies on the biological properties of a prostaglandin analogue, SC-29333, a potent inhibitor of gastric secretion. Abstract. *International Conference on Prostaglandins*, Florence, May 26–30, 160

Dessy, F. and Weiss, M. J. (1975). Broncholytic activity of some PGE_1 and PGE_2 derivatives in the guinea-pig. Abstract. *International Conference on Prostaglandins*, Florence, May 26–30, 185

Flint, A. P. F. and Hillier, K. (1975). Prostaglandins and reproductive processes in the female sheep and goat. In: *Advances in Prostaglandin Research: Prostaglandins and Reproduction*. Karim, S. M. M. (ed.), pp. 271–308 (Lancaster: Medical and Technical Publications)

Ford, S. H. and Fried, J. (1969). Smooth muscle activity of rac-8-oxa prostaglandin $F_{1\alpha}$ and related substances. *Life Sci.*, **8**, 983

Fried, J., Lin, C., Mehra, M., Kao, W. and Dalven, P. (1971). Synthesis and biological activity of prostaglandin antagonists. *Ann. N.Y. Acad. Sci.*, **180**, 38

Fung, W. P. and Karim, S. M. M. (1974). Treatment of peptic ulcer pain with prostaglandin 15 (R) 15 methyl E_2 methyl ester. *J. Int. Res. Commun. System*, **2**, 1001

Fung, W. P. and Karim, S. M. M. (1976a). Effect of 15 (R) 15 methyl prostaglandin E_2 on the healing of gastric ulcers: A double blind endoscopic trial. *Prostaglandins* (In press)

Fung, W. P. and Karim, S. M. M. (1976b). Prostaglandin deficiency as a cause of gastric ulcers in man—healing effect of PGE_2. *Aust. N.Z. J. Med.* In press

Fung, W. P., Karim, S. M. M. and Tye, C. Y. (1974a). Effect of 15 (R) 15 methyl prostaglandin E_2 methyl ester on healing of gastric ulcers, controlled endoscopic study. *Lancet*, **ii**, 10–12

Fung, W. P., Karim, S. M. M. and Tye, C. Y. (1974b). Double-blind trial on 15 (R) 15 methyl prostaglandin E_2 methyl ester in the relief of peptic ulcer pain. *Ann. Acad. Med. Singapore*, **3**, 375

Fung, W. P., Lee, S. K. and Karim, S. M. M. (1974). Effect of prostaglandins 15 (R) 15 methyl E_2 methyl ester on the gastric mucosa in patients with peptic ulceration—an endoscopic and histological study. *Prostaglandins*, **5**, 564

Greenberg, R. (1975). A comparison of the bronchodilator activity of an 11-deoxy prostaglandin (AY-23578) with its 15-methyl analogue (AY-24559). Abstract. *International Conference on Prostaglandins*, Florence, May 26–30, 186

Horton, E. W., Main, I. H. M., Thompson, C. J. and Wright, P. M. (1968). Effect of orally administered prostaglandin E_1 on gastric secretion and gastrointestinal motility in man. *Gut*, **9**, 655

Impicciatore, M., Bertaccini, G. and Usardi, M. M. (1975). Effect of a new synthetic prostaglandin on acid gastric secretion in different laboratory animals. Abstract. *International Conference on Prostaglandins*, Florence, May 26–30, 162

Kadowitz, P. J. and Hyman, A. L. (1974). Effects of prostaglandins 15-methyl $F_{2\alpha}$ and 15-methyl E_2 on canine pulmonary circulation and isolated lobar arteries and veins. *Fed. Proc.*, **33**(3), 576

Karim, S. M. M. and Adaikan, P. G. (1974). (Unpublished results.)

Karim, S. M. M. and Adaikan, P. G. (1975). (Unpublished results.)

Karim, S. M. M., Adaikan, P. G. and Lo, P. Y. (1976). Pharmacological activities of 16-methylene PGE_2 methyl ester β-cyclodextrin clathrate (ONO-481CD). In press

Karim, S. M. M. and Amy, J. J. (1973). Effect of prostaglandin 16, 16 dimethyl E_2 methyl ester on the pregnant human uterus. *Prostaglandins*, **4**, 581

Karim, S. M. M. and Amy, J. J. (1975). Interruption of pregnancy with prostaglandins. *Advances in Prostaglandin Research*: *Prostaglandins and Reproduction*. Karim, S. M. M. (ed.), pp. 77–148 (Lancaster: Medical and Technical Publications)

Karim, S. M. M., Carter, D. C., Bhana, D. and Ganesan, P. A. (1973a). Effect of orally and intravenously administered prostaglandins 15 (R) 15 methyl E_2 on gastric secretion in man. *Adv. Biosci.*, **9**, 255

Karim, S. M. M., Carter, D. C., Bhana, D. and Ganesan, P. A. (1973b). Effect of orally administered prostaglandin E_2 and its 15-methyl analogues on gastric secretion. *Br. Med. J.*, 1, 143

Karim, S. M. M., Carter, D. C., Bhana, D. and Ganesan, P. A. (1973c). Inhibition of basal and pentagastrin induced gastric acid secretion in man with prostaglandin 16,16-dimethyl E_2 methyl ester. *Int. Res. Commun. System*, (73-3) 8-3-2

Karim, S. M. M., Carter, D. C., Bhana, D. and Ganesan, P. A. (1973d). The effect of orally and intravenously administered prostaglandin 16, 16 dimethyl E_2 methyl ester on human gastric acid secretion. *Prostaglandins*, 4, 71

Karim, S. M. M. and Fung, W. P. (1975a). Effect of 15 (R) 15 methyl prostaglandin E_2 on gastric secretion and a preliminary study on the healing of gastric ulcers in man. *Int. Res. Commun. System*, 3, 348

Karim, S. M. M. and Fung, W. P. (1976). Effects of some naturally occurring prostaglandins and synthetic analogues on gastric secretion and ulcer healing in man. In *Prostaglandin and Thromboxane Research*, Vol. 1, Samuelsson, B. and Paoletti, R. (eds.) (New York: Raven Press)

Karim, S. M. M. and Ratnam, S. S. (1976). Termination of pregnancy with prostaglandin analogues. In *Prostaglandin and Thromboxane Research*, Vol. 2, Samuelsson, B. and Paoletti, R. (eds.) (New York: Raven Press)

Karim, S. M. M. and Sharma, S. M. (1972). Termination of second trimester pregnancy with 15-methyl analogues of prostaglandins E_2 and $F_{2\alpha}$. *J. Obstet. Gynaecol. Br. Commonw.*, 79, 737

Karim, S. M. M., Sivasamboo, R. and Ratnam, S. S. (1974). Abortifacient action of orally administered 16, 16-dimethyl prostaglandin E_2 and its methyl ester. *Prostaglandins*, 6, No. 4, 349

Karim, S. M. M., Sharma, S. D., Filshie, G. M., Salmon, J. A. and Ganesan, P. A. (1973). Termination of pregnancy with prostaglandin analogues. *Adv. Biosci.*, 9, 811

Kawasaki, A., Ishii, K., Ishii, M. and Tatsumi, M. (1975). Hypotensive and other pharmacological activities of prostaglandin analogue ONO-464. Abstract. *International Conference on Prostaglandins*, Florence, May 26–30, 130

Kirton, K. T. and Forbes, A. D. (1972). Activity of 15 (S) 15 methyl prostaglandin E_2 and $F_{2\alpha}$ as stimulants of uterine contractility. *Prostaglandins*, 1, 319

Kirton, K. T. (1975). Prostaglandins and reproduction in sub-human primates. In: *Advances in Prostaglandin Research: Prostaglandins and Reproduction*. Karim, S. M. M. (ed.), pp. 229–240 (Lancaster: Medical and Technical Publications)

Konturek, S. J., Kwiecien, N., Swierczek, J., Sito, E., Oleksey, J. and Robert, A. (1975). Inhibition of pentagastrin-induced gastric secretion by orally administered 15-methyl analogues of PGE_2 in man. Abstract. *International Conference on Prostaglandins*, Florence, May 26–30, 161

Labhsetwar, A. P. (1975). Effects of prostaglandins on the reproductive system of laboratory animals. In *Advances in Prostaglandins Research: Prostaglandins and Reproduction*. Karim, S. M. M. (ed.), pp. 241–270 (Lancaster: Medical and Technical Publications)

Lee, Y. W. and Bianchi, R. G. (1972). The antisecretory and antiulcer activity of a prostaglandin analogue SC-24665 in experimental animals. Abstr. *5th Int. Congr. Pharmacol. San Francisco*, 136

Lippman, W. (1969). Inhibition of gastric acid secretion in the rat by synthetic prostaglandins. *J. Pharm. Pharmacol.*, 21, 335

Lippman, W. (1970). Inhibition of gastric acid secretion by a potent synthetic prostaglandin. *J. Pharm. Pharmacol.*, 22, 65

Lippman, W. (1971). Oral antigastric acid secretory activity of synthetic prostaglandin analogues (9-oxaprostanoic acids). *Experientia*, 29, 990

Lippman, W. (1974). Inhibition of indomethacin-induced gastric ulceration in the rat by perorally-administered synthetic and natural prostaglandin analogues. *Prostaglandins*, 7, 1

Lippman, W. and Seethaler, K. (1973). Oral antiulcer activity of a synthetic prostaglandin analogue (9-oxaprostanoic acid: AY-22469). *Experientia*, 29, 993

Lo, P. Y., Karim, S. M. M. and Adaikan, P. G. (1976). Effects of some prostaglandin analogues on human and guinea pig tracheo-bronchial muscle *in vitro* and *in vivo*. In press

Magerlein, B. J., DuCharme, D. W., Magee, W. E., Miller, W. L., Robert, A. and Weeks, J. R. (1973). Synthesis and biological properties of 16-alkylprostaglandins. *Prostaglandins*, 4, 143

Magerlein, B. J. and Miller, W. L. (1975). 16-Fluoroprostaglandins. *Prostaglandins*, **9**, 527

Main, I. H. M. (1973). Prostaglandins and the gastrointestinal tract. In *The Prostaglandins*, Cuthbert, M. F. (ed.), (London: William Heinemann Medical Books Ltd., 287

McDonald-Gibson, R. G., Flack, J. D. and Ramwell, P. W. (1973). Inhibition of prostaglandin biosynthesis by 7-oxa and 5-oxa prostaglandins analogue. *Biochem. J.*, **132**, 117

Main, I. H. M. and Whittle, B. J. R. (1974). Methyl analogues of prostaglandin E_2 and gastrointestinal function in the rat. *Br. J. Pharmac.*, **52**, 113P

Miller, W. L., Weeks, J. R., Lauderdale, J. W. and Kirton, K. T. (1975). Biological activities of 17-phenyl-18, 19, 20 trinor prostaglandins. *Prostaglandins*, **9**, 9

Nakano, J. (1969). Cardiovascular effect of a prostaglandin isolated from a gorgonian *Plexaura homomalla*. *J. Pharm. Pharmacol.*, **21**, 782

Nakano, J. and Kessinger, J. M. (1970a). Effect of 15(R)PGA$_2$ on the cardiovascular responses to PGA$_2$ in dogs. *Clin. Res.*, **18**, 117

Nakano, J. and Kessinger, J. M. (1970b). Effects of 8-iso prostaglandin E_2 on the systemic and pulmonary circulations. *Clin. Res.*, **18**, 322

Nylander, B. and Andersson, S. (1975a). Gastric secretion inhibition by two 16-methylated analogues of prostaglandin E_2 given intragastrically to patients with duodenal ulcer disease. *Scand. J. Gastroent.*, **10**, 217

Nylander, B. and Andersson, S. (1975b). Gastric secretory inhibition induced by certain methyl analogs of prostaglandin E_2 in healthy male volunteers and in patients with duodenal ulcer disease. Abstract. *International Conference on Prostaglandins*, Florence, May 26–30, 171

Obrien, P. E. and Carter, D. C. (1975). Effect of gastric secretory inhibitors on the gastric mucosal barrier. *Gut*, **16**, 437

Ojima, M. and Fujita, K. (1975). Inhibition of platelet aggregation and white thrombus formation by prostaglandin analogue ONO-747. Abstract. *International Conference on Prostaglandins*, Florence, May 26–30, 65

Ramwell, P. W., Shaw, J. E., Corey, E. I. and Andersson, N. (1969). Biological activity of synthetic prostaglandins. *Nature (Lond.)*, **221**, 1251

Robert, A. (1968). Antisecretory property of prostaglandins. *Prostaglandin Symp. of Worcester Found. for Exp. Biol.* Ramwell, P. W. and Shaw, J. E. (eds.), p. 47 (New York: Interscience)

Robert, A. (1973). Prostaglandins and gastric secretion. Research in prostaglandins. *Worcester Foundation for Experimental Biology*, **2(4)**, 1–4

Robert, A. (1974). Effects of prostaglandins on the stomach and the intestine. *Prostaglandins*, **6**, 523

Robert, A., Lancaster, C., Nezamis, J. E. and Badalamenti, J. N. (1973). A gastric antisecretory and antiulcer prostaglandin with oral and long acting activity. *Gastroenterology*, **64**, 790

Robert, A., Lancaster, C. and Nezamis, J. E. (1975). Inhibition of gastric secretion after intravaginal administration of prostaglandins. Abstract. *International Conference on Prostaglandins*, Florence, May 26–30, 162

Robert, A. and Magerlein, B. J. (1973). 15-methyl PGE$_2$ and 16, 16-dimethyl PGE$_2$: potent inhibitors of gastric secretion. *Adv. Biosci.*, **9**, 247

Robert, A., Nezamis, J. E. and Phillips, J. P. (1967). Inhibition of gastric secretion by prostaglandins. *Am. J. Dig. Dis.*, **12**, 1073

Robert, A., Nylander, B. and Andersson, S. (1974). Marked inhibition of gastric secretion by two prostaglandin analogues given orally to man. *Life Sci.*, **14**, 533

Robert, A. and Standish, W. L. (1973). Production of duodenal ulcers in rats with one injection of histamine. *Fed. Proc.*, **32**, 322

Robert, A., Stowe, D. F. and Nezamis, J. E. (1971 . Prevention of duodenal ulcers by administration of prostaglandin E_2 (PGE$_2$). *Scand. J. Gastroenterol.*, **6**, 303

Robert, A. and Yankee, E. W. (1976). Gastric antisecretory effect of 15 (R) 15 methyl PGE$_2$ methyl ester and of 15 (S) 15 methyl PGE$_2$ methyl ester. *Proc. Soc. Exp. Biol. Med.* (In Press)

Rosenberg, R., Robert, A., Gonda, M., Dreiling, D. A. and Rucick, J. 1974). Synthetic prostaglandin analogues and pancreatic secretion. *Gastroenterology*, **66**, 767

Rudick, J., Gonda, M., Dreiling, D. A. and Janowitz, H. D. (1971). Effects of prostaglandin E_2 on pancreatic exocrine function. *Gastroenterology*, **60**, 272

Salmon, J. A., Karim, S. M. M., Carter, D. C., Adaikan, P. G. and Bhana, D. (1975). Effect of 15 (R) 15 methyl prostaglandin E_2 methyl ester on basal and pentagastrin stimulated pepsin secretion in man. *Int. Res. Commun. System*, **3**, 83

Sanner, J. H. and Eakins, K. E. (1976). Prostaglandin antagonists. In *Advances in Prostaglandin Research: Prostaglandins—Chemical and Biochemical Aspects*. Karim, S. M. M. (ed.), pp. 137–187 (Lancaster: Medical and Technical Publications)

Schneider, W. P. (1976). The chemistry of the prostaglandins. In *Advances in Prostaglandin Research: Prostaglandins—Chemical and Biochemical Aspects*, Karim, S. M. M. (ed.), pp. 1–23 (Lancaster: Medical and Technical Publications)

Schölkens, B. A. and Babej, M. (1975). Effect of prostaglandin antagonists on smooth muscle contraction. *Arch. Pharmacol.*, **287**, Suppl. 4

Sekhar, N. C., Weeks, J. R. and Kupiecki, F. P. (1968). Antithrombotic activity of a new prostaglandin 8-iso PGE_2. *Circulation*, **38** (Suppl. VI) VI–23

Smith, A. P. (1974). Effects of three prostaglandin analogues on airway tone in asthmatics and normal subjects. *Int. Res. Commun. System*, **2**, 1457

Smith, A. P. (1976). Prostaglandins and the respiratory system. In *Advances in Prostaglandin Research: Physiological, pharmacological and pathological aspects*, Karim, S. M. M. (ed.), pp. 83–102 (Lancaster: Medical and Technical Publications)

Sokoloff, J. and Berk, R. N. (1973). The effect of prostaglandin E_2 on bile flow and the biliary excretion of iopanoic acid. *Invest. Radiol.*, **8**, 9

Strand, J. C., Miller, M. P. and McGiff, J. C. (1974). Biological activity of the methyl esters of prostaglandin E_2 and its (15 S)-methyl analogue. *Eur. J. Pharmacol.*, **26**, 151

Wada, T. and Ishizawa, M. (1970). Effects of prostaglandin on the function of the gastric secretion. *Jap. J. Clinic.*, **28**, 2465

Weeks, J. R. and DuCharme, D. W. (1975). The cardiovascular pharmacology of 16, 16 dimethyl prostaglandin E_2 in the rat and dog. Abstract. *International Conference on Prostaglandins*, Florence, May 26–30, 133

Weeks, J. R., DuCharme, D. W., Magee, W. E. and Miller, W. L. (1973). The biological activity of the (15 S)-15-methyl analogues of prostaglandin E_2 and $F_{2\alpha}$. *J. Pharmacol. Exp. Ther.*, **186**, 67

Weeks, J. R., Sekhar, N. C. and Kupiecki, F. P. (1968). Pharmacological profile of a new prostaglandin 8-iso-prostaglandin E_2. *The Pharmacologist*, **10**, 329

Weir, E. K., Reeves, J. T., Droegemueller, W. and Grover, R. F. (1975a). 15-methylation augments the cardiovascular effects of prostaglandin $F_{2\alpha}$. *Prostaglandins*, **9**, 369

Weir, E. K., Silvers, G. W., Greer, B. E., Droegemueller, W., Reeves, J. T. and Grover, R. F. (1975b). Bronchoconstriction induced by 15-methyl prostaglandin $F_{2\alpha}$ in pregnant women. *Clin. Res.*, **23**, 118A

Whittle, B. J. R. (1975 – Gastric antisecretory and antiulcer activity of prostaglandin E_2 methyl analogues. Abstract. *International Conference on Prostaglandins*, Florence, May 26–30, p. 165

Wilson, D. E., Phillips, C. and Levine, R. A. (1971 – . Inhibition of gastric secretion in man by prostaglandin A_2. *Gastroenterology*, **61**, 201

Wiqvist, J. N., Martin, M., Bygdeman, M. and Green, K. (1975). Prostaglandin analogues and uterotonic potency: A comparative study of seven compounds. *Prostaglandins*, **9**, 255

Yankee, E. W., Ayer, D. E., Bundy, G. L. and Lincoln, F. H. (1975). Synthesis and biological activities of new prostaglandins. (In Press)

Youngdale, G. A. and Lincoln, F. H. (1974). $PGF_{2\alpha}$ 15-methyl ether methyl ethyl ester. *Prostaglandins*, **6**, 207

Index

Acetylcholine
  reduction of cAMP formation by 170
  role in thermoregulation 12–17
Adenylate cyclase
  and anaphylaxis 95
  and inotropic actions of prosta-
    glandins 120
  and metabolically induced coronary
    vasodilatation 145, 146
  and myocardial metabolism 126
  and sedative action of prosta-
    glandins 12
  and thermoregulation 12, 14, 16, 17
  effect of morphine on 17
    prostaglandins on 20, 21, 23
      in tumours 320–322
  sensitivity to E and F prostaglandins 8
  stimulation by cholera toxin 266
    by prostaglandins 295, 306
      in gastrointestinal tract 261, 264,
        265
      in platelets 284, 285
    by vasoactive hormones 230
Adrenergic transmission, effect of
    prostaglandins on 12, 23, 38–50
  in heart 39–41
  in kidney 41, 42
  in spleen 38, 39
  in the central nervous system 12,
    23
  in vascular tissue 42–45, 151, 156–
    170
  in vas deferens 45, 46
  in other tissues 46, 47
Alimentary tract, prostaglandins and
    247–276
  actions of prostaglandins on gastric
    secretion 254–260
    on gut muscle 250–254
    on motility in vivo 253, 254
    on peristalsis in vitro 252, 253
  distribution, release and metabolism
    of prostaglandins in 248–250
  gastric bleeding with aspirin-like
    drugs 260
  prostaglandins in intestinal absorp-
    tion, secretion and ulceration
    260–262
    in gut diseases 265–269
    in pancreatic secretion 262–264
    in salivary secretion 262
    in the biliary tract 264, 265
Anaphylaxis, role of prostaglandins in
    94, 95, 96, 97
Angiotensin
  effect attenuated by prostaglandins
    215
    mediated by cholinergic nerves 52
  in pregnancy 139, 140
  interaction with prostaglandins
    in alimentary tract 252
    in cardiovascular system 144, 146,
      147, 148, 149, 150, 151, 152, 164
    in kidney 206, 212, 213, 215–218,
      229, 230, 235–237
  production inhibited by PGAs 235
  tachyphylaxis to 216, 217
Antipyretics
  blockade of prostaglandin synthesis
    by 12
  lack of effect on normal body
    temperature 16
Arachidonic acid 2–6, 205
  and neurotransmission 41, 42, 47, 53,
    167
  conversion of in tumour tissues 317
  decreased conversion of by indo-
    methacin in vivo 153
  hyperthermic effect of 13
  hypotensive effect of, 153

Arachidonic acid—*contd.*
  increase in angiotensin production by
      235
    renal perfusion pressure by 155,
      235
    uterine blood flow by 139
  occurrence of 64, 65, 169
    in kidney 231
    in lung 84, 85
    in the eye 75, 76, 77, 78
    in tumour tissue 313
  release of by 5-HT 9
    by PGEs in lung 94
  stimulation of platelet aggregation by
      286
Aspirin
  antagonism of hypotensive effect of
      arachidonic acid by 154
  osteolysis by breast tumours 312,
      323
  platelet aggregation by 286
  $PGF_{2\alpha}$ in human bronchus 88
  release of prostaglandins from
      cardiovascular tissue 163
    from spleen 165, 299
  X-ray induced diarrhea 268
  effect of blood flow in the kidney
      236
  metabolically induced coronary
      vasodilatation 145, 146
  prostaglandin biosynthesis 6, 94, 203
    in gut 253
    in platelets 298, 299
    in the eye 75–78
    in tumours 314, 315
  gastric bleeding and 260
  gastric mucosal permeability and 335
  reduction of metabolism of prosta-
      glandins by 91
Asthma
  15-epi PGA_2 in 354
  prostaglandins in 84, 86–89, 90, 96,
      97, 98

Benzydamine, facilitation of PGE_2
    synthesis by 203
Blood coagulation, role of prosta-
    glandins in 277–291
  see also platelets
Bone resorption
  by dental cysts 313, 314
  stimulation of by prostaglandins 269,
      304, 305, 322, 323
  from mouse fibrosarcoma 314

Calcium, interaction with prosta-
    glandins
  in kidney 219, 220
  in neurotransmission 48–50
  in the cardiovascular system 120,
      121, 143, 152, 153, 156, 160,
      161, 162
Carcinoma, role of prostaglandins in
    265, 266, 268, 303–325
Cardiovascular system
  effects of prostaglandins on 103–200
    adrenergic transmission 156–170
    blood pressure 104–117
    cardiac output 117, 118
    chronotropic effects 121–124
    circulation
      carotid 136, 137
      cerebral 137–139
      coronary 124–126
      forearm, hindlimb and cutane-
        ous 133–136
      pulmonary 127, 128
      reproductive organs 139, 140
      splanchnic 128–132
    inotropic 118–121
    isolated vascular smooth muscle
        141–143
    myocardial metabolism 126, 127
    reactivity to other vasoactive sub-
        stances 144–153
  role of prostaglandins in hyper-
      tension 153–156, 220
  in human cardiovascular system
      170–183
Cholinergic transmission
  and cyclic GMP 23
  and hyperthermic effect of prosta-
      glandins 16
  and prostaglandins 169, 170
    in gastrointestinal tract 52, 53, 251
    in other tissues 53
  and sedative effect of prostaglandins
      12
Cyclic AMP
  and anaphylaxis 95
  and gastric acid secretion 255, 256
  and inotropic actions of prosta-
      glandins 120
  and messenger theory 20
  and metabolically induced coronary
      vasodilatation 145, 146
  and myocardial metabolism 126
  effect of prostaglandins on 20, 21,
      304

in blood coagulation 284, 285
in the biliary tract 264, 265
in the eye 75
in tumours 321, 322
generation of by vasoactive hormones 230
hyperthermic effect of 16
occurrence in tumours 316
opposition by cyclic GMP 295
role in cell differentiation 21, 22
in cholera 266, 267
in pancreatic secretion 263, 264
in prostaglandin-induced fever 16, 17
in synaptic transmission 22, 23, 164, 170
in tumours 318-322
Cyclic GMP
and cholinergic transmission 23
opposition by cyclic AMP 295

Dehydrogenase, 15-hydroxy, 7, 8, 12, 329
and prostaglandin analogues 350, 353
in the eye 71
in the gastrointestinal tract 253, 254
in the kidney 204, 205, 206, 222
in the lung 91, 94, 169
specificity for A and E prostaglandins 110
turnover 210
dexamethasone, lack of effect on prostaglandin synthesis in the eye 77, 78
Disodium cromoglycate 89, 96

Eicosatetraynoic acid
and neurotransmission 39, 41, 43, 46, 47, 167
effect on bronchial muscle tone 90
platelet aggregation 286
prostaglandin release from cardiovascular tissue 163, 166
prostaglandin synthesis 95
Endoperoxides 3, 6
activity of 8, 9, 206, 235
in kidney 206, 207, 223
in the central nervous system 10
release during platelet aggregation 286
Eye
prostaglandin antagonists and 73-75
prostaglandins and 63-81, 296, 298

effect on aqueous humour
dynamics 67-69
intraocular pressure 65, 67
other effects 72, 73
in aqueous humour
of animals 69, 70
of glaucoma patients 70, 71
of patients with ocular inflammation 71
removal of from intraocular fluids 71, 72
prostaglandin synthesis inhibitors and 75-78

Fever, prostaglandins in 12-17, 25, 267, 295
in the c.s.f. 11, 14

Ganglionic transmission, effect of prostaglandins on 50, 51

Haemostasis, platelets in 278, 279
5-Hydroxytryptamine
effect antagonized by PGEs 127, 128, 144
potentiated by PGE₁ 152
liberation in inflammation 298
in platelet aggregation 279
in tumours 307, 309, 310
releases fatty acids in brain synaptosomes 9, 15
in lung 94
role in thermoregulation 12-17
turnover increased by prostaglandins 12

Imidazole
antagonism of the effects of PGs in the eye 75
in the gut 253
potentiation of effect of PGE₂ on vascular smooth muscle 152
Indomethacin
antagonism of cholera-induced intestinal secretion 267
hypotensive effect of arachidonic acid 153, 154
increased renal perfusion pressure after arachidonic acid 155, 235
nerve-stimulated prostaglandin release from kidney and cardiovascular system 163
osteolysis in Walker carcinosarcoma 312

Indomethacin, antagonism—*contd.*
prostaglandin release from spleen
165
effect on cerebral blood flow 25
epinephrine infusion into spleen
147, 299
exercise-induced asthma 97
kidney blood flow 236
lipolysis 47
metabolically induced coronary
vasodilatation 145
mucosal blood flow 129
neurotransmission 39, 41, 42, 43,
46, 47, 50, 52, 53, 167, 251,
252
plasma renin activity 235
resting tone of lung tissues 90
uterine blood flow 139, 140
gastric bleeding and 260
hypertensive effect in dogs 220
in rabbits 153
in anaphylaxis 96, 97
in cholera 266, 267
increases sphincter pressure 254
in endotoxin shock 268
inhibits prostaglandin biosynthesis 6,
94
by dental cysts 313
in gastrointestinal tract 252, 253
in inflammation 298
in kidney 215, 220, 232, 233, 234
in the eye 75–78
in the lung 95, 96
in tumours 314, 315, 316, 317,
320–322
in medullary carcinoma of the
thyroid 266, 308
in peridontal disease 269
lack of effect on PGA biosynthesis
208
mucosal permeability and 335
ulcerogenic effect 255, 256, 260, 261,
334, 335
used to determine 'basal' levels of
prostaglandin in tissue 248
treat hypercalcaemia 311, 323
treat peridontal disease 314
Indoxole, inhibits prostaglandin synthesis in the eye 77, 78
Inflammation 293–302
in gut 269
in rheumatoid arthritis 297
in skin 136, 294, 295, 296, 297
in the eye 64, 69–71, 73, 78

Irin
discovery of 63, 64
release following trauma to the eye
69, 296
Isomerase in prostaglandin synthesis 3,
6, 112, 208

9-Keto reductase 3, 6, 8, 169, 206, 222,
223, 225, 231, 238
Kinins
in inflammation 298
interactions with prostaglandins in
kidney 210, 213, 221–223, 225–231,
237, 238
release from tumours 307, 309

Lipolysis
effect of indomethacin on 47
inhibition of by PGE_1 126
by 8-iso PGE_1 345

Meclofenamic acid
antagonism of PGF_{2x} on human
bronchus 88
on rabbit cardiovascular system
113, 114
effect on lipolysis 47
neurotransmission 39, 42, 44, 46
inhibition of prostaglandin biosynthesis by 169, 232, 233, 234
Medullin
characterization of 202
isolation of 202
Migraine, involvement of prostaglandins in 11, 25
Morphine
antagonism of PG-induced stimulation of brain adenylate cyclase by
17
effect on cholinergic transmission 53,
251

Naproxen, inhibits prostaglandin synthesis in the eye 77
Neurotransmission, effects of prostaglandins on
at adrenergic junctions 38–50
at cholinergic junctions 51–53
at ganglia 50, 51
Norepinephrine
and cAMP levels in brain 22, 23
and regulation of food intake 17
effect of prostaglandins on, *see*
adrenergic transmission

interaction with prostaglandins in
the eye 76
release of prostaglandins in kidney
by 217–219
role in thermoregulation 12–17

7-Oxa-prostynoic acid
and prostaglandins in the eye 74
antagonism of effect of oxygen on
the ductus arteriosus 143
as prostaglandin antagonists 351,
352, 353
inhibition of prostaglandin synthetase by 349
Oxyphenbutazone, inhibits prostaglandin synthesis in the eye 77

Papaverine, antagonism of effect of
PGE_2 on vascular smooth muscle
by 152, 155
Paracetamol
inhibition of 5-HT and epinephrine
hyperthermia 15
prostaglandin synthesis 6, 299
lack of effect on prostaglandin synthesis in the eye 77
Phenylbutazone
antagonism of hypotensive effect of
arachidonic acid by 154
gastric bleeding and 260
inhibition of prostaglandin synthesis
in the eye by 77
lack of effect on PGD_2 synthesis 203
Phosphodiesterase
activation of by prostaglandins 21,
264
enhanced activity of in isolated
aorta of SHR 156
role in prostaglandin-induced platelet
aggregation 284
stimulation by imidazole 75
Phosphodiesterase inhibitors
and cAMP levels 21, 23, 146, 152
and cell differentiation 21, 320, 321
and intestinal secretion 261
and pancreatic secretion 263, 264
potentiation of effect of PGE on
cAMP production in vitro 319
role in prostaglandin-induced
platelet aggregation 284, 285
Phospholipase
in brain 4
in inflammation 299, 300

inhibition by mepacrine 221, 230
in prostaglandin biosynthesis 2, 3,
164, 205, 230, 231
Phosphorylase, activation of by PGE_1
120, 126
Pirprofen, inhibits prostaglandin synthesis in the eye 77, 78
Platelets, aggregation of
ADP in 279, 285
5-HT and catecholamines in 279
inhibition of by PGE_2 44, 278, 279,
280, 281, 304
by other PGs 282, 283
by prostaglandin analogues 345
inhibition/stimulation of by PGE_2
281, 282, 283
in vitro 279, 280
in vivo 280, 281
mechanism of action of prostaglandins in 284–286
Plexaura homomalla, isolation of PGA_2
from 112, 340
Polyphloretin phosphate
antagonism of effects of prostaglandin analogues 353
prostaglandins
in dental cysts 269, 313
in the eye 73–75
on smooth muscle 73, 90, 113,
249, 250, 251, 353
inhibition of prostaglandin dehydrogenase by 249, 353
lack of effect on PG-stimulated
respiration 90
production of diarrhea by 254
reduction of dehydrogenase activity
in lung by 94
effects of anaphylaxis by 95, 96
stimulation of food intake by 17
Prostaglandin analogues
activity of 343
as antagonists 351, 352
as synthesis inhibitors 352, 353
effects of
antithrombotic 345
antiulcer 334–337
cardiovascular 340–347
increased mucosal blood flow
338
on bile production 338
on gastrin production 339, 340
on gut motility 339
on reproductive system 354
on respiratory system 353, 354

Prostaglandin analogues—*contd.*
  inhibition of gastric secretion by 257,
      259, 329–334, 338
    pancreatic secretion by 338
    pepsin production by 338, 339
  metabolism of in gut 250
  possible use in inhibition of gastric
      secretion 256, 355
    in peptic ulcer disease 259, 260,
        261, 355
    in pregnancy termination 345,
        354, 355
    in prevention of esophageal
        reflux 254
    gastric bleeding 260
  smooth muscle stimulation by 348–
      351
  structure of 330, 331, 332
Prostaglandins
  actions of 11–20
    on behaviour 11, 12
    on cardiovascular system 103–200
    on cerebral circulation 24, 25
    on the alimentary tract 247–276
    on the respiratory system 83–101
  and blood coagulation 277–291
  and cyclic AMP 20, 21, 75, 264, 265,
      284, 285, 304, 319–322
  and food intake 17
  and 5-HT 12, 15
  and hypertension 220, 238, 239
  and kinins 210, 215, 221–223, 237,
      238
  and the eye 63–81
  anti-inflammatory actions of 295
  as hyperthermic agents 13–16
  assay of 211–214, 250
  as tissue hormones 207–211, 233, 234
  as venous hormones 233, 238
  biosynthesis of 2–6, 298–300
    in gut 248–250
    inhibition of 6
      by anti-inflammatory drugs 73,
          94, 211, 215, 221, 236, 298–
          300
      by antipyretics 12
      by prostaglandin analogues 352,
          353
      by steroids 299
    in kidney 203–206
    in the eye 64
      inhibition of 73, 75–77
    stimulation of 229–231
      in dental cysts 313

  in tumours 268, 304–322
  facilitation of neurotransmission by
      168, 252
  15-hydroxy dehydrogenase *see*
      dehydrogenase
  in blood coagulation 277–291
  in brain 4
  in cerebrospinal fluid 10, 11
  in fever 11–17
  inflammatory actions of 293–295
  in inflammation 293–302
  interaction with cAMP in the central
      nervous system 20–24
  in the central nervous system 1–36
    brain stem 17, 18
    hypothalamus 12–17
    neurons 19, 20
    spinal cord 18, 19
  leukotactic actions of 294
  messenger role of 21
  metabolism of 6–9
    by the lungs 91–95
    in gut 248–250
  prejunctional inhibition by 47–50,
      169
  receptors 251, 253, 351
  release of 9–11
    from cardiovascular tissues 163,
        164
      inhibition of 163
    from lung tissues 94–97
    in anaphylaxis 94
    in gut 248–250
  renal 201–245
  role in bone resorption 269, 304,
      305
    in gut diseases 265–269
  use of as antithrombotic agents 287
    in gastric ulcer therapy 255
    in pregnancy termination 355
    in preservation of blood for trans-
        fusion 186, 287
  in von Willebrand's disease 282
Prostaglandin synthetase 3, 169
  differential sensitivity of to inhibitors
      in different tissues 77, 169, 267,
          299, 308
  inhibition of 75, 203
    by hydroquinone 77
    by nutmeg 308, 309
    by 5- and 7-oxa prostaglandins
        349, 352, 353
    by sulphasalazine 269
  in hypothalamus 13

in kidney 203–205, 231, 237
in other tissues 64, 65, 168, 169, 203, 204, 233, 298
in platelets 298
in tumour tissues 317
role in inflammation 298, 299, 300

Renal prostaglandins
and the renal circulation 231–237
assay of 211–214
degradation of 203–211
identification of 202
mechanism of basal output of 237, 238
range of activities of 214–231
synthesis of 203–211
Δ^{13} Reductase
in the central nervous system 7, 8, 12
in the lung 91
respiratory system
effect of prostaglandin analogues on 353, 354
prostaglandins on 83–101
bronchial muscle tone 84–89
pulmonary circulation 89, 90
ventilation 90
metabolism of prostaglandins in 91–95
release of prostaglandins in 95, 96–98
in asthma 96, 97
in pulmonary embolization 97

Salicylate, inhibition of prostaglandin production by in tumours 314, 315

SC-19220
and prostaglandins in the eye 74
in the gastrointestinal tract 251
in the isolated vas deferens 45
effect on bronchial muscle tone 90

Thermoregulation 12–17
Thromboxanes 36, 298
Tumours 303–325
animal 306, 314–317
BP8/P_1 tumours 316, 317
chondrosarcoma 317
Moloney sarcoma 315, 316
mouse fibrosarcoma 314, 315
sarcoma 180 317
human 305–314
breast cancer 312, 313
carcinoid 309–311
dental cyst 312, 313
ganglioneuroma 312
increased prostaglandin synthesis by 250, 309
Kaposis sarcoma 311, 312
medullary carcinoma of thyroid 266, 307–309
neuroblastoma 312
phaeochromocytoma 311
renal cell carcinoma 311, 323
tissue culture 317–321

Vasopressin, cardiovascular effects modified by prostaglandins 144, 148, 149